FOURTH EDITION

EMERGENCY CARE AND TRANSPORTATION

OF THE SICK AND INJURED

FOURTH EDITION

EMERGENCY CARE AND TRANSPORTATION

OF THE SICK AND INJURED

BY THE
AMERICAN ACADEMY OF ORTHOPAEDIC SURGEONS

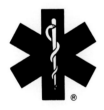 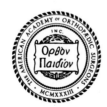

This textbook is intended solely as a guide to the appropriate procedures to be employed when rendering emergency care to or transporting the sick or injured. It is not intended as a statement of the standards of care required in any particular situation, since circumstances and patients' physical condition can vary widely from one emergency to another. Nor is it intended that this textbook shall in any way advise emergency personnel concerning legal authority to perform the activities or procedures discussed. Such local determinations should be made only with the aid of legal counsel.

CREDITS

Book design and production: The Book Department, Inc.

Contributing editor: Margaret Kearney

Medical illustration: Laurel Cook

Technical illustration: Boston Graphics, Inc.

Cover design: Richmond Jones

Photography: Curtis P. Clogston, MD, *Director, Low Tech, Inc.*
Dennis A. Havel, RBP, *Chief Photographer*
Thomas Vermersch
Andras Schoffer
John McGregor
William B. Love
Martha Hartzog

FOURTH EDITION
Copyright © 1987 by American Academy of Orthopaedic Surgeons

Emergency Care and Transportation of the Sick and Injured
Third Edition © 1981, Second Edition © 1977, First Edition © 1971

ISBN 0-89203-012-7

Library of Congress Catalog Card Number 86-071640

D E F 0 8 9

Published and distributed by:
American Academy of Orthopaedic Surgeons
222 S. Prospect Ave., Park Ridge, IL 60068
Telephone 1-800-626-6726

Printed in the United States of America

Table of Contents

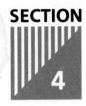
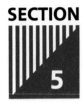
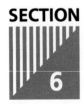

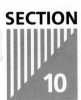

Board of Editors

James D. Heckman, MD, *Chairman*
San Antonio, Texas

Ronald E. Rosenthal, MD
New Hyde Park, New York

Robert A. Worsing, Jr., MD
Wichita, Kansas

Arthur S. McFee, MD, *Special Consultant*
San Antonio, Texas

Dedication

This textbook is dedicated to the men and women engaged in emergency medical services whose unselfish devotion has improved, without measure, the quality and effectiveness of prehospital care.

We especially recognize the numerous valuable contributions made by the late Joseph D. (Deke) Farrington, MD (1909–1982), called by many the "father" of emergency medicine in the United States. For over forty years he worked diligently to improve the quality of prehospital care in America. His accomplishments were many: He helped to develop the list of "Essential Equipment for Ambulances"; he was a distinguished member of the National Academy of Sciences panel that developed the national training criteria for emergency medical technicians; and he founded the National Association of Emergency Medical Technicians and was the first editor-in-chief of *The EMT Journal.* Most significantly for us, he was a major contributor to the first three editions of this textbook. Many of the ideas presented in this text were the product of his knowledge and experience. His vision, concern, and enthusiasm provide a continuing stimulus for the creation of this edition dedicated to him.

Contributors

Literally thousands of individuals have contributed to the content of this and previous editions of this textbook. It is impossible to list everyone, but the Board of Editors wishes especially to thank the following for their substantial input:

Cecil Arnold
Washington, D.C.
William Auchterlonie, EMT-P I/C
Wichita, Kansas
Mark D. Baker, EMT
Wichita, Kansas
Marvin Birnbaum, MD
Madison, Wisconsin
C. Robert Clark, MD
Lookout Mountain, Tennessee
Ewell Clarke, MD
San Antonio, Texas
Curtis P. Clogston, MD
San Antonio, Texas
Nancy Colley, BSE, EMT
Riverside, Missouri
Richard O. Cummins, MD
Seattle, Washington
Lorraine J. Day, MD
San Francisco, California
Ralph J. DiLibero, MD
Palos Verdes Estates, California
Donna C. Dowd, MD
San Antonio, Texas
Carol L. Dunetz, MD
New Hyde Park, New York
Mickey Eisenberg, MD
Seattle, Washington
Michael F. French, NREMT-A
Madison, Wisconsin
Charles E. Garoni, BA, EMT-P
San Antonio, Texas
Charles B. Gillespie, MD
Albany, Georgia
John C. Goll, EMT-P
Indianapolis, Indiana
Donald J. Gordon, MD, Ph.D.
San Antonio, Texas
James Gosselin, EMT-I
New Britain, Connecticut
Judith R. Graves, RN
Seattle, Washington
Walter A. Hoyt, Jr., MD
Akron, Ohio

Diana Jansen, RN
Madison, Wisconsin
Jerald Jansen, EMT-A
Madison, Wisconsin
George L. Johnson, EMT
Albany, New York
Lou Jordan, PA
Baltimore, Maryland
Richard L. Judd, Ph.D.
New Britain, Connecticut
J.G. Kendrick, MD
Wichita, Kansas
Russell Kulp
Braintree, Massachusetts
Denny Kurogi, NREMT-A
Overland Park, Kansas
John H. Littlefield, Ph.D.
San Antonio, Texas
Brian D. Mahoney, MD
Minneapolis, Minnesota
Dennis Mauk, EMT-P
Wichita, Kansas
Ernest C. McClellan, MD
Wichita, Kansas
Newton McCollough, MD
Tubac, Arizona
William McManus, MD
Fort Sam Houston, Texas
Norman E. McSwain, MD
New Orleans, Louisiana
Kathleen K. Mechler, RN
San Antonio, Texas
T.A. Don Michael, MD
Bakersfield, California
William J. Mills, Jr., MD
Anchorage, Alaska
Rocco Morando, NREMT-A
Columbus, Ohio
H. George Nurnberg, MD
Jamaica, New York
Jeanne O'Brien, RN, NREMT-P
Omaha, Nebraska
James O. Page, JD
Carlsbad, California

Judith A. Pankratz, RN, EMT-A
Madison, Wisconsin
Basil A. Pruitt, Jr., MD
Fort Sam Houston, Texas
Donald J. Ptacnik, REMT-A I/C
Bend, Oregon
Ruby J. Ruffin, RN
San Antonio, Texas
Ernest Ruiz, MD
Minneapolis, Minnesota
Nels Sanddal, REMT-A
Boulder, Montana
Joe L. Smetana
Waco, Texas
Paul J. Smith, EMT
Indianapolis, Indiana
John Stafford, MD
Phoenix, Arizona
John D. States, MD
Rochester, New York
Ronald D. Stewart, MD
Pittsburgh, Pennsylvania
Luther M. Strayer, III, MD
Neenah, Wisconsin
Douglas Stutz
Silver Spring, Maryland
John Suelzer, MD
Indianapolis, Indiana
Olin Tapley, EMT-P
Wichita, Kansas
Michael V. Vance, MD
Phoenix, Arizona
Richard Vomacka
Sioux City, Iowa
Diana M. Walter, RN
San Antonio, Texas
Katherine H. West, RN
Springfield, Virginia
Roger D. White, MD
Rochester, Minnesota
Richard Withington, MD
Watertown, New York
Robert Zickler
Indianapolis, Indiana

Reviewers

Many thanks to the following individuals who, throughout the production stages, either reviewed the complete manuscript or examined the selected chapters of *Emergency Care and Transportation of the Sick and Injured, Fourth Edition.* Their suggestions and feedback were extremely helpful.

Allan Braslow, Ph.D.
Champaign, Illinois
Patrick Cote
State EMS Training Coordinator
Augusta, Maine
Kenneth D. Cross
Firemedic Lieutenant
Montgomery, Alabama
S. Gail Dubs
EMS Training Coordinator
Harrisburg, Pennsylvania
Deane Edmond
Supervisor, EMS Training
Concord, New Hampshire
M. Brian Evans, REMT-P
EMS Program Director
Birmingham, Alabama
Michael J. Fagel, LT, EMT-A
North Aurora, Illinois
Ann Feddersen, RN, NREMT-P
Albuquerque, New Mexico
Larry Fountain, RN, EMT
Mc Allister, Oklahoma
Jeraldine M. Frey, EMT I/C
Benton, Illinois
Helen L. Guilford, RN
EMT Instructor
Baxter, Kentucky
Janet Head, RN, REMTA, MS
Kansas City, Kansas

William J. Hollis
EMS Training Supervisor
Olympia, Washington
Peter G. Leary
EMS Training Coordinator
Providence, Rhode Island
Mary Elaine Makris, EMT-P
ALS Training Program Consultant
Phoenix, Arizona
Eddie Manley
EMS System Coordinator
Oklahoma City, Oklahoma
Mary Beth Michos, *Captain*
Montgomery County Fire &
Rescue
Rockville, Maryland
Gary Morgan, EMT I/C
Buffalo, New York
Jeffrey L. Nelson
EMS Coordinator
Champaign, Illinois
Thomas Olson
Educational Chairperson, EMS
Department
Oak Creek, Wisconsin
Nickolas J. O'Neil, RN, EMT-P
Director of EMS Training
Boston, Massachusetts
Michael Reckage, *Captain*
South River Rescue Squad
South River, New Jersey

Carolyn R. Schmidt
EMS Administrator/Certification
Little Rock, Arkansas
D. Terry Shorr
EMS Training Director
Charleston, West Virginia
Charlene M. Skaff, NREMT-P
Fargo, North Dakota
Alonzo W. Smith, BA, EMT-P
Columbia, South Carolina
Joseph L. Stevenson, *Supervisor*
EMS Training & Certification
Nashville, Tennessee
Mary Ann Talley, BSN, MPA
Mobile, Alabama
William C. Wade
Rescue Lieutenant
Tampa, Florida
Michael S. Wataha, EMT I/C
Murray Hill, New Jersey
Jason T. White, *Chief*
Paramedic Training
Jefferson City, Missouri
Vaughn Whitehead, EMT I/C
Tampa, Florida
The Prepublication Review
Committee
National Council of State EMS
Training Coordinators
Boulder, Montana

Technical Consultants

Bexar County Hospital District

Boston EMS

Bulverde/Spring Branch EMS

City of Austin EMS

Clayton Volunteer Fire Department

Creighton University

Department of Epidemiology, School of Aerospace
  Medicine (USAF)

Entomological Society of America

Florida Chapter of the American College
  of Emergency Physicians

Guilfoyle Ambulance Service Inc.

Hudson Bend Fire Department

Life Watch of Wichita

New York City EMS

New York State EMS

NNR Publishing Company

Office of EMS of Massachusetts

Office of the Chief Medical Examiner
  of Massachusetts

Omaha Fire Division

Don Ptacnik's EMS Consulting

Santa Rosa Children's Hospital

Southern Berkshire Volunteer Ambulance Squad

Southern Pacific Transportation Company

Texas Department of Health, Bureau of Emergency
  Management

Travis County Fire Control

Watertown Ski Patrol

Wesley Medical Center

Westlake Fire Department

Wichita Fire Department

Wichita-Sedgwick County EMS

Witte Museum of San Antonio

Foreword

THE AMERICAN ACADEMY OF ORTHOPAEDIC SURGEONS IS proud of being a part of the growth of Emergency Medical Services in the United States. In 1971, at the time of the printing of the first edition of this text, the concepts of emergency medical technicians, paramedics, and emergency medical services were just becoming recognized. Now, during the printing of this fourth edition, well-developed emergency medical services are routine in the cities and towns of the United States. In some cities, emergency medical services has become a third city service along with police and fire departments.

Just as there have been many changes and improvements in EMS since 1971, the Academy has worked diligently to keep pace with the changes in our new editions of the "Orange Book." The Board of Editors have really outdone themselves with this fourth edition by not only extensively revising and updating all of the chapters but also by adding four-color photographs and an appendix dealing with the specifics of intravenous therapy, airway management, and cardiac defibrillation. James D. Heckman, MD, Professor of Orthopaedics of the University of Texas Health Science Center in San Antonio, served as the Chairman of the Board of Editors for the third edition and now the fourth edition of this text. Two of his associates, Arthur S. McFee, MD of San Antonio, Texas, and Ronald E. Rosenthal, MD of New Hyde Park, New York, are both well known to the readers of the text because they have been a part of all of the previous editions. The third member of the editorial board, Robert Worsing, MD, of Wichita, Kansas, has brought many new concepts and insights to this edition.

On behalf of the Board of Directors of the American Academy of Orthopaedic Surgeons and all of the fellows of our Academy, it is my pleasure to congratulate the Board of Editors for this state-of-the-art text on emergency medical care.

Charles A. Rockwood, Jr., MD
Department of Orthopaedic Surgery
University of Texas Health Science Center
San Antonio, Texas

The EMT Code of Ethics

PROFESSIONAL STATUS AS AN EMERGENCY MEDICAL TECHnician and Emergency Medical Technician-Paramedic is maintained and enriched by the willingness of the individual practitioner to accept and fulfill obligations to society, other medical professionals, and the profession of Emergency Medical Technician. As an Emergency Medical Technician at the basic level or an Emergency Medical Technician-Paramedic, I solemnly pledge myself to the following code of professional ethics:

A fundamental responsibility to the Emergency Medical Technician is to conserve life, to alleviate suffering, to promote health, to do no harm, and to encourage the quality and equal availability of emergency medical care.

The Emergency Medical Technician provides services based on human need, with respect for human dignity, unrestricted by consideration of nationality, race, creed, color, or status.

The Emergency Medical Technician does not use professional knowledge and skills in any enterprise detrimental to the public well being.

The Emergency Medical Technician respects and holds in confidence all information of a confidential nature obtained in the course of professional work unless required by law to divulge such information.

The Emergency Medical Technician, as a citizen, understands and upholds the law and performs the duties of citizenship; as a professional, the Emergency Medical Technician has the never-ending responsibility to work with concerned citizens and other health care professionals in promoting a high standard of emergency medical care to all people.

The Emergency Medical Technician shall maintain professional competence and demonstrate concern for the competence of other members of the Emergency Medical Services health care team.

An Emergency Medical Technician assumes responsibility in defining and upholding standards of professional practice and education.

The Emergency Medical Technician assumes responsibility for individual professional actions and judgment, both in dependent and independent emergency functions, and knows and upholds the laws which affect the practice of the Emergency Medical Technician.

An Emergency Medical Technician has the responsibility to be aware of and participate in matters of legislation affecting the Emergency Medical Technician and the Emergency Medical Services System.

The Emergency Medical Technician adheres to standards of personal ethics which reflect credit upon the profession.

Emergency Medical Technicians, or groups of Emergency Medical Technicians, who advertise professional services, do so in conformity with the dignity of the profession.

The Emergency Medical Technician has an obligation to protect the public by not delegating to a person less qualified, any service which requires the professional competence of an Emergency Medical Technician.

The Emergency Medical Technician will work harmoniously with and sustain confidence in Emergency Medical Technician associates, the nurse, the physician, and other members of the Emergency Medical Services health care team.

The Emergency Medical Technician refuses to participate in unethical procedures, and assumes the responsibility to expose incompetence or unethical conduct of others to the appropriate authority in a proper and professional manner.

The National Association
of Emergency Medical Technicians

Preface

FIVE YEARS HAVE ELAPSED SINCE PUBLICATION OF THE third edition of this textbook. During that time significant advances have occurred in the emergency care field. There is a greater basic core of knowledge, many refinements in skills, and perhaps, most important, a significantly greater scientific basis upon which evaluation and treatment plans can be made in a logical and informed way. For these reasons, this fourth edition has been extensively rewritten. As with previous editions of this text, the information has been collected from many sources. Numerous experts have been called upon to contribute to all stages of the project. The most current and correct information has been distilled from these many sources to provide a consistent and medically accurate textbook. Where controversy exists regarding the best approach to a specific emergency problem, the alternative methods are presented, or a synthesis of those methods designed to provide a practical and useful approach is described. With each revision of this text, critiques of the previous editions are sought, considered carefully, and addressed. Because of the constantly changing nature of the emergency care field, the editorial committee will continue to respect and respond to any criticism of this edition to assure continued currency and appropriateness of its contents.

New technical improvements have been made in this edition to enhance the student's ability to comprehend and retain the critical basic information. Most notably, color has been added to the text with four-color illustrations throughout. In addition, great effort has been made to improve the readability of the text without compromising the quality of the critical medical content. To further enhance the student's ability to get the most out of this text, a section on study and reading skills has been added to the first chapter. A new chapter has been added on mechanisms of injury to provide the student with an overview of the injury process.

In 1984, the United States Department of Transportation, National Highway Traffic Safety Administration revised its national standard curriculum for the EMT-A. The Course Guide for that curriculum has been used as the working outline for the preparation of this fourth edition. This text covers all of the material in the DOT curriculum in the order in which it is presented in the Course Guide. This format will assure consistency and completeness in coverage of all of the essential elements of education and training at the EMT-A level.

To expand the usefulness of the text and to address the various needs of training programs throughout the country, three appendices have been added to cover the intermediate skills of intravenous therapy, advanced airway management, and cardiac defibrillation by EMTs. It is hoped that these appendices can be used by instructors as one resource for training EMTs beyond the basic level in any one, or all three of these areas.

The successful completion of this edition could not have been accomplished without the extraordinary voluntary efforts of the members of the Board of Editors who have devoted innumerable hours to this task. I express my sincere appreciation to each member for his outstanding contribution. We have received excellent administrative support and technical assistance from Robert Napolitano and Pat Becker of the American Academy of Orthopaedic Surgeons. And the continuing support of the Academy office staff has provided direction and incentive for the successful completion of this work.

Special thanks must be extended to The Book Department, Inc. of Boston, and especially to Greg Johnson, director of production for this book, for their tolerance, excellent design, and technical assistance. I wish to extend special thanks to Margaret Kearney for her outstanding editorial work, to Laurel Cook whose fine illustrations have added significant clarity and visual appeal to the text, and to Dr. Curtis Clogston and Dennis Havel who are responsible for the excellent and clinically accurate photography throughout the book.

Personally, I wish to thank Charles A. Rockwood, Jr., MD for his continuing encouragement, guidance, and support during the entire project; the Board of Directors of the Academy for their confidence, encouragement, and support; Mary Fuentes for her tolerance, her editorial and secretarial skills, and her continuing positive attitude throughout the entire project; and especially, Susan, Coleman, and Betsy Heckman for their love and patient understanding over the past two years.

James D. Heckman

James D. Heckman, MD
San Antonio, Texas, 1986

The EMT Oath

Be it pledged as an Emergency Medical Technician, I will honor the physical and judicial laws of God and man. I will follow that regimen which, according to my ability and judgment, I consider for the benefit of patients and abstain from whatever is deleterious and mischievous, nor shall I suggest any such counsel. Into whatever homes I enter, I will go into them for the benefit of only the sick and injured, never revealing what I see or hear in the lives of men unless required by law.

I shall also share my medical knowledge with those who may benefit from what I have learned. I will serve unselfishly and continuously in order to help make a better world for all mankind.

While I continue to keep this oath unviolated, may it be granted to me to enjoy life, and the practice of the art, respected by all men, in all times. Should I trespass or violate this oath, may the reverse be my lot. So help me God.

Adopted by The National Association of
Emergency Medical Technicians, 1978

SECTION 1

INTRODUCTION

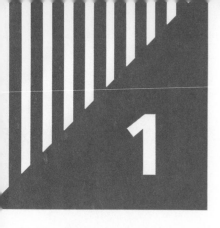

Orientation

THE EMERGENCY MEDICAL SERVICES (EMS) SYSTEM

For years there has been a wide gap between what is possible and what in fact has been delivered in emergency medical care. The knowledge and hardware necessary to develop an **emergency medical services (EMS) system** existed long before such services became available to the public. In reality, EMS as we know it today, had its beginnings twenty years ago in 1966. In that year, the Committees on Trauma and Shock of the National Academy of Sciences National Research Council jointly published "Accidental Death and Disability: The Neglected Disease of Modern Society." This report brought public attention to the inadequate emergency medical care being provided to the sick and injured in many areas of the country.

Two federal agencies initiated reform measures. The National Highway Traffic Safety Administration of the Department of Transportation (DOT), through the Highway Safety Act of 1966, and the Department of Health, Education, and Welfare (HEW), through the Emergency Medical Services Act of 1973, created funding sources to develop improved prehospital emergency care. Thousands of dedicated individuals, assisted by a number of professional organizations and guided by regulatory input from various levels of government, organized and established local EMS systems in the early 1970s.

By the 1980s, the focus changed from establishing EMS systems to developing educational programs to provide consistent levels of quality care to the sick and injured. The programs included additional classroom training and "hands-on" skills sessions, as well as programs for certification, continuing education, and mandatory retraining. Despite the improvements in prehospital care seen today, a great deal remains to be done. The gap between available services and the people who need them is narrowing but still exists in many areas of the country. Likewise, the gap between what is theoretically feasible and what is realistically available is also narrowing.

The EMS system is made up of various parts that work together to provide the sick and injured with the best possible emergency medical care in the shortest possible time. The EMS system represents the combined efforts of the first responder, the EMT with basic life-support skills, the EMT-intermediate or EMT-paramedic with advanced life-support skills, emergency department personnel, physicians, allied health personnel, hospital administration, EMS system administration, and the overseeing governmental agencies.

The way an EMS system functions varies widely, depending on the geographic area and population served. Regardless of whether it is in a rural area, a large city, or a vast metropolitan complex, the EMS system requires the following 13 essential elements:

1. An advisory council on emergency medical service
2. Physician-directed medical control, including quality control review
3. EMT training programs, including continuing education programs
4. Instructor training programs
5. A communications system, including system access

6. Dispatch center(s)
7. Ambulance service(s)
8. EMT and emergency department personnel rapport and trust
9. Reports and records
10. Disaster plans
11. Public information and education programs
12. Categorized hospital emergency capabilities
13. Funding

THE EMERGENCY MEDICAL TECHNICIAN (EMT)

The cornerstone of the EMS system is the **emergency medical technician (EMT).** EMTs have the greatest opportunity of perhaps any group in society to relieve suffering and to reduce injury severity and death at the scene of an accidental injury or sudden illness and during transportation to a medical facility. To become a valued member of the prehospital emergency medical care team, the EMT needs the following:

1. Proper training and experience
2. Ready availability of the proper equipment and supplies
3. A properly designed vehicle to meet the needs of the sick and injured
4. Radio communication with emergency department personnel
5. Ready availability of physician-directed medical control

Roles and Responsibilities of the EMT

EMTs have to earn the respect and recognition of the community in which they live and work. They must be viewed as responsible members of the emergency medical care team. To these ends, the attitude and conduct of EMTs must at all times reflect a sincere dedication to serve mankind. The moral and ethical standards of EMTs must be of the highest order. EMTs must take pride in their personal appearance, as well as in their technical knowledge and skills used to render care to the sick and injured. Such knowledge and skills, however, must be continually expanded and updated. EMTs must strive for perfection in job performance, with full recognition of personal limitations. EMTs must accept and benefit from constructive criticism and advice.

EMTs are expected to perform under pressure with composure and self-confidence. Emotions have to be controlled through self-discipline. The abnormal or exaggerated actions of patients and families under stress need to be handled with understanding and sympathy. These are the qualities of responsible leadership, which EMTs must provide to ensure the health, survival, safety, comfort, and confidence of their patients from the time the EMTs arrive on the scene until they transfer patient care to other medical professionals.

No matter how severe the circumstances, EMTs have a moral obligation to provide the best emergency medical care possible until relieved by a physician or other qualified person at the scene or at the hospital. The EMT's primary responsibilities to the patient are to:

1. Carefully assess and evaluate all signs and symptoms.
2. Give prompt and efficient medical care.
3. Provide safe and efficient transportation.
4. Arrange the orderly transfer of patient care at the receiving medical facility.
5. Communicate with all parties and agencies involved.

In addition to the patient-care responsibilities, EMTs have additional responsibilities, including

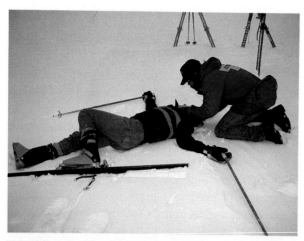

FIGURE 1.1 The first responder is the first person present at the scene of sudden illness or injury. By using their hands, lungs, mouth, and brain, first responders can sustain life until a trained EMT or other professional emergency medical personnel arrive.

maintaining control at the scene, gaining access to and disentangling patients, keeping accurate records, and operating and maintaining the emergency vehicle and its equipment and supplies. Last, but just as important, EMTs have a responsibility to themselves and others at the scene to perform their duties with due regard for their own safety as well as the safety of those around them.

Prehospital Care Personnel and the EMT

In the structure of emergency medical service systems throughout the country, there are recognized differences among basic first-aid training, a DOT first-responder training course, and a DOT-approved EMT training course. Basic first-aid and the slightly more advanced first-responder training programs incorporate basic life-sustaining measures that members of the general public should learn in order to recognize the many hazards encountered during their daily activities. Ideally, basic first-aid training should begin at the fifth-grade level. All EMTs should actively participate as instructors in these community training programs. Ideally, this training should be made available to as many citizens as possible, but especially to those individuals who through their jobs or recreational interests are likely to encounter situations that might require the use of emergency medical techniques. First-aid and first-responder training should be under the direction of and taught in part by knowledgeable physicians. Professional emergency medical care, on the other hand, is administered at the scene of an accident or illness and during transport to a medical facility by highly trained EMTs. These individuals might be volunteers, employees of a commercial ambulance service, or members of a municipal ambulance operation.

The term "first responder" needs further clarification in order to prevent confusion as to its true meaning. This clarification is important because the first responder plays an important role in the EMS system. The **first responder** is the first person present at the scene of sudden illness or injury (Figure 1.1). That first person could be a firefighter, police officer, safety engineer, occupational health or school nurse, coach or trainer, lifeguard, youth leader, or many others in public places. The first responder may or may not have had first-aid or first-responder training. Ideally, these individuals should be trained to the level of the First Responder Curriculum, which has been developed by the Department of Transportation. This training includes **cardiopulmonary resuscitation (CPR).** First responders may have little or no equipment, and in reality they need none to sustain life until a trained EMT arrives on the scene. By using their hands, lungs, mouth, and brain, first responders can assess the injury or illness, provide air to the lungs, blood to the brain, and control bleeding. In other words, they can provide **basic life support.**

Just as it is essential that the first responder do enough for the patient, it is essential that the first responder does not try to do too much. One of the greatest mistakes the general public and first responders make is to remove the injured victim from a vehicle or accident scene. Many additional injuries, including permanent paralysis, have been caused by such well-intentioned, but potentially dangerous, actions. At the scene of an injury accident, an unwarranted fear of fire is frequently the cause for such intervention.

A first responder should attempt to gain access to the patient if possible and provide necessary, life-sustaining CPR, control accessible bleeding using pressure, comfort the patient, and await the arrival of the EMT. Only if the patient's position prevents necessary life-sustaining care or if some circumstances exist that pose an immediate threat to the life of the patient or first responder — for example, fire or imminent collapse of a structure — should the first responder attempt to move the patient before the EMT arrives with appropriate equipment.

Upon arrival, the EMT assumes responsibility immediately but tactfully. The quality and effectiveness of the care rendered by the first responders is assessed, and the first responders are asked to continue assistance as needed. The EMT should give credit for what was done and graciously suggest improvements for subsequent care, keeping in mind that the scene of an accident is not the place to be openly critical of the skills or techniques of a first responder. The training of first responders, especially in rural areas, is currently one of the weakest elements of EMS systems nationwide. The EMT must therefore be actively involved not only in promoting such training programs for the general public and first responders, but also in the instruction process. In addition, the EMT must promote the continuing education and evaluation process for first responders

and EMTs. It is very possible that the life the first responder saves might very well be the EMT's own.

The EMT may come in contact with two additional groups of prehospital emergency medical care personnel, the EMT-paramedic and the EMT-intermediate. The **EMT-paramedic (EMT-P)** has completed an extensive course of training in advanced life support, including intravenous therapy, pharmacology, cardiac monitoring, and defibrillation; advanced airway maintenance, including intubation; and other advanced assessment and treatment skills. Some states have established an intermediate level of training between the EMT and the EMT-paramedic. The **EMT-intermediate (EMT-I)** has training in specific aspects of advanced life support. This training is generally limited to a very specific area, such as intravenous therapy, cardiac defibrillation, or advanced airway management. Whenever an EMT-I or EMT-P arrives on the scene, the EMT should give a brief account of the situation, transfer the responsibility for patient care, and stand by to assist as requested.

Hospital Personnel and the EMT

There is no better way for the EMT to understand how prehospital care influences full recovery or aids in reducing permanent physical impairment than to observe the continuation of emergency medical care by the staff of the emergency department. How much is learned depends on the EMT's sincerity of purpose, eagerness for self-improvement in knowledge, techniques, and skills, and willingness to accept advice and constructive feedback. An EMT with these attributes can enjoy a close working relationship with the hospital staff (Figure 1.2). It is for this reason that in-hospital observation programs are built into the EMT training program.

Although legal restrictions or local and hospital rules may prevent the EMT from participating actively in all procedures in the emergency department, much can be learned through direct observation, instruction, demonstration, and assisting to the extent permitted. As an observer, the EMT will become familiar with hospital equipment and its use, the functions of staff members, and the policies and procedures in all emergency areas of the hospital. In addition, the EMT will keep abreast of advances in emergency care as well as in the use of new equipment. The experience gained from participation

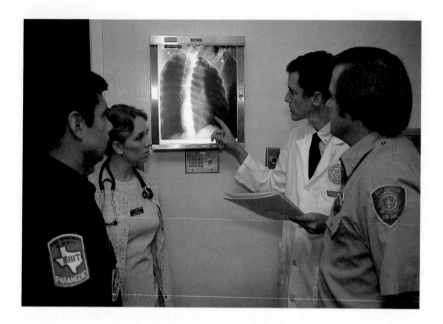

FIGURE 1.2 One of the best ways for an EMT to understand how important prehospital emergency care is in aiding full recovery and reducing permanent impairment is to observe the continuation of medical care in the hospital emergency department.

serves to emphasize the importance and benefits of proper initial emergency care and efficient transportation, as well as the consequences of delay, inadequate care, or poor judgment.

Rarely is a physician present at the scene of an accident or at the onset of unexpected illness to give on-the-spot directions to the EMT. Consultation and advice are usually given to the EMT over the radio through established medical control procedures. In addition to acting as an instructor for the medical subjects taught in this book, the emergency department physician can effectively train the EMT in the emergency department by demonstrating assessment and treatment techniques on actual patients. With such instruction, the EMT becomes more comfortable using medical terminology, is better able to interpret the signs and symptoms of injury and disease, and develops needed patient management skills. At the same time, the physician becomes familiar with the capabilities of the EMT and develops a degree of trust in the EMT's skills so there will be no hesitation in allowing the EMT to proceed with patient care protocols if and when radio communication fails. Such prior face-to-face communication improves radio communication between the EMT and the physician.

The people who staff the emergency departments of most hospitals are eager and willing to help improve the skills and efficiency of EMTs, not only during the initial phase of training, but throughout their careers. A close rapport among all involved in providing emergency medical care not only assures optimal patient care; it also affords the EMTs and emergency department staffs the opportunity to discuss their mutual problems, benefit from each other's experiences, and better fulfill their respective roles as members of the emergency medical care team.

Emotional Stress and the EMT

The EMT needs great willpower when confronted with horrifying events or life-threatening illness or injury that makes it difficult to remain calm and perform effectively. The kind of self-control that is needed to respond effectively to the suffering of others can only be developed through proper training, through gaining experience in dealing with all degrees of physical and mental distress, and especially through an unswerving dedication to serve humanity. At times, even the most experienced physician or combat-hardened medic may find it difficult to overcome personal reactions and proceed without hesitation to release patients from life-endangering situations, to administer life-support measures to the mutilated, or to recover the remains of those mangled in highway accidents, aircraft disasters, or explosions. The EMT must learn to face these situations calmly and to act responsibly as a member of the emergency medical care team. The EMT must also realize that feelings which must be kept under control are normal. They are experienced by all who have to deal with such situations, and they contribute to the emotional stress of an EMT's job.

A high percentage of the patients the EMT treats will be rational and cooperative. Their concerns will generally be relieved by calm and efficient care and a simple explanation of what the EMT is doing and why. Often the EMT will realize that a given condition is not a true medical emergency, but for the patient it might seem to be truly serious. Neither by action nor word should the EMT fail to take the patient's concern seriously. This means being extremely careful about what is said at the scene. During periods of great stress, words that seem immaterial or are uttered in jest might become fixed in the patient's mind and cause untold harm. Conversations at the scene must be appropriate. Statements such as "Everything will be all right" or "There is nothing to worry about" are inappropriate. A person who is trapped in a wrecked car, hurting from head to foot, and worrying about the condition of a loved one or about the payments on the car knows very well that all is not well. What will reassure the patient is that a trained EMT is present. The EMT must explain briefly the emergency actions to be taken and discuss to which medical facility the patient wishes to be transported.

When the EMT is not sure whether or not a case is an actual emergency, the point to remember is that while a physician may examine and decide to dismiss a patient, the EMT does not have that option. For both ethical and medicolegal reasons, a physician must examine all patients treated by an EMT and judge the degree of medical need of every "emergency" patient. The EMT must also realize that the most subtle of symptoms may be early signs of catastrophe, and that symptoms of many illnesses may be similar to those of alcohol and drug abuse or withdrawal, hysteria, or other conditions. The EMT must not only accept the patient's complaints at face value, but also provide appropriate care for the injury or illness reported until able to transfer the care of the patient to a hospital or physician.

A patient's reaction to acute injury or illness may be influenced by certain personality traits. Members of some ethnic groups may be highly emotional and demonstrative over what may seem to be a minor problem, whereas those of other groups show little or no emotion, even in the face of serious injury or illness. Many factors, such as social and economic background, dependence on others, level of maturity, fear of medical personnel, senility, mental disorders, alcoholism, drug addiction, reaction to medication, nutritional status, and chronic disease, may influence how a patient reacts.

Although the EMT cannot be expected to know the underlying causes that might trigger unusual emotional responses, a quick, calm appraisal of the actions of the patient and of relatives and bystanders will help to gain the confidence and cooperation of all concerned. Courtesy, calmness, proper tone of voice, sincere concern, and efficient action during the examination and treatment will go far to relieve anxiety, fear, and insecurity. Calm reassurance rather than abrupt dismissal, chiding, or accusation will inspire confidence and gain cooperation. Compassion is a notable attribute, but the EMT must be careful that it does not overrule reason. For example, a screaming toddler with no obvious life-threatening injuries, yet covered with another victim's blood, can appeal to the EMT's compassion and attention, while an unconscious, nonbreathing adult nearby dies from lack of care.

Patients must be given the opportunity to express their fears and concerns, many of which may easily be relieved on the spot. The usual concerns are for the safety or well-being of others involved in the accident, and for the damage or loss of personal property. The EMT's response must be discreet and diplomatic, giving reassurance when possible and waiting for the appropriate time and place to disclose the death or critical injury of loved ones. If possible, the EMT should wait until an experienced person such as a minister or emergency department nurse can tell the patient of the death or critical injury of a loved one so that the psychological support the person may need is available.

Some patients, especially children and the confused or aged, may be terrified or feel rejected when separated from family members. Other patients may not want family members to share their stress or witness their disability or pain. The extent to which relatives participate in patient care, including whether or not they go with the patient to the hospital, must be decided on the basis of the best interests of the patient. It is usually best if parents go with their children and if relatives accompany confused, elderly patients.

The religious customs or needs of the patient must also be respected. Many people have strong convictions against the administration of drugs and blood and blood products. Some people will cling to religious medals or amulets, especially if an attempt is made to remove them. Others will express a strong desire for religious counsel, baptism, or last rites if death is imminent at the scene. The EMT must try to accommodate these requests.

In the case of death, the body of the deceased must be handled with respect and dignity. It must be exposed as little as possible. The EMT must be aware of local restrictions about moving the body or changing its position, especially if there is a possibility of a criminal investigation. Even under these circumstances, CPR and appropriate treatment must be instituted unless there are obvious signs of death, such as rigor mortis, decapitation, or other massive injuries not compatible with life.

The care of the handicapped patient presents special problems. This is particularly true of the deaf, the deaf-mute, and the blind. The deaf patient who does not have a functioning hearing aid will have difficulty in understanding verbal questions about symptoms. The deaf-mute will be able to respond only with sign language or in writing. Unless pertinent information is needed at the scene, obvious problems should be treated. The patient can be placated with efficient action and brief written notes. Detailed questioning may be delayed until the patient is transferred to a medical facility where relatives or others may act as interpreters.

Similar problems will occur with patients who do not speak English. In communities with large non-English-speaking populations, the EMT will find it helpful to carry a card with frequently used medical words and their translations (Figure 1.3).

The blind patient, of course, will be able to talk with the EMT, but the EMT must be careful to explain what is occurring, the actions to be taken, and the qualifications of the EMT performing these actions. While the majority of blind people are very self-reliant, they behave like any other patient when disoriented and confused. Such situations can be avoided by keeping them fully informed.

Personal Safety of the EMT

The personal safety of all those involved in an emergency situation is very important — so impor-

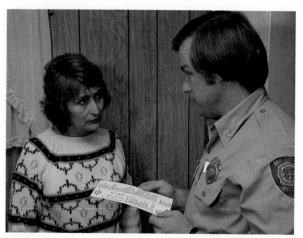

FIGURE 1.3   Language translation cards list frequently used medical words and their translations into English. EMTs who work in communities with large non-English-speaking populations should carry these cards.

tant, in fact, that the steps the EMT takes to preserve personal safety must become automatic. A second accident at the scene or an injury to an EMT compounds the problems, delays emergency medical care for the patients, increases the burden on the remaining EMTs, and may result in unnecessary fatalities.

Perhaps the easiest and most effective way in which EMTs can protect themselves is by using seat belts. Seat belts should be worn at all times unless patient care makes it impossible. Many EMS units have instituted mandatory seat-belt policies for the driver at all times, for all EMTs during transit to the scene, and for anyone riding with a patient.

The scene of an accident must be well marked since a second accident often results in damage to the ambulance and injury to the EMTs. If the police have not already done so, proper warning devices should be placed at a sufficient distance from the scene to alert motorists coming from both directions. The ambulance should be parked at a safe, yet convenient, distance from the scene; the exact location will be determined by factors discussed later in the text. Before any attempt is made to access patients trapped in vehicles, the vehicle's stability should be checked and any necessary measures taken to secure it. A vehicle's stability should not be determined by pushing or rocking, as this may be all that is needed to overturn the vehicle or send it crashing into a ditch.

The risk of injury to an EMT who is working at the scene of a wreck can be greatly reduced by wearing protective clothing. For example, a firefighter's helmet or hard hat, turnout gear, goggles or face shield, and leather gloves are all designed to decrease the risk of injury from broken glass or jagged metal during disentanglement of the patient (Figure 1.4).

To work effectively at night, the EMT must have plenty of light. Poor lighting increases the risk of further injury to both the patient and the EMT and results in poor emergency medical care for the patient. Proper lighting is included in the equipment requirements for ambulances. Reflective emblems or clothing help make the EMT more visible at night and decrease the risk of injury to the EMT (Figure 1.5).

The EMT should never enter an unstable accident scene. Fires, poisonous gas, downed electrical wires, or hazardous materials require preliminary action by other public safety personnel. Unstable situations also include civil disturbances such as shootings, brawls, hostage situations, and riots. The EMT must recognize hazardous situations and call for additional specialized assistance to stabilize the scene before entering and rendering care; failure to do so may seriously jeopardize the EMT's personal safety. The EMT should rely on the advice of police or other public safety officials for the appropriate pro-

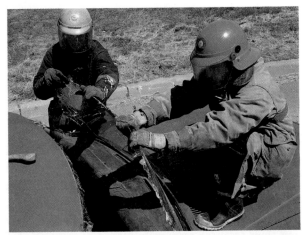

FIGURE 1.4 Wearing protective clothing, including a helmet or hard hat, turnout gear, goggles or a face shield, and leather gloves, will greatly reduce the risk of injury to the EMT.

tective measures to take under these circumstances. Again, the general rule is that the EMT not enter an unsecured or unstable incident scene.

Training for the EMT

Emergency medical technology is an exciting field of study. Few areas offer more direct application of theory and skills. Everything that is taught in an EMT class will be important when it comes to saving lives and lessening human suffering.

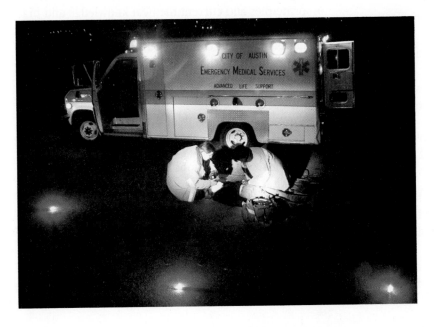

FIGURE 1.5 Adequate lighting is essential for providing emergency care. Poor lighting increases the risk of further injury to both the EMT and the patient. Reflective emblems or clothing also help make the EMT more visible at night.

Emergency medical technology combines theoretical information, practical skills, and common sense. Becoming an effective EMT means mastering the information in this textbook, becoming competent in the technical skills taught in laboratory sessions, and developing common sense. The EMT must also possess a great deal of compassion and understanding.

The Department of Transportation's Emergency Medical Technician-Ambulance: National Standard Curriculum specifies that training consist of a minimum of 110 hours; most EMT courses run from 110 to 140 hours. During their training program, EMTs will develop the capabilities necessary to carry out their required responsibilities. The training may be divided into three main categories. The first and most important category is the care of life-threatening conditions. For such situations, the EMT must learn to:

1. Establish and maintain an open airway.
2. Provide adequate pulmonary ventilation.
3. Perform cardiopulmonary resuscitation.
4. Control accessible bleeding.
5. Treat shock.
6. Care for cases of poisoning.

The second category of training covers conditions that, while not life-threatening, must be cared for before the patient is transported to a medical facility. To handle these situations, the EMT must learn to:

1. Dress and bandage wounds.
2. Splint fractures and dislocations.
3. Deliver a baby.
4. Care for newborn infants, including premature infants.
5. Cope with the psychologic stresses on patients, families, colleagues, and the EMT.

The third training category covers important nonmedical requirements. The EMT must develop competence in the following areas:

1. Verbal and written communications skills
2. Defensive and emergency driving skills
3. Maintenance and use of supplies and equipment
4. Proper extrication techniques and equipment
5. Avoiding or coping with medicolegal problems

Licensure, Certification, and Continuing Education for the EMT

Licensure, certification, recertification, and continuing education policies and procedures vary from state to state, although efforts are being made to establish a national standard. It is important for each EMT to understand and conform to the local requirements. EMT training is not a one-time effort. In order to maintain, update, and broaden needed knowledge and skills, the EMT must continue to study. This responsibility for continuing educational effort exists whether the EMT is affiliated with a full-time paid ambulance service or a rural volunteer rescue squad. In fact, rural volunteers probably have a greater need for continuing education in that they will not have as many opportunities to refresh their knowledge and skills in actual patient-handling situations.

Four major national organizations that are concerned with the education, licensure, and certification of EMTs are the National Council of State EMS Training Coordinators, Inc., the National Registry of Emergency Medical Technicians, the International Society of Fire Service Instructors, and the National Association of Emergency Medical Technicians.

The National Council of State EMS Training Coordinators, Inc.

The purpose of the National Council of State EMS Training Coordinators is to promote the training of EMS personnel based on sound educational principles and current medical knowledge and practice. The council seeks acceptance of a standardized national EMT training curriculum, certification/recertification policies and procedures, and the reciprocity of certification from state to state. Public recognition and trust of the EMT as a health care professional is a major goal of the National Council. Forty-seven states are represented on the council, in addition to numerous liaison appointees from professional organizations that are involved in prehospital care.

The National Registry of Emergency Medical Technicians

The National Registry of EMTs is the recognized national agency for certifying EMTs and documenting their level of competence according to recommended standards. The goals of the Registry are to promote and improve the delivery of emergency medical services by:

1. Assisting in the development and evaluation of educational programs to train EMTs.
2. Establishing qualifications for eligibility in applying for certification.
3. Preparing and conducting examinations designed to assure the competence of EMTs.
4. Establishing a system of recertification every two years.
5. Establishing procedures for revocation of certification for cause.
6. Maintaining a national directory of registered EMTs.

The Registry also develops guidelines and programs to assist registered EMTs raise their level of competence, thereby assuring the provision of improved emergency medical services. Finally, the Registry will do any and all things necessary or desirable for the attainment of these goals.

The three levels of national certification available through the National Registry are basic (EMT-ambulance and EMT-nonambulance), intermediate (EMT-intermediate), and advanced (EMT-paramedic). The shoulder patch of the National Registry of EMTs has been copyrighted, and rockers attesting to the EMT's level of competence are available (Figure 1.6).

The International Society of Fire Service Instructors

The International Society of Fire Service Instructors has approximately 6,000 members in all 50 states and 10 foreign countries. Its EMS section is designed to meet the training and education needs of persons providing emergency medical services training. It serves as a communication link for its members through newsletters, meetings, and other clearinghouse activities.

The National Association of Emergency Medical Technicians

The National Association of Emergency Medical Technicians (NAEMT) was formed in 1975 by a representative group of nationally registered EMTs from existing state EMT organizations, national EMS leaders, and the National Registry of EMTs to serve the needs of EMTs throughout the coun-

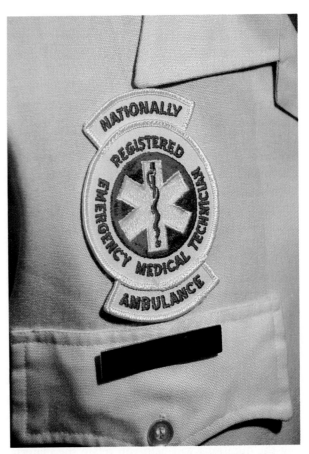

FIGURE 1.6 Rockers are small patches that are positioned below the National Registry patch. They indicate an EMT's level of competence and any specialized training.

try. The association has a membership in excess of 10,000 in 26 affiliated EMT associations. It sponsors continuing education programs on a national, regional, and local level. It provides a total of 17 other membership programs and services. The association's goals are to promote the professional status of the EMT, encourage the constant upgrading of the education and abilities of the EMT, and strive for a national standard of recognition for the skills and abilities of the EMT.

USING *EMERGENCY CARE AND TRANSPORTATION OF THE SICK AND INJURED,* 4th ed.

For many of you, this may be the first time you have been a student in several years. For others, this course is part of an ongoing educational process. Whatever group you fall into, the editors have strived to ease your learning tasks. The content and objectives of this textbook conform to the EMT National Standard Curriculum developed by the United States Department of Transportation in 1984. The format of each chapter has been modified from previous editions to enhance student retention of the information presented. Each chapter begins with an overview of the topic to be covered and a list of educational objectives that outline the core material. Important new words are printed in **bold-faced type.** A simple definition of these words usually follows. Should you have forgotten the meaning of a word when it is used in later chapters, there is a glossary of these key words at the end of the textbook. The end of each chapter contains a few thought-provoking questions under the heading "You Are the EMT." They should help you apply the principles within the chapter to the types of situations you will encounter as an EMT.

The student workbook is divided into sections that correspond to the chapters in the text. Each section contains questions on the material covered in the chapter. The questions are multiple-choice, fill-in-the-blank, true-false, or label the diagram. Answering the questions will help you retain the material that you have just studied. The end of each section in the workbook contains a series of multiple-choice questions. In addition to having been designed to review the material that you have just covered, these questions will also provide you with some practice in the testing format used in the written portion of most licensure and certification examinations.

To assist you in successfully completing the EMT course you have undertaken, the "SURVIVE" study technique was developed. Its purpose is to help you gain and retain more from your reading assignments and workbook activities. Take a few minutes to review this "lifesaving" study technique.

S - SKIM

Read the chapter overview and objectives. Briefly skim the chapter. Look at all the headings, pictures, charts, and diagrams.

U - UNDERLINE

Underline or highlight any unfamiliar words or medical terms that you have been asked to define. Do not highlight long sentences or passages. The purpose of highlighting is to allow the quick location of key information within the text. Excessive highlighting defeats this purpose.

R - READ

Read the objectives at the beginning of the chapter again. Read the workbook questions and any questions distributed by your instructor. This will allow you to direct your reading toward the specific goals of the chapter. Now, read the chapter.

V - VERBALIZE

Answer the questions from the workbook and your instructor out loud. This technique will help you to remember in two ways. First, it turns a written stimulus into an auditory response. At the same time, it holds the answer in your brain long enough for it to be transferred to long-term memory.

I - INTEGRATE

Integrate the new information with the information you have previously learned in the textbook as well as in your lab sessions. Using the information helps make it meaningful and is an excellent way to increase memory retention.

V - VARY

Vary your activity. Take a break from your studies so the newly acquired information can "sink in." Stop frequently to review the material you have just covered.

E - EVALUATE

Evaluate the newly presented information. Does it conflict with previously presented materials? Do the lecturers say the same thing as the textbook? Were all of your questions answered? If not, you need to get those questions cleared up as soon as possible.

One of the most important tasks for the EMT student is learning to study effectively. Hopefully, the SURVIVE format will provide the structure needed to sharpen your study skills. The following additional study hints will not only help you SURVIVE but also EXCEL!

1. Do not miss any classroom lectures or lab sessions.
2. Take advantage of any extra study or practical lab sessions.

3. Form a study group with classmates who are serious about doing well.
4. If your class is offered at a college, especially a community college, find out if a learning resource center is available and take advantage of programs offered.
5. Be sure that your life status is at a stable point.
6. Come to class with a positive attitude. Plan to do better than just getting by.
7. Always act in a professional manner.
8. Be good to yourself and show pride in your accomplishments by treating yourself to something special when you have achieved your goals.

After you have successfully completed your EMT course and passed your certification and/or Registry exams, remember that the learning process for the EMT never ends. Eagerly pursue recertification and continuing educational opportunities as time permits.

YOU ARE THE EMT...

1. Right now you have passed a first responder course. What additional skills must you acquire to become an EMT? An EMT-P?
2. You will receive much of your EMT training in the hospital emergency department. Besides having the opportunity to practice assessment and treatment techniques on actual patients, what other benefits will you derive from this kind of experience? What benefits can emergency room physicians derive from teaching you?
3. Perhaps the most important step you can take to preserve your personal safety is to wear a seat belt. What other precautions should EMTs take when responding to an automobile accident?
4. Describe an unstable accident scene. How would you go about stabilizing the situation?

2 Legal Responsibilities

OVERVIEW

An EMT involved in an emergency response situation may become involved in a variety of potential legal problems. One type of legal problem occurs when an individual is dissatisfied with the quality of emergency care rendered. Unskilled assessment or treatment performed by the EMT which worsens the patient's condition, or failure to protect the patient from further injury, may raise the question of negligence. And if negligence did occur, does the patient deserve a legal remedy or settlement? This type of potential legal problem is the focus of this chapter, as well as the concepts of consent and immunity.

Chapter 2 begins with a discussion of standard of care and how it is established — that is, whether standards are imposed by local custom, by law, or as a measure against professional or institutional standards. The chapter next explains the doctrine of negligence and the law of consent. The last part of the chapter discusses forms of immunity, duty to respond, and types of records and reports.

OBJECTIVES

The objectives of Chapter 2 are to
- understand the basis of legal responsibility — the standard of care — and how standard of care can be established.
- become knowledgeable concerning the doctrine of negligence.
- become informed of the law of consent, including implied consent, consent to treat minors, consent of the mentally ill, and the right to refuse treatment.
- identify the various forms of immunity granted by the law.
- distinguish between duty to respond and response on a volunteer basis.
- appreciate the importance of keeping accurate records and reports, especially regarding cases of child abuse, injuries during felonies, drug-related injuries, childbirth, crimes, and death.

STANDARD OF CARE

Regardless of the activity one is involved in, the law requires an individual to act or behave toward other individuals in a certain, definable way. Under given circumstances, the individual has a duty to act or refrain from acting. Generally speaking, the individual must be concerned about the safety and welfare of other individuals when his or her behavior or activities have the potential for causing others injury or harm. The manner in which the individual must act or behave is called a **standard of care.**

Standard of care is established in many ways, among them being local custom, statutes, ordinances, administrative regulations, and case law. In addition, professional or institutional standards have a bearing on determining the adequacy of an EMT's conduct.

Standards Imposed by Local Custom

The conduct of an individual is to be judged in comparison with the conduct of other (hypothetical) persons of similar training and experience. For example, the conduct of an EMT employed by an ambulance service is to be judged in comparison with the expected conduct of EMTs from comparable ambulance services. Such standards are often based on locally accepted protocols. In the first place, the EMT will not be held to the same standard of care as a physician or other more highly trained individual. Further, the EMT's conduct must be judged in the light of the given emergency situation, taking into consideration the general confusion at the scene of the emergency, the needs of other patients, and the type of equipment available. Therefore, the prevailing custom of the community is an important element in determining the standard of emergency care required. Specifically, the standard of care is how a reasonably prudent person with similar training and experience would act under similar circumstances, with similar equipment, and in the same place.

Standards Imposed by Law

In addition to local customs, standards of emergency medical care may be imposed by statutes, ordinances, administrative regulation, or case law. In many jurisdictions, violating one of these standards is said to create **presumptive negligence.** Therefore, EMTs must familiarize themselves with the particular legal standards that may exist in their state. In many states, this may take the form of published treatment protocols by a state agency.

Professional or Institutional Standards

In addition to the standards imposed by the force of law, professional or institutional standards may be admitted as evidence in determining the adequacy of an EMT's conduct. **Professional standards** include published recommendations of organizations and societies involved in emergency medical care. **Institutional standards** include specific rules and procedures of the ambulance service or organization to which the EMT is attached.

Two words of caution are important. First, EMTs should familiarize themselves with the published standards of their organizations. Second, an EMT who is involved in formulating standards for a particular agency should attempt to make the standards reasonable and realistic so that they do not impose an unreasonable burden on the EMTs. Optimum emergency medical care should be every EMT's goal, but it is not realistic to have institutional standards that *demand* optimum care.

In legal terms, the standard of care for an EMT may be stated as follows: "To perform as a reasonable, prudent, properly trained EMT would perform under the same or similar circumstances." A reasonably skillful, good faith effort to apply the information and skills that are presented in this book would generally meet the standard of care expected of a basic EMT.

THE DOCTRINE OF NEGLIGENCE

Potential legal problems occur when the standard of care is not met. Failure to perform an important or necessary technique, or performing such a technique in a careless or unskilled manner, would violate the standard of care. When that violation of the standard of care causes further injury to the patient, a court may find the EMT negligent. The doctrine of **negligence** is the basis for legal responsibility. Legal negligence results in a civil liability in those instances where the actions or behavior of the individual, who had a duty to act, did not conform to the standard of care, and injury resulted.

When charged with negligent actions or behavior, the individual cannot be found liable before the facts of the case have been presented and weighed carefully. The performance of the individual must be weighed against the applicable standard of care. In the case of an EMT, if the actions or performance of the EMT were those that might be expected of a reasonable, prudent, properly trained EMT operating in the same or similar circumstances, there would be no negligent action or behavior and, therefore, no liability. On the other hand, if the actions or performance of the EMT were reckless, careless, or lacking in skill, the standard of care would have been violated, and the EMT might be found negligent. However, before the EMT can be found liable, it must be shown that the violation of the standard of care was the actual cause of the injury or loss suffered by the patient.

This last requirement for proof of causation may be the major reason why very few lawsuits for negligence have been filed against EMTs. In most instances, EMTs are called to assist an individual who has a preexisting illness or injury. Because the illness or injury existed before the EMT arrived at the scene, the EMT cannot be held responsible for the preexisting condition. The EMT may, however, be held responsible for an aggravation or worsening of the condition that results from a violation of the standard of care.

It is important to recognize that the civil law of negligence is a system for evaluating an individual's behavior against a standard of behavior. If the behavior is found inappropriate, legal remedies may be awarded. Regardless of the field of human activity, every individual has the right not to be subjected to undue harm. When the individual is subjected to undue harm and an injury or aggravation of a preexisting injury occurs, the person who caused that injury or aggravation is expected to compensate the injured individual.

Abandonment

Having begun to provide care, the EMT must follow through with all necessary and appropriate treatment. The EMT must continue to provide care until responsibility for patient care is transferred to another medical professional of an equal or higher level of skill, or until the patient is transferred to a medical facility. Failure to continue the treatment is referred to as **abandonment.** Abandonment is legally and ethically the most serious act an EMT can commit.

THE LAW OF CONSENT

The law of **consent** has confronted every experienced EMT. It is a long-established legal right that an individual is entitled to be free from intentional touching or interference by another person without his or her consent.

Without consent, the intentional touching of an individual is said to constitute a technical battery. However, not every touching without consent results in possible exposure to legal action. People often enter situations in which a reasonable person could expect touching. For example, bumping in crowds at a sporting event does not result in legal action. Consent to such contact is implied from the fact that the individual voluntarily entered the situation. This type of **implied consent** is applicable to emergency situations. Just as a person voluntarily entering a crowd implies consent for bumping, emergency situations create an implication that the person consents to receive emergency medical care and to be transported to a medical facility.

In addition to implied consent, the EMT will be frequently involved with another type of consent — **actual consent.** Actual consent occurs where the patient expressly authorizes the EMT to provide care or transportation. Actual consent may take the form of words, a nod of agreement, or other expression of approval or consent.

The EMT should attempt to obtain actual consent if possible. At the same time, for consent to be effective, it should also be informed consent. **Informed consent** means that the patient must understand the nature and extent of any procedure before agreeing to it. The patient should also have sufficient mental and physical capacity to make such a judgment.

Hospitals normally obtain a patient's consent by requiring a signature on a printed document. The signed document is useful as evidence that the pa-

tient was informed of what was to take place and willingly agreed to permit these activities. Most often, in field situations encountered by the EMT, obtaining written consent from the patient is not practical. Instead, oral consent will be obtained from the patient. Oral consent is valid and binding, although it may be difficult to prove.

Implied Consent

The law assumes that an individual who needs immediate emergency medical care to prevent death or permanent physical impairment would consent to such care and transportation to a medical facility. However, this doctrine of implied consent is limited to true emergency situations. Generally, implied consent is appropriate when the patient is unconscious, delusional, or otherwise physically incapable of giving informed consent. In these cases, as well as in those where prompt action is necessary to prevent death or serious physical impairment, the EMT may proceed with the required care and transportation without obtaining consent.

When the patient is unable to express consent but another responsible person or relative is present, it is advisable to obtain permission from that person or relative to proceed with care. The law in most instances recognizes the right of a spouse, close relative, or next of kin to give consent for injured persons unable to consent for themselves.

Consent to Treat Minors

The law recognizes that a minor may not have the wisdom, maturity, or judgment to give valid consent for emergency medical care. Therefore, the authority to consent for the minor is given to the parents or individuals who are so close to the minor as to be treated as the equivalent of parents. Despite this rule, the consent given by a minor may in some cases be valid, depending on the age and maturity of the individual. For example, the consent of a 17-year-old is more likely to be valid than that of a 4-year-old. Many states have enacted laws that permit minors to give a binding consent to receive medical care. The laws of many states also allow emancipated, married, or pregnant minors to be treated as adults for the purposes of consenting to medical treatment.

The laws and principles related to consent of minors merely determine who has the right to consent — not whether consent is needed. If a true emergency exists, the consent to treat the minor is implied. However, the consent of the parents should be obtained if possible.

Consent of the Mentally Ill

A mentally incompetent person is not capable of giving an informed consent to receive medical treatment. However, unless the individual has been legally judged incompetent, there may be a question as to his or her capabilities. When a legal determination of incompetence has occurred, another individual, such as a guardian or conservator, usually possesses the right to consent on behalf of the patient.

In many field situations, EMTs will encounter patients who may appear confused or in mental distress. These symptoms should be considered in deciding whether the patient can give a knowing or informed consent to medical treatment. When a true emergency situation exists, the doctrine of implied consent applies.

The Right to Refuse Treatment

Mentally competent adults have the right to refuse treatment. Injured or ill people who refuse treatment or transportation present EMTs with a dilemma: Do they care for such people against their will and risk being accused of battery or do they leave them alone and risk a worsening of the condition and being accused of negligence or abandonment? Just as the consent to receive treatment must be informed, the refusal of treatment or transportation must also be informed. That means that if the refusing patient is delusional or confused, the EMT cannot assume that the refusal of treatment is a knowing refusal. On the other hand, competent adults who for religious reasons refuse specific kinds of treatment generally have a legal right to refuse such treatment.

When an individual refuses treatment, the EMT must try to determine whether the individual's mental condition is impaired. When in doubt, it is always best to assume that there is mental impairment and to proceed with treatment. When compared to the decision to abandon a patient and having that patient's condition worsen, the decision to provide treatment is defensible from both legal and medical points of view.

A special situation occurs when a parent refuses to permit treatment of an ill or injured child. The EMT has an obligation to consider the emotional impact of the emergency on the parent's judgment. In this, and virtually all cases of refusal to receive treatment, the EMT usually can resolve the situation through patience and calm persuasion. When refusal is adamant, however, and no amount of persuasion can resolve the situation, it is essential that the refusing individual, guardian, conservator, or parent of the patient be asked to sign an official release form that acknowledges refusal. This form should be witnessed and stored with the run report and the medical incident report that are compiled by the ambulance personnel. It is advisable to include a comment about the refusal on the medical incident report and on the run report forms as well. In those instances in which the individual also refuses to sign the refusal form, the circumstances of the incident and the refusal should be thoroughly documented and the record stored for future reference.

The requirement for consent and the problem of refusing patients are related. Emergency medical care may be rendered only with the consent of the patient, and a mentally competent adult has the right to refuse treatment. These matters become more complex in cases involving minors or in cases where the patient appears to be delusional or confused. The EMT should try to err on the side of rendering treatment rather than withholding it. Failure to render treatment to an individual invites much greater exposure to legal liability than rendering treatment to an individual who has failed to give consent or who expresses a refusal to be treated or transported. In most instances, the law is on the side of emergency medical care personnel. Also, in most cases, the problem of a refusing patient can best be resolved by the persuasive skills of the EMT in the field.

FORMS OF IMMUNITY

As stated earlier, the civil law of negligence is intended to provide legal remedies to persons who suffer injury or damage as a result of the negligent actions or behavior of another. Throughout the history of law, however, there have been limited situations where the law has granted **immunity** from the burdens of compensating the injured or damaged individual. Most of the forms of immunity have been based on the special status of the individual to whom the immunity applies.

For example, in English common law, the doctrine of **sovereign immunity** meant, in essence, that the king could do no wrong. Under that principle, injured or damaged individuals were deprived of a remedy when their injury or damage was caused by the negligence of the king or other member of the royal family. The resulting injustice eventually caused the doctrine to be abandoned.

Later, the doctrine of **governmental immunity** was adopted throughout the United States. Under this rule, government agencies were held to be immune from the legal consequences of their actions. Persons injured or damaged by the negligent actions, behaviors, or omissions of a government agency or its employees were deprived of a remedy. Injustice commonly resulted from this form of immunity, and it has been substantially eroded in recent years. In fact, more than half of the states have abandoned the doctrine of governmental immunity.

A relatively new form of immunity has been created in recent years. Adopted by statute in virtually all states, this new immunity seeks to protect citizens and emergency medical care workers from legal liability. These **"Good Samaritan" laws** attempt to assure that someone who voluntarily helps an injured or suddenly ill person at the scene is not legally liable for errors or omissions in rendering good faith emergency care. Most of these statutes do not provide immunity for gross negligence or willful and wanton misconduct that results in an injury.

Another group of laws, currently in effect in every state, seeks to grant immunity from liability to official emergency medical care providers, such as EMTs. The provisions of these laws vary widely from state to state. As with the "Good Samaritan" laws, most do not provide immunity when injury or damage is caused by gross negligence or willful and wanton misconduct.

In considering immunities, EMTs should recognize that any immunity granted to one individual has the potential for injustice to another. Making one person unaccountable for his or her negligence can mean that an individual injured by that negligence may have no legal recourse. Generally throughout the history of law, efforts to grant immunity to individuals with special standing or status have been relatively short-lived.

The current trend toward providing immunity to citizens and emergency care personnel has not been thoroughly tested by the courts, largely because few legal conflicts arise from emergency medical care and transportation in the field. Most legal scholars agree that the immunities granted by the various state laws are not absolute by any means. Furthermore, in order to determine whether an immunity applies in a particular case, it would be necessary to initiate a lawsuit and evaluate the relevant evidence and testimony. Though the immunity laws may provide some protection, it is clear that much better protection is provided by rendering top-quality emergency medical care.

Emergency Medical Technician Statutes

Most states have adopted specific statutes that grant special privileges to EMTs. These statutes frequently authorize the performance of certain specified medical procedures. Many also grant a partial immunity to the EMT and the physicians and nurses who give emergency instructions to EMTs, EMT-intermediates, or EMT-paramedics via radio or other forms of communication.

Exemptions from the Medical Practices Act

Nearly every state exempts emergency medical care from the licensure requirements of the Medical Practices Act for nonmedical personnel. Since many emergency medical care procedures may be construed to be the performance of a medical act, the EMT is protected in those situations. Such exemption is, however, not all-inclusive, since there are specific licensure or certification requirements for EMTs in all states. A state's requirement for specific licensure or certification of the EMT affects the exemption from the Medical Practices Act.

The Effect of Licensure or Certification

By definition, **licensure** is formal permission to perform certain acts. **Certification** is formal notice of certain privileges and abilities after the completion of certain training and testing. In those states that require licensure or certification by a specified state agency, these requirements frequently are interpreted as necessary conditions to the rendering of emergency medical care on a regular or continuing basis. Furthermore, the possession of a license or certificate obligates the individual to conform to the standard of care of other licensed or certified emergency medical care personnel. In those states that might not require licensure or certification, individuals rendering emergency medical care on a regular or continuing basis may nonetheless be held to the same standard of care expected of certified EMTs.

DUTY TO RESPOND

The primary distinction between an ambulance service attached to a government agency and one that is volunteer or commercial lies in the **duty to respond.** A municipal ambulance service, being part of a governmental service, may have a duty to respond to a call within its jurisdiction, while a commercial or volunteer service may not be so obligated unless such care is advertised or is a requirement of its licensure. However, once a response has been made by any type of ambulance service, the principles of duty to act and the standards of care are equally applicable to both types of emergency personnel.

RECORDS AND REPORTS

Society through its government has formulated a policy to protect its people by health regulations and statutes. Because certain individuals are in a position to observe and gather information about diseases, injuries, and emergency events, an obligation to compile such information and report it to certain agencies may be imposed. Even where there is no such requirement, it is advisable for EMTs to compile a complete and accurate record of all incidents when they come in contact with sick or injured individuals. Most medical and legal experts believe that a complete and accurate record of an emergency medical incident is an important safeguard against legal complications. The absence of a record, or a substantially incomplete record, may mean the EMT has to testify to the events, their findings, and their actions relying on memory alone. Reliance on one's memory can prove to be wholly inadequate and embarrassing in the face of aggressive cross-examination.

Two rules of thumb relating to reports and records should be followed by the EMT. Typically applied in the courtroom setting, the first rule suggests that if an action or procedure is not recorded on the written report, it was not done. The second rule of thumb generally suggests that an incomplete

or untidy report is evidence of incomplete or inexpert emergency medical care. Both of these potentially dangerous presumptions can be avoided by compiling and maintaining accurate reports and records of all events and patients.

Special Reporting Requirements

Child Abuse

All states and the District of Columbia have enacted laws to protect abused children, and some have added other protected groups such as the elderly. Most states have a reporting obligation for certain individuals, whose definition may range from "physician" to "any person." EMTs must be aware of the requirements of law in their state. Such statutes frequently grant immunity from liability for libel, slander, or defamation of character to the person obligated to report, if the reports are made in good faith.

Injury during the Commission of a Felony

Many states have laws requiring the reporting of an injury likely to have occurred during the commission of a criminal act or other specific injuries such as gunshot or knife wounds or poisonings. Again, EMTs must be familiar with the legal requirements of their state.

Drug-Related Injuries

In some instances, drug-related injuries must be reported. These requirements may affect the EMT. However, it should be stressed that the United States Supreme Court has held that drug addiction, as opposed to drug possession or sale, is an illness and not a crime. Hence, an injury as a result of a drug overdose may not be within the definition of an injury resulting from a felonious act.

Some states, by statute, specifically establish confidentiality and excuse certain specified individuals from reporting drug cases, either to a government agency or a minor's parents, if, in the discretion of those individuals, withholding reporting is necessary for the proper treatment of the patient. Once again, EMTs must be familiar with the legal requirements of their state.

Childbirth

Many states require that anyone in attendance at a live birth in any place other than a licensed medical facility report the birth. As before, the EMT must be familiar with state requirements.

Other Reporting Requirements

Other reporting requirements may include attempted suicides, dog bites, certain communicable diseases, assaults, and rapes.

Scene of a Crime

If there is evidence at an emergency scene that a crime may have been committed, the EMT must notify the dispatcher immediately so that proper authorities can be informed. Provided that there is no active criminal activity occurring at the scene that renders the scene hazardous or unstable, such circumstances should not deter the EMT from providing necessary emergency medical care to the patient and transporting the patient to the hospital, if necessary, before the authorities arrive. While emergency medical care is being provided, the EMT must be careful not to disturb the scene of the crime any more than absolutely necessary. Notes and drawings should be made of the position of the patient and of the presence and position of any weapon or other objects that may be valuable to the investigating officers. The EMT should confer periodically with local authorities and be aware of their wishes as to any actions the EMT should take at the scene of a crime. It is best if these guidelines can be established by protocol.

The Deceased

In most states, EMTs do not have the authority to pronounce an individual dead. If there is any chance that life exists or that the patient can be resuscitated, the EMT must make every effort to preserve that life at the scene and during transport to medical facilities. At times, however, death is obvious; rigor mortis has set in, decapitation has occurred, the body is consumed by fire, or there is a massive head injury with parts missing. In such instances, there is no urgent reason to move the body. The only immediate action required of the EMT is to cover the body and prevent its disturbance. Local rules and protocols from the medical examiner or coroner will determine the ultimate action of the EMT in these instances.

Occasionally an EMT will respond to a call for assistance because a patient has died from some disease and the family members present decide that they do not wish any resuscitative efforts to be made but no written documentation to that effect has been initiated. This places the EMT in a very difficult position and one that will be occurring more frequently with the development of terminal nursing home placement, hospice, and home health programs. Each ambulance service, in consultation with its medical director and legal counsel, must develop a protocol to follow in such circumstances.

It must be emphasized that only general legal principles have been discussed here, since state laws differ widely. Even though medical-legal responsibilities must be taken seriously, they should not intimidate EMTs and prevent them from doing their job. In very few cases has liability been imposed on EMTs because of their conduct. The liability for not performing is at least as great as the liability of performing improperly. The best legal defense is proper training, continuing education, skillful rendering of required emergency care, and careful written documentation.

YOU ARE THE EMT...

1. Before you can be accused of negligence, what has to be proved?
2. Your patient, a middle-aged man, is unconscious and requires oxygen. You begin treatment, based on implied consent. What does that mean? A few minutes later his wife arrives. What kind of consent will you seek from her?
3. You have responded to a bicycle accident in which a 14-year-old boy appears to have suffered a severe concussion. You realize he should be transported to the hospital for x-rays and examination by a doctor. He refuses to go and will not tell you his name. He says he's OK and will get in terrible trouble if his parents find out he was skipping school. What will you do?
4. You are a certified EMT. How does certification differ from licensure?

SECTION 2

PATIENT ASSESSMENT

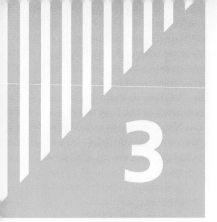

3

General and Topographic Anatomy

OVERVIEW

A working knowledge of human anatomy is essential for all medical personnel, including EMTs. Even though EMTs are not expected to diagnose every injury or illness, they can aid emergency department personnel by conveying correct information using medical terminology. Such information is gathered after examination of a patient at the scene of an accident or sudden illness.

Topographic anatomy refers to how the superficial landmarks on the surface of the body are used as guides to locate the internal structures that lie beneath them. The language of topographic anatomy refers to the names of the principal regions of the body and the way the locations of these regions are described in relationship to one another.

Chapter 3 begins by defining the terms used to describe topographic anatomy when the body is in the anatomic position. The chapter then describes the topographic features of the seven major regions of the body. The last section of the chapter discusses arterial pulse points, or where on the body the major arteries can be palpated.

OBJECTIVES

The objectives of Chapter 3 are to

- define the common terms used in topographic anatomy.
- describe the major topographic features of the head, neck, thorax, abdomen, pelvis, lower extremity, shoulder girdle, and upper extremity.
- identify the major arterial pulse points.

THE LANGUAGE OF TOPOGRAPHIC ANATOMY

The surface of the body has many definite, visible features that serve as guides or landmarks to structures that lie beneath them. These external features, or **topography,** give clues to the general anatomy of the body. A sharp awareness of the superficial landmarks of the body — its **topographic anatomy** — will help the well-trained examiner to evaluate the ill or injured patient. Visual inspection of the body is the simplest step in the primary and secondary surveys. Because so much information regarding the extent of injury or illness can be obtained through inspection, the importance of critical visual inspection of the patient cannot be overemphasized. In fact, many important facts about a patient's injury or disease might be missed because of inadequate visual inspection.

All medical personnel must be familiar with the language of topographic anatomy. The use of the proper terms will assure that correct information is transmitted with the least possible confusion. The terms used to describe the topographic anatomy are applied to the body when it is in the **anatomic position,** or the position of the patient standing erect, facing the examiner, arms at the sides, and palms forward (Figure 3.1). When the terms *right* and *left* are used, they refer to the patient's right and left. The principal regions of the body are the head, neck, thorax (chest), abdomen, and extremities (arms and legs).

The front surface of the body, facing the examiner, is the **anterior surface.** The surface of the patient away from the examiner is the **posterior surface.** An imaginary vertical line drawn from the midforehead through the nose and the **umbilicus** (navel) to the floor is termed the **midline** of the body. This imaginary line divides the body into two halves, which are mirror images of each other. Parts of the body that lie at some distance from the midline are

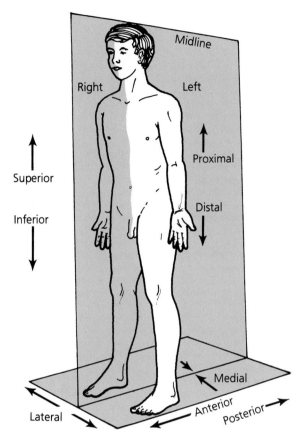

FIGURE 3.1 The terms used to describe the topographic anatomy are applied to the body in its anatomic position — that is, standing erect, facing the examiner, palms forward.

termed **lateral structures.** Parts that lie closer to the midline are termed **medial structures.** For example, we speak of the medial (inner) and lateral (outer) aspects of the knee or the eye. The **superior portion** of the body, or any body part, is that portion nearer the head, while a portion nearer the feet is the **inferior portion.** We also use these terms to describe the relationship of one structure to another. For example, the nose is superior to the mouth and inferior to the forehead.

The terms *proximal* and *distal* are used to describe the relationship of any two structures on a limb. **Proximal** describes structures that are closer to the trunk. **Distal** describes structures that are nearer to the free end of the extremity. For example, the elbow is distal to the shoulder yet proximal to the wrist and hand.

The EMT should be familiar with all of these terms and be able to use them when describing the

location of an injury or other physical findings. In this way any other examiner will know immediately where to look and what to expect. Visual inspection of the body should be systematic, thorough, and performed in exactly the same sequence for all patients. A specific examination routine should be developed so that the examiner will not overlook a significant but perhaps subtle sign of injury or disease.

Whenever possible, the injured part should be compared to the corresponding uninjured part on the opposite side of the body. While body structure varies significantly from individual to individual, the mirror image opposite side provides an excellent reference point for comparison. The usefulness to the examiner of comparing a given injured region with the corresponding uninjured location on the opposite side cannot be overemphasized (Figure 3.2).

THE HEAD

The head is divided into two parts: the cranium and the face. An imaginary horizontal plane passing across the top of the ears and eyes separates these two portions of the head (Figure 3.3, left). The area above the imaginary plane is the **cranium.** It contains the brain, which connects to the spinal cord through a large opening at the base of the skull (the **foramen magnum**). The most posterior portion of the cranium is called the **occiput.** On each side of the cranium, the lateral portions are called the **temples** or **temporal regions.** Between the

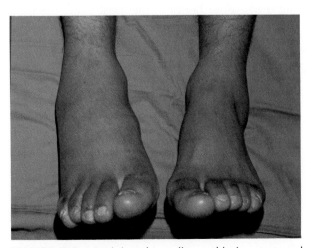

FIGURE 3.2 An injured, swollen ankle is compared with the uninjured ankle.

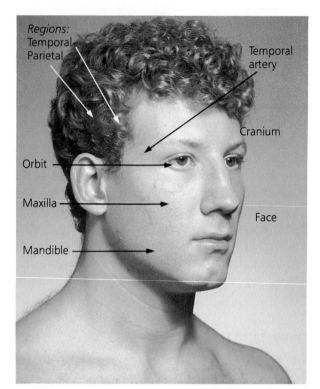

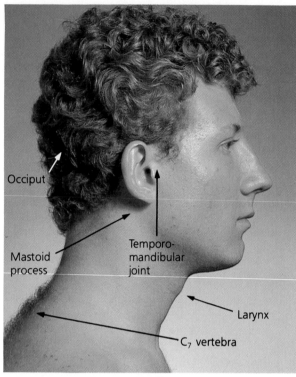

FIGURE 3.3   (left) The major topographic features of the head; (right) lateral view of the head and neck.

temporal regions and the occiput lie the **parietal regions.** The forehead is called the **frontal region.** Just anterior to the ear, in the temporal region, one can feel the pulse of the temporal artery. The skin covering the cranium and usually bearing hair is called the **scalp.**

Below the imaginary plane lies the face, which is composed of the eyes, ears, nose, mouth, cheeks, and jowls. Four bones — the nasal bone, the right and left **maxilla** (cheekbone), and the **mandible** (jawbone) — are the major bones of the face.

The **orbit** of the eye is composed of the lower edge of the frontal bone of the skull, the maxilla, and the nasal bone. The bony orbit protects the eye from injury. By viewing the face from the side (Figure 3.3, right), one can observe the eyeball recessed in the orbit.

Only the proximal one-third of the nose — the **bridge** — is formed by bone. The remaining two-thirds of the nose is a framework made of cartilage. Unlike the nose, the exposed portion of the ear is composed entirely of cartilage that is covered by skin. The **pinna** is the name given to the ear itself. The earlobes are dependent fleshy portions at the bottom

of each ear. The **tragus** is a small rounded fleshy bulge immediately in front of the ear canal. The temporal artery can be palpated just anterior to the tragus. One centimeter posterior to the tip of the lobe of the ear is a prominent bony mass at the base of the skull called the **mastoid process.**

The mandible forms the jaw and chin. Motion of the mandible occurs at a joint (the **temporomandibular joint**), which lies just in front of the ear on either side of the face. Below the ear and in front of the mastoid process, the angle of the mandible is easily palpated.

THE NECK

The neck contains many structures. It is supported by the **cervical spine,** or the first seven vertebrae in the spinal column. The **spinal cord** exits from the foramen magnum and lies within the **spinal canal** formed by the vertebrae. The upper part of the **esophagus** and the **trachea** (windpipe) lie in the midline of the neck. The carotid arteries may be found on either side of the trachea, along with the jugular veins and several nerves (Figure 3.4).

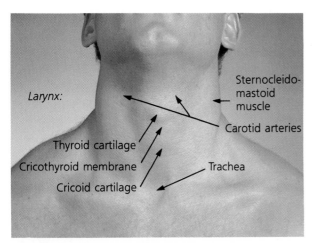

FIGURE 3.4 Anterior view of the neck.

Several useful landmarks can be palpated and seen in the neck. The most obvious is the firm prominence in the center of the anterior surface commonly known as the "**Adam's apple.**" Specifically, this prominence is the upper part of the **larynx,** the **thyroid cartilage.** It is more prominent in men than women. The other portion of the larynx is the **cricoid cartilage,** a firm ridge of cartilage inferior to the thyroid cartilage, which is somewhat more difficult to palpate. Between the thyroid cartilage and the cricoid cartilage in the midline of the neck is a soft depression, the **cricothyroid membrane.** This is a thin sheet of connective tissue (**fascia**) that joins the two cartilages. The cricothyroid membrane is covered at this point only by skin. The larynx is composed of three structures: the thyroid cartilage, the cricothyroid membrane, and the cricoid cartilage.

Inferior to the larynx, several additional firm ridges are palpable. These ridges are the cartilage rings of the trachea. The trachea connects the larynx with the main air passages of the lungs, or the **bronchi.** On either side of the lower larynx and the upper trachea lies the **thyroid gland.** Unless it is enlarged, this gland is usually not palpable.

Pulsations of the carotid arteries are easily palpable 1 to 2 centimeters lateral to the larynx. Lying immediately adjacent to these arteries, but not palpable, are the internal jugular veins and several important nerves. Lateral to these vessels and nerves lie the **sternocleidomastoid muscles.** These muscles originate from the mastoid process in the cranium and insert into the medial border of each collarbone at the base of the neck.

A series of bony prominences lie posteriorly, in the midline of the neck. They are the spines of the **cervical vertebrae.** The lower spines are more prominent than the upper ones. They are more easily palpable when the neck is in flexion. At the base of the neck posteriorly, the most prominent spine is the seventh cervical vertebra (see Figure 3.3, right).

THE THORAX

The **thorax,** or chest, is the cavity that contains the heart, lungs, esophagus, and the great vessels (the aorta and two venae cavae). It is formed by the 12 **thoracic vertebrae** and their 12 pairs of ribs. The **clavicle** (collarbone) overlies its upper boundaries in front and articulates with the **scapula** (shoulder blade), which lies in the muscular tissue of the thoracic wall posteriorly (Figure 3.5). The lower boundary of the thorax is the **diaphragm,** which separates the thorax from the abdomen.

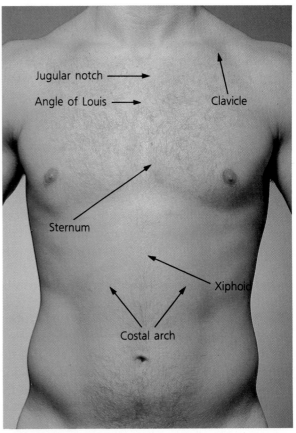

FIGURE 3.5 Anterior aspect of the thorax demonstrating the bony landmarks.

The dimensions of the thorax are defined by the **bony rib cage** and its attachments. Anteriorly, in the midline of the chest is the **sternum** (breastbone). The superior border of the sternum forms the easily palpable **jugular notch.** There are three components of the sternum: the manubrium, the body, and the xiphoid process. The upper quarter of the sternum is called the **manubrium.** The **body** comprises the rest of the sternum except for a narrow, cartilaginous tip inferiorly, which is called the **xiphoid process.** The junction of the manubrium and the body forms a very prominent ridge on the sternum, called the **angle of Louis.** The angle of Louis lies at the level where the second rib is attached to the sternum; it provides a constant and reliable bony landmark on the anterior chest wall.

In the midline of the upper back, the spines of the 12 thoracic vertebrae can be palpated. Twelve **ribs** on each side form small joints with their respective thoracic vertebrae and extend around to the front to create the walls of the **thoracic cage.** The upper five ribs connect to the sternum through a short bridge of cartilage. The sixth through tenth ribs insert into the costal arch. The **costal arch** is a bridge of cartilage that connects the ends of the sixth through tenth ribs with the lower portion of the sternum. The eleventh and twelfth ribs are called **floating ribs** because they do not attach to the sternum through the costal arch. The costal arch is easily palpable and represents the boundary between the lower border of the thorax and the upper border of the abdomen.

On a male chest, the nipples lie at the level of the interspace between the fourth and fifth ribs. In females, breasts obviously vary in size, and consequently nipple position may vary. The center of the breast, however, still lies in the interspace between the fourth and fifth ribs.

On the posterior chest wall the scapulae overlie the thoracic wall and are surrounded by large muscles (Figure 3.6). When the patient is standing or sitting erect, the two scapulae should lie at approximately the same level, with their inferior tips at about the level of the seventh thoracic vertebra. In the lower part of the thorax on each side an angle called the **costovertebral angle** is formed by the junction of the spine and the tenth rib. The kidneys lie deep to (beneath) the back muscles in the costovertebral angle.

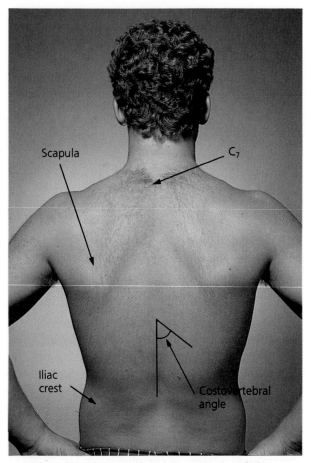

FIGURE 3.6 The topographic anatomy of the posterior view of the thorax. Major bony landmarks are also shown.

The diaphragm is a muscular dome that forms the undersurface of the thorax, separating the chest from the abdominal cavity. Anteriorly it attaches to the costal arch, and posteriorly it attaches to the **lumbar vertebrae.** The diaphragm cannot be seen or palpated.

Within the thoracic cage (Figure 3.7), the largest structures are the heart and lungs. The **heart** lies immediately under the sternum. It extends from the second to the sixth ribs anteriorly and from the fifth to the eighth thoracic vertebrae posteriorly. The lower border of the heart extends into the left side of the chest, normally to the midclavicular line. Diseased hearts may be larger or smaller.

The major blood vessels that travel to and from the heart also lie in the chest cavity. On the right side of the spinal column, the **superior** and **inferior venae cavae** carry blood to the heart. Just beneath

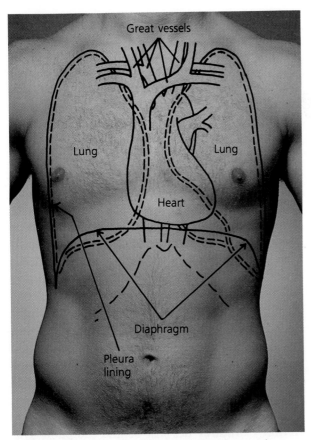

FIGURE 3.7 Anterior aspect of the thorax showing the relative positions of the major thoracic organs beneath the surface.

tion of the sternum. The angle of Louis is readily palpable in the upper portion of the sternum at the level of the space between the second and third ribs (the second intercostal space). Inferiorly, the costal arch is readily palpable on both sides of the anterior chest wall. In the midline, the tip of the xiphoid process is a tender and easily palpated landmark.

THE ABDOMEN

The **abdomen** is the second major body cavity. It contains the major organs of digestion and excretion. The diaphragm separates the thorax from the abdomen. Anteriorly and posteriorly, thick muscular abdominal walls create the boundaries of this space. Inferiorly, the abdomen is arbitrarily separated from the pelvis by an imaginary plane that extends from the **symphysis pubis** through the **sacrum.** Many organs lie in both the abdomen and the pelvis, and the primary distinction between these two cavities is their external appearance.

The simplest and most common method of describing the portions of the abdomen is by quadrants. In this system the abdomen is divided into four equal parts by two imaginary lines that intersect at right angles at the umbilicus. On the anterior abdominal wall the quadrants thus formed are right upper, right lower, left upper, and left lower (Figure 3.8). The

the manubrium of the sternum, the arch of the **aorta** and the **pulmonary artery** exit the heart. The arch of the aorta passes to the left and lies along the left side of the spinal column as it descends into the abdomen. The esophagus lies behind the great vessels and directly on the anterior aspect of the spinal column as it passes through the chest into the abdomen.

All space within the chest not occupied by the heart, great vessels, and esophagus is occupied by the **lungs.** Anteriorly, the lungs extend down to the surface of the diaphragm at the level of the xiphoid process. Posteriorly, the lungs extend farther inferiorly to the surface of the diaphragm at the level of the twelfth thoracic vertebra.

The major palpable landmarks in the chest are obviously the ribs. Most of them can be easily felt except for the first, which is hidden under and behind the clavicle. Both clavicles and the sternum can be easily palpated. The jugular notch is the top por-

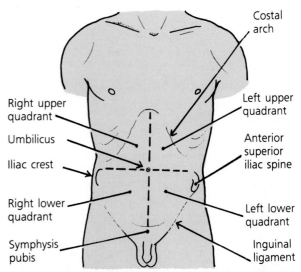

FIGURE 3.8 In the abdomen, quadrants are the easiest system for identifying areas. Major bony landmarks are also shown.

terms *right* and *left* refer to the patient's right and left and not the observer's. Pain or injury in a given quadrant usually arises from or involves the organs that lie in that quadrant. This simple means of designation will allow the examiner to identify injured or diseased organs that require emergency attention.

In the right upper quadrant the major organs are the **liver, gallbladder,** and a portion of the **colon** (Figure 3.9). Most of the liver lies in this quadrant almost entirely under the protection of the eighth to twelfth ribs. The liver fills the entire anteroposterior depth of the abdomen in this quadrant. Thus injuries in this area are frequently associated with injuries of the liver. Tenderness without injury in the right upper quadrant usually is a result of gallbladder disease.

In the left upper quadrant the principal organs are the **stomach,** the **spleen,** and a portion of the

colon (Figure 3.9). The stomach and the spleen are almost entirely under the protection of the left rib cage. The spleen lies in the lateral and posterior portion of this quadrant, under the diaphragm and immediately in front of the ninth to eleventh ribs. The spleen is frequently injured, especially when these ribs are fractured. Tenderness or pain in the left upper quadrant following an injury often points to a ruptured spleen.

The right lower quadrant contains two portions of the large intestine: the **cecum** and the ascending colon (Figure 3.9). The **appendix** is a small tubular structure that is attached to the lower border of the cecum. Appendicitis is the most frequent cause of tenderness and pain in this region. In the left lower quadrant lie the descending and the sigmoid portions of the colon (Figure 3.9).

Several organs lie in more than one quadrant. The **small intestine,** for instance, occupies the central part of the abdomen around the umbilicus, and parts of it lie in all four quadrants. The **large intestine** also encircles the abdomen, beginning in the right lower quadrant and ending in the left lower quadrant as it circles through all four quadrants. The **urinary bladder** lies just behind the pubic symphysis in the middle of the abdomen and, therefore, lies in both lower quadrants. The **pancreas** lies just behind the abdominal cavity on the posterior abdominal wall in both upper quadrants. The **kidneys** also lie behind the abdominal cavity. They are above the level of the umbilicus, extending from the eleventh rib to the third lumbar vertebrae on each side. They are approximately 5 inches long and lie just in front of the costovertebral angle (Figure 3.6).

The chief topographic landmarks in the abdomen are the costal arch, the umbilicus, the anterior superior iliac spines, the iliac crest, and the pubic symphysis. The costal arch, as noted earlier, is the fused cartilages of the sixth through the tenth ribs. It forms the superior arching boundary of the abdomen. The umbilicus, a constant structure, is in the same horizontal plane as the fourth lumbar vertebra and the superior edge of the **iliac crest,** the rim of the pelvic bone. The **anterior superior iliac spines** are the hard bony prominences at the front on each side of the lower abdomen just below the plane of the umbilicus. In the midline in the lowermost portion of the abdomen is another hard bony prominence, the symphysis pubis. Between the

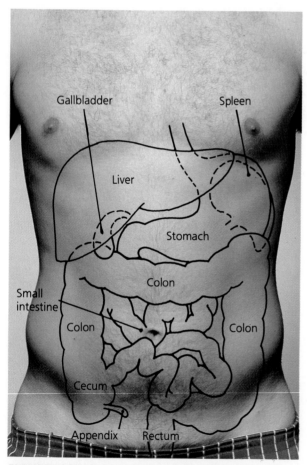

FIGURE 3.9 Anterior view of the abdomen showing the position of the major abdominal organs.

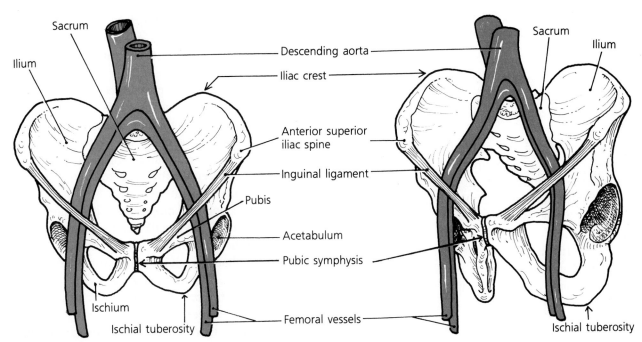

FIGURE 3.10 The pelvis, a very strong, closed bony ring, is composed of several separate elements and bears the sockets for the hip joints. The inguinal ligament lies just above the femoral vessels and helps protect them.

lateral edge of the pubic symphysis and the anterior superior spine on each side the examiner can palpate the tough **inguinal ligament,** which stretches between these two structures. Below the ligament lie the femoral vessels.

Posteriorly, one does not usually refer to abdominal quadrants. The posterior portion of the iliac crest can be palpated, as can the spines of the five lumbar vertebrae in the midline. The lowermost rib on either side forms the costovertebral angle with the spines of the vertebrae.

THE PELVIS

The **pelvis** is a closed bony ring that consists of three bones: the sacrum and the two pelvic bones. Much like the skull, each pelvic bone is formed by the fusion of three separate bones. These three bones are called the **ilium,** the **ischium,** and the **pubis** (Figure 3.10). The pelvic cavity is bounded superiorly by an imaginary plane that runs from the symphysis pubis to the top of the sacrum. Its lateral walls are formed by the inner borders of the pelvic bone, and its inferior boundary is the **pelvic outlet,** a layer of muscles with openings for the gastrointestinal tract

(the **rectum**), the female reproductive system (the **vagina**), and the urinary tract (the **urethra**). The pelvis contains the lower portion of the gastrointestinal tract (the **rectosigmoid colon**), the female reproductive organs, and the urinary bladder.

The prominent anterior bony landmarks of the pelvis are the symphysis pubis in the midline and the anterior superior iliac spines. The inguinal ligament attaches to these two bony prominences and can be palpated in thin persons. Just distal to the midpoint of the inguinal ligament the femoral artery can be palpated as it enters the thigh. From the anterior superior iliac spine, the ilium extends laterally and posteriorly to form the rim of the pelvis. This bony ridge is called the iliac crest.

Posteriorly, the pelvis has a flattened appearance, and in the middle third, the firm bony sacrum can be palpated. Just lateral to the sacrum on either side is a joint with the iliac portion of the pelvic bone (the **sacroiliac joint**). In the sitting position, a bony prominence is easily felt in the middle of each buttock. These prominences are the **ischial tuberosities.** The **sciatic nerve** — the major nerve to the lower extremity — lies just lateral to the tuberosity as it enters the thigh.

THE LOWER EXTREMITIES

The three major portions of the lower extremity are the thigh, the leg, and the foot. The joint between the thigh and pelvis is called the hip. The joint between the thigh and the leg is the knee joint, and the joint between the leg and the foot is the ankle joint.

On the lateral side of the thigh just below the hip joint is a bony prominence called the **greater trochanter** (Figure 3.11). In examination, the position of this prominence should always be compared with that on the opposite side as a guide to fracture or dislocation of the hip.

The **femur** is the supporting bone of the thigh. It is surrounded by large muscles, and thus proximally, the only part of the femur that can be palpated is the greater trochanter. Near the knee, the medial

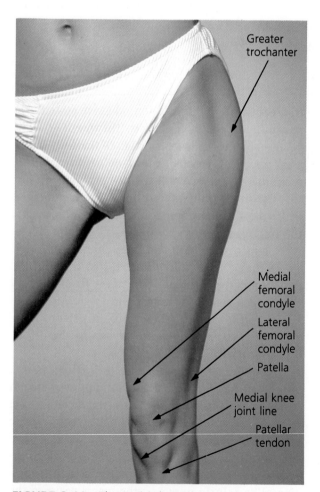

FIGURE 3.11 The major bony landmark in the upper portion of the lower extremity is the greater trochanter of the femur.

and lateral **femoral condyles** can be palpated. Anteriorly, the large muscle of the thigh is called the **quadriceps;** the **hamstring muscles** lie posteriorly.

The **patella** (kneecap) is a specialized bone that lies within the tendon of the quadriceps muscle. It provides protection for the anterior aspect of the knee joint. The patella normally glides smoothly in a groove on the anterior surface of the femur. This groove lies between the rounded condyles that make up the distal end of the femur.

The knee joint is composed of the femoral condyles superiorly, the patella anteriorly, and the upper end of the tibia distally. The actual joint line of the knee is about 1 inch inferior to the lower margin of the patella. This joint line can be palpated on either side of the patellar tendon when the knee is flexed to 90 degrees.

The leg is that portion of the lower extremity that extends from the knee joint to the ankle joint (Figure 13.12). The bones of the leg are the **tibia** (shin bone) and the **fibula.** The upper end of the tibia is called the **tibial plateau,** and it forms the inferior surface of the knee joint. The tibia is palpable throughout its entire length, extending from the medial tibial plateau, through the **tibial tuberosity** (the point of insertion of the quadriceps tendon), and along the **tibial crest** down to the ankle joint. The entire length of the tibia can be palpated on the anterior surface of the leg just under the skin.

The fibula lies on the lateral side of the leg. The rounded head of the fibula (the fibular head) can be easily palpated on the lateral side of the knee when the knee is flexed to 90 degrees. Lying immediately below the head of the fibula is the **peroneal nerve.** This nerve controls movement at the ankle and supplies sensation to the top of the foot. Injury to the fibula in this region or excessive pressure from a splint may cause permanent paralysis of this nerve.

The ankle joint is formed by the prominent distal ends of the tibia and the fibula. The end of the tibia forms the **medial malleolus,** and the end of the fibula forms the **lateral malleolus.** These two bony prominences form the socket of the ankle joint. Both are usually visible and easily palpated. The two malleoli form a socket for the **talus,** or ankle bone. The undersurface of the talus has an articular surface for the **calcaneus** (heel bone), which forms the prominence of the heel. The calcaneus is also called in any secondary survey of the injured limb to identify points of localized tenderness.

THE SHOULDER GIRDLE

The **shoulder girdle** is composed of the clavicle anteriorly, the scapula posteriorly, and the upper end of the **humerus** laterally. The clavicle, or collarbone, is firmly attached medially to the upper part of the sternum at the **sternoclavicular joint** (Figure 3.13). The clavicle is palpable throughout its entire length from the sternum to its attachment to the scapula. The **acromion process** of the scapula makes up the rounded lateral border of the shoulder girdle and forms a joint with the lateral end of the clavicle, the **acromioclavicular joint,** also called the **A/C joint.**

The scapula is a large, broad flat bone that overlies the posterior wall of the thorax and is surrounded by large muscles. Because of the presence of the muscles, only small portions of this bone are palpable. The acromion process can be palpated around the lateral edge of the shoulder girdle. It continues on as the spine of the scapula across the back (see Figure 3.6).

The external appearance of the shoulder girdle is that of a gently rounded area without significantly noticeable prominences. The rounded appearance is produced by the head of the humerus (the humeral head), the upper end of the bone of the arm that articulates with a portion of the scapula to form the true shoulder joint.

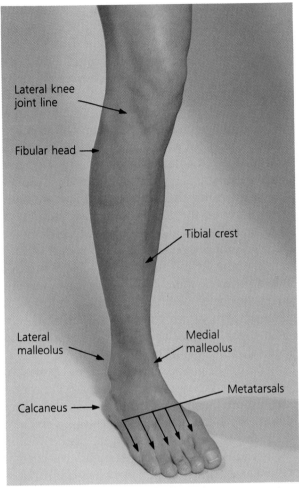

FIGURE 3.12 Anterolateral view of the leg and foot with the bony prominences labeled.

the **os calcis** and can be palpated through the skin of the heel. The talus and calcaneus, along with five other bones, make up the rear portion of the foot. These seven bones are called **tarsal bones.** Five **metatarsal bones** form the substance of the foot. The five toes are formed by fourteen **phalanges** (singular form is phalanx): two in the great toe and three in each of the smaller toes.

Inspection of the lower extremity will identify injury in many instances. The examiner should always compare the injured limb to the opposite, uninjured one. Any difference in the shape or appearance of the injured limb should make the examiner suspicious of injury. Palpation of the bony landmarks (great trochanter, femoral condyles, patella, medial tibial plateau, fibular head, tibial crest, malleoli, calcaneus, and metatarsal heads) should be included

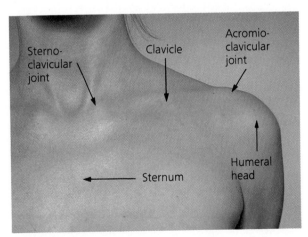

FIGURE 3.13 The rounded prominence of the shoulder girdle laterally is created by the humeral head, covered by muscle.

THE UPPER EXTREMITY

The upper extremity extends from the shoulder girdle to the fingertips. It is composed of the arm, elbow, forearm, wrist, hand, and fingers. The arm extends from the shoulder to the elbow. The supporting bone of the arm is the humerus. Just like the thigh, there are few bony landmarks in the arm because it is covered by large muscles — the **biceps muscle** in the front and the **triceps muscle** in the back. Near the elbow joint, the medial and lateral **humeral condyles** form the medial and lateral borders of the upper portion of the elbow joint. These bony prominences are easily palpable when the elbow is flexed (Figure 3.14). The elbow is the joint between the distal end of the humerus and the two forearm bones, the ulna and the radius. The **olecranon process** of the ulna forms a third prominence easily seen and palpated on the posterior portion of the elbow.

The forearm is composed of two bones, the **ulna** and the **radius.** The ulna is larger in the proximal forearm, and the radius is larger in the distal forearm. The olecranon process of the ulna forms most of the elbow joint. The entire **ulna shaft** from the tip of the olecranon process distally can be palpated, as it lies just under the skin on the posterior surface of the forearm. The radius is covered by muscles and cannot be palpated except in the lower third of the forearm where it enlarges to form a major portion of the wrist joint. Just as the two bones of the leg form a socket for the ankle joint, there are bony prominences on the ends of the radius and ulna to form the socket for the wrist joint. Here they are called **styloid processes.** Both the **radial styloid** and the **ulnar styloid** are easily palpable. The radial styloid is on the thumb side of the wrist, and the ulnar styloid is on the little finger side. Simultaneous palpation of these two processes will reveal that the radial styloid process usually lies about one centimeter distal to that of the ulna.

There are eight bones, called **carpal bones,** in the wrist. At the base of each finger lies a **metacarpal bone.** The metacarpals form the substance of the palm. The thumb has two phalanges, and each of the fingers has three phalanges (Figure 3.15).

As in the lower extremity, careful inspection of the upper extremity, especially when compared to the opposite limb, will often reveal an abnormality. Palpation of the bony landmarks (clavicle, acromion process, humeral condyles, olecranon process, ulnar

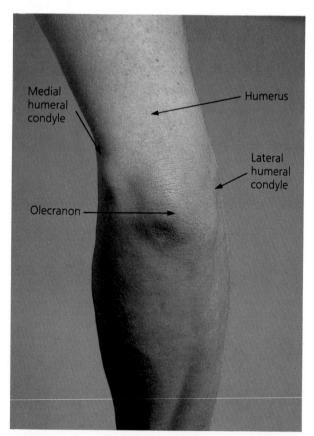

FIGURE 3.14 Posterior view of the elbow showing the three bony prominences: the medial and lateral condyles of the humerus and the olecranon process of the ulna.

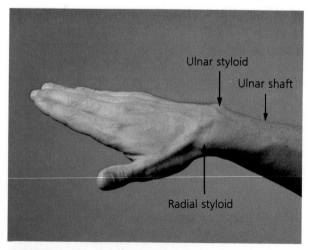

FIGURE 3.15 Dorsal view of the forearm, wrist, and hand.

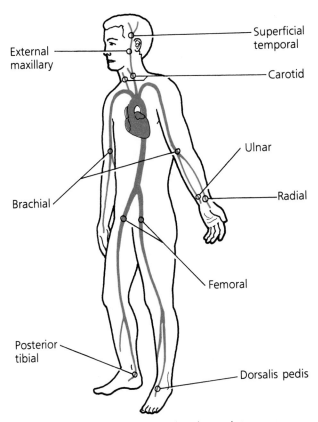

External maxillary

Superficial temporal

Carotid

Ulnar

Radial

Brachial

Femoral

Posterior tibial

Dorsalis pedis

FIGURE 3.16 Major arterial pulse points.

shaft, styloid processes, metacarpals, and phalanges) will identify points of local tenderness following injury.

ARTERIAL PULSE POINTS

An artery can be palpated wherever it passes over a bony prominence or lies close to the skin. At these points the arterial pulse can be taken. These points have been called **arterial pressure points** because in the past it was believed that compression at one of these points would help control hemorrhage distal to it. Although the theory behind this principle is sound, applying pressure over any single artery will rarely completely stop circulation distal to that point because there is always more than one artery supplying blood to an injury site. Therefore, local pressure on the wound is the best method for con-

trol of hemorrhage. Pressure on the arterial pulse points can be used on occasion to supplement the control of rapid, severe bleeding. Major arterial pulse points are shown in Figure 3.16. Palpation at these points will allow the examiner to ascertain the presence of cardiac activity. In addition, following injury, decrease or absence of the pulse may indicate damage to the artery proximal to the pulse point.

Anterior to the upper portion of the ear, just over the temporomandibular joint, lies the superficial **temporal artery.** Anterior to the angle of the mandible on the inner surface of the lower jaw the **external maxillary artery** can be palpated. It contributes much of the blood supply to the face. The **carotid arteries** may be palpated anteriorly in the neck just lateral to the larynx. On the inner surface of the arm, about 5 centimeters above the elbow, the **brachial artery** can be palpated. Arterial pulsations may be felt in both the **radial** and **ulnar arteries** at the wrist just proximal to the styloid processes. The **femoral artery** may be palpated as it passes beneath the inguinal ligament in the groin. Just posterior to the medial malleolus is the **posterior tibial artery.** On the anterior surface of the foot between the first and second metatarsals is the **dorsalis pedis artery.** This artery is not always present. When it is present, its pulsations may be felt easily.

YOU ARE THE EMT...

1. The costovertebral angle is formed by the spine and tenth rib. What organs lie deep to the back muscles in the costovertebral angle?
2. Is the patella distal or proximal to the tibia? Is the patella in the superior portion of the body or the inferior portion?
3. Name three abdominal organs that lie in more than one quadrant and identify the quadrants they share.
4. The lungs take up a good portion of the thorax. What other structures lie in the thorax? What organ separates the thorax from the abdomen?

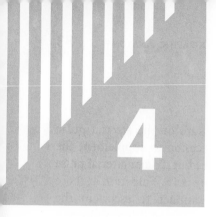

4 Patient Assessment

OVERVIEW

The most important function of the emergency medical technician is to identify and treat any life-threatening conditions first, and then to assess the patient carefully for other complaints or findings that may require emergency treatment or transportation to a hospital. The importance of this function is stressed over and over again because failure to perform patient assessment correctly will result in improper patient care and possibly permanent impairment or even death.

Chapter 4 begins by distinguishing between signs and symptoms. Then ten basic diagnostic signs are described. The second half of Chapter 4 explains how patient assessment is carried out using these diagnostic signs. The sequence of assessment and treatment priorities is especially important and thus the order in which topics are presented is significant.

OBJECTIVES

The objectives of Chapter 4 are to

- distinguish between signs and symptoms.
- describe the four vital signs (pulse, respiration, blood pressure, and temperature) and six other diagnostic signs (skin color, capillary refill, pupil size and response to light, level of consciousness, ability to move, and reaction to pain).
- understand the sequence of assessment and treatment priorities, including the first assessment, arrival at the scene, the primary survey, the chief complaint, vital signs, history of present illness, and the secondary survey.

SIGNS AND SYMPTOMS

The words "sign" and "symptom" are often used incorrectly, even by experienced medical personnel. A **symptom** is something that the patient tells the EMT, such as, "My arm hurts," or "I feel dizzy." A **sign** is something that the EMT observes in a patient, such as deformity or bleeding in a fractured arm or the patient's blood pressure. Because they are actually observed by the EMT, signs are considered to be more reliable than symptoms (Figure 4.1).

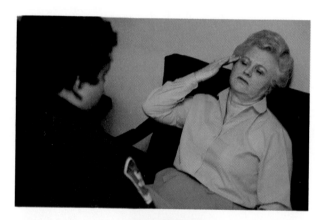

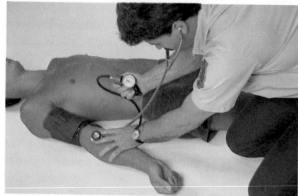

FIGURE 4.1 A *symptom* is a complaint that the patient relates to the EMT. The patient (top) is telling the EMT that she feels dizzy. A *sign* is something the EMT observes. The EMT (bottom) is taking the patient's blood pressure. Both symptoms and signs should be recorded.

DIAGNOSTIC SIGNS

There are many signs the EMT should *look, listen, and feel* for. To elicit these signs the EMT must have the proper tools, the most important of these being eyes, ears, and hands. Above all, the EMT must have the ability to use these "tools" in a calm manner in a stressful environment. An EMT who panics at the scene will be unable to perform a proper assessment or set the right priorities for treatment. Other tools that are useful are a penlight, a wrist watch with a second hand, a stethoscope, and a blood-pressure cuff. The stethoscope is easily misused — the earpieces should be placed *facing forward* in the ears (Figure 4.2).

Patient assessment requires the EMT to look (inspect), listen (**auscultate**), and feel (**palpate**) for four **vital signs** (pulse, respiration, blood pressure, and temperature) and six other diagnostic signs (skin color, capillary refill, pupil size and response to light, level of consciousness, ability to move, and reaction to pain).

Pulse

The **pulse** is the wave of pressure that is felt as the heart contracts and propels blood through the arteries. It is a useful indication of the condition of the heart, the blood vessels, and the blood itself. The EMT measures the pulse by palpating an artery at a **pulse point,** which is where an artery lies close to the surface of the skin. It is better felt where there is a bone lying behind the artery. While the pulse can be palpated at any of the pulse points described in Chapter 3, the most common place to palpate for the pulse is in the wrist, along the path of the radial artery (Figure 4.3, top).

If the pulse cannot be palpated in either arm, the EMT should attempt to find it in the neck along the path of the carotid artery (Figure 4.3, bottom). The **carotid pulse** is more accurate than the radial pulse and is easier to feel in an emergency situation. If the heart is beating weakly, the carotid pulse may be present while the radial pulse may be impossible to feel. The carotid pulse is found in the neck under the anterior edge of the sternocleidomastoid muscle. When taking the carotid pulse, the EMT should first make sure that the patient is in a lying or sitting position. The EMT should never try to feel both carotid

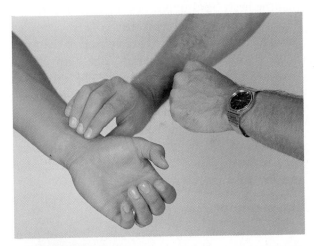
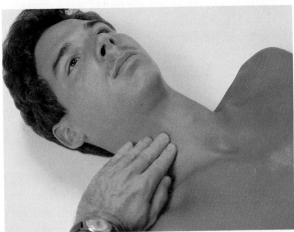

FIGURE 4.3 Palpation of the radial pulse at the wrist (top) and of the carotid pulse in the neck.

FIGURE 4.2 The earpieces of a stethoscope should be placed facing forward in the ears.

pulses at the same time because excessive pressure on the two arteries might cut off circulation to the brain.

The EMT must assess the rate, strength, and regularity of the pulse. The normal **pulse rate** in the typical adult is 60 to 80 beats per minute and is a reflection of the heart rate. In a child, the normal rate is 80 to 100 beats per minute. The pulse rate is obtained by counting the number of beats that occur over a 15-second period and multiplying that number by 4.

The **pulse volume** is a rough indicator of the strength of the heart's contractions. After palpating the pulse in many patients, the EMT will develop a sense of the pulse volume. A rapid, weak pulse can indicate shock from loss of blood. A "bounding" pulse is present in fright or with high blood pressure. If the pulse is absent, it may mean that the artery being palpated is blocked from disease or injury or that the heart has stopped beating or is undergoing decreased strength of contractions.

The third important characteristic of the pulse is the **regularity** of its rhythm. The pulse should have a regular frequency of beats. The absence of beats, called "skipped beats," or irregularity of beats usually signals significant cardiac disease.

The pulse is an instantaneous indicator of the condition of the patient and should be taken *and recorded* (rate, volume, and regularity) frequently during any emergency encounter.

Respirations

Normal breathing occurs easily, without pain, noise, or effort. Although the rate of respirations can vary widely, it is usually between 12 and 20 breaths per minute. Interestingly, well-trained athletes may breathe only 6 to 8 times per minute. Normal respirations are not unusually shallow or deep. A record should be made of the rate and character of respirations when a patient is first seen, and any change should be observed and recorded.

Rapid, shallow respirations are associated with shock. Deep, gasping, labored breathing may indicate partial airway obstruction or lung disease. With respiratory depression or respiratory arrest, there will be little or no movement of the chest and abdomen and little or no airflow felt or heard at the nose and mouth. A choking patient can be identified by the inability to cough or talk and the instinctive, nearly

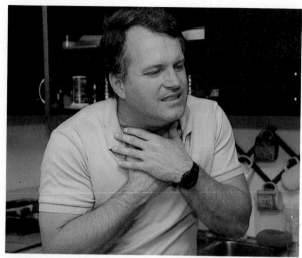

FIGURE 4.4   Nearly every choking person will grasp the throat.

universal gesture of clutching the throat that characterizes the choking victim (Figure 4.4).

Sputum is matter that is expectorated from the lungs. It is produced by injury or disease of the lungs. Injury to the chest may cause the patient to cough up blood or frothy (foamlike) sputum. Heart failure can also cause the production of a frothy sputum. Patients with pneumonia and bronchitis may cough up thick sputum of various colors. The EMT should note the volume, color, and other characteristics of any sputum that is produced.

Occasionally, the EMT can learn something about the patient by smelling the patient's breath. For example, the breath of patients with severe diabetic acidosis often gives off a sweet or fruity odor. Obviously, the intoxicated patient may smell of alcohol. However, the EMT must not be misled by the smell of alcohol into thinking that the patient is "just drunk" when something much more serious might be going on. Any particularly obvious odor of the breath should be noted and recorded.

Blood Pressure

Blood pressure is the pressure of the circulating blood against the walls of the arteries. In the normal person, the arterial system is a closed system attached to a pump (the heart) and completely filled with blood. Changes in the blood pressure indicate changes in the blood volume, in the capacity of the vessels to contain the blood, or in the ability of the heart to pump the blood. Changes in the blood pressure, like those in the pulse, can occur rapidly. Blood pressure changes are not as rapid as pulse changes, however, because normal protective mechanisms exist to maintain blood pressure even in the face of injury or disease.

Blood pressure can fall markedly after severe bleeding, following a heart attack, or in other states of shock. Low blood pressure means there is insufficient pressure in the arterial system to supply blood to all the organs of the body. As a consequence, the organs may be severely damaged. The causes of low blood pressure must be identified promptly and treated aggressively. The treatment of low blood pressure that is caused by severe bleeding requires emergency control of the source of such bleeding if it is accessible.

If the blood pressure is abnormally high, damage to or rupture of the vessels in the arterial circuit may occur. It is equally important that the cause of elevated blood pressure be found and treated. The treatment of elevated blood pressure is complex and may require hospitalization.

Blood pressure can change rapidly during transport of a patient to the hospital. It is important that emergency department personnel should be notified of the status of the blood pressure as early as possible in the course of the prehospital evaluation and also be made aware of any changes before arrival at the hospital. Therefore, during the course of emergency medical care, the EMT should check and record the blood pressure at frequent intervals, along with the time it was taken.

Blood pressure is recorded at systolic and diastolic levels. **Systolic pressure** is the level present in the artery at the moment the heart contracts. **Diastolic pressure** is the level present during relaxation of the heart. Systolic pressure is the maximum pressure to which the arteries are subjected, while diastolic pressure represents the minimum amount of pressure that is always present in the arteries. With most diseases or injuries, these pressures change in a parallel fashion — in other words both rise or both fall. Two exceptions to this rule occur with brain injury and cardiac tamponade. Head injury at times causes a rise in the systolic pressure with a stable or falling diastolic pressure. A fall in systolic pressure, accompanied by a rising diastolic pressure, occurs in **cardiac tamponade,** a condition in which the sac around the heart fills with blood.

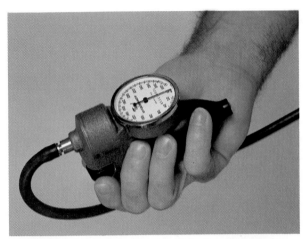

FIGURE 4.5 A blood pressure cuff, or sphygmomanometer. The EMT's thumb and index finger operate the knob that controls the release of air from the cuff, while the rest of the hand inflates the cuff using the bulb.

Blood pressure is measured by one of two methods or a combination of the two, which is recommended for the EMT in the field. Both methods require the use of the blood pressure cuff, called the **sphygmomanometer** (Figure 4.5). It is important to select a cuff that is the appropriate size for the patient. The sphygmomanometer has a rubber bladder inside of it; this bladder should be long enough to encircle the patient's arm completely. The width of the bladder should be at least 20 percent greater than the diameter of the arm (Figure 4.6). Narrow cuffs are made for taking the blood pressure of

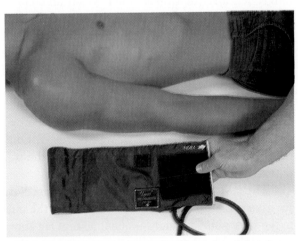

FIGURE 4.6 It is important to use the right size cuff — one that is at least 20 percent wider than the diameter of the arm.

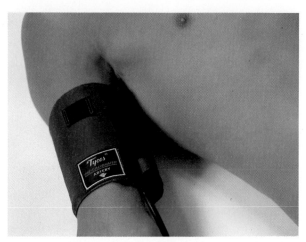

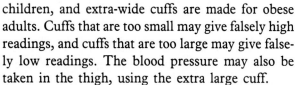

FIGURE 4.7   The cuff is wrapped securely around the arm about 1 inch above the elbow.

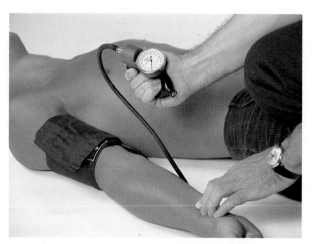

FIGURE 4.8   The pressure is first taken by palpation.

children, and extra-wide cuffs are made for obese adults. Cuffs that are too small may give falsely high readings, and cuffs that are too large may give falsely low readings. The blood pressure may also be taken in the thigh, using the extra large cuff.

The cuff should be wrapped snugly around the patient's upper arm, with the lower edge of the cuff about 1 inch above the inside of the patient's elbow (Figure 4.7). The center of the inflatable bladder, usually marked with an arrow on the cuff, should cover the patient's brachial artery.

The EMT should first take the blood pressure by palpation. This is done by finding the patient's radial pulse. Then, with the other hand, the EMT inflates the blood pressure cuff until the pulse is no longer felt and then for another 30 millimeters of mercury (mm Hg) on the gauge of the blood pressure cuff. Then the EMT deflates the cuff slowly until the pulse returns (Figure 4.8). The reading on the gauge when the pulse returns is the patient's systolic blood pressure, by palpation. Since the blood pressure determined by palpation is less accurate than if determined by auscultation, it should be recorded with the word "palpation" written beside it. Only the systolic pressure can be measured using the palpation method.

The EMT should then take the blood pressure by **auscultation.** That means reinflating the cuff to the same point as before — about 30 mm Hg above the systolic blood pressure as determined by palpation — and placing the stethoscope in the patient's **antecubital fossa,** located at the front of the elbow

over the brachial artery (Figure 4.9). The cuff should be gradually deflated while the EMT listens for the sound of the pulse in the artery. The sound first heard is recorded as the systolic pressure. The EMT continues to deflate the cuff until the sounds disappear. The pressure at which the sounds disappear is the second reading, or the diastolic pressure. The blood pressure should be recorded in the form systolic/diastolic, for example, 120/80 mm Hg. The position of the patient (sitting, standing, or lying) and the extremity in which the pressure is taken should also be recorded.

Blood pressure levels vary with age and sex. A useful rule of thumb for estimating the normal systolic blood pressure in the male is to add 100 to the age of the patient, up to the level of 150 mm Hg. Normal diastolic pressure in the male ranges between 65 and 90 mm Hg. Both pressures are about 10 mm Hg lower in the female. Sounds at the elbow are at times impossible to hear in a moving ambulance, and often the EMT must rely on measuring the blood pressure by palpation during transport. Only rarely can the upper extremities not be used to determine blood pressure. In such circumstances, the blood pressure may be taken in the thigh, using an extra large cuff and palpating for the pulse in the posterior tibial artery.

Temperature

Normal body temperature is 98.6 degrees Fahrenheit (37.0 degrees Centigrade). The skin is largely responsible for regulation of body tempera-

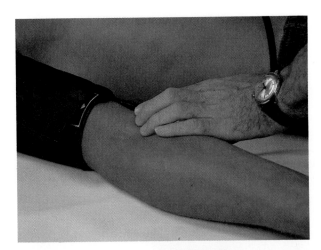

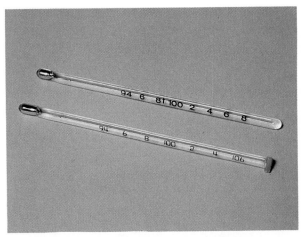

FIGURE 4.10   An oral (top) and a rectal thermometer.

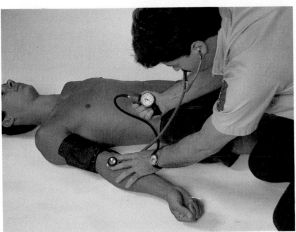

FIGURE 4.9   The brachial pulse (top) is palpated to determine where the stethoscope will be placed. The stethoscope (bottom) is placed over the brachial artery and the blood pressure is taken by auscultation.

ture, by radiation of heat from skin blood vessels and the evaporation of sweat.

Changes in temperature result from illness or injury. A cool, clammy (damp) skin is indicative of a general response of the sympathetic nervous system to an insult, such as blood loss (shock) or heat exhaustion. As a result of nervous stimulation, sweat glands are hyperactive and skin blood vessels contract, resulting in cold, pale, wet, or clammy skin. These signs are often the first indication of shock, and they must be recognized as such. Exposure to cold will produce a cool, dry skin. Dry, hot skin may be caused by fever or by exposure to excessive heat, as in heatstroke.

A patient's temperature is usually taken by mouth, with the bulb of the thermometer placed be-

neath the tongue. The thermometer should be left in place with the patient's mouth closed for 3 minutes. In a child or uncooperative patient, the thermometer can be placed in the axilla (armpit), keeping the patient's arm at the side. Axillary temperatures are notoriously inaccurate, take a long time to register accurately (10 minutes), and should be used only as a last resort. Rectal temperature is very accurate and is usually taken, if necessary, in the emergency department. The rectal temperature is routinely one-half to 1 degree above oral temperature and is taken with a rectal thermometer left in place for 1 minute (Figure 4.10).

Skin Color

Skin color depends primarily on the presence of circulating blood in the vessels of the skin. In deeply pigmented people, skin color depends primarily on the skin pigment. The presence of such pigment may hide skin color changes that result from illness or injury. In patients with deeply pigmented skin, color changes may be apparent in the fingernail beds, in the **sclera** (the "whites") of the eye, or inside the mouth. In lightly pigmented patients where changes are seen more easily, the skin colors of medical importance are red, white, and blue.

A red color may be present with high blood pressure, fever, certain stages of carbon monoxide poisoning, and heatstroke. The patient who has severe high blood pressure may sometimes be **plethoric** (dark, reddish-purple skin color due to filling of all visible blood vessels). The patient who has

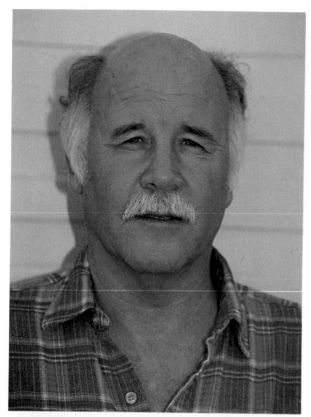

FIGURE 4.11 Red skin color may indicate high blood pressure, heat stroke, or carbon monoxide poisoning.

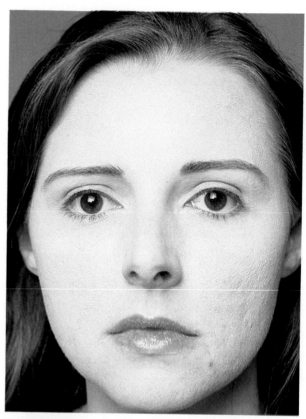

FIGURE 4.12 Pale skin color may indicate insufficient circulation.

carbon monoxide poisoning is usually cherry red, as is the heatstroke patient (Figure 4.11).

A pale, white, ashen, or grayish skin is indicative of insufficient circulation and is seen in patients who are in shock, in certain stages of fright, or suffering from cold exposure. In these circumstances, there is literally not enough blood circulating in the skin (Figure 4.12).

A bluish color, **cyanosis,** results from poor oxygenation of the circulating blood. As a result, blood is very dark and the overlying tissue appears blue. Cyanosis is caused by respiratory insufficiency due to airway obstruction or inadequate lung function. It is usually first seen in the fingertips and around the mouth. Cyanosis always indicates a significant lack of oxygen and demands rapid correction of the underlying respiratory problems (Figure 4.13).

Chronic illness may also produce color changes such as the yellow color, called **jaundice,** seen in liver disease (See Chapter 33). In this condition, bile pigments that are normally present in the liver and

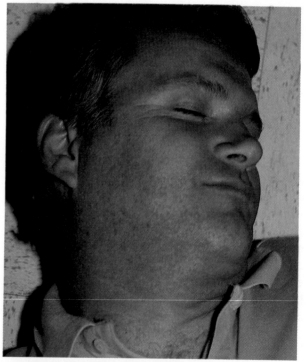

FIGURE 4.13 Blue skin color is characteristic of the lack of oxygen in the blood.

the gastrointestinal tract are deposited in the patient's skin.

Assessment of the patient's color can lead to an immediate decision about the need for treatment. Oxygen may be necessary, arrest of bleeding may be required, or full resuscitation may be indicated. Sometimes a glance at the patient is all that is necessary for the EMT to identify treatment priorities.

Capillary Refill

Capillary refill is the ability of the circulatory system to restore blood to the capillary blood vessels after it has been squeezed out by the examiner. Customarily, the capillary bed under the fingernails is the most reliably tested area. Capillary refill should be both prompt and pink — that is, the normal pink color underneath the nail bed should return within 2 seconds after gentle compression is released. It may be delayed or completely absent. This test is not valid if the returning color is blue, since this may indicate that the capillaries are refilling from the veins, rather than from the arteries, with fresh, oxygenated blood (Figure 4.14).

Pupil Size and Response to Light

The pupils of the eye, when normal, are regular in outline and usually of the same size. Changes and variation in size of one or both pupils are important signs in emergency medical care. In a small percentage of normal persons, **anisocoria** (unequal pupil size) is found. The incidence of this phenomenon is so small, however, that in the injured patient variation in pupil size is regarded as a reliable sign of brain damage (Figure 4.15).

Constricted pupils are often present in a drug addict or a patient with a central nervous system disease (Figure 4.16). Variation in the size of the two pupils is seen in patients with head injuries or strokes. Dilated pupils indicate a relaxed or unconscious state; such dilation of the pupils usually occurs rapidly (within 30 seconds) after cardiac arrest (Figure 4.17). Head injury or prior drug use, however, may cause

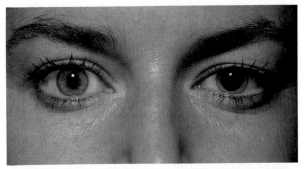

FIGURE 4.15   Variation of pupil size may indicate head injury or stroke.

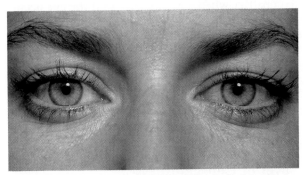

FIGURE 4.16   Constricted pupils in a dark environment may indicate drug usage or central nervous system disease.

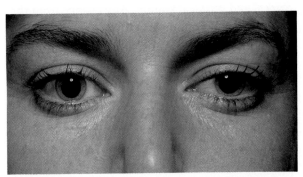

FIGURE 4.17   Dilated pupils in a bright environment or when being examined with a penlight may indicate a relaxed or unconscious state.

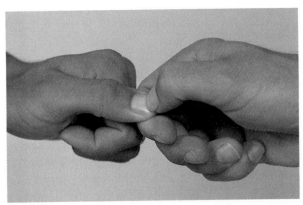

FIGURE 4.14   One important method of assessing the circulation is by observing the capillary refill.

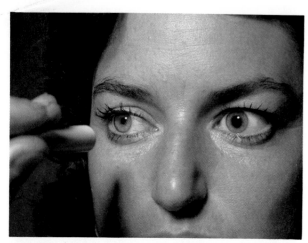

FIGURE 4.18   Normally, the pupil should constrict when light is shined into it.

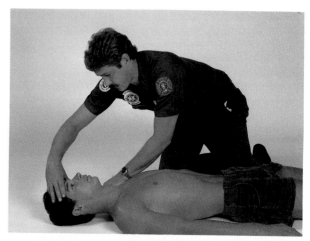

FIGURE 4.19   Increasing difficulty in rousing a patient indicates a need for urgent attention at the hospital. This EMT is guarding the patient's cervical spine with his right hand while using his left hand to try to rouse the patient.

the pupils to remain constricted, even in patients with cardiac arrest.

Ordinarily, pupils constrict promptly when light shines into the eye. This is a normal protective reaction of the eye (Figure 4.18). Failure of the pupils to constrict when a light shines into the eye occurs in disease, poisoning, drug overdose, and injury. In death, the pupils are widely dilated and fail to respond to light.

The state of the pupils, especially progressive changes, is a rapid reflection of central nervous system injury or disease. Any such changes should be noted, reported, and recorded early in the examination of all patients.

Level of Consciousness

Normally a person is alert, oriented (knows the time, his location, his name, and the circumstances surrounding the medical emergency), and responsive to vocal and physical stimuli. Any change from that state is indicative of illness or injury. Recording such a change is extremely important in emergency medical care. Such changes may vary from mild confusion in an alcoholic or mental patient to deep coma in a poisoned or head-injured person. The patient's level of consciousness is probably the single most reliable sign in assessing the status of the central nervous system (Figure 4.19).

It is extremely important for the EMT to note the level of consciousness of a patient early in the course of evaluation. All subsequent changes must also be noted and recorded. Progressive deteriora-tion in the level of consciousness or increasing difficulty in rousing a patient are signs that indicate an urgent need for prompt attention at the hospital. This is especially true with a patient who is unconscious following an injury, then rouses and seems normal for a period of time (lucid interval), but suddenly becomes unconscious again. Such a patient is probably experiencing bleeding inside the skull and is in need of immediate surgery. A specific place on the ambulance form should be reserved for a neurological checklist to record the reactive changes of the patient and the specific time at which the observation was made.

Ability to Move

The inability of a conscious patient to move voluntarily is known as **paralysis.** It may occur as a result of illness or injury. Paralysis of one side of the body (**hemiplegia**) may occur as a result of bleeding or blood-clot formation within the brain (**stroke**). Certain drugs, if used over long periods of time, may also cause paralysis.

Inability to move the legs or arms after an injury indicates damage to the spinal cord until proved otherwise. Inability to move the legs while the arms remain normal indicates a spinal cord injury below the neck level. Paralysis is a particularly important sign, and its presence and the time of onset must be recorded (Figure 4.20).

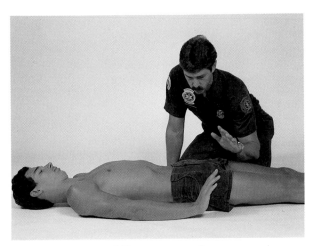

FIGURE 4.20 Inability to move the arms or legs can be a sign of spinal cord injury.

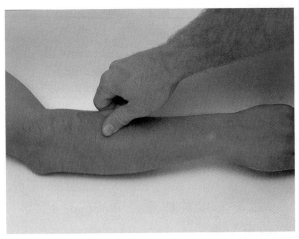

FIGURE 4.21 A gentle pinch is used to test the patient's reaction to pain.

Reaction to Pain

Reaction by vocal response or body movement to a painful physical stimulation is a normal function of the body. But just because the patient is not screaming or clutching "where it hurts" does not mean that significant injury has not occurred. Changes in the normal reaction to pain may result from loss of sensation following an injury or illness. The EMT should test the patient's reaction to pain by gently pinching the skin. Extreme force or pressure should not be used (Figure 4.21). The loss of voluntary movement of the extremities after an injury, or paralysis, is usually accompanied by loss of sensation in the affected extremities. Occasionally, however, movement is retained, and the patient complains only of numbness or tingling in the extremities. It is important that this fact be recognized as a sign of probable injury of the spinal cord so that mishandling does not aggravate the condition.

Severe pain in an extremity with loss of skin sensation may be the result of **occlusion,** or blockage, of the main artery of the extremity. In such a case, the pulse in the extremity is absent. The ability to move the extremity is usually retained, although it is often held immobile because of pain.

Frequently, patients suffering from hysteria, violent shock, or excessive drug or alcohol use may feel no pain from an injury for several hours. This loss of pain sensation is not accompanied by paralysis, and the patient may continue to try to use the injured limb.

Use of the Diagnostic Signs

The alert EMT, using eyes, ears, hands, and a few simple instruments, can obtain a great deal of information about the patient by assessing the diagnostic signs just listed. The four vital signs (pulse, respiration, blood pressure, and temperature) can be used to identify most critically ill patients. The other diagnostic signs will provide many clues as to the cause of the patient's injury or illness and help to assess the severity of the problem. Accurate assessment of the diagnostic signs is essential for proper management of every patient. Periodic reassessment of the pertinent diagnostic signs at least every 10 to 15 minutes will allow the EMT to determine if the patient's condition is improving or deteriorating. It is essential that all observations be recorded and that the time of each observation be recorded as well. A written record of the patient's course is the information of value to the emergency department personnel.

ASSESSMENT AND TREATMENT PRIORITIES

The rest of this chapter addresses the sequence of assessment and treatment that should be undertaken by the EMT. The highest priorities must, of course, be addressed first, both in terms of assessment and treatment, before proceeding to less important priorities. The following procedures should be carried out in the order in which they are presented.

The First Assessment

The first assessment of the patient is not performed by the emergency medical technician in the field; rather, it is performed by the dispatcher who first receives the call. The dispatcher should obtain important information from the caller and relay this information to the EMT. The EMT in the field should use this information to prepare mentally for the type of emergency to be encountered and to determine what equipment will be needed. The function of the dispatcher is extremely important and is covered in detail in Chapter 49 (Figure 4.22).

Arrival at the Scene

Upon arriving at the scene, the EMT should begin to assess the patient and the environment even before getting out of the ambulance. The presence of police cars may indicate the possibility of violence or trauma. Having been called to a restaurant may arouse suspicions of a choking victim. A patient who is lying outside on a cold or rainy day could be suffering from exposure to the elements. Any circumstances that relate to the event should always be mentally recorded because they may provide clues to the nature of the patient's problem or condition.

It is especially important for the EMT to assess the scene for possible personal danger or danger to uninvolved bystanders. It is foolhardy to enter a dangerous scene without taking self-protective measures. For example, when called to the scene of a shooting, the EMT should wait for clearance from police of-

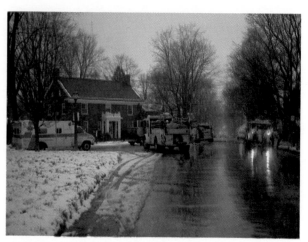

FIGURE 4.23 The initial assessment of the environment is an important source of information.

ficers at the scene before approaching the patient. And, if the EMT arrives before the police, waiting for them is still the best policy. Until the police have secured the area, the EMT can keep bystanders from accidentally approaching the scene. Likewise, if the patient is on fire, the EMT should put out the fire before doing anything else, again being careful to take self-protective measures (Figure 4.23).

For the patient who has been in a motor vehicle accident, the mechanism of injury must be noted as well. Is the windshield cracked or the steering wheel bent? Has the car rolled over? Was the patient thrown from the vehicle? Knowledge about the mechanism of injury will guide the thoughtful EMT to certain specific injuries and patterns of injury (see Chapter 12).

To avoid further injuries, the safety of the patient should be considered next. For example, if a patient has suffered a heart attack while crossing a busy street, it may be necessary to divert the flow of traffic before starting to work on the patient. Or, in this situation, the patient could be moved quickly to a safer place before the necessary assessment and treatment begins. Upon approaching the scene, the EMT will notice many obvious findings at once — for example, bleeding, unconsciousness, or extreme agitation. Any obvious findings such as these should be noted, but they should not distract the EMT from proceeding with a further orderly assessment of the patient.

The EMT must also, at this point, be able to identify patients who are obviously dead at the scene.

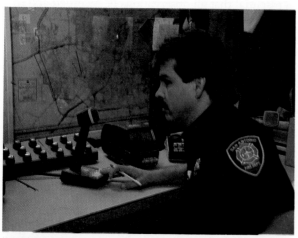

FIGURE 4.22 The EMS dispatcher provides the EMT in the field with important information.

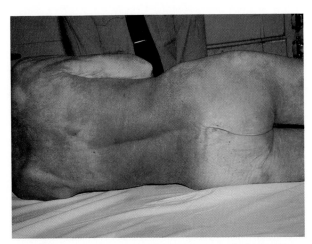

FIGURE 4.24   Dependent lividity, an obvious sign of death, is caused by blood settling to the lower parts of the body. This body was found in a supine position, with the lividity seen as purple discoloration of the back, except in those areas of firm contact with the ground (white areas across back at scapulae and buttocks).

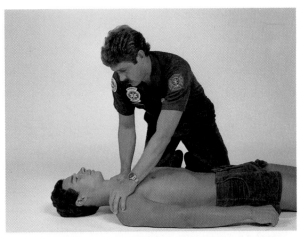

FIGURE 4.25   The EMT assesses airway, breathing, and circulation in the seemingly unconscious person by first attempting to rouse the patient.

Lividity is the redness caused by blood pooling in the dependent parts of the body and is seen 15 to 30 minutes after death (Figure 4.24). Several hours later, **rigor mortis** will be noted by the resistance felt from the patient's body when an attempt is made to move it. Rigor mortis is best seen by trying to straighten a flexed extremity. Decomposition and decapitation are other obvious signs of death.

The Primary Survey

The purpose of the **primary survey** is to find and treat the most life-threatening emergencies first. This is accomplished by assessing and stabilizing the following systems in this order of importance:

1. Airway
2. Breathing
3. Circulation
4. Disability

The assessment of airway, breathing, and circulation in the seemingly unconscious patient begins by attempting to rouse the patient (Figure 4.25). If the patient cannot be aroused, breathing and circulation are assessed (Figure 4.26) and resuscitation, if necessary, is begun as described in Chapters 6 and 8.

If the patient is conscious or is unconscious but breathing, the assessment of airway, breathing, circulation, and disability continues with the following steps, which can be done in nearly one motion.

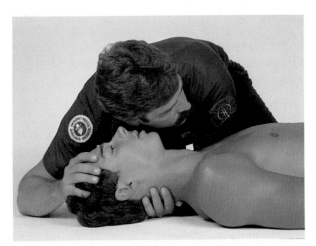

FIGURE 4.26   If the patient cannot be roused, the EMT should "look, listen, and feel" for breathing.

1. Place your face squarely in front of the patient's face while grasping the patient's nearest wrist with your hand.
2. Ask the patient "Are you okay?" while you take the pulse (Figure 4.27).

Observe the patient's response closely and continue assessment of the following four critical factors:

Airway

In assessing the airway, the EMT asks the obvious: Is the patient breathing? Does the patient

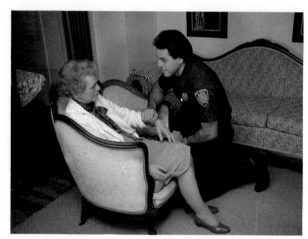

FIGURE 4.27 The EMT squarely faces the patient and asks, "Are you okay?" while examining the patient's face and neck for signs of distress.

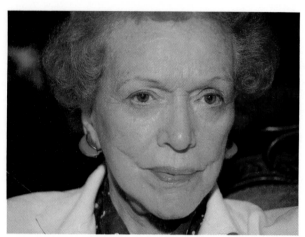

FIGURE 4.28 The face and neck of the patient should be examined for the patient's overall level of distress, for difficulty in breathing, for cyanosis around the mouth, for distended neck veins, and for level of consciousness. Abnormal findings in these areas would indicate immediate administration of oxygen and possible ventilatory support.

have an adequate airway? If the patient does not appear to be breathing or has an inadequate airway, airway management must be started immediately (see Chapter 6).

Breathing

In determining if the patient is having difficulty breathing, the EMT should notice the character of the respirations — are they shallow or deep? Does the patient appear to be choking? Is the patient cyanotic, suggesting poor oxygenation? If the patient appears to have any difficulty breathing, the EMT should immediately begin support of the patient's breathing as described in Chapter 6 (Figure 4.28).

Circulation

The next step is to check to see if the pulse is present. Using one hand, the EMT can assess the rate and quality of the radial pulse. If the radial pulse is absent, the EMT should palpate for the carotid pulse in the neck or, if the patient is alert, the radial pulse in the other wrist. If the pulse is absent in both wrists and in the neck, immediate circulatory support should be given. If the patient has been injured, circulatory support should be provided by antishock trousers, which are described in Chapter 11. If the patient has not been injured, full cardiopulmonary resuscitation (CPR) should be carried out as described in Chapter 8.

If the pulse is present, the EMT should next assess the patient's skin color, temperature, and moisture. While looking at the patient's face, the EMT should note color changes and excessive sweating. While taking the pulse, the EMT can palpate the skin and identify abnormalities in skin temperature and moisture (Figure 4.29).

After assessing the patient's pulse, skin temperature, and color, the EMT should further assess the circulation by squeezing one of the patient's fingernails to check capillary refill (Figure 4.30). Any sources of external bleeding should be sought and quickly controlled, as described in Chapter 10. In cases of significant trauma, all the patient's clothing should be removed to find all sources of bleeding to complete the assessment of the circulation. If the trauma patient has signs of diminished circulation, the chest, abdomen, and thighs should be examined because they may reveal evidence of internal bleeding.

Disability

Once the airway, breathing, and circulation have been assessed, the EMT moves on to assess the patient's level of consciousness. The patient's neurological status is assessed by noting the quality of the patient's response to the question, "Are you okay?" and by noting if the patient's extremities move spontaneously. The patient's level of consciousness or

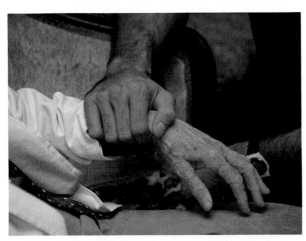

FIGURE 4.29 The EMT first notes the warmth, moisture, and color of the extremity. Then the radial pulse is assessed for rate and quality. If the radial pulse is not obtainable, the other wrist is checked. If both radial pulses were absent, the EMT would check the carotid pulse and begin immediate circulatory support, if indicated.

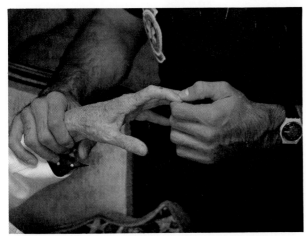

FIGURE 4.30 As a final check of the patient's circulatory status, the capillary refill is assessed.

"mental status" can be described using one of the following four terms.

1. *Alert.* The patient's eyes open spontaneously and she answers questions in a clear manner. She knows the date, where she is, and her own name. If the patient knows the date, location, and her name, she is said to be "oriented."

2. *Responsive to verbal stimulus.* The patient's eyes do not open spontaneously, and he may not be oriented to time, place, and person, but he responds in some meaningful way when spoken to.

3. *Responsive to pain.* The patient does not respond to verbal stimuli, but she moves or cries out in response to pain. The response to a painful stimulus is tested by gently, but firmly, pinching the patient's skin. An appropriate response is withdrawal from this painful stimulus. If the patient is paralyzed in an extremity, this examination is not valid in that extremity. Extremely painful stimuli should never be applied to the patient.

4. *Unresponsive.* The patient does not respond to the painful stimulus.

These four terms describing the patient's mental status are referred to as the **AVPU scale.**

If the patient has been injured and is unconscious, complains of pain in the head or neck, or is having difficulty moving any extremity, or if the mechanism of injury suggests significant trauma, all assessment and treatment should be done while another person guards the stability of the cervical spine. Injuries to the cervical spine caused by rough handling of the patient can produce immediate paralysis and death.

If the patient is unconscious or unable to respond, the patient's clothes, wallet, wrist, and neck should be checked for an **emergency medical identification card or tag** (Figure 4.31). These usually bear warning of any serious medical problem.

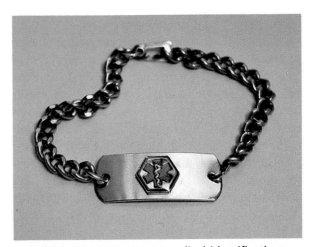

FIGURE 4.31 Emergency medical identification cards or tags may alert the EMT that the patient has a known, life-threatening condition.

Except for the desire to obtain information of medical importance that can be found in wallet cards, there is no reason for the EMT to search the patient. If police are present, it is best that any search be done by them or in their presence and so recorded.

The primary assessment up to this point has been concerned with identifying life-threatening conditions. This concern must be primary in the mind of the EMT. When an abnormality in airway, breathing, or circulation is identified, treatment must be instituted immediately and the deficit corrected to assure adequate performance of the patient's vital functions. The airway, breathing, and circulation must be stabilized as a first priority, and they must be continuously supported until the patient is delivered to the emergency department.

Only after adequate performance of the patient's vital functions has been assured should the EMT proceed with further evaluation of the patient's problem. In rare instances, when the patient is critically ill or injured, the necessity for resuscitation and immediate transport may mean that no further assessment is done.

The Chief Complaint

Until now, the EMT has been concerned primarily with signs, or those things that can actually be observed. When asking the patient "Are you okay?" the EMT has been concerned with the response only in terms of its quality. That is, the response was not assessed for content — only for an indication of the patient's ability to breathe and respond to a verbal stimulus. Now the EMT must address the patient's symptoms.

Usually the first words out of the patient's mouth in response to a general question such as "What's wrong?" or "What happened?" is called the **chief complaint** (Figure 4.32). Despite what has already been observed, the EMT should not jump to any conclusions about what is troubling the patient. Now is the time to listen. It is important to understand the patient's problems in the patient's own terms. Generally, the chief complaint is recorded in a few of the patient's own words, along with the duration of the symptoms: "I fell and hurt my arm 2 hours ago." "I have had pain in my chest since last night." If the patient is not capable of giving a chief complaint, it should be elicited from a family member or bystander (Figure 4.33). The informant's relation-

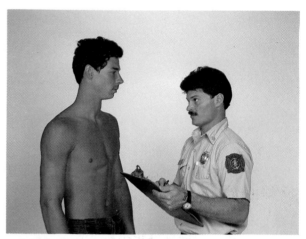

FIGURE 4.32   The patient's initial response to the EMT's question "What's wrong?" is the *chief complaint.*

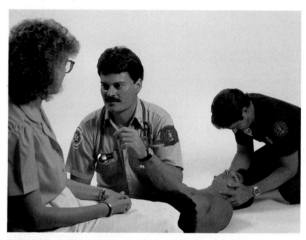

FIGURE 4.33   If the patient is unresponsive, the chief complaint and any other pertinent history should be obtained from bystanders.

ship to the patient should be indicated on the ambulance form. For example,

Wife: "He passed out and stopped breathing" — 4 minutes

Vital Signs

The vital signs (pulse, respirations, blood pressure, and, if indicated, temperature) should be determined at this point in the assessment of the patient. Generally, one EMT can do this while the other takes the history of present illness as described next (Figure 4.34).

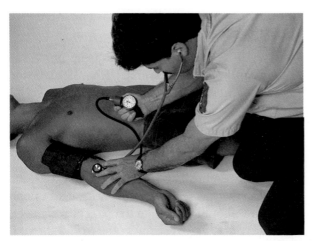

FIGURE 4.34 Determining the patient's vital signs is part of the patient assessment.

History of Present Illness

If time permits, it is valuable to learn the events leading up to the current episode. This information is obtained by the EMT's asking the patient or an informed bystander questions that shed light on the patient's current problem as it relates to the patient's overall medical state. It is important for the EMT to know about any major medical problems such as diabetes or heart disease, the medications the patient takes, any allergies the patient may have, when the patient last ate, and the events that led up to the current illness or injury. This information can be easily remembered through the use of the word "AMPLE":

A — Allergies
M — Medications
P — Previous illness
L — Last meal or drink
E — Events preceding the illness or injury

One of the most common chief complaints is pain. Pain can, and will, be described in many different ways. It is important to question the patient about the nature and extent of the pain that is present. The questions relating to pain can be remembered by the letters PQRST:

P — *Provoke.* What causes the pain? What makes the pain worse? What makes the pain better?

Q — *Quality.* What does the pain feel like? Sharp? Dull? Burning? Stabbing? Crushing?

R — *Radiation.* Does the pain travel from one area to another? For example, does the patient's chest pain seem to go up into his jaw?

S — *Severity.* Does the patient think the pain is mild, moderate, or severe?

T — *Time.* Is the pain constant or intermittent? Has the pain occurred before? When did it start? Does it change in severity (get better, then worse)?

Following trauma, the mechanism of injury should be recorded, since it may give a clue to significant hidden injuries. Patients who have been in automobile wrecks should also be asked about the path of their vehicle before and after impact, their position inside the car, and which parts of their body were struck during the impact. Certainly, if the patient has been thrown from the vehicle or if the vehicle has rolled over, this information should be indicated on the patient's record. Often this information can be indicated by diagram (Figure 4.35).

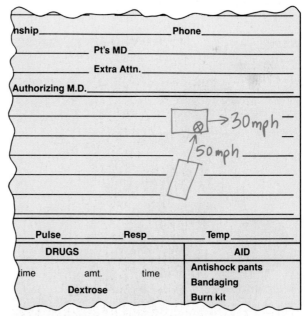

FIGURE 4.35 The mechanism of injury after an automobile accident can be easily illustrated with simple drawings. This diagram represents the patient as the passenger (indicated by the X) in a car that was going 30 miles per hour and was struck on the passenger's side by another vehicle traveling at 50 miles per hour. The circle around the symbol for the patient indicates that he was wearing his seat belt.

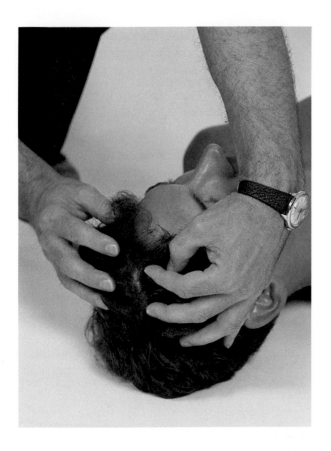

Secondary Survey (Head-to-Toe Examination)

The final step in the assessment process is examining the patient carefully from head to toe, looking for wounds and deformities, and observing whether the patient feels pain and has sensation. This head-to-toe examination is called the **secondary survey.** If the patient has been found to have life-threatening injuries during the primary survey, the necessity for immediate resuscitation and transport may mean that the secondary survey cannot be done. The EMT should explain to the patient what is being done and why. By reassuring the patient throughout the examination, the EMT can establish rapport and ensure better cooperation. The secondary survey is represented pictorially in Figures 4.36 through 4.77.

FIGURE 4.36 The EMT should look for lacerations or bruises of the scalp.

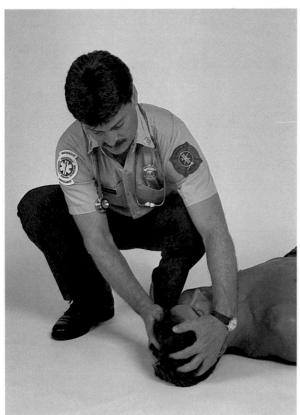

FIGURE 4.37 Tenderness, depressions of the skull, and any deformities should be noted. Care should be taken not to press firmly over areas of skull depression.

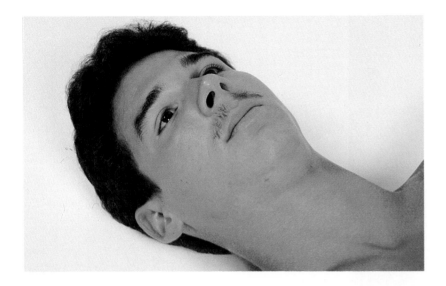

FIGURE 4.38 Lacerations, bruises, and deformities of the face should be noted.

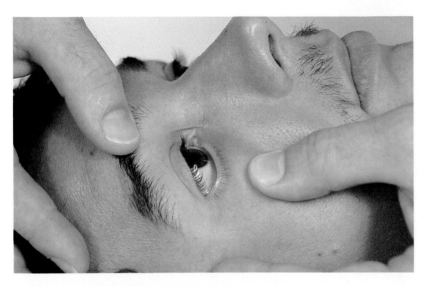

FIGURE 4.39 The eyes and lids should be inspected in more detail.

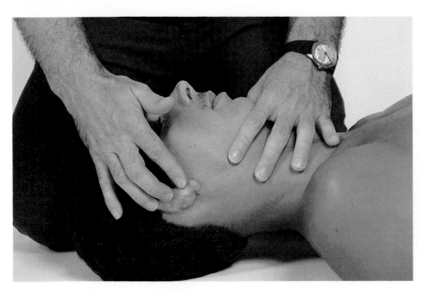

FIGURE 4.40 The EMT is pulling the patient's ear forward to search for bruising of the mastoid process. Mastoid bruising is characteristic of a basilar skull fracture. See Chapter 19.

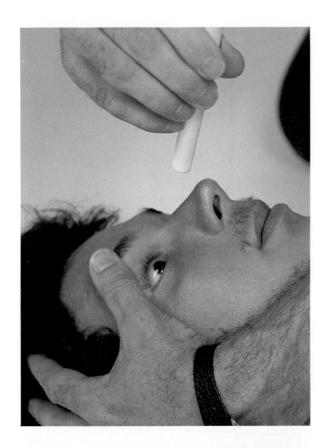

FIGURE 4.41 The eyes are examined for redness and for contact lenses, and the pupils are assessed.

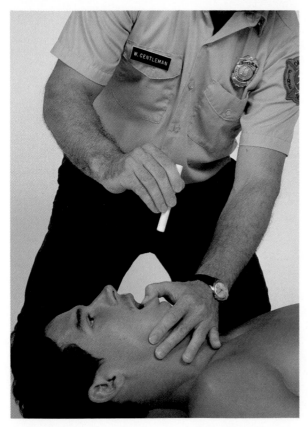

FIGURE 4.42 The nose is examined for drainage or bleeding, and the mouth is examined for cyanosis, foreign bodies (including loose teeth or dentures), bleeding, lacerations, or deformities.

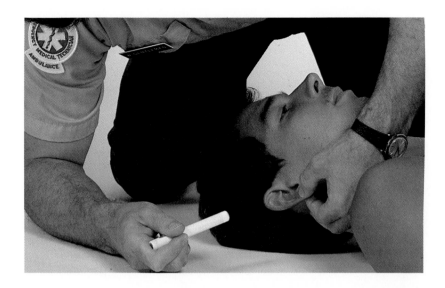

FIGURE 4.43 The penlight is used to look for drainage or blood in the ears.

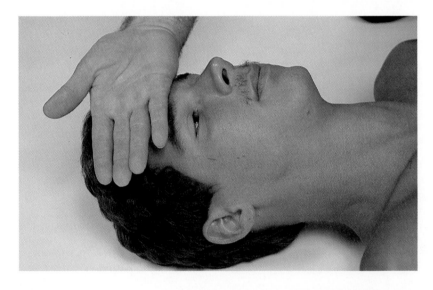

FIGURE 4.44 The forehead is felt for temperature and moisture.

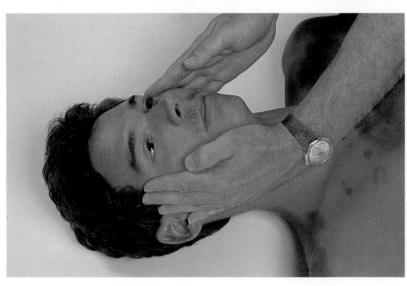

FIGURE 4.45 The zygomas (bones forming the lateral wall of the orbit of the eye) are palpated for tenderness or instability.

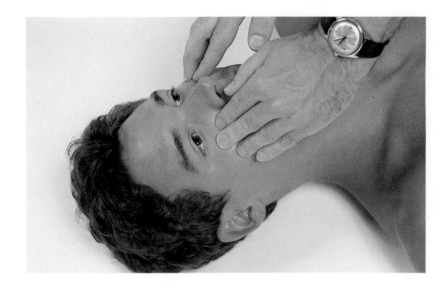

FIGURE 4.46 The maxillae (cheek bones) are palpated.

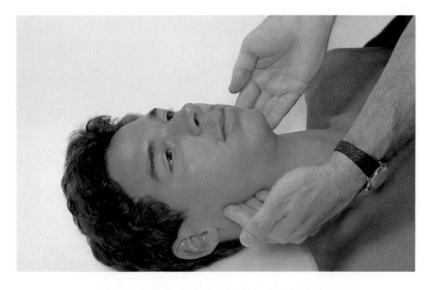

FIGURE 4.47 The mandible (jawbone) is palpated.

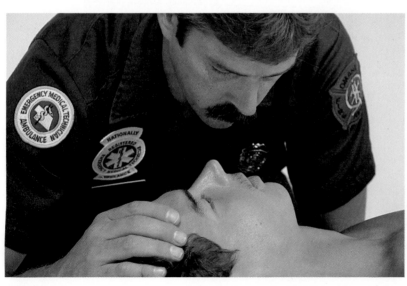

FIGURE 4.48 The EMT should check for unusual odors on the patient's breath.

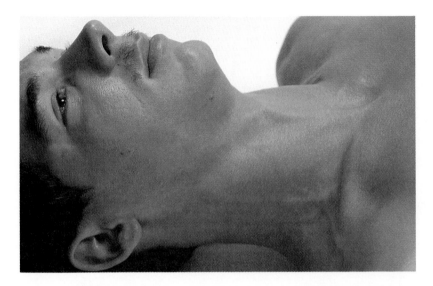

FIGURE 4.49 The EMT looks for distended neck veins, lacerations, bruises, and deformity. These neck veins are distended. Distended neck veins are not necessarily significant when the patient is lying down. Veins that are distended when the patient is in the sitting position, however, may indicate cardiac or other thoracic problems.

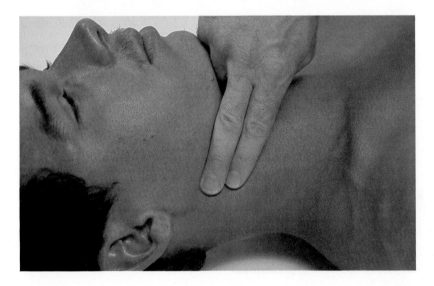

FIGURE 4.50 If the neck veins are distended, it may be significant to note that they refill from below after all the blood has been expressed from them by the EMT's examining hand.

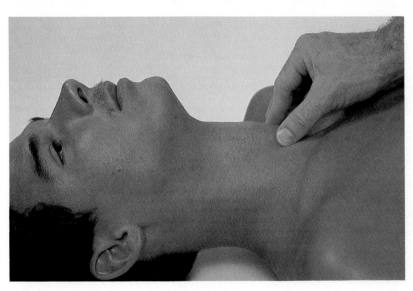

FIGURE 4.51 The trachea is noted to be in the midline at the suprasternal notch. Deviation of the trachea may indicate pneumothorax.

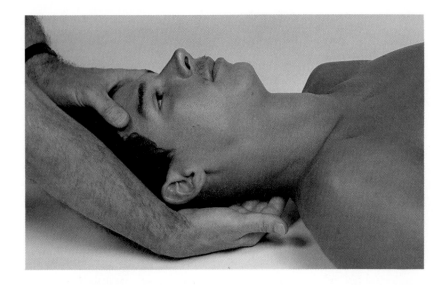

FIGURE 4.52 The cervical spine is gently palpated for deformity or tenderness.

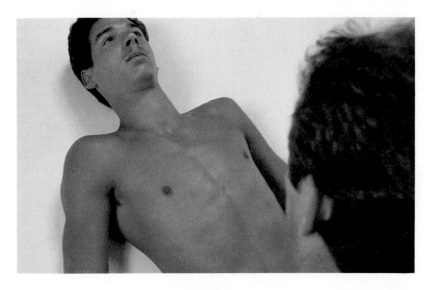

FIGURE 4.53 The EMT looks carefully for signs of injury before laying hands on the patient's trunk. Movement of the chest with respiration is also important to observe.

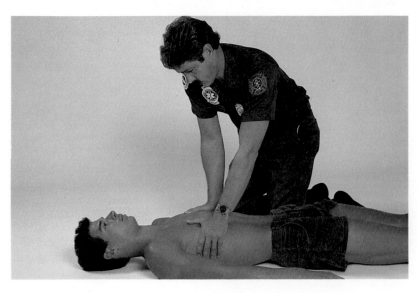

FIGURE 4.54 The EMT presses on the ribs to elicit tenderness. This should be done gently, and the EMT should avoid pressing over obvious bruises or fractures. The EMT should also note the presence of subcutaneous emphysema, a crackling sensation caused by air bubbles trapped in tissues beneath the skin.

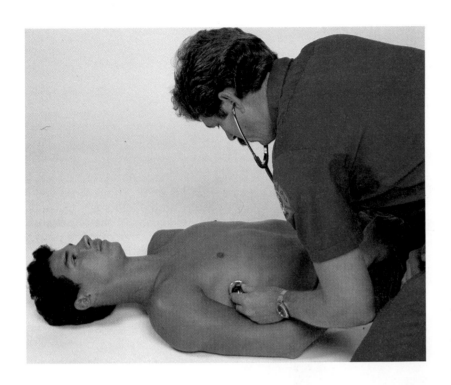

FIGURE 4.55 The EMT listens at the nipple level in the mid-axillary line to compare the equality of the breath sounds on the two sides of the chest.

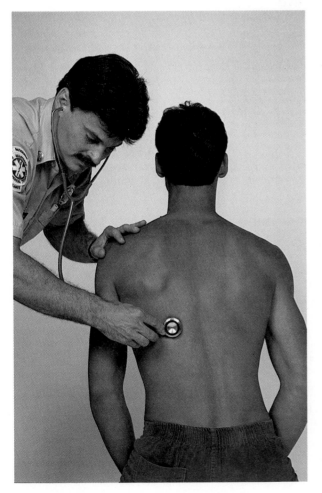

FIGURE 4.56 (left) The breath sounds should be examined from the back as well. Although the patient is shown here in the sitting position, this examination can usually be performed when the patient is in the supine position. Comparison of the two sides is helpful in determining if an abnormality exists.

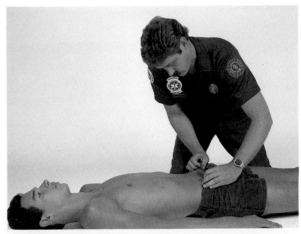

FIGURE 4.57 The EMT looks to see if the patient's abdomen is distended as well as examines for wounds, bruises, or other obvious signs of injury. If the patient has sustained trauma to the genital area, this should also be examined.

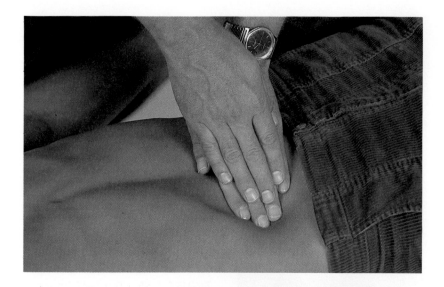

FIGURE 4.58 The EMT presses gently on the abdomen and notes any tenderness. If the muscles of the patient's abdomen are unusually tense, this finding is called "rigidity" and is extremely significant.

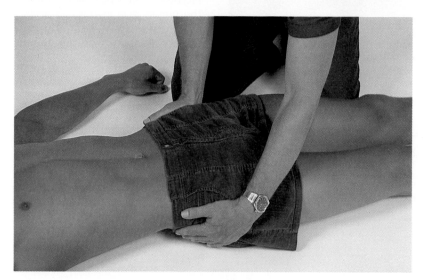

FIGURE 4.59 The pelvis is compressed from the sides to determine if it is tender.

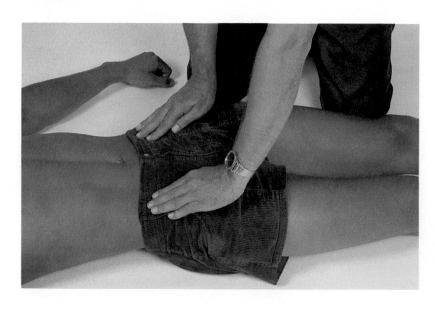

FIGURE 4.60 The EMT is pressing the patient's iliac crests to elicit signs of instability, tenderness, or crepitus.

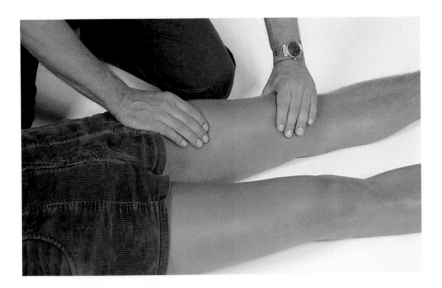

FIGURE 4.61 The lower extremities are inspected for lacerations, bruises, edema, or deformity. Then they are palpated for tenderness, except over obvious fracture sites.

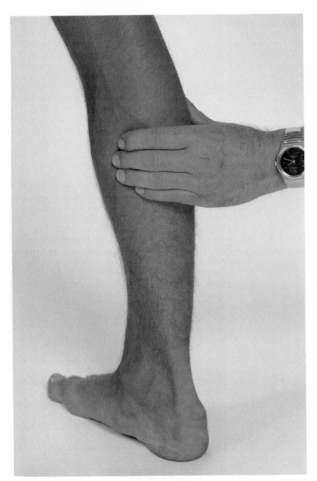

FIGURE 4.62 Tenderness elicited by squeezing the calves may indicate clots in the legs which may travel through the circulation to the lungs, where they can be fatal. This examination should be performed gently and, if it is positive, not repeated, since the examination itself may dislodge clots.

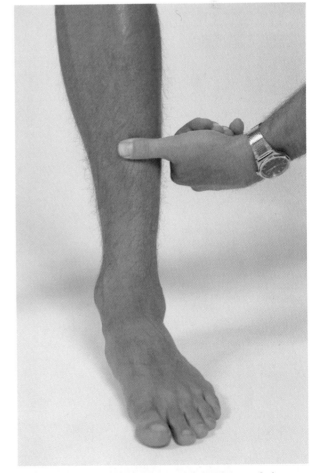

FIGURE 4.63 Pressing against the front of the shin is done to determine the presence of pretibial edema (swelling). When the swelling is extreme, the imprint of the examining finger will remain even after the finger is removed; this is called "pitting edema."

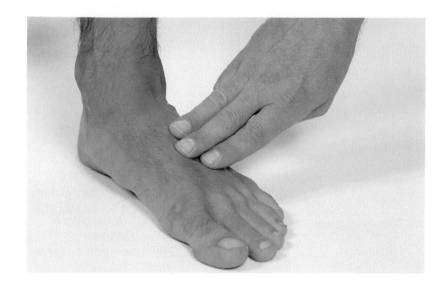

FIGURE 4.64 The dorsalis pedis pulse is checked in each foot.

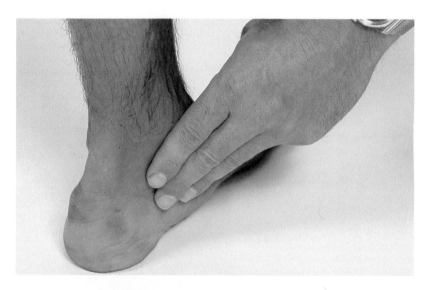

FIGURE 4.65 The posterior tibial pulse is examined on the medial side of each ankle.

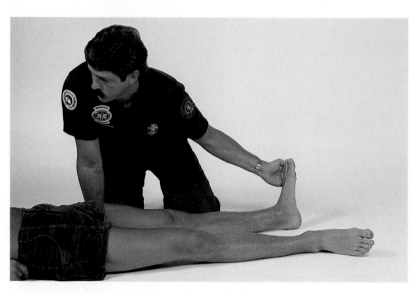

FIGURE 4.66 The strength of the foot is tested by having the patient press his foot against the EMT's hand. This is compared to the opposite side. The presence of sensation and movement should be noted.

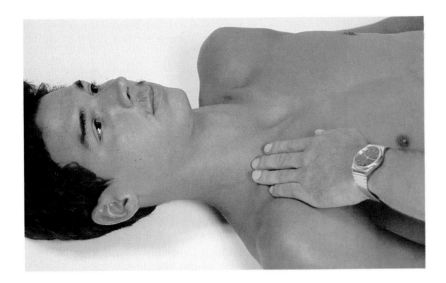

FIGURE 4.67 Inspection and palpation of the clavicles should be included when checking the upper extremities.

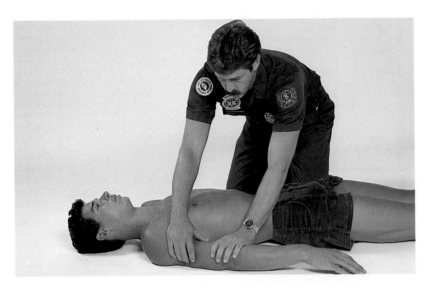

FIGURE 4.68 Squeezing the extremities may reveal hidden fractures by eliciting tenderness.

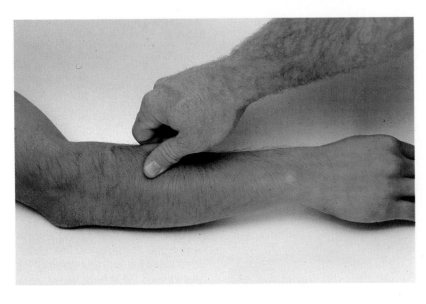

FIGURE 4.69 Gentle pinching is used to test reaction to pain. This need not be done if the patient is able to identify the sensation of light touch in the extremities.

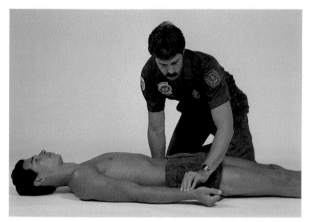

FIGURE 4.70 The pulses are checked in each upper extremity.

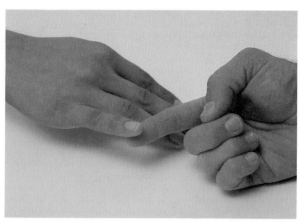

FIGURE 4.71 The EMT is testing the patient's sensation of light touch by gently stroking the palmar surface of the tip of the little finger.

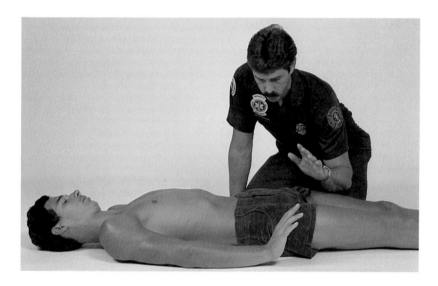

FIGURE 4.72 The EMT is testing the patient's ability to move his hand. He may also ask the patient to open and close his fist as an additional means of testing neurological function. This is also a test of the patient's ability to follow commands.

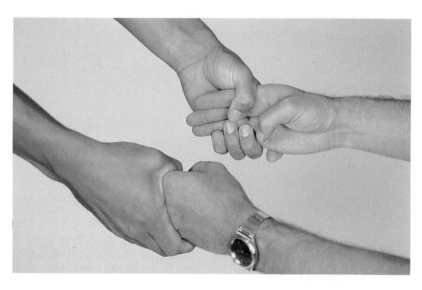

FIGURE 4.73 Comparing the patient's grip strength on the two sides is useful for determining the presence of weakness.

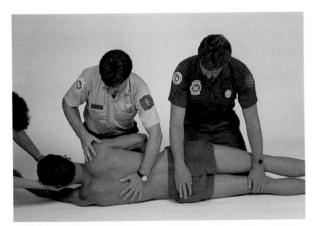

FIGURE 4.74 If spinal cord injury is suspected, the patient should be carefully log-rolled to inspect the back.

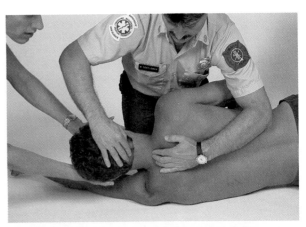

FIGURE 4.75 The cervical spine is carefully palpated for tenderness or deformity.

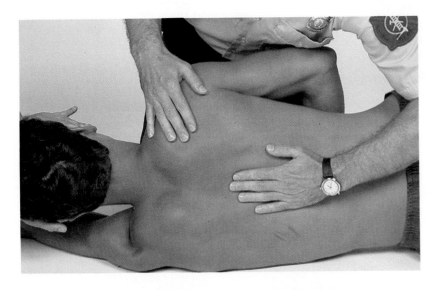

FIGURE 4.76 The thoracic spine is likewise examined for possible injury.

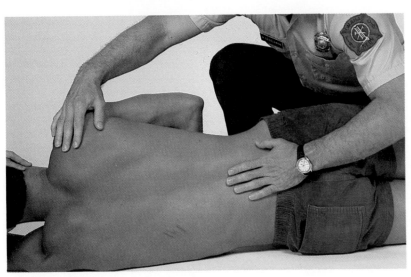

FIGURE 4.77 The lumbar spine is similarly examined.

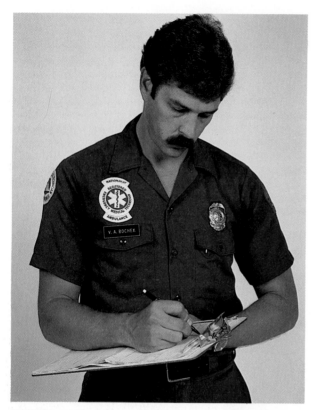

FIGURE 4.78 Document, document, document! A famous lawyer once said, "If it isn't written down, you didn't do it."

Once the secondary survey is completed, the EMT will have compiled a mental list of all the patient's serious disorders. Then the EMT can pro-

ceed in a systematic way to stabilize all serious injuries while continuing to assure adequacy of the patient's vital functions through periodic monitoring of the vital signs. Finally, the EMT should make a careful recording of all findings and treatments. Repeat assessments should also be documented. The progression of vital signs and neurological status are especially important to hospital personnel and should be carefully recorded (Figure 4.78).

YOU ARE THE EMT...

1. The patient tells you she has been vomiting all day and is worried because now she is vomiting blood. She began to have stomach pains the night before. Her temperature is 101 degrees F, and she is dizzy when she walks. She has a fierce headache. Her pulse is rapid, and blood pressure is 120/85. Which of these are signs and which are symptoms?
2. Your patient is a 50-year-old male. His blood pressure is 150/95. Which number is the diastolic pressure? The systolic? Is this blood pressure in the normal range? Why or why not?
3. You have taken the patient's pulse, respiration, and blood pressure. What is the fourth vital sign? Name four additional diagnostic signs.
4. Why is it so important to assess the level of consciousness? Describe the AVPU scale.

SECTION 3

CARDIOPULMONARY RESUSCITATION

5

The Respiratory System

OVERVIEW

The respiratory system consists of the structures of the body that contribute to respiration, or breathing. The function of the respiratory system is to provide the body with oxygen and dispose of carbon dioxide. The exchange of oxygen and carbon dioxide takes place in the lungs and in the tissues. It is a complicated process that occurs automatically unless the airways or the lungs become diseased or damaged. In order to provide the lifesaving treatment required when a patient is not breathing effectively, the EMT must be able to locate the structures of the respiratory system and understand their function.

Chapter 5 begins with a description of the breathing process, including the exchange of oxygen and carbon dioxide that takes place. The airways and lungs are also described in this section. The chapter next discusses the mechanics of breathing and the role of the diaphragm and intercostal muscles. The last section of Chapter 5 explains how breathing is controlled by the brain and is stimulated by the level of carbon dioxide present in the arterial blood.

OBJECTIVES

The objectives of Chapter 5 are to

- describe the breathing process, including the exchange of oxygen and carbon dioxide and the role of the airways and lungs.
- understand the mechanics of breathing, or how the diaphragm and intercostal muscles contract and relax during inhalation and expiration.
- realize that breathing is controlled by the brain's response to levels of carbon dioxide and oxygen present in the arterial blood.

THE BREATHING PROCESS

The **thorax,** or chest, is the more superior (upper) of the two major body cavities. It is bounded by the rib cage anteriorly, superiorly, and posteriorly, and by the diaphragm inferiorly. The clavicles pass anterior to its uppermost portion. The thorax contains the lungs — one in each half, or **hemithorax.** Between the lungs, in a space called the **mediastinum,** lie the heart, the great arteries and veins, the esophagus, the trachea and major bronchi, and many nerves (Figure 5.1).

The **respiratory system** consists of all the structures of the body that contribute to normal respiration, or the process of breathing. Strictly speaking, it includes the nose, mouth, throat, larynx, trachea, and bronchi, which are all air passages or airways. It also includes the lungs, where oxygen (O_2) is passed into the blood and carbon dioxide (CO_2) is removed from the blood to be exhaled. Finally, it includes the diaphragm, the muscles of the chest wall, and the accessory muscles of breathing, which permit normal respiratory movement (Figure 5.2).

In this text, the term **airway** usually refers to the **upper airway** or the passage above the larynx (voice box). "Clearing the airway" means removing obstructing material or tissue from the nose, mouth, or throat (Figure 5.3). The **lower airway** includes the larynx, the trachea, the major bronchi, and the other air passages within the lung.

The Exchange of Oxygen and Carbon Dioxide

All living cells of the body are engaged in a series of chemical processes by which the energy needed for life is extracted from food. The name given to the sum total of these processes is **metabolism.** In the course of metabolism, each cell uses oxygen and produces carbon dioxide and other waste substances.

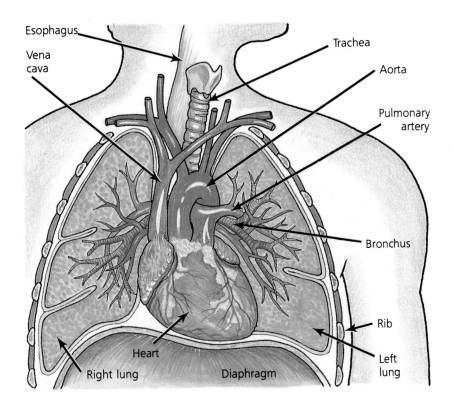

Esophagus

Vena cava

Trachea

Aorta

Pulmonary artery

Bronchus

Rib

Heart

Left lung

Right lung

Diaphragm

FIGURE 5.1 The important anatomic structures of the chest cavity.

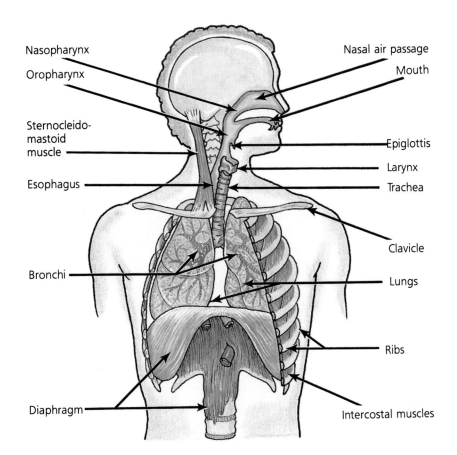

Nasopharynx

Oropharynx

Sternocleido-mastoid muscle

Esophagus

Bronchi

Diaphragm

Nasal air passage

Mouth

Epiglottis

Larynx

Trachea

Clavicle

Lungs

Ribs

Intercostal muscles

FIGURE 5.2 The respiratory system includes airways, lungs, and muscles. Some passages — the mouth and pharynx — are shared in common with the digestive system.

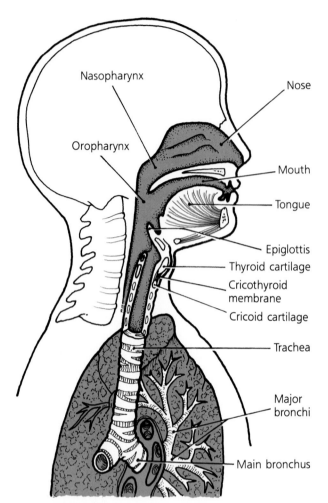

FIGURE 5.3 The upper airway includes the air passages above the larynx, or the nose, mouth, and throat. The lower airway includes the larynx, trachea, major bronchi, and other air passages within the lungs.

This basic chemical reaction occurs in all cells:

$$C_6H_{12}O_6 + 6O_2 \longrightarrow 6CO_2 + 6H_2O + Energy$$
$$\text{(Glucose)} \quad \text{(Oxygen)} \quad \text{(Carbon} \quad \text{(Water)}$$
$$\text{Dioxide)}$$

Cells not able to participate in metabolic processes are dead or dying.

Each living cell in the body requires a regular supply of oxygen; some cells are more dependent on a constant oxygen supply than others. Cells in the heart will be damaged if the oxygen supply is interrupted for more than a few seconds. Cells in the brain and nervous system may die after 4 to 6 minutes without oxygen. These cells can never be replaced, and permanent changes result from the damage. Other cells in the body are not as critically dependent upon a constant oxygen supply. They can withstand short periods without oxygen and still survive. The respiratory system, which delivers oxygen to body tissues and removes carbon dioxide, is thus a very important part of the body. Normally, the air that we breathe contains 20 percent oxygen and 79 percent nitrogen. Minute amounts of other gases make up the final 1 percent.

Blood that has passed through the body has given up oxygen to the tissues and absorbed carbon dioxide produced by cellular metabolism. Venous blood is collected in the right atrium of the heart and is pumped into the lungs by the right ventricle. In the lungs, it passes into a fine network of **pulmonary capillaries,** which are in close contact with the **alveoli** (air sacs) of the lungs. In these air sacs, the blood gives up carbon dioxide and absorbs new oxygen. The refreshed blood is collected from the lungs into the left atrium. It is passed into the strong left ventricle and is pumped into the aorta, and then throughout the body to carry oxygen again to all tissues.

The capillaries in the lungs are located in the walls of the alveoli. The walls of the capillaries and the alveoli are extremely thin. Air in the alveoli and blood in the capillaries are thus separated only by two very thin layers of tissue. Oxygen and carbon dioxide can move rapidly across these layers between the alveoli and capillaries. Figure 5.4 is a schematic representation of the exchange of gases and nutrients in tissues and of gases in the lung. Oxygen passes from the lung across the capillary walls into the blood, and from the blood across the capillary walls into the cells of body tissues. In the reverse of this process, carbon dioxide passes from tissues in the body across the capillary walls into the blood. It passes from the blood across the capillary walls and enters the alveoli in the lung. It is then dispersed in the air exhaled from the lung.

Not all inhaled oxygen is extracted from the blood as it passes through the body. Exhaled air contains 16 percent oxygen and 5 percent carbon dioxide. The remainder is nitrogen. This 16 percent concentration of oxygen is sufficient to support artificial ventilation. That is, even though the EMT is "exhaling" breaths of air in mouth-to-mouth resuscitation, the patient receives the 16 percent concentration of oxygen contained in each exhaled breath from the EMT.

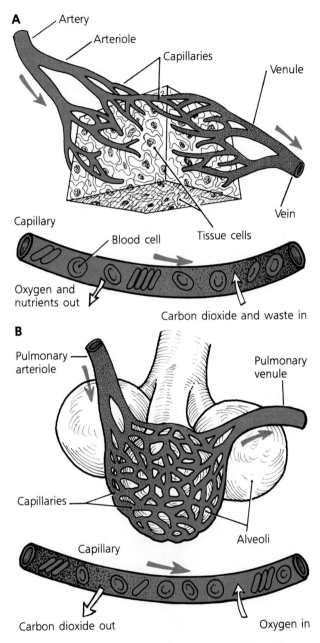

FIGURE 5.4 The exchange of oxygen and carbon dioxide in respiration. (a) Oxygen (O_2) passes from the blood through capillaries to tissue cells. In the reverse process, carbon dioxide (CO_2) passes from tissue cells through capillaries to the blood. (b) In the lung, oxygen is picked up by the blood and carbon dioxide is given off.

The Airways

The upper airway includes the nose, mouth, and throat. The nose and mouth lead to the **pharynx** (throat). At the bottom of the pharynx are two

passageways: the **esophagus** behind and the **trachea** (windpipe) in front. Food and liquids enter the pharynx and pass into the esophagus, which carries them to the stomach. Air and other gases enter the trachea and go to the lungs (Figure 5.3).

Guarding the opening of the trachea is a thin, leaf-shaped valve called the **epiglottis** (Figure 5.3). This valve allows air to pass into the trachea but prevents food or liquid from entering. Air moves past the epiglottis into the larynx and the trachea. The first part of the lower airway is the **larynx** (voice box), which consists of a rather complicated arrangement of tiny bones, cartilage, muscles, and the two vocal cords. The larynx is unable to tolerate any foreign solid or liquid material. A violent episode of coughing and spasm of the vocal cords will result from contact with solids or liquids. The "**Adam's apple**," or **thyroid cartilage,** prominent in the neck, is the anterior portion of the larynx. Tiny muscles open and close the vocal cords. Sounds are created as air is forced past the vocal cords, making them vibrate. These vibrations make the sound. The pitch of the sound changes as the cords open and close. You can feel these vibrations if you place your fingers lightly on the larynx as you speak or sing. Words and other understandable sounds are formed by the tongue and muscles of the mouth.

Immediately inferior to the thyroid cartilage is the palpable **cricoid cartilage.** Between these two prominences lies the **cricothyroid membrane,** which can be felt as a depression in the midline of the neck just inferior to the thyroid cartilage (Figure 5.3). Below the cricoid cartilage is the trachea. Approximately 5 inches long, it is a semirigid tube made up of partial rings of cartilage that are completed posteriorly by strong connective tissue. The cartilaginous rings keep the trachea from collapsing when air is moved in and out of the lungs. The trachea ends by dividing into smaller tubes, called the right and left **main bronchi,** which enter each lung. Each main bronchus immediately branches within the lung into smaller and smaller airways. Within the right lung, three major **bronchi** are formed; within the left, there are only two.

There are two **lungs,** one on each side of the thoracic cage (Figures 5.1 and 5.2). The lungs are suspended within the thoracic cage by the trachea, by the arteries and veins that run to and from the heart, and by the pulmonary ligaments. The airways divide further and finally end in millions of tiny alveoli in each lung (Figure 5.5). Healthy lungs contain about 700 million alveoli. The combined surface area of these alveoli is equal to about one-fourth that of a basketball court. Within these alveoli, the exchange of oxygen and carbon dioxide takes place: Oxygen is given to the blood and carbon dioxide is given off by the blood (Figure 5.4b).

The Lungs

The lungs hang freely within the chest cavity. Although they have no intrinsic capacity for expansion or contraction themselves since they have no muscle, there is a very definite mechanism to ensure

that they follow the motion of the chest wall and expand or contract with it. Covering each lung is a layer of very smooth, glistening tissue called **pleura** (Figure 5.6). Another layer of pleura lines the inside of the chest cavity. The two layers are called **parietal pleura** (lining the chest wall) and **visceral pleura** (covering the lungs).

Between the parietal pleura and the visceral pleura is the **pleural space,** which is not a space in the usual sense because normally these layers are everywhere in close contact. In fact, the layers are sealed tightly against one another by a thin film of fluid. When the chest wall expands, the lung is pulled with it and made to expand by the force exerted through these closely applied pleural surfaces. The pleural space is thus a potential one. Normally the pleural space is quite small and contains only the thin film of pleural fluid as each lung entirely fills its chest cavity.

The potential space between the pleural surfaces can enlarge when the pleural surfaces are separated by blood from a lacerated chest wall or lung, or by air from a torn lung or a hole in the chest wall. If the surfaces are separated, the mechanism for normal expansion of the lungs is lost. If enough blood

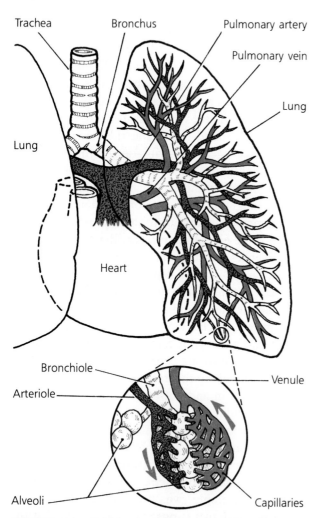

FIGURE 5.5 Within the lung, millions of air sacs (alveoli) lie at the ends of the air passages. Several alveoli are shown in the enlargement of a small area of the lung. Pulmonary capillaries are in very close contact with the alveolar wall.

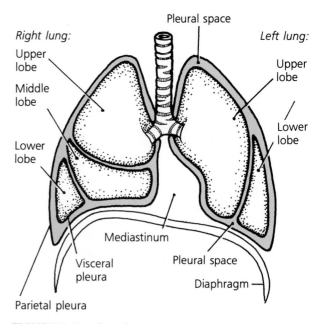

FIGURE 5.6 The pleura lining the chest wall and covering the lungs is an essential part of the breathing mechanism. The pleural space is not an actual space until blood or air leaks into it, causing the pleural surfaces to separate.

or air collects, the lung can be compressed to the extent that it cannot expand at all during inspiration, and insufficient oxygen is taken in to maintain life. Patients with this type of injury may die from lack of oxygen.

The smooth, lubricated pleural surfaces allow the lungs to move perfectly freely within the chest when one is breathing. If the pleural surfaces are injured or become diseased, they no longer have a friction-free, lubricated surface. Then, as the lungs move in breathing, the surfaces rub together, causing friction and pain. This condition is called **pleurisy.**

THE MECHANICS OF BREATHING

Since the lungs contain no muscular tissue and cannot themselves move, expansion and contraction must be provided by other tissues. Movement of the thorax and diaphragm permits air to enter the lungs through the trachea and into the alveoli. The thoracic cage is a semirigid muscular and bony frame enclosed by skin. Contraction of the diaphragm and the intercostal and accessory muscles of breathing causes it to expand in three dimensions: anteroposterior, transverse, and infero-superior. Because of their attachments through the pleural surfaces, the lungs follow the chest wall motion exactly.

The **diaphragm** is one of the specialized muscles of the body. It is skeletal muscle in that it is attached to the costal arch and the vertebrae (Figure 5.7). It is striated (marked by streaks or lines under the microscope) like all other skeletal muscle. It is voluntary muscle in that one can take a deep breath, cough, or override breathing at will. However, unlike other skeletal or voluntary muscle, the diaphragm performs an automatic function. Breathing continues while we sleep and at all other times. The function and control of breathing can be overridden by conscious will; and an individual can temporarily breathe faster, slower, or hold one's breath. However, these variations in breathing pattern cannot be continued indefinitely. Ultimately, when critical balances of carbon dioxide and oxygen in the body are close to being disturbed, automatic regulation of breathing resumes. Thus, although the diaphragm looks like voluntary skeletal muscle and is attached to the skeleton, it behaves, for the most part, like involuntary muscle.

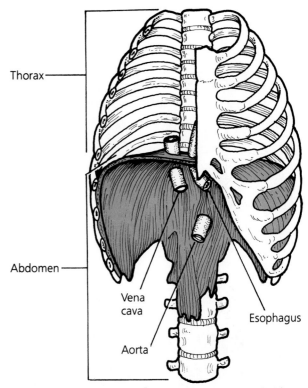

FIGURE 5.7 The dome-shaped diaphragm divides the thorax from the abdomen. It is pierced by the great vessels and the esophagus.

The chest cage can be compared to a bell jar in which the lungs are suspended. The base is the movable diaphragm. The ribs maintain the shape of the chest. The only opening into the chest is the trachea. Air can move only through the trachea, to and from the interior of the lungs, to fill and empty the alveoli (Figure 5.8). When the diaphragm and chest wall muscles contract, the volume that the jar can hold is increased, causing a slight vacuum. Normally, the pressure within the chest cavity is slightly less than atmospheric pressure. Contracting the diaphragm and intercostal muscles enlarges the thorax; intrathoracic pressure declines still further. This respiratory motion (**inspiration** and chest expansion) causes the higher air pressure outside to drive air through the trachea, filling the lungs (Figure 5.8a). When the air pressure outside equals the air pressure inside, air stops moving. Any gas will move from a higher to a lower pressure area until the pressure in each area is equal. When equalization occurs, movement of air ceases and inspiration stops. When the diaphragm and intercostal muscles relax

A. Inhalation and chest expansion

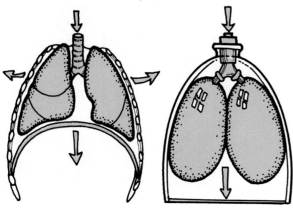

B. Exhalation and chest contraction

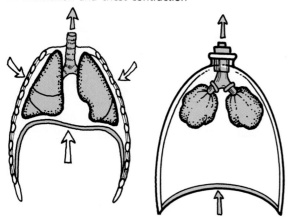

FIGURE 5.8 Inhaling and exhaling can be visualized through the use of a bell jar containing balloons and closed at the end by a diaphragm. (a) When the diaphragm is depressed, pressure in the jar decreases and the balloons fill. (b) When the diaphragm is elevated, pressure increases in the jar and the balloons empty. Movement of the diaphragm causes movement of air in and out of the balloons, as in the lungs.

(**expiration** and chest contraction), pressure inside the thorax becomes higher than that outside, and air is expelled (Figure 5.8b).

The active muscular part of breathing is inspiration. During inspiration (inhaling), the diaphragm and intercostal muscles contract. When the diaphragm contracts, it moves downward and enlarges the thoracic cavity from top to bottom. When the intercostal muscles contract, they raise the ribs. These actions combine to enlarge the chest cavity in all dimensions. Pressure within the cavity falls, and air

rushes into the lungs. Take a deep breath to see how the chest increases in size with inspiration.

During expiration (exhaling), the diaphragm and the intercostal muscles relax. As they relax, all dimensions of the chest cavity decrease. When the volume of the chest cavity decreases, air in the lungs is compressed into a smaller space. Pressure is increased, and air is pushed out through the trachea. The actual decrease in the size of the chest cavity after relaxation is accomplished largely by the action of elastic tissue in the lung which stretches during inhalation and recoils after relaxation of the muscular chest wall. In this situation, the chest wall, because of the pleural surface adhesion, follows the elastic recoil of the lung. There is also an inherent tendency for the chest wall (ribs and muscles) to assume a normal resting position, which aids in exhalation. As opposed to inspiration, expiration does not normally require muscular effort. It represents relaxation of effort and the assumption of a normal resting position.

It is important to remember that there is only one normal opening into the chest cavity. This opening is the trachea. While air may readily pass into the chest cavity if there is any other opening, it will not proceed to the interior of the lung or to the alveoli; rather it comes to lie in the pleural space, compressing the lung.

THE CONTROL OF BREATHING

The brain controls breathing. The center for this control is in the brain stem, one of the best-protected areas of the nervous system. When more oxygen is needed, the brain stem sends stimuli along nerves to muscles of the chest and diaphragm, causing them to work faster and more forcefully. Breathing is largely involuntary, but it can be controlled up to a point. Thus, when you want to hold your breath, you can override automatic impulses from the brain for a short while. Similarly, if you want to breathe more rapidly or more deeply, you can do so for a period of time. The brain, however, is acutely and automatically aware of the levels of oxygen and carbon dioxide in the arterial blood. When these levels change significantly, it responds and regains control of the rate and depth of respiration.

The principal stimulus for respiration is the level of carbon dioxide (CO_2) in the arterial blood. It is normally maintained within very strict limits. Very slight rises in the carbon dioxide level stimulate more rapid breathing; very slight falls depress it. A backup system also exists. The brain is sensitive to diminished arterial oxygen (O_2) as a stimulus to breathe. This oxygen drive is much less sensitive than the quickly responding carbon dioxide drive. If the arterial levels of carbon dioxide or oxygen become abnormal, the brain will automatically control respiration. For these reasons, you cannot hold your breath indefinitely or breathe rapidly and deeply indefinitely. There are direct nervous connections from the brain to the lung and the muscles of respiration through which this control is exerted. Control of respiration by arterial carbon dioxide concentration is so sensitive that normally it is adjusted on a breath-to-breath basis.

YOU ARE THE EMT...

1. Where are the pulmonary capillaries located? What is their function?
2. Everyone knows that you inhale oxygen and exhale carbon dioxide. Why is it, then, that mouth-to-mouth resuscitation can revive a patient when the rescuer is "exhaling" into the patient's lungs?
3. What is pleurisy?
4. The diaphragm is described as a skeletal muscle that acts like an involuntary muscle. What can it do as a voluntary muscle? Why is it described as acting like an involuntary muscle?

6 Basic Life Support: Airway and Ventilation

OVERVIEW

Basic life support is an emergency lifesaving procedure that is carried out without mechanical equipment or aids to treat respiratory arrest, cardiac arrest, or both. It is a method of providing artificial ventilation and circulation. It depends for its effectiveness on prompt recognition of respiratory or cardiac arrest and the immediate start of treatment. The EMT is expected to be able to recognize cardiac or respiratory arrest without difficulty and to institute proper basic life support measures forthwith.

Several methods exist for opening the airway and providing artificial ventilation. Each has specific applications in conscious or unconscious patients, with or without head or spinal injury. Similarly, specific techniques must be used for removing foreign bodies that obstruct the airway. Again, all steps must be carried out as quickly as possible. Time is critical.

Chapter 6 begins with a discussion of basic life support — why it is lifesaving, how it came to be introduced, and the role of the EMT in instituting it. The chapter next describes the methods of opening the airway in adults, providing artificial ventilation in adults, and relieving foreign body obstruction in adults. The last section adapts all of these techniques of basic ventilatory support to infants and children.

OBJECTIVES

The objectives of Chapter 6 are to

- comprehend the need for basic life support, the urgency surrounding its institution, the responsibilities of the EMT in beginning and terminating CPR, and the proper way to position a patient to receive basic life support.
- describe the four techniques for opening the airway in adults.
- learn how to perform mouth-to-mouth, mouth-to-nose, and mouth-to-stoma ventilation in adults and how to relieve gastric distention that sometimes occurs with artificial ventilation.
- learn how to distinguish foreign body obstruction from other conditions that cause respiratory failure and become familiar with the techniques for dislodging foreign objects that are obstructing the airway.
- know how to adapt basic ventilatory support procedures to children and infants.

GENERAL CONSIDERATIONS

Oxygen, present in the atmosphere at a concentration of about 20 percent, is essential for the life of all tissues and cells. The heart develops dangerous arrhythmias (irregular beats) within seconds after being deprived of oxygen. The brain undergoes potentially irreversible damage after the absence of oxygen for as little as 4 to 6 minutes (Figure 6.1).

The delivery of oxygen from the atmosphere to individual body cells of all types requires two necessary actions: breathing and circulation. Breathing means moving air from the atmosphere into and out of the lungs. Oxygen can then pass from the pulmonary alveoli to the capillaries to enrich the blood as it passes through the lungs. At the same time, carbon dioxide, produced by cells in the normal course of metabolism, moves from the blood into the alveoli and is exhaled. The blood, enriched with oxygen, is delivered (circulated) to every part of the body by the pumping action of the heart. Any profound disturbance of the airway, breathing, or circulation can promptly produce disturbed heart function, brain damage, or death.

Basic life support is an emergency lifesaving procedure to treat failure of the respiratory or car-

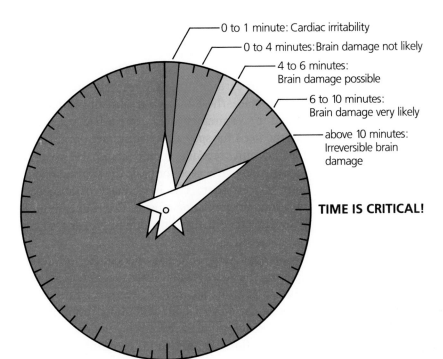

0 to 1 minute: Cardiac irritability

0 to 4 minutes: Brain damage not likely

4 to 6 minutes:
Brain damage possible

6 to 10 minutes:
Brain damage very likely

above 10 minutes:
Irreversible brain
damage

TIME IS CRITICAL!

FIGURE 6.1 Time is critical. If the brain is deprived of oxygen for 4 to 6 minutes, brain damage is likely to occur. After 6 minutes without oxygen, brain damage is extremely likely.

diovascular systems. It is prompt treatment without the use of complex mechanical equipment that must be started as soon as possible after respiratory or cardiac arrest has occurred. The principles of basic life support were introduced in 1960. The specific techniques for life support have been reviewed and revised as necessary at national conferences on **cardiopulmonary resuscitation (CPR)** and **emergency cardiac care (ECC)** held every six years since then. The recommendations are published periodically in the *Journal of the American Medical Association.* The most recent gathering was the "1985 National Conference on Standards and Guidelines for Cardiopulmonary Resuscitation and Emergency Cardiac Care." Recommendations in this text follow those that were adopted at this conference. In many instances significant changes have been introduced since 1980.

One of the most important findings in the evaluation of effectiveness of basic life support measures over the past five years has dealt with EMTs themselves. It has been noted that EMT competence in giving basic life support is good immediately after training. However, it declines rapidly thereafter unless the EMT receives periodic retraining or is required to use the skills frequently. Techniques not regularly used tend to be performed sloppily. The

EMT must understand the urgent need to institute basic life support promptly and the absolute necessity for its being carried out properly. Poorly done, it is useless, of no benefit to the patient, and exhausting to the EMT. Retraining and maintenance of skills are absolutely necessary for effective performance of these lifesaving techniques.

As can be seen in Figure 6.2, prompt basic life support is indicated for:

A   Airway obstruction
B   Breathing (respiratory) arrest
C   Circulatory (cardiac) arrest

Basic life support is not the same as advanced life support, which requires the use of complex equipment and steps in treatment: cardiac monitoring devices, defibrillation, the maintenance of an intravenous line, and the infusion of appropriate drugs. Basic life support, on the other hand, can be provided by one EMT alone or two together, without equipment. It can also be provided by alert and well-trained first responders at the scene. It is the first line of treatment for respiratory or cardiac arrest. The correct application of basic life support can maintain life until the patient recovers sufficiently to be transported to a hospital or until advanced life support can be delivered.

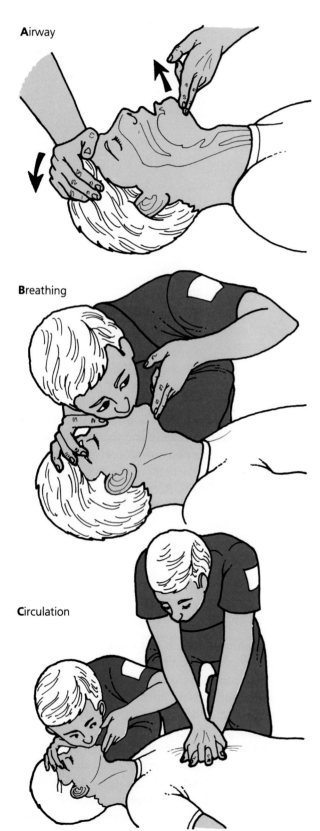

Airway

Breathing

Circulation

FIGURE 6.2 The ABC steps of cardiopulmonary resuscitation: **A**irway, **B**reathing, and **C**irculation are the essential components of basic life support.

Urgency in Instituting CPR

There must be a maximum sense of urgency in instituting basic life support. The outstanding advantage of cardiopulmonary resuscitation is that it permits the earliest possible treatment of airway obstruction, respiratory arrest, or cardiac arrest without the need for specialized equipment or material. Ideally, only seconds should elapse between the recognition of the need for basic life support and the start of treatment. The inadequacy or absence of breathing or circulation must be determined promptly to allow the timely institution of proper resuscitative procedures.

If breathing alone is inadequate or absent, opening the airway with or without **artificial ventilation** may be all that is necessary. Frequently, clearing the airway alone will allow resumption of normal respiration. If there is no evidence of effective heart function, **artificial circulation** must be instituted in combination with artificial ventilation. If breathing ceases before the heart stops, enough oxygen will be available in the lungs to maintain life for several minutes. However, if cardiac arrest occurs first, delivery of oxygenated blood to the heart and brain ceases immediately. Significant cardiac arrhythmias occur seconds after depriving the heart of oxygen, and the heart then fails to pump blood effectively to the brain. Permanent brain damage may occur when it is without oxygen for 4 to 6 minutes. After 6 minutes without oxygen, brain damage is almost certain. Therefore, speed is essential in determining the need for beginning basic life support.

Primary Assessment

Because of the urgent need to start CPR, a prompt primary assessment, as described in Chapter 4, must be performed on all patients. The primary assessment is specifically designed to evaluate the need for CPR: to assess the adequacy of the airway, the quality of breathing, the quality of circulation, and the level of consciousness. The level of consciousness will be a good guide to the extent of basic life support required by the patient. For example, the patient who is alert and oriented will not require cardiopulmonary resuscitation, whereas patients who are not fully conscious frequently do require at least some degree of basic life support. Not all unconscious patients require full cardiopulmonary resuscitation, but virtually all patients who are in need of CPR are unconscious.

In the unconscious patient in need of CPR, the EMT should try to discover the cause of unconsciousness. Specifically, the EMT must determine if the unconscious state was caused by a head or cervical spine injury. In those injury cases, care must be taken during CPR to protect the spinal cord from injury. The presence of a head or spinal injury is not a contraindication to CPR. It simply indicates that basic life support must be carried out within certain specific physical limits.

Beginning and Terminating Basic Life Support

It is the responsibility of the EMT to institute basic life support in virtually all patients who have sustained a cardiopulmonary arrest. Only two exceptions exist to this general rule. First, CPR should not be administered if obvious signs of irreversible death are present. These signs include putrefaction of the body and rigor mortis. Second, CPR is not indicated for certain persons in cardiopulmonary arrest who are known to have been in the terminal stage of an incurable disease. In this situation, CPR serves only to prolong the death of the patient.

In all other circumstances, CPR is given to any individual who has sustained a partial or complete cardiopulmonary arrest. Even if a substantial amount of time has passed since the patient's collapse, it is impossible to know when the last instant of effective perfusion with oxygenated blood occurred. Extrinsic factors, such as the temperature of the environment, or intrinsic factors, such as the hardiness of the individual patient's tissues and organs, may affect the patient's ability to survive. Therefore, CPR should be instituted promptly in virtually all patients who have sustained a partial or complete cardiopulmonary arrest.

When resuscitation is started in the absence of a physician, it must be continued until one of the following events occurs:

1. Effective spontaneous circulation and ventilation are restored.
2. Resuscitation efforts are transferred to another responsible person who takes charge and continues basic life support.

3. A physician assumes responsibility.
4. The EMT is too exhausted to continue the resuscitation efforts.

It is *not* the responsibility of an EMT to terminate CPR unless the individual technician(s) can no longer physically provide the support. In general, this decision to terminate CPR will not have to be made by an EMT since resuscitation should always be continued until the patient's care is transferred to a physician at the emergency department.

Positioning the Patient

For cardiopulmonary resuscitation to be effective, the patient must be horizontal (lying down), supine (face up), and on a firm surface. Even when faultlessly performed, external chest compression will produce no blood flow to the brain if the body is vertical. Optimal airway management and artificial ventilation require that the patient be supine. It is imperative, therefore, to place immediately in a supine position a patient who requires basic life support. If the patient is crumpled up or face down, repositioning will be necessary. Considerable caution is necessary when a neck or back injury is suspected. The patient must be rolled as a single unit, including head, neck, and back. Elevating the lower extremities about 12 inches while keeping the rest of the body horizontal will promote venous blood return and assist artificial circulation if external chest compression is required.

For proper positioning, the EMT kneels beside the patient, but not in bodily contact. The EMT must be sufficiently far away so that when rolled toward the EMT, the patient does not come to rest in the EMT's lap (Figure 6.3a). The EMT then rapidly straightens the patient's legs and moves the nearer arm above the head (Figure 6.3b). Then, he places one of his hands behind the back of the head and neck of the patient and the other on the distant shoulder (Figure 6.3c). The patient can then be turned toward the EMT by pulling on the distant shoulder with the head and neck controlled so that they turn with the rest of the torso as a unit (Figure 6.3d). In this way, the head and neck remain in the same vertical plane as the back. Aggravation of any spinal injury is minimized. When the patient is flat on his or her back, the EMT brings the patient's farther arm back to the side (Figure 6.3e). When it

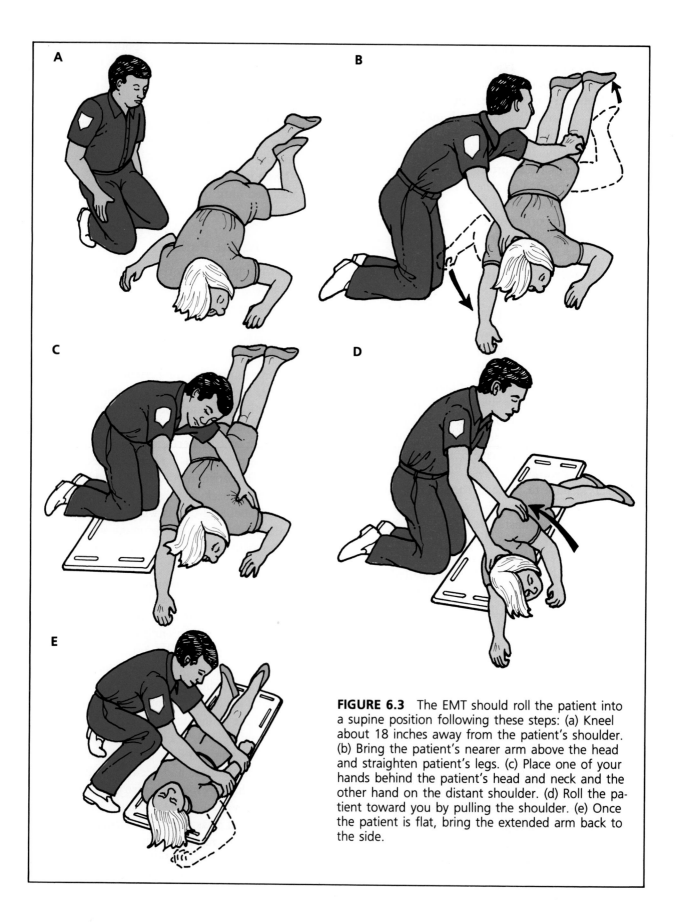

FIGURE 6.3 The EMT should roll the patient into a supine position following these steps: (a) Kneel about 18 inches away from the patient's shoulder. (b) Bring the patient's nearer arm above the head and straighten patient's legs. (c) Place one of your hands behind the patient's head and neck and the other hand on the distant shoulder. (d) Roll the patient toward you by pulling the shoulder. (e) Once the patient is flat, bring the extended arm back to the side.

is possible, the patient should be rolled onto a long spine board, which will provide support during transport and emergency room care. Once the patient is properly positioned, the adequacy of airway, breathing, and circulation should be reassessed and basic life support started if there is any degree of deficiency in these basic functions.

OPENING THE AIRWAY IN ADULTS

Immediate opening of the airway is the most important factor in successful cardiopulmonary resuscitation. Without a patent airway, artificial ventilation will not succeed. Far and away, the most common cause of airway obstruction in the semiconscious or unconscious patient is relaxation of the muscles of the throat and tongue. The airway is obstructed by its own tissues, which tend to fall back into the throat to create the block (Figure 6.4). Dentures, blood clots, vomitus, mucus, food, or other foreign bodies may also cause obstruction. Obstruction of the airway from an aspirated foreign body is discussed later in this chapter. A variety of maneuvers exist to establish a patent airway when it is obstructed by relaxation of the muscles of the throat and tongue.

Head-Tilt / Chin-Lift Maneuver

Opening the airway to relieve an obstruction caused by relaxation of the tongue often can be accomplished easily and quickly by tilting the patient's head backward as far as possible (Figure 6.5). This procedure is known as the **head-tilt maneuver.**

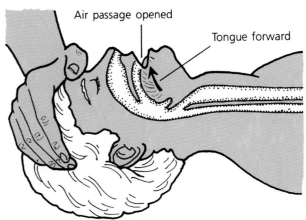

FIGURE 6.5 The head-tilt maneuver. The airway is opened by extending the neck with firm pressure applied to the forehead. The maneuver causes an anterior motion of the tongue to raise it from the posterior pharyngeal wall.

Sometimes this simple maneuver is all that is required to cause the patient to resume breathing spontaneously. For the head tilt to be performed, the patient must by lying supine. Kneeling close to the patient, the EMT places a hand on the patient's forehead and applies firm backward pressure with the palm. This results in movement of the patient's head as far back as possible. This extension of the neck will move the tongue forward, away from the posterior pharynx, clearing the airway. An effective head tilt may be difficult to obtain with only one hand on the forehead. In this instance, the other hand can be used to apply a chin lift. The head tilt is the initial and often the most important general step in opening the airway.

Having achieved the head tilt, the EMT can open the airway further with the **head-tilt/chin-lift maneuver.** EMTs must be familiar with the chin-lift technique and be able to perform it well. The tips of the fingers of the hand not on the forehead are placed under the bony part of the chin. The chin is lifted forward, bringing the entire lower jaw with it, and helping to tilt the head back (Figure 6.6). The fingers must not compress the soft tissue under the chin, thereby obstructing the airway. The forehead hand continues to maintain the backward tilt of the head. The chin should be lifted so that the teeth are nearly brought together; however, the EMT should avoid closing the mouth completely.

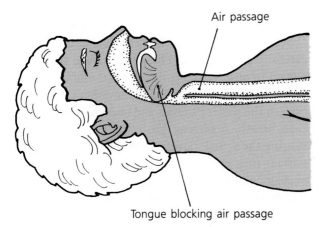

FIGURE 6.4 Muscular relaxation in the unconscious individual may allow the tongue to fall back into the airway and obstruct it.

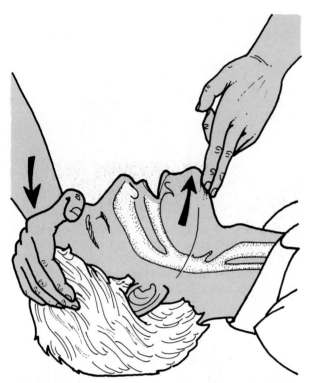

FIGURE 6.6 The head-tilt/chin-lift technique. While the head is tilted backward with one hand, the fingers of the other hand lift the chin forward, as indicated by the arrow.

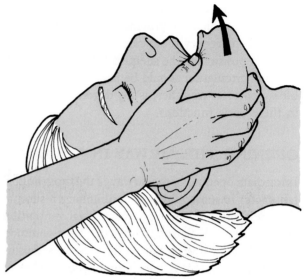

FIGURE 6.7 In the jaw-thrust maneuver, the EMT places the fingers behind the angle of the patient's jaw and forcefully brings it forward.

The jaw thrust is performed best with the EMT kneeling by the patient's head (Figure 6.7). When a cervical spine injury is suspected, this simple maneuver can be modified to keep the head in a neutral position while thrusting the jaw forward and opening the mouth as described.

ARTIFICIAL VENTILATION IN ADULTS

Once the airway has been opened by one of the techniques described above, the patient may start to breathe spontaneously. To assess whether breathing has returned, the EMT places an ear about 1 inch above the nose and mouth of the patient and listens carefully (Figure 6.8). The EMT's head should be turned to observe the patient's chest and abdomen. If the EMT can feel and hear movement of air and can see the patient's chest and abdomen move with each breath, breathing has returned. Feeling and hearing the actual movement of air are far more important than seeing body movements. With airway obstruction, it is possible that there will be no air movement, even though the chest and abdomen rise and fall considerably with the patient's frantic attempts to breathe. In addition, observing chest and abdominal movement often is difficult with a fully clothed patient. Finally, there may be very little or

If the patient has loose dentures, they can be held in position with the chin lift, making obstruction by the lips less likely. If artificial ventilation is needed, a mouth-to-mouth seal is much more easily achieved when dentures are in place. If dentures cannot be managed in place, they should be removed.

Jaw-Thrust Maneuver

The two methods just described are effective for opening the airway in most patients. If not, an additional forward movement of the lower jaw — the **jaw-thrust maneuver** — may be required. The jaw thrust is a triple maneuver in which the EMT places his fingers behind the angles of the patient's lower jaw and then:

1. Forcefully moves the jaw forward;
2. Tilts the head backward without significantly extending the cervical spine;
3. Uses his thumbs to pull the patient's lower lip down, to allow breathing through the mouth as well as the nose.

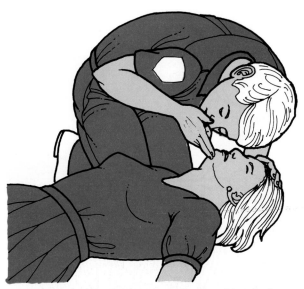

FIGURE 6.8 Respiration is determined by feeling the movement of air on the cheek, by hearing it, and by seeing the chest and abdomen move with each breath.

no perceptible chest movement, even with normal breathing, particularly in some patients with chronic lung disease. Once the EMT is satisfied that there is no movement of air, artificial ventilation must be started promptly.

In respiratory arrest, death results from a lack of oxygen (**anoxia**) combined with the accumulation of an excess of carbon dioxide. These changes cannot be corrected without good ventilation to get rid of carbon dioxide and provide a generous supply of oxygen. Adequate ventilation requires a cycle of inspiration/expiration lasting 1 to 1½ seconds. Ventilations must be given slowly and deliberately, with inspiration taking at least half of each cycle. Ventilation should be given during pauses if cardiac compression is being done simultaneously. Either one ventilation after every 5 compressions (12 per minute) or two after every 15 compressions (8 per minute) are required.

No equipment is needed to give effective artificial ventilation. It should never be delayed to obtain devices for ventilatory assistance. Once the need is identified, rescue breathing should be started immediately and should continue along with efforts to support the circulation and correct cardiac problems. Rescue breathing, whether mouth-to-mouth, mouth-to-nose, or mouth-to-stoma, will deliver exhaled gas

from the rescuer. This gas contains 16 percent oxygen, sufficient to maintain the patient's life.

Mouth-to-Mouth Ventilation

To perform **mouth-to-mouth ventilation,** the EMT opens the airway with the head-tilt/chin-lift maneuver. While the EMT continues to exert pressure on the forehead to maintain the backward tilt of the head, the patient's nostrils are pinched together using the thumb and index finger of this hand (Figure 6.9a). With this technique, the thumb of the hand lifting the chin could be used to depress the lower

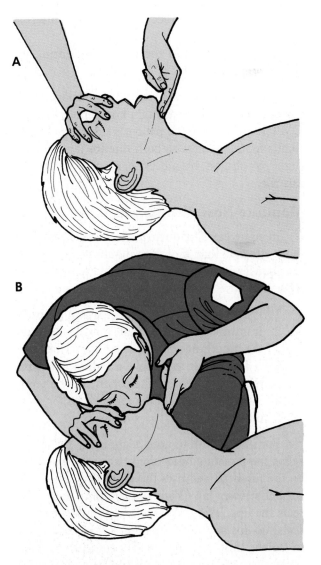

FIGURE 6.9 Mouth-to-mouth ventilation. (a) The EMT seals off the patient's nose, and (b) after encircling the patient's open mouth with his own, exhales deeply into it.

lip to help keep the mouth open during mouth-to-mouth ventilation. The EMT then opens the patient's mouth widely, takes a deep breath, makes a tight seal with his mouth around the patient's mouth, and exhales into it (Figure 6.9b). The EMT then removes his mouth and allows the patient to exhale passively, turning slightly to watch for movement of the patient's chest. Breaths are given slowly in a cycle lasting 1½ seconds for each. Maximum ventilation of the lung is thereby assured.

Adequate ventilation is ensured if with every breath, the EMT:

1. Sees the patient's chest rise and fall.
2. Feels the resistance of the patient's lungs as they expand.
3. Hears and feels the air escape during exhalation.

When giving mouth-to-mouth ventilation and using the jaw thrust to maintain an open airway, the EMT must move to the patient's side, keep the patient's mouth open with both thumbs, and seal the nose by placing his cheek against the patient's nostrils.

Mouth-to-Nose Ventilation

In some cases, **mouth-to-nose ventilation** is more effective than mouth-to-mouth ventilation. It is a good alternative to mouth-to-mouth ventilation. Mouth-to-nose ventilation is recommended when:

1. It is impossible to open the patient's mouth.
2. It is impossible to ventilate a patient through the mouth because of severe facial injuries.
3. It is difficult to achieve a tight seal around the mouth because the patient has no teeth.
4. The EMT prefers the nasal route for some other reason.

For the mouth-to-nose technique, the EMT keeps the patient's head tilted back with one hand on the forehead and uses the other hand to lift the patient's lower jaw (Figure 6.10). This maneuver seals the lips. The EMT then takes a deep breath, seals his lips around the patient's nose, and blows in slowly until the lungs are felt to expand. Then, he removes his mouth and allows the patient to exhale passively. The EMT can see the chest fall when the patient exhales. It may be necessary to open the patient's mouth or separate the patient's lips to allow

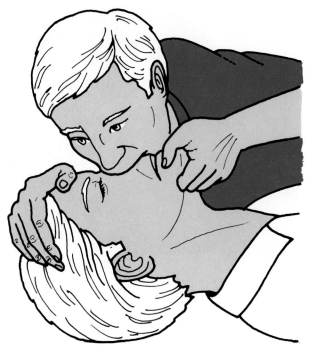

FIGURE 6.10 Mouth-to-nose ventilation using the chin-lift maneuver.

air to escape during exhalation. When using the jaw thrust to maintain the airway, the EMT uses his cheek to seal the patient's mouth and does not use his thumbs to retract the lower lip when giving mouth-to-nose ventilation.

Mouth-to-Stoma Ventilation

Direct **mouth-to-stoma** ventilation must be used for patients who have had surgical removal of the larynx (a **laryngectomy**). These patients have a permanent **tracheal stoma** (an opening in the neck that connects the trachea directly to the skin). It may be seen as an opening at the center, at the front and the base of the neck. In many of these patients, there will be other openings in the neck, according to the type of operation done. Any opening other than the midline tracheal stoma should be ignored. The midline opening is the only one that can be used to put air into the patient's lungs. In general, other neck openings will lie to one side or the other, but not in the midline (Figure 6.11).

Neither head-tilt/chin-lift nor jaw-thrust maneuvers are required for mouth-to-stoma ventilation. If the patient has a tube in the stoma, the EMT should ventilate through the tube. Standard practice

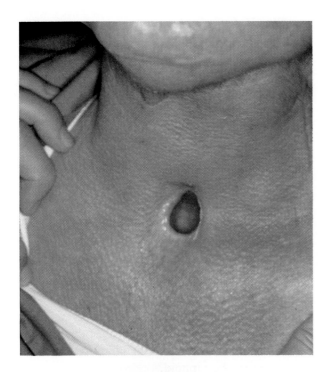

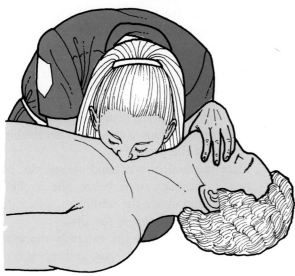

FIGURE 6.11 (top) A tracheal stoma lies in the midline of the neck. (bottom) Mouth-to-stoma ventilation.

is to seal the patient's mouth and nose with one hand to prevent a leak of air up the trachea when ventilating through a tracheal tube or stoma. Release the patient's mouth and nose for exhalation.

Gastric Distention

Artificial ventilation frequently causes distention of the stomach (**gastric distention**). It appears most often in children, but it is also common in adults. It is most likely to appear when excessive pressures are used for ventilation or when the airway is obstructed. Slight gastric distention may be disregarded. Marked inflation of the stomach is dangerous because it causes regurgitation of gastric contents during CPR; the distended stomach can also reduce the lung volume by elevating the diaphragm.

Gastric distention has been found by investigators to occur when high ventilatory pressures are used or when several rapid breaths are administered quickly in succession. Slower periodic ventilations at lower pressures are more likely to produce air that finds its way to the lungs.

Acute, massive gastric distention that interferes with adequate ventilation must be relieved promptly. Frequently, this can be done by exerting moderate pressure on the patient's abdomen between the umbilicus and the rib cage with the flat of the hand. The EMT must be alert to the fact that regurgitation will include air, gastric juice, and food. Pulmonary aspiration of the gastric contents must be prevented during this maneuver. The patient's entire body should be turned to one side, and a suction device should be used promptly to remove any regurgitated material.

FOREIGN BODY AIRWAY OBSTRUCTION IN ADULTS

There can be several causes of airway obstruction: muscular relaxation in an unconscious patient; vomited or regurgitated stomach contents; blood clot, bone fragments, or damaged tissue after an injury; dentures; or foreign bodies. The maneuvers to open the obstructed airway that has been caused by muscle relaxation have been discussed. Loose dentures and large pieces of vomited food, mucus, or blood clots should be swept forward and out of the mouth with the EMT's index finger. Once it becomes available, suctioning should be used to maintain a clear airway. On occasion, a large foreign body will be aspirated and block the upper airway.

Recognition of Foreign Body Obstruction

Sudden airway obstruction by a foreign body in an adult usually occurs during a meal. In a child, it occurs during mealtime or at play (sucking small objects).

Early recognition of airway obstruction is the key to successful management. The EMT must learn to differentiate between primary airway obstruction and other conditions resulting in respiratory failure or arrest, such as fainting, stroke, or acute myocardial infarction.

The EMT may be faced with two situations in which upper airway obstruction is present: The patient may be conscious when discovered, and become unconscious, or the patient may be unconscious when discovered.

Conscious Patient

Sudden upper airway obstruction is usually recognized when the patient who is eating or has just finished eating is suddenly unable to speak or cough, grasps the throat, appears cyanotic, and demonstrates exaggerated efforts to breathe. Air movement is either absent or not detectable. Initially, the patient will remain conscious and be able to indicate quite clearly the nature of the problem. A standard simple question such as "are you choking?" will frequently be answered by the patient nodding "yes." Doubt about the diagnosis is then removed. If the obstruction is not removed in a short period of time, oxygen in the lungs will be used up, and unconsciousness and death will follow.

Unconscious Patient

When a patient is discovered unconscious, the cause is initially unknown. The unconsciousness may have been caused by airway obstruction, cardiac or cardiopulmonary arrest, or a number of other problems. Any patient found unconscious must be managed as a patient with cardiopulmonary arrest. The obstructed airway must be dealt with when discovered. The obstruction should be suspected in the unconscious patient when the standard airway maneuvers and ventilation efforts do not result in effective ventilation of the patient's lungs.

Maneuvers to Relieve Upper Airway Obstruction

Two manual maneuvers are recommended for relieving foreign body airway obstruction: (1) the Heimlich or subdiaphragmatic thrust maneuver (abdominal thrusts), and (2) finger sweeps and manual removal of the object.

The Heimlich Maneuver

The **Heimlich** or **subdiaphragmatic thrust maneuver,** also called the **abdominal thrust maneuver,** is the preferred initial treatment to dislodge an aspirated foreign body in adults and children. Dislodging the object requires that energy be imparted to it to make it move. The subdiaphragmatic or abdominal thrust maneuver imparts the greatest energy for the longest period of time in the proper direction to force the object out of the airway.

A series of six to ten abdominal thrusts is applied until the obstructing body is dislodged. With the patient sitting or standing, the EMT follows these steps:

1. Stand behind the patient, with arms wrapped around the patient's waist.
2. Grasp one fist with the other hand and place the thumb side of the fist against the patient's abdomen, just above the umbilicus and well below the xiphoid.
3. Press your fist into the patient's abdomen with a quick upward thrust (Figure 6.12).
4. Repeat the maneuver 6 to 10 times.

With the patient supine, the EMT must modify the technique as follows:

1. Position the patient supine and kneel close to the patient's hips or straddle either the hips or legs of the patient.
2. Place the heel of one hand against the patient's abdomen well below the xiphoid process and above the umbilicus; place the second hand on top of the first.
3. Press the hand into the patient's abdomen with a quick upward thrust and repeat 6 to 10 times (Figure 6.13).

This maneuver can be accomplished safely in all adults and children with good results. Pregnancy and obesity do not contraindicate its use, however, the chest thrust is recommended for patients in advanced stages of pregnancy, or for the markedly obese.

Manual Removal of a Foreign Body

If at any time the foreign body causing an airway obstruction appears in the mouth, or is believed to be in the mouth, it should be removed cautiously with the EMT's fingers. Abdominal thrusts may dis-

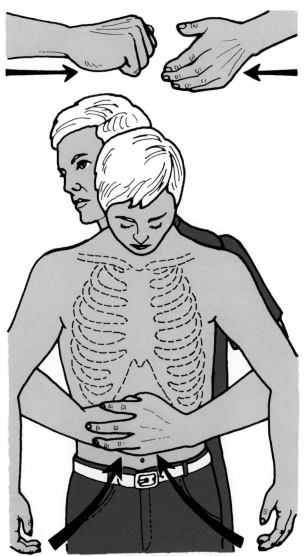

FIGURE 6.12 Proper positioning of the hands for applying abdominal thrusts in an adult who is standing or sitting.

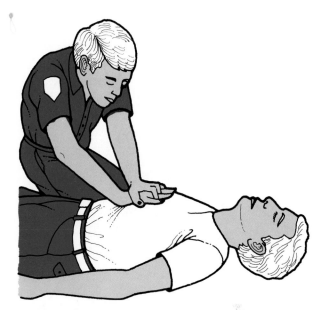

FIGURE 6.13 Proper positioning of the hands for applying abdominal thrusts in the supine patient.

The **tongue-jaw-lift** maneuver for opening the mouth includes these steps:

1. Keep the head in the neutral position.
2. Open the patient's mouth by grasping both the tongue and the lower jaw between your thumb and fingers and lifting them forward (Figure 6.14c). This action will help pull the tongue back away from the throat and away from the foreign body that may be lodged there.

Finger probes to remove foreign bodies include these steps:

1. Hold the patient's mouth open using either the cross-finger or tongue-jaw-lift technique.
2. Use the index finger of your opposite hand as a hook to sweep down inside the patient's cheek to the base of the tongue.
3. Dislodge any impacted foreign body up into the mouth.
4. When the foreign body comes up within reach, grasp it and carefully remove it (Figure 6.14d).

Care should be taken when finger probes are attempted that the dislodged foreign body is not pushed farther back into the airway.

lodge the foreign body but not expel it. The EMT can use either a cross-finger technique or a tongue-jaw lift combined with a finger probe to remove the foreign material.

The **cross-finger technique** for opening the mouth includes these steps:

1. Cross your thumb under your index finger.
2. Brace your thumb and index finger against the patient's lower and upper teeth, respectively (Figure 6.14a).
3. Use your fingers to force the patient's jaws open (Figure 6.14b).

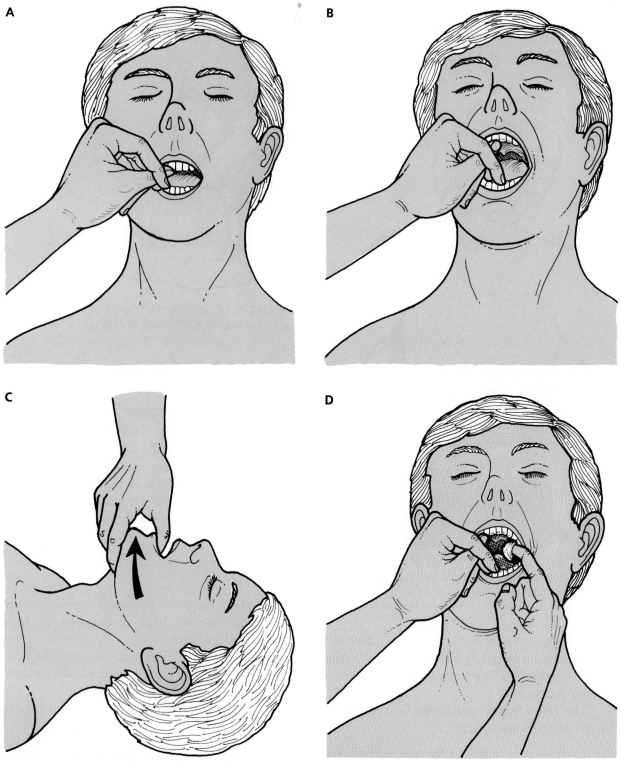

FIGURE 6.14   Manual removal of a foreign body. (a) Using the cross-finger technique, the EMT braces the thumb and index finger on the patient's teeth and (b) forces the jaws apart. (c) Using the tongue-jaw-lift maneuver, the EMT can pull the tongue and jaw to open the mouth and to help visualize the foreign body. (d) A finger probe is used to sweep the foreign body out of the mouth.

Partial Airway Obstruction

On occasion, a partial airway obstruction will be present. The patient will be able to exchange some air but will still have some degree of respiratory distress. Great care must be taken with this patient to prevent a partial airway obstruction from becoming a complete airway obstruction. Abdominal thrusts generally will be ineffective in dislodging the partially obstructing object, and manual manipulation is dangerous because the object could be forced farther down the airway and completely obstruct it. In the case of a partial airway obstruction, the airway maneuvers (head-tilt/chin-lift or jaw-thrust) should be used in order to support the airway in its most efficient position, and supplemental 100 percent oxygen should be administered promptly. The patient should be transported promptly to the hospital for removal of the partially obstructing foreign body.

BASIC VENTILATORY SUPPORT IN INFANTS AND CHILDREN

The basic principles of CPR are the same whether the patient is an infant, child, or adult. The differences in CPR for the infant and child relate to the different underlying causes of emergencies in infants and children and the smaller size of infants and children. In the great majority of instances, full cardiopulmonary arrest in infants and children results from respiratory arrest. In adults cardiac arrest usually occurs first. The causes of respiratory arrest in infants and children are numerous. If uncorrected, respiratory arrest will lead to cardiac arrest and death. Some of the major crises that necessitate resuscitation in infants and children include:

1. Aspiration of foreign bodies into the airway: peanuts, candy, small toys
2. Poisonings and drug overdose
3. Airway infections such as croup and epiglottitis
4. Near drowning
5. Sudden infant death syndrome (SIDS)

For the purposes of CPR, anyone under one year of age is considered an infant. A child is between the ages of one and eight years. Above eight years of age, techniques used for adults can generally be applied. These definitions are to be considered guidelines only. The fact is that variations do occur among infants and children in size relative to age. Small children may well be treated best as infants, and large ones as adults.

Opening the Airway

In children and infants, attention first must be directed by the EMT, or any first responder, to clearing the airway and to proper ventilation. In many instances, opening the airway and adequate rescue breathing are all that is needed for effective resuscitation.

After the primary assessment, the EMT will have established whether the infant or child is unresponsive, is in acute respiratory distress, or is cyanotic. The next step is to secure an open airway. In children (one to eight years of age), the preferred technique is the chin-lift maneuver (Figure 6.15). The head-tilt technique, because of the suppleness of the child's neck, may result in excessive extension of the neck that itself can produce obstruction. In general, it is best to maintain the child's neck in a neutral position and to use the chin lift to open the airway.

The jaw-thrust maneuver without head tilt may be used as an alternative technique to open the child's airway and is the preferred method when neck injury is suspected. It should be performed in the same manner as in an adult.

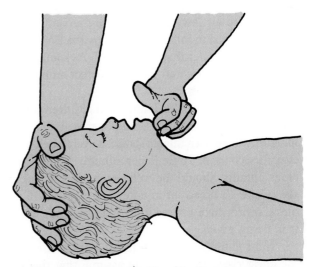

FIGURE 6.15 The chin-lift technique is used to open the airway in the infant or child. The tips of one or more fingers lift the lower jaw forward while the other hand maintains the head in a neutral position.

As soon as the airway is opened, the adequacy of breathing should be assessed. The EMT should place an ear over the patient's mouth and nose and look toward the chest and abdomen. The patient is breathing if the EMT:

1. Sees the chest and abdomen rise and fall.
2. Feels the air move from the mouth and nose.
3. Hears air move during exhalation.

Artificial Ventilation

If the patient is not breathing, or is struggling to breathe, or has cyanosis, rescue breathing must be started. For infants, the preferred technique of artificial ventilation is **mouth-to-nose-and-mouth ventilation.** The EMT must cover both the mouth and the nose with his mouth and make a seal. If the child is large enough so that a tight seal cannot be made over both mouth and nose together, mouth-to-mouth ventilation is performed as in the adult.

Once an airtight seal has been established, two gentle breaths are delivered over 3 to 4 seconds. The initial breaths serve as a means of checking for airway obstruction as well as expanding the lungs. The lungs of a child, and especially an infant, are much smaller than those of an adult. Therefore, the volume of air needed for effective ventilation will be less than in an adult and should be limited to the amount needed to cause the chest to rise. On the other hand, the smaller air passages of the child provide a greater resistance to airflow, and therefore the ventilatory pressure needed to inflate the lungs by the EMT will probably be greater than anticipated. As soon as the chest is seen to rise and fall, the correct amount of force is being used.

Ventilatory rates for infants and children under conditions of resuscitation should be more rapid than for adults. Newborn infants should be ventilated once every 3 seconds or 20 times per minute; children and older infants should be ventilated once every 4 seconds or 15 times per minute. These rates will require appropriate pauses in cardiac compression if it is being given.

If air enters freely with the initial breaths and the chest rises, the EMT can assume that the airway is clear. The EMT can then proceed to check the pulse. If air does not enter freely, the airway must be checked for obstruction. The maneuvers (chin-lift or jaw-thrust) to open the airway should be repeated, and if air still does not enter freely, an obstruction must be suspected. The airway must be cleared.

Gastric Distention

Artificial ventilation can cause stomach distention, especially if high respiratory pressures are used. Massive distention can interfere with artificial ventilation by elevating the diaphragm, decreasing lung volume, and posing a threat of gastric regurgitation. Instances of gastric distention can be minimized by limiting ventilation volumes to the point at which the chest rises. Attempts at relieving gastric distention by pressure on the abdomen should be made when the abdomen is so tense that ventilation is ineffective. Gastric decompression is accomplished by turning the infant's entire body to one side, head down, and applying firm manual pressure to the abdomen. The danger of aspiration of stomach contents into the lungs is such that pressure maneuvers should be done when the EMT is prepared to suction regurgitated material out of the throat promptly.

Foreign Body Airway Obstruction

As has been pointed out, primary airway obstruction is a common problem in infants and children. Airway obstruction is usually caused by a foreign body or an infection, such as croup or epiglottitis, resulting in swelling and narrowing of the airway. The differentiation between a foreign body and an infectious cause is important. With infection, the steps for dislodging a foreign body will not be helpful, can be dangerous, and will cause a delay in transporting the child to the hospital.

The signs of croup or epiglottitis develop in a child who has been ill with a fever, has a barking cough, and develops progressive airway obstruction. The patient should be given oxygen and transported promptly to the hospital. This child will require treatment for the infectious disease causing airway obstruction.

A previously healthy child who, while eating, playing with small toys, or crawling about the house, has sudden difficulty breathing has probably aspirated a foreign body. As in adults, foreign bodies may cause partial or complete airway obstruction. With a partial airway obstruction, air exchange can be either good or poor. With good air exchange, the patient can cough forcefully, although there may be wheezing between coughs. As long as good air exchange continues (the patient can breathe, cough, or talk), the EMT should not interfere with the patient's attempts to expel the foreign body. Oxygen should be given, and the child should be transported promptly to the hospital. The emergency department personnel should be notified of the problem and the expected time of arrival.

Poor air exchange may be present when the child is first seen, or good air exchange may progress to poor air exchange. Poor air exchange is characterized by an ineffective cough, high pitched noises while inhaling, increased respiratory difficulty, and, especially, cyanosis of the nail beds and skin. When

available, oxygen should be given to the patient with poor air exchange. When oxygen is unavailable, or when oxygen administration does not convert poor air exchange into good air exchange, partial obstruction with poor air exchange must be managed as a complete obstruction.

Relief of foreign body obstruction in children is achieved with the use of the Heimlich or subdiaphragmatic thrust maneuver. Six to 10 thrusts should be delivered until the foreign body is expelled. If the foreign body is not expelled, the mouth should be opened, the jaw and tongue lifted forward, and a finger sweep of the mouth performed to remove the object. In the rare instance when the foreign body

FIGURE 6.16 (a) The proper position for delivering back blows to relieve airway obstruction in the infant. (b) After giving four back blows, the EMT should turn the infant over and give four chest compressions.

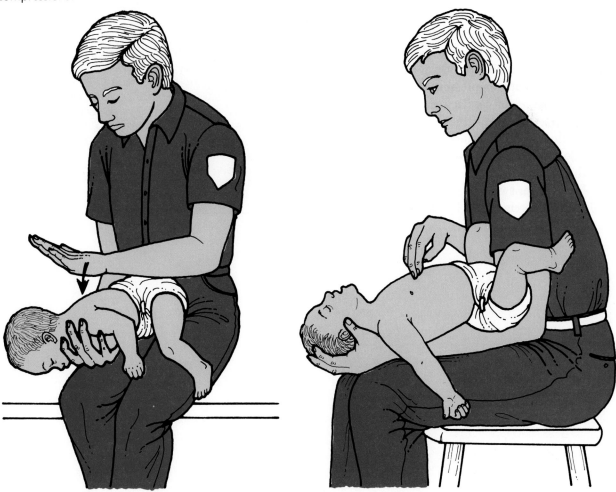

cannot be retrieved, mouth-to-mouth ventilation should be attempted while the patient is transported rapidly to the hospital.

The actual technique for delivering the abdominal thrust may vary with the size of the child. Ordinarily, it will be convenient to administer it with the child supine. In the older child (over eight) the technique with the patient erect may be similar to that for adults.

Some concern exists that the abdominal thrust might injure the liver of an infant. For this reason, the EMT should deliver a series of four quick back blows and then a series of chest thrust maneuvers when clearing the airway of an infant that has become obstructed by a foreign body.

To deliver chest thrusts or back blows to an infant, the EMT should place one hand on the infant's back and neck and the other supporting the chest, jaws, and face. The infant thus is sandwiched between the EMT's hands and arms. While the EMT's arm continues to provide support for the head and neck, the infant is placed with the head lower than the trunk. Four back blows can then be delivered in rapid succession (Figure 6.16a). External chest compressions are subsequently done by turning the child face up and compressing the sternum in the same manner as for cardiac resuscitation except at a slower rate (Figure 6.16b). The EMT must be careful that his hands when surrounding the small child do not compress the upper abdomen and damage the liver.

Blind finger sweeps done prior to attempting to dislodge the foreign body by back blows or thrusts should be avoided in infants and children since the foreign body can easily be pushed farther back in the throat and cause further obstruction. In the unconscious pediatric patient, immediately after the chest or abdominal thrusts, the tongue and the lower jaw are lifted forward and the mouth opened. This maneuver is done by placing the thumb in the patient's mouth, over the tongue, with the fingers wrapped around the lower jaw. If the foreign body is seen, it can be removed with a finger sweep of the other hand.

If the patient has not started breathing after these maneuvers, the airway should again be opened and another attempt made to deliver artificial ventilation. If the chest does not rise, obstruction persists. The above techniques should be repeated in an attempt to relieve the obstruction.

YOU ARE THE EMT...

1. When should you give CPR? When should you *not* give CPR?
2. You have started CPR on an unconscious patient in complete cardiopulmonary arrest. How long should you continue CPR?
3. What is the difference between cardiac arrest and respiratory arrest? Which occurs more frequently in children? Why?
4. You have been called to treat a 2-year-old who is having trouble breathing. The mother thinks her daughter may have choked on a penny. What will you do?

The Circulatory System

OVERVIEW

The circulatory system is what keeps the "human machine" running. It delivers oxygen and nutrients to the brain and to the cells of all of the body tissues. It takes away cellular wastes and carbon dioxide. It works as a closed circuit — that is, blood is continuously pumped by the heart from the left ventricle through the aorta, into the arteries, into the arterioles, into the capillaries, into the venules, into the veins, and back into the heart. It is a long route, but in only one minute the body's entire blood volume of 5 to 6 liters is circulated through all these vessels.

Problems occur whenever something interferes with this complicated circulation system. Illness such as heart attack or stroke or injuries in which vessels are lacerated can be of life-threatening proportions within minutes because the human machine will not run if the blood cannot deliver oxygen and glucose to the brain. In order to administer lifesaving treatment, the EMT must understand how the circulatory system works.

Chapter 7 begins with an explanation of how blood circulates in the body. It then describes the elements that make up the circulatory system. These include blood, the heart, arteries, and veins. The last section is about pulse and blood pressure, both of which relate to how blood is pumped through the circulatory system.

OBJECTIVES

The objectives of Chapter 7 are to

- learn how blood circulates in the body.
- describe the components of the circulatory system — blood, the heart, the arteries, and the veins.
- become familiar with pulse and blood pressure and understand how loss of blood pressure can bring on shock.

HOW BLOOD CIRCULATES

The **circulatory (cardiovascular) system** is a complex arrangement of connected tubes that include arteries, arterioles, capillaries, venules, and veins. At the center of the system, and providing its driving force, is the heart. Blood circulates throughout the entire body under pressure generated by the two sides of the heart. The **systemic circulation,** sometimes called the greater circulation, carries oxygenated blood from the left ventricle of the heart throughout the body and back to the right atrium of the heart. The **pulmonary circulation,** sometimes called the lesser circulation, carries unoxygenated blood from the right ventricle through the lungs and back to the left atrium. In the greater circuit, as blood passes through the tissues and organs it gives up oxygen and nutrients and absorbs cellular wastes and carbon dioxide. In the lesser circuit, as blood passes through the lungs it gives up carbon dioxide and absorbs oxygen.

Oxygenated blood flows out from the left ventricle of the heart through the **aorta** to pass to the body in general (Figure 7.1). It leaves the aorta through **arteries.** The arteries gradually become smaller (**arterioles**) until the blood finally passes into and through small **capillaries.** Capillaries are small thin-walled vessels in which individual red blood cells can make close contact with the individual cells of the body. Blood passes through capillaries into small veins (**venules**), which unite and become larger the closer they get to the heart. **Veins** deliver blood to the right atrium of the heart through the **superior** and **inferior venae cavae** (Figure 7.2). The blood then passes to the right ventricle, where it is pumped to the lungs. The blood passes through the pulmonary capillary system. Then it returns to the left side of the heart to complete the circuit.

The circulatory system is entirely closed, with two sets of capillaries that connect arterioles and venules — one in the lungs and one in the tissues of the rest of the body. No one part of the circulatory system is the most important. The capillaries are the network that delivers the nutrients and oxygen in the blood to the individual tissue cells and picks up cellular waste products. The life of the organism as a whole depends on the life of each cell

within it. **Capillary perfusion** of tissues, the process whereby oxygen and nutrients are brought to every cell and waste and carbon dioxide are removed, is the key to continuous healthy existence.

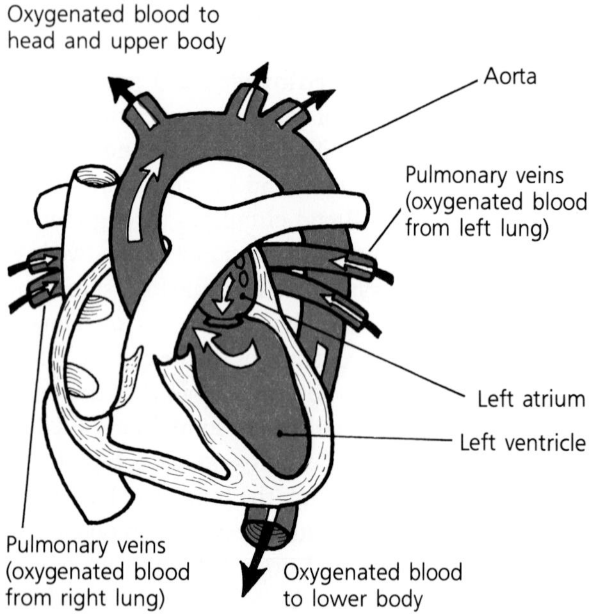

Perfusion must be very clearly understood. It means that blood is entering an organ or tissue through its arteries and leaving through the veins. To do so, it must pass through the appropriate capillary bed and provide tissue nourishment and waste removal. Adequate perfusion means adequate oxygen and nutrition for each cell in the body. It also means adequate removal of waste and carbon dioxide. Perfusion of an organ can fail because of local vessel injury, shock, heart failure, or a number of more complex causes. With inadequate perfusion, cells and tissues die.

COMPONENTS OF THE CIRCULATORY SYSTEM

Blood

Blood is a complex, thick, red fluid composed of **plasma,** red blood cells called **erythrocytes,** white blood cells called **leukocytes,** and **platelets** (Figure 7.3). Plasma is a sticky, yellow fluid that carries the blood cells and nutrients. It also transports cellular waste material to the organs of excretion. It contains most of the compounds needed to produce a blood clot. Red cells give color to the blood and carry oxygen. White cells play a role in the body defense mechanisms against infection. Platelets are tiny, disc-shaped elements that are much smaller than the cells; they are essential in the initial formation of a blood clot, the mechanism that stops bleeding.

Blood under pressure will gush or spurt intermittently from an artery and is bright red. From a vein, it will flow in a steady stream and is dark bluish-red. From capillaries, it will ooze at many tiny individual points. Clotting normally takes from 6 to 10 minutes.

The Heart

The **heart** is a hollow muscular organ approximately the size of an adult's clenched fist. A wall called the **septum** divides the heart down the middle into right and left sides. Each side of the heart is divided again into an upper chamber (**atrium**) and a lower chamber (**ventricle**).

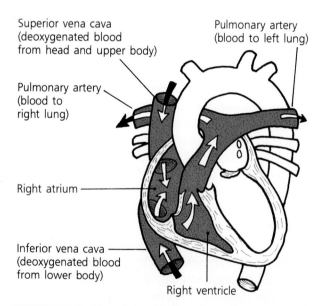

FIGURE 7.1 The left-sided, or higher-pressure, pump of the heart circulates oxygenated blood to all parts of the body.

Oxygenated blood to head and upper body

Aorta

Pulmonary veins (oxygenated blood from left lung)

Left atrium

Left ventricle

Pulmonary veins (oxygenated blood from right lung)

Oxygenated blood to lower body

Superior vena cava (deoxygenated blood from head and upper body)

Pulmonary artery (blood to left lung)

Pulmonary artery (blood to right lung)

Right atrium

Inferior vena cava (deoxygenated blood from lower body)

Right ventricle

FIGURE 7.2 The right-sided, or lower-pressure, pump of the heart circulates blood from the body to the lungs.

normal individual, the heartbeat may range from 50 to 95 beats per minute. A very well conditioned athlete may have a rate of 50 to 55 beats per minute; but this slow beat is not frequently seen. The usual adult heart rate is 60 to 80 beats per minute. At each beat, 70 to 80 milliliters of blood are ejected from the adult heart. In one minute, the entire blood volume of 5 to 6 liters is circulated through all the vessels.

The heart is made of a unique, adapted tissue called **cardiac muscle.** It is actually two pumps of unequal force but equal capacity. It must function

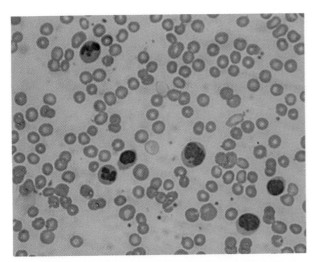

FIGURE 7.3 The microscopic appearance of the three major elements of the blood: red blood cells, white blood cells, and platelets.

The heart works as two paired pumps. The right side of the heart collects blood from the veins of the body. The blood enters through the venae cavae into the right atrium, where the heart pumps it through the pulmonary artery and into the lungs from the right ventricle (Figure 7.2). The left side receives oxygenated blood from the lungs through the pulmonary veins into the left atrium and pumps it through the aorta and arteries to all parts of the body from the left ventricle (Figure 7.1).

The exit of each of the four heart chambers is guarded by a one-way valve. The valves prevent the back flow of blood and keep it moving through the circulatory system in the proper direction. When a valve controlling the filling of a heart chamber is open, the other valve allowing it to empty is shut and vice versa. Normally, blood moves in only one direction through the entire circuit.

When a ventricle (lower chamber) contracts, the valve to the artery opens, and the valve between the ventricle and atrium (upper chamber) closes. Blood is forced from the ventricle out into the artery (pulmonary artery or aorta). At the end of contraction, the ventricle relaxes. The valve to the artery closes, and the valve to the ventricle opens. Blood flows from the atrium to fill the ventricle. When the ventricle is stimulated to contract, the cycle is repeated.

The complete cycle that a blood cell makes in the circulatory system is shown in Figure 7.4. In the

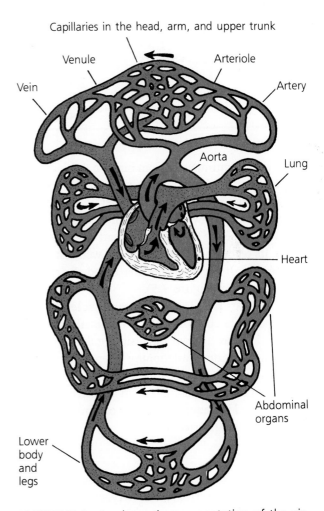

FIGURE 7.4 A schematic representation of the circulatory system, including the heart, arteries, veins, and interconnecting capillaries. The capillaries, the smallest vessels, connect arterioles with venules. In the capillaries an exchange of nutrients and waste products occurs between tissues and blood. In the lung an exchange of gases takes place between blood and air in the alveoli.

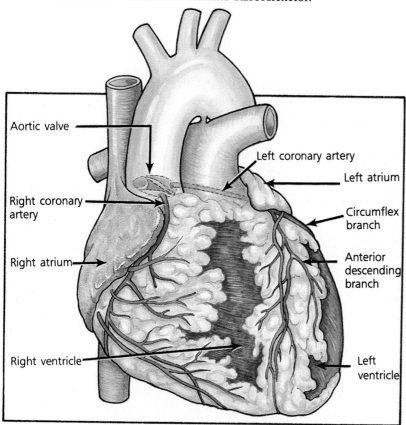

Aortic valve

Right coronary artery

Right atrium

Right ventricle

Left coronary artery

Left atrium

Circumflex branch

Anterior descending branch

Left ventricle

FIGURE 7.5 The coronary arteries are the first branches of the aorta. They provide a rich supply of blood to the cardiac muscle.

as a muscle continuously from birth to death and has developed special adaptations to meet the needs of this continuous function. It can tolerate a serious interruption of its own blood supply for only a very few seconds before the signs of a heart attack develop. Thus, its blood supply is as rich and well distributed as possible. It receives the first blood distribution from the aorta (Figure 7.5).

The heart is an **involuntary muscle.** As such, it is under the control of the **autonomic nervous system.** It has its own intrinsic regulatory system and will continue functioning even if its central nervous system control is lost. It is distinct from skeletal or smooth muscle both in its microscopic appearance and its requirement for a continuous supply of oxygen and nutrients.

The Arteries

The aorta is the major artery leaving the left side of the heart. It carries freshly oxygenated blood to the body. This blood vessel is found just in front of the spine in the chest and abdominal cavities. The aorta has many branches that supply the heart, head, neck, arms, and abdominal and thoracic organs before it ends in the lower abdomen. It divides at the level of the umbilicus into the two common **iliac arteries** that lead to the lower extremities (Figure

7.6a). Each of these arteries divides into smaller and smaller arterioles, finally forming the thin-walled tiny capillaries.

In the body there are billions of cells and billions of capillaries. Capillary vessels are fine end divisions of the arterial system that allow contact between cells of the body tissues and the red blood cells. At this level, each individual cell of the body lives. Oxygen and other nutrients pass from blood cells and plasma in the capillaries to the individual tissue cells through the very thin wall of the capillary (Figure 7.7a). Carbon dioxide and other metabolic waste products pass in a reverse direction from the tissue cells to the blood to be carried away. Blood in arteries is characteristically bright red because it is rich in oxygen. Blood in the veins is dark bluish red, since it has passed through a capillary bed and given up its oxygen to the tissues. Capillaries connect directly at one end with the arterioles and at the other with the venules.

The Veins

Blood from the capillary system returns to the heart through the veins. Capillaries form small venules that join to form the larger veins. The veins of the entire body ultimately join to form two major vessels, the superior vena cava and inferior vena cava (Figure 7.6b). Blood returning from the head, neck,

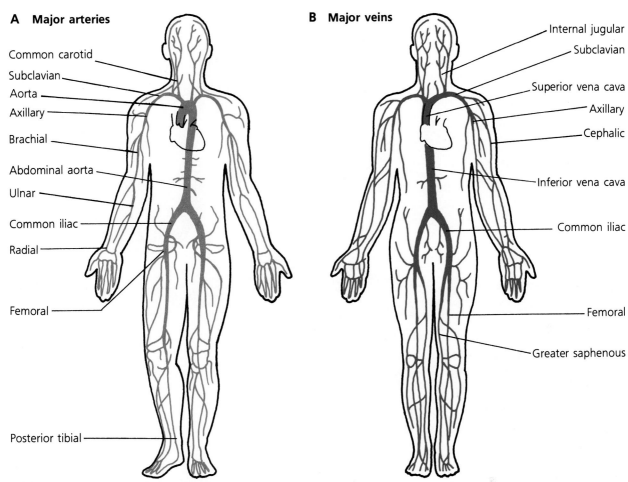

A   Major arteries

Common carotid
Subclavian
Aorta
Axillary
Brachial
Abdominal aorta
Ulnar
Common iliac
Radial
Femoral
Posterior tibial

B   Major veins

Internal jugular
Subclavian
Superior vena cava
Axillary
Cephalic
Inferior vena cava
Common iliac
Femoral
Greater saphenous

FIGURE 7.6   (a) The major named arteries of the body distribute oxygenated blood from the heart to the principal organs or regions of the body. The name of each artery corresponds to the organ or region served. (b) The major veins are named to correspond to the regions of the body they drain. Blood is returned by these veins to the heart, which pumps it through the lungs for oxygenation.

shoulders, and upper extremities passes through the superior vena cava. Blood from the abdomen, pelvis, and lower extremities passes through the inferior vena cava. The superior and inferior venae cavae join to form the right atrium of the heart. The right ventricle receives blood from the right atrium and pumps it into the lungs through the pulmonary arteries.

Circulation in the Lungs

The general plan of circulation through the lungs is essentially the same as that in the rest of the body. Blood vessels from the right side of the heart branch and rebranch, finally forming capillaries. The **pulmonary capillaries** lie close to the **alveoli** (air sacs) of the lungs. The exchange of oxygen and carbon dioxide between air in the lung and blood in the capillaries is rapid (Figure 7.7b). The oxygenated blood from the lungs enters the four **pulmonary veins** that unite to form the left atrium. It then passes to the left ventricle and is pumped to the body again.

PULSE AND BLOOD PRESSURE

The Pulse

The **pulse,** which is palpated most easily at the neck, wrist, or groin, is created by the forceful pumping of blood out the left ventricle and into the major arteries. It is present throughout the entire arterial system. It can be felt most easily where the larger

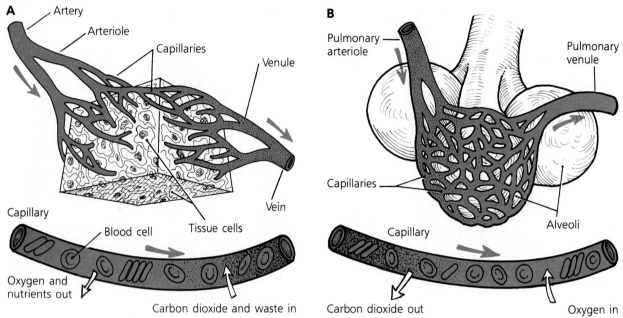

FIGURE 7.7 The exchange of oxygen and carbon dioxide between blood in vessels and tissue cells. The capillary is no larger than a single blood cell. (a) Oxygen (O_2) passes from the blood through capillaries to tissue cells. In the reverse process, carbon dioxide (CO_2) passes from tissue cells through capillaries to the blood. (b) In the lung, O_2 is picked up by the blood and CO_2 is given off.

arteries are near the skin. The **carotid artery pulse** can be felt at the upper portion of the neck; the **radial artery pulse** is felt at the wrist, just at the base of the thumb; the **femoral artery pulse** is felt in the groin. (Pulse points are discussed in Chapter 3.) The normal pulse can range from 50 to 95 beats per minute. The average adult pulse is 60 to 80 beats per minute, and in infants and children, it is a bit higher, at 80 to 100 beats per minute.

Blood Pressure

Blood pressure is the pressure that the blood exerts against the walls of the arteries as it passes through them. When the cardiac muscle of the left ventricle contracts, it pumps blood from the ventricle into the aorta. This muscular contraction is called **systole.** When the muscle of the ventricle relaxes, the ventricle fills with blood. This phase is called **diastole.** The intermittent forceful ejection of blood from the left ventricle of the heart into the aorta is transmitted through the arteries as a repeated pressure wave. This pressure wave keeps the blood moving through the body. The high and low points of

the wave can be measured with a **sphygmomanometer** (blood pressure cuff) and expressed numerically in millimeters of mercury (mm Hg). The high point is called the **systolic blood pressure** (the heart muscle is contracting). The low point is called the **diastolic blood pressure** (the heart muscle is relaxed).

Normal adult arterial blood pressure is usually 120/80 mm Hg. In infants and children it is less. Normal blood pressure in children is 90/60 mm Hg; in infants it is 70 to 80/50 mm Hg. Because diastolic pressure is the level to which arteries are subjected constantly, it is regarded as very important in patients with hypertension. Sustained high diastolic blood pressure is more dangerous for patients than an intermittent high systolic reading.

Both the wave and the flow of blood can be stopped by applying pressure on an artery. Applied pressure must exceed the pressure of the blood that flows through the artery. Several factors control **arterial pressure.** They include the blood volume itself, the state of the arteries and arterioles (whether they are dilated or constricted), the capacity of the

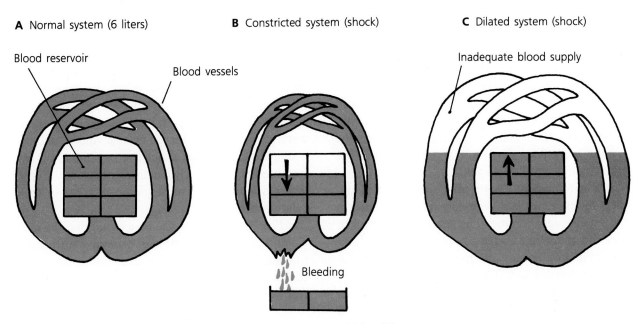

A Normal system (6 liters)   **B** Constricted system (shock)   **C** Dilated system (shock)

Blood reservoir

Blood vessels

Inadequate blood supply

Bleeding

FIGURE 7.8 A schematic representation of the volume of blood in the body under varying circumstances. (a) The normal blood volume in an adult is 6 liters. (b) When bleeding occurs, the blood volume in the veins and arteries decreases, and the blood vessels constrict. If severe bleeding causes the volume of blood in circulation to be reduced rapidly, the patient may go into shock. (c) If the walls of the blood vessels become relaxed, the peripheral vascular system enlarges to hold more blood, thereby reducing the amount of blood in circulation as effectively as if bleeding to the outside of the body had occurred. It is possible, therefore, for shock to be produced in a patient without any loss of blood from the body.

heart muscle to contract normally, and the normal elasticity of the arteries.

Pressure of blood in the veins (**venous pressure**) is much less than that in the arteries. This low pressure aids in the return of blood to the heart. If the venous pressure falls below normal, insufficient blood is returned to the heart, and a failure in the circulatory system occurs. Normal venous pressure is expressed in centimeters of water and not millimeters of mercury since it usually is measured differently. The normal venous pressure is 8 to 15 cm of water. The two values, centimeters of water and millimeters of mercury, are almost equivalent. They can be closely related by multiplying the reading in mm Hg by 1.3 to approximate the value in centimeters of water. Two factors control the venous pressure: **blood volume** (the amount of blood within the circulatory system) and the capacity of the veins (**vascular volume**).

The average adult has approximately 6 liters of blood in the system. Children have less — 2 to 3 liters depending on their age and size; infants have only about 300 milliliters. The loss of an amount of blood that may be negligible for an adult could be fatal for a baby.

In all healthy people, the circulatory system is automatically adjusted and readjusted constantly so that 100 percent of the capacity of the arteries, veins, and capillaries holds just 100 percent of the blood at that moment. Never are all the vessels fully dilated or constricted (Figure 7.8). The size of arteries and veins is controlled by the nervous system, according to the amount of blood available and many other factors to keep blood pressure normal at all times. Under the condition of normal pressure, with a system that can hold just 100 percent of the blood available, all parts of the system will be perfused all of the time.

Loss of normal blood pressure is an indication that the blood can no longer circulate efficiently to every organ in the body. There are many reasons for loss of blood pressure. The end result in each case is the same: organs, tissues, and cells are no longer adequately perfused or supplied with oxygen and food, and wastes can accumulate. Under these conditions, cells, tissues, and whole organs may die. The state of inadequate perfusion, when it involves the entire body, is called **shock.**

When a patient loses a small amount of blood, the arteries, veins, and heart automatically adjust to the smaller new volume. The adjustment occurs in an effort to maintain adequate pressure throughout the circulatory system and thereby maintain circulation for every organ. The adjustment occurs very rapidly after the loss, actually within minutes. Specifically, the vessels contract to provide a smaller bed for the reduced volume of blood to fill. And the heart pumps more rapidly to circulate the remaining blood more efficiently. The reciprocal relationship of pulse and blood pressure (as the latter declines, the pulse rises to compensate) is almost always seen as shock develops. If the loss of blood is too great, the adjustment fails and the patient goes into shock.

The change in the size of arteries and veins is brought about by muscles in their walls. These muscles can contract or relax in response to changes in blood volume, heat, cold, fright, an injury, or an infection. The contraction or relaxation of the muscle causes a change in the diameter of the artery or vein. These muscles do not act as pumps; they only change the diameter of the vessels and hence their

volume. A normal process of continuous adjustment is maintained by the autonomic nervous system. If the muscles of the arteries and veins contract, the vessel diameters decrease; the system therefore holds less fluid. If these muscles relax, then the vessels dilate and the system can hold a larger volume of blood. Massive dilation of the vessels can produce a system far too large for the normal volume of blood available. Once again, shock occurs, and all organs, because they are poorly perfused, are at risk. Figure 7.8 is a schematic representation of some of these relationships.

Finally, shock can also be a signal that the muscle of the heart is incapable of pumping sufficiently to maintain circulation. This condition is seen in the patient with a **myocardial infarction** (heart attack) from direct damage of the muscle itself.

YOU ARE THE EMT...

1. Where does the systemic circulation carry oxygenated blood? Where does the pulmonary circulation carry blood? Does the pulmonary circulation carry oxygenated or unoxygenated blood?
2. What is capillary perfusion? Why is it so important?
3. What is the difference between venous pressure and arterial pressure? What two factors control venous pressure?
4. Does shock occur when the arteries and veins contract or relax? Explain.

Basic Life Support: Artificial Circulation

8

OVERVIEW

The patient is in cardiac arrest. Time is critical. Only minutes separate life and death. Before CPR training was offered in schools and communities, death usually won out. Now, however, more and more people know how to perform cardiopulmonary resuscitation and take advantage of those few life-and-death minutes. Thus the EMT is apt to arrive at the scene and find someone has already begun CPR on a cardiac arrest patient. The EMT must then evaluate the patient, assess the technique, and assist the rescuer, without ever interrupting the stride. Or, the EMT may arrive and discover there is no assistance available. In this situation, the EMT must use the few precious minutes that are available to institute one-rescuer CPR. In any cardiac arrest emergency, the EMT's role is critical.

Chapter 8 begins by defining cardiac arrest and naming its major causes. The chapter next focuses on the techniques of providing artificial circulation to adults, including external chest compression with a single rescuer, with the entry of a second rescuer, and with two rescuers. The last section describes the modifications necessary when artificial circulation is administered to infants and children.

OBJECTIVES

The objectives of Chapter 8 are to

- define cardiac arrest and identify its causes.
- become knowledgeable in the techniques of administering artificial circulation to adults.
- recognize the adjustments that have to be made when providing artificial circulation to children or infants.

CARDIAC ARREST

Cardiac arrest means the failure of the heart to generate an effective and perceptible blood flow. In cardiac arrest, pulses are not palpable, even in the major vessels (the carotid and femoral arteries). Effective blood flow is nonexistent. Cardiac arrest does not mean that the heart is without any muscular or electrical activity. Indeed, the heart can consume a great deal of energy during cardiac arrest and demonstrate much muscular activity. However, uncoordinated or excessively rapid beating does not produce effective blood flow. Indeed, in situations in which muscular activity remains but is uncoordinated and produces no blood flow, the heart continues to consume energy while cut off from perfusion itself. The consumption of energy will ultimately cause more damage to the heart tissue, in part because of the accumulation of waste products. The four major causes of cardiac arrest are asystole, ventricular fibrillation, ventricular tachycardia, and electromechanical dissociation.

In **asystole,** the heart is essentially without any electric or muscular activity. It is not beating. No pulses are felt. There is no electrical activity to record on an electrocardiogram. This stage is the end point to which all other cardiac arrest states come.

In **ventricular fibrillation,** the major pumping chambers of the heart undergo continuous, uncoordinated muscular quivering (**fibrillation**). This is the most common **arrhythmia** (abnormal heart rhythm) causing cardiac arrest. No effective blood flow comes out of the heart because the ventricles do not contract. This state may come about because of loss of blood supply to the heart muscle, a result of coronary artery disease. Since the heart itself is not perfused, no oxygen and nutrients reach it to support the muscular activity. In the absence of oxygen, the muscle contractions rapidly deplete the heart of its own energy stores and produce waste products that further damage the heart muscle.

Ventricular tachycardia (rapid heart rate) is another type of arrhythmia in which the heart beats so fast that there is not enough time for the pumping chambers to fill adequately between beats. When tachycardia persists, effective body perfusion declines. The heart itself becomes more **ischemic** (lacking oxygen), and ventricular fibrillation can rapidly ensue. In ventricular tachycardia, the EKG tracing shows recognizable waves. They disappear as this arrhythmia degenerates further into fibrillation.

Electromechanical dissociation is that form of cardiac arrest in which the **electrocardiogram (ECG or EKG)** displays an apparently adequate heart rate and rhythm, but the heart is incapable of generating a palpable pulse and blood pressure in the circulation. The heart rate may be slow or fast, depending on the underlying cause of this form of cardiac arrest. Electromechanical dissociation can be caused by a variety of disorders: massive blood loss, cardiac tamponade, tension pneumothorax, acute pulmonary embolism, anaphylactic shock, or a severe heart attack. Obviously, in these situations it is necessary to identify the most likely cause of the electromechanical dissociation and proceed rapidly with attempts to correct it. Meanwhile, since the heart is not beating effectively, it is necessary to institute **cardiopulmonary resuscitation (CPR).**

The conditions leading to electromechanical dissociation often progress rapidly. They must be treated promptly to avoid this outcome. Dissociation itself can develop rapidly. These considerations underscore the need for prompt treatment of the underlying cause and for *absolutely prompt* restoration of circulation. Rapid CPR is mandatory to restore adequate perfusion and oxygenation of the heart so that it can continue to function while proper definitive care is directed at the cause of the arrest.

ARTIFICIAL CIRCULATION IN ADULTS

Disturbances of the regular electrical rhythm and activity of the heart may prevent adequate cardiac muscular contraction and result in the failure of the heart to generate blood flow and produce a pulse. Any significant damage of the heart muscle itself from acute myocardial infarction or various muscle diseases may render the heart unable to contract properly. The absence of a strong, palpable central pulse, such as the carotid or femoral, indicates no blood flow and hence the presence of cardiac arrest.

Assessment of Circulation

Unconsciousness almost always exists in cardiac arrest states since the brain is not being properly perfused. Loss of consciousness may take some time to develop after respiratory arrest or airway obstruction. After determining the patient's level of consciousness, turning the patient if necessary, noting the patient's respiratory status, opening the airway, and starting artificial ventilation, if needed, the EMT must assess the circulation. Cardiac arrest is determined by the absence of a palpable pulse in a large artery, such as the carotid. The carotid artery is close to the heart, large, and readily palpable in the neck. It is found most easily by locating the larynx at the front of the neck and then sliding two fingers toward one side. The pulse is felt in the groove between the larynx and the sternocleidomastoid muscle, with the pulp of the index and long fingers held side by side (Figure 8.1). Light pressure is sufficient to palpate the pulse.

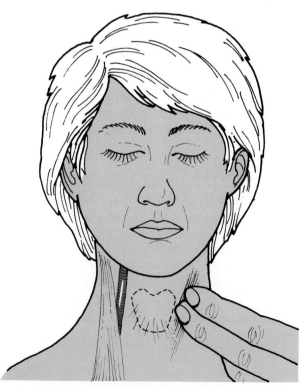

FIGURE 8.1   The carotid pulse is felt in the groove between the larynx and the sternocleidomastoid muscle.

Excessive pressure must not be applied because it can obstruct the carotid circulation, dislodge blood clots, or produce marked reflex slowing of heart activity.

Another conveniently felt large artery near the skin is the femoral artery in the groin. When pulses are not palpable, the EMT can confirm the absence of heart activity by listening over the left chest using an ear or the stethoscope.

If the patient has been positioned for artificial ventilation, the hand on the forehead that has been maintaining backward head tilt can be left in position to maintain the airway. The other hand can be used for locating the carotid pulse. If the pulse is present but breathing is absent, the EMT should ventilate the patient twice for 1 to 1½ seconds each breath. Then the patient should be ventilated once every 5 seconds slowly and fully until adequate breathing resumes. If the pulse is absent, the EMT should ventilate the patient twice and start **external chest compression,** which adds artificial circulation to the already initiated artificial ventilation.

External Chest Compression

The heart lies slightly to the left of the middle of the chest between the sternum and the spine (Figure 8.2). Rhythmic pressure and relaxation applied to the lower half of the sternum will compress the heart between it and the spine and produce an artificial circulation.

In any patient with cardiac arrest, the carotid artery flow resulting from external chest compression, even flawlessly performed, is only about one-quarter to one-third that of the normal volume. For this volume to be achieved, the patient must be on a firm, flat surface. It may be the ground, the floor, or a spine board on an ambulance litter. The patient who is in bed must be placed rapidly on the floor. This step is quicker than looking for some type of firm support and minimizes the delay in starting cardiac compression. External chest compression is always accompanied by artificial ventilation.

With a Single Rescuer

If working alone, the EMT first positions the patient properly. Then the EMT kneels close to the patient's side, with one knee at the level of the head and the other at the level of the upper chest. The heel of one hand should be placed on the lower half

of the body of the sternum. Great care must be taken *not* to place the hand on either the xiphoid process, which extends downward over the upper abdomen, or beside the sternum onto the ribs or costal cartilages (Figure 8.3).

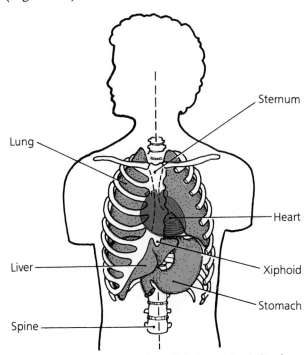

FIGURE 8.2 The heart lies slightly to the left of the middle of the chest, between the sternum and the spine, with the lungs on either side and with the liver and stomach below.

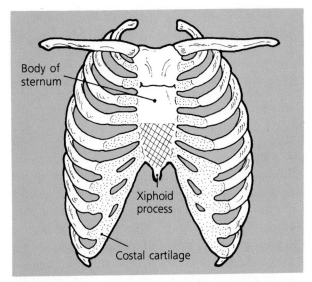

FIGURE 8.3 The xiphoid process is at the lower tip of the sternum and extends downward over the upper abdomen. The shaded area of the sternum is compressed.

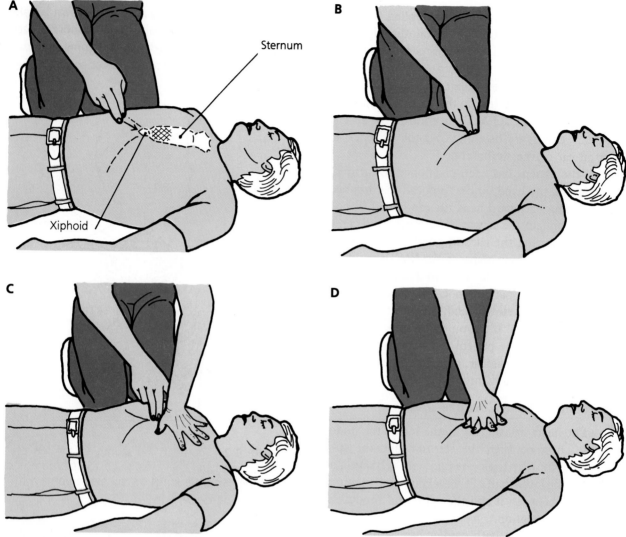

FIGURE 8.4 The correct hand position for chest compression: (a) Slide your index finger and your long fingers nearest the patient's feet along the center of the patient's rib cage to the notch in the center of the chest. (b) Push the long finger high into the notch, and lay the index finger on the lower portion of the sternum. (c) Then place the heel of the second hand on the lower half of the sternum, touching the index finger of your first hand. (d) Remove your first hand from the notch and place it over and parallel to the hand on the sternum.

Correct positioning of the hands is achieved by sliding the index and long fingers of the hand nearer the patient's feet along the edge of the rib cage until they reach the xiphoid notch in the center of the chest (Figure 8.4a). The long finger is pushed as high as possible into the notch, and the index finger is then laid on the lower portion of the sternum with the two fingers touching (Figure 8.4b). The heel of the other hand is then placed on the lower half of the sternum (Figure 8.4c) so that it touches the index finger of the first hand. The first hand is then re-moved from the notch in the center of the rib cage and applied over and parallel to the hand now resting on the patient's lower sternum (Figure 8.4d). *Only the heel of one hand is in contact with the lower half of the sternum.* The technique may be improved or made more comfortable for the EMT if the fingers of the lower hand are interlocked with the fingers of the upper hand and pulled slightly away from the chest wall.

Pressure is exerted vertically downward through both arms to depress the adult sternum 1½ to 2 inches. A rocking motion by the EMT, rising gently upward, allows pressure to be delivered vertically down from the shoulders while the elbows are kept straight (Figure 8.5). Vertical downward pressure produces a compression that must be followed immediately by a period of relaxation. The time spent in compression is a crucial factor in determining blood flow. At least 50 percent of the compression-relaxation cycle must be spent in compression.

The actual motions must be smooth, rhythmic, and uninterrupted. Short, jabbing compression strokes are absolutely ineffective in producing artificial blood flow. The heel of the EMT's hand should not be removed from the chest during relaxation, but pressure on the sternum must be com-

pletely released so it can return to its normal resting position between compressions. Compression and relaxation must be rhythmic. The EMT's hand must not bounce or come away from the patient's chest during compression (Figure 8.6). Considerable attention must be given to the actual technique of compression since, even well done, it carries some risk. Complications of cardiac compression have included fractured ribs, lacerated liver, ruptured spleen, or fracture of the sternum. While they cannot be entirely avoided, their occurrence can be minimized with a good, smooth technique.

When alone, the EMT must pause to give artificial ventilation. Then cardiac compressions must be resumed at a rate of 80 to 100 per minute. After every 15 cardiac compressions, the EMT delivers 2 ventilations (ratio 15:2). The 15 compressions are delivered in 10 to 11 seconds. Two full ventilations are delivered in the next 4 to 5 seconds using at least 1½ seconds for inspiration.

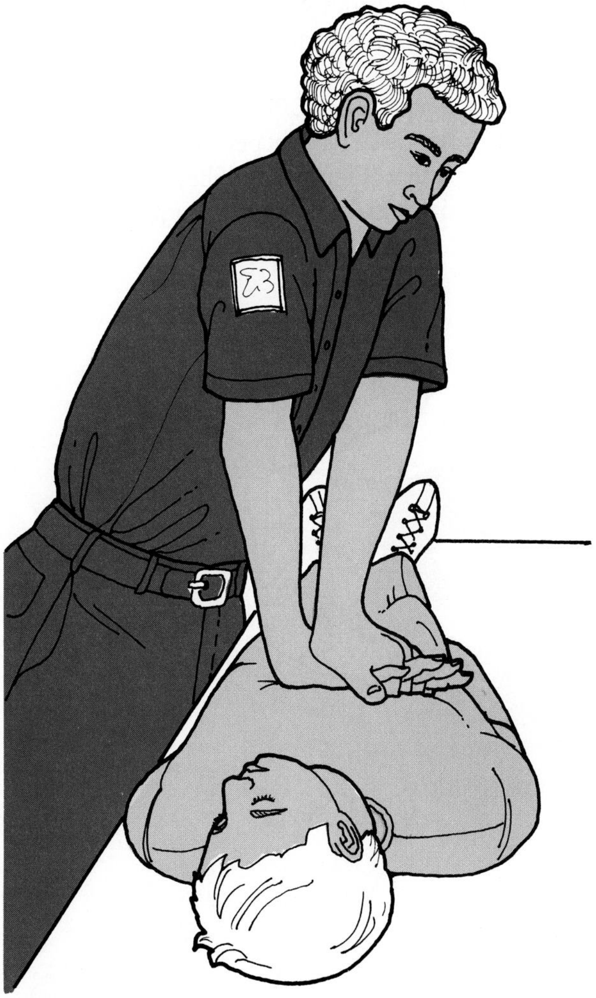

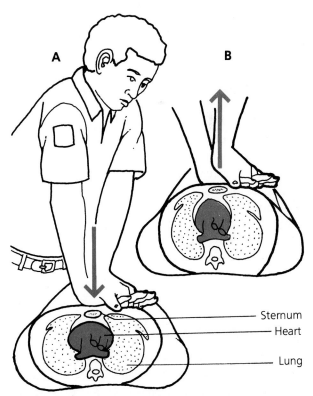

FIGURE 8.5 External chest compression is produced by vertical downward pressure through both extended arms to depress the adult sternum 1½ to 2 inches.

FIGURE 8.6 (a) Compression and relaxation should be rhythmic and of equal duration. The heel of the hand should not be removed from the sternum. (b) Pressure on the sternum must be released so it can return to its normal resting position between compressions.

With Entry of a Second Rescuer

When the second EMT becomes available after single-EMT CPR has been started and is in progress, the recommended procedure for entry into the resuscitation is simple. Without stopping CPR, the original EMT announces clearly that everything is ready for a switch to two-EMT CPR. The logical point of entrance is after a sequence of 15 compressions and 2 breaths. The new EMT should kneel down on the side of the patient opposite to the original EMT, in position to perform artificial ventilation. First, the new EMT should check the patient's pulse to make sure that the first EMT has correctly diagnosed the patient's condition and that the first EMT's efforts at artificial circulation are effective. If cardiac compressions are adequate, a carotid pulse should be palpable after each compression; if no pulse is felt, the compressor's technique should be evaluated. If a pulse is felt with each compression, the new EMT should say "Stop compression." The original EMT should stop compressing for 5 seconds so the second EMT can check for a spontaneous pulse. If none is found, two-EMT CPR is started.

Immediately after confirming the absence of a pulse, the second EMT should open the airway and deliver two breaths. The entire process, from the moment the new EMT arrives to the point when the breaths are delivered, should be done within 10 seconds to ensure that effective CPR continues. As soon as these first two breaths are delivered, CPR continues, with one breath being delivered after every 5 compressions. For artificial ventilation to be delivered effectively, a pause of 1 to 1½ seconds after every 5 cardiac compressions is required. Therefore, the compression rate must be at least 80 to 100 per minute.

With Two Rescuers

All professional rescuers (rescue squad members, EMTs, medical and paramedical professionals) should be proficient in both one- and two-rescuer techniques. Two-rescuer CPR provides an opportunity for a coordinated effort that is less fatiguing and more effective. The two-rescuer technique allows better treatment of the patient and should be used whenever possible.

When two EMTs arrive to treat one patient, both must act promptly. One rescuer goes to the head of the patient and performs a primary survey, while the second EMT gets in position to give chest compression. The EMT at the head checks for absence of breathing and pulse. If both are absent, he gives two breaths and CPR begins.

Two-EMT CPR should be performed with the EMTs on opposite sides of the patient (Figure 8.7). They can then switch positions when necessary without significant interruption in the ventilation-compression sequence. To switch, the EMT who is providing ventilation, after giving a breath, moves into position to begin cardiac compression. The EMT performing compression, after the fifth compression, moves to the patient's head and checks the pulse for 5 seconds but no longer. If no pulse is felt, the EMT at the head ventilates the patient twice and says, "Continue CPR."

When performing CPR on a litter in an ambulance, both EMTs must perform from the same side of the patient (Figure 8.8). They can then switch positions using the following technique. The EMT

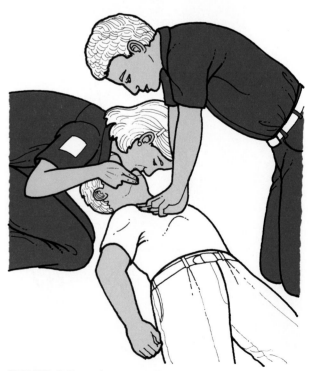

FIGURE 8.7 When two EMTs perform CPR, one is on each side of the patient. Here, one EMT performs mouth-to-mouth ventilation while the other delivers external chest compression.

ventilating the patient rapidly moves behind the EMT doing chest compressions and assumes that role. The other EMT moves to the head of the patient to continue ventilation.

Effectiveness of CPR

It is appropriate to monitor the effectiveness of cardiopulmonary resuscitation. The carotid pulse must be palpated periodically for no more than 5 seconds during CPR to check the effectiveness of chest compression or the return of a spontaneous, effective heartbeat. Palpation should be done after the first minute of CPR and every 5 minutes thereafter. Pupils and pulse are checked by the EMT performing the ventilation, particularly just before switching positions during CPR. The reaction of the pupils to light should be checked periodically, since pupil constriction provides a good indication of the delivery of oxygenated blood to the patient's brain. Pupils that constrict when exposed to light indicate adequate oxygenation and blood flow to the brain. If the pupils remain widely dilated and do not react to light, serious brain damage may be imminent or may have

occurred. Dilated but reactive pupils are a less ominous sign. However, it must be emphasized that normal pupillary reactions may be altered in the elderly and frequently are drastically changed by the use of drugs.

CPR Interruption

CPR should not be interrupted for more than 5 seconds for any reason, except when it is necessary to move a patient up or down a stairway. It may be impossible to continue effective resuscitation under these circumstances. When a patient has to be moved, it is best to perform CPR at the head or foot of the stairs, then interrupt at a given signal and move quickly to the next level, where effective activity can be resumed. Interruptions should not exceed 15 seconds. Nor should the patient be moved until all transportation arrangements are set and the EMTs are ready to provide uninterrupted CPR during transport.

Without advanced life support (monitoring, an intravenous line, drugs, and defibrillation), basic life support will rarely be sufficient for patient survival, regardless of how well it is performed. If advanced life support modalities cannot be brought to the scene, the patient must be moved promptly to the hospital. Two-person CPR should be continued during transport to the hospital.

ARTIFICIAL CIRCULATION IN INFANTS AND CHILDREN

The basic principles of CPR are the same whether the patient is an infant, child, or adult. The differences in performing CPR on an infant and child relate to the different underlying causes of emergencies in infants and children and the need for techniques that apply to variations in size.

In the majority of instances, cardiopulmonary arrest in infants and children begins with respiratory arrest. Secondary cardiac arrest results from hypoxia. Therefore, the EMT must direct major initial attention to the airway and ventilation. In many cases restoration of an open airway and adequate ventilation of the lungs is all that is needed for resuscitation.

For the purposes of CPR, anyone under one year of age is considered an infant. A child is classified as being between the ages of one and eight years.

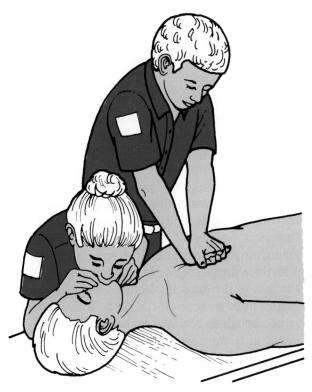

FIGURE 8.8 In an ambulance, two EMTs perform CPR from the same side of the patient.

Above eight years, techniques for adults can generally be applied. These definitions are guidelines only. Variations can occur frequently among infants and children in size relative to age.

Assessment of Circulation

Once the airway and ventilation have been assessed and problems corrected as needed, the EMT can direct attention to the circulation. As in the adult, this routine begins with a check for a palpable pulse. As in the adult, too, absence of a palpable major pulse defines the need for external chest compression to circulate the blood.

The pulse in a child can be felt over the carotid artery in a manner similar to that described for the adult. Palpating this pulse in an infant may present a problem. Unfortunately, the very short and, at times, fat neck of an infant makes the carotid pulse difficult to palpate. **Precordial** (chest wall over the heart) **cardiac activity** represents a transmitted impulse rather than an arterial pulse and, therefore, is not reliable. In contrast, some infants with good cardiac activity may have a very quiet precordium, leading to the incorrect impression that the heart is in arrest. Because of this difficulty, in infants, the brachial artery should be palpated to assess the quality of the peripheral pulse.

The brachial artery is located on the inner side of the arm, midway between the elbow and shoulder (Figure 8.9). The EMT's thumb is placed on the outer surface of the arm between the elbow and shoulder. The tips of the index and long fingers are then positioned to press lightly toward the bone, on the medial side of the biceps, to palpate the pulse.

External Chest Compression

It is in the technique of external chest compression that differences among infants, children, and adults become most apparent. The differences are related to the small size of the chest, the faster heart rate of the infant and the child, and the relative fragility of the surrounding organs.

Position of the Heart. As the chest grows, the portion occupied by the heart diminishes. The heart in the infant and child is situated at approximately the same level as in adults. If an imaginary line is drawn between the nipples, the proper area for compression lies one finger's breadth below this line on the sternum. The index finger is placed just below the line as it crosses the sternum. The adjacent long finger identifies the most superior point for compression (Figure 8.10). Using the same technique as described for the adult, the xiphoid notch in the center of the chest can be located with the long finger. The area just under the index finger is then the appropriate place for compression. The sternum of the child is only 6 to 7 cm long. The thickness of two fingers of an adult EMT is 3 to 4 cm. Two fingers will easily cover the lower half of the sternum.

Chest Size. The chest of an infant or child is smaller and more pliable than that of an adult. Two hands are not necessary for effective compression. In an infant, two fingers are adequate. With the fingers on the lower sternum, it is depressed ½ to 1 inch. As in adults, the patient must be on a hard surface for optimal results. With a child, more force may need to be exerted, but the use of two or three fingers is usually adequate. If the child is large enough so that the sternum will not easily compress with three fingers, the heel of one hand is used. Only the heel of the hand is placed on the sternum; the fingers must be kept off the chest. If the patient is large enough to require the heel of the hand, the depth of compression should be 1 to 1½ inches.

Heart Rate. Because of the faster heart rate in infants and children, the compression rate must also be faster. In infants the minimal compression rate is 100 per minute; for children it is 80 to 100 per minute.

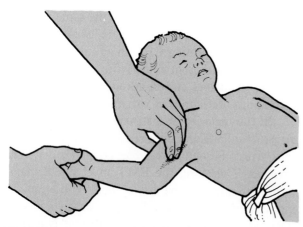

FIGURE 8.9 Checking the brachial pulse in an infant. This major pulse is located on the inner aspect of the upper arm, midway between elbow and shoulder. The tips of the index and middle fingers are used to locate and palpate the brachial pulse.

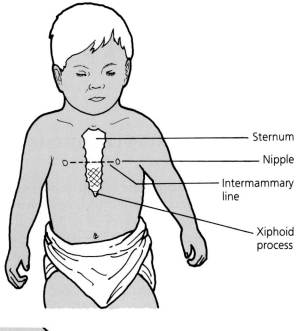

Fragility of Organs. Especially in infants, the liver is relatively large, immediately under the right diaphragm, and very fragile. The spleen on the left is much smaller and much less fragile than in adults. Each, however, may be injured by carelessly applied CPR. The compressing fingers must be placed in the midline of the chest.

External chest compression on a child must be coordinated with ventilation, as in the adult. The rate of compression to ventilation is 5:1, both for single-EMT and dual-EMT rescue. When only one EMT is present, after each fifth compression the EMT opens the airway and ventilates the patient once. If two EMTs are present, the ventilation is given during a pause after the fifth compression. For infants, one ventilation (1 to 1.5 seconds per breath) should be given after every fifth compression.

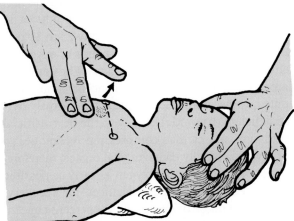

FIGURE 8.10 The proper area for cardiac compression in a child is in the midline, one finger's breadth below the intermammary line.

YOU ARE THE EMT...

1. How does ventricular fibrillation differ from ventricular tachycardia? Why are both called arrhythmias?
2. You have been told that the patient you are about to treat is in cardiac arrest. How will you confirm this report?
3. Why must external chest compression be accompanied by artificial ventilation?
4. You and your partner have been performing two-EMT CPR on a patient for 10 minutes. How do you monitor the effectiveness of your efforts?

9

Ventilation Equipment and Oxygen Therapy

OVERVIEW

Although basic life support for a patient with respiratory or cardiac arrest is carried out without any mechanical aids, the EMT should take advantage of equipment as it becomes available. The EMT should also know how to provide oxygen-enriched air because the inherent inefficiency of artificial circulation makes the provision of supplemental oxygen mandatory.

The various means of providing oxygen and regulating the delivery to patients who require supplementary oxygen are standard in the United States. Several precautionary systems exist to ensure that patients do not receive wrong gases by error. Of course, it is imperative that the EMT become skilled in the use of all artificial ventilation equipment because incorrect or inefficient use could cause a patient's condition to worsen.

Chapter 9 begins with a definition of hypoxia (oxygen deficiency) and its effects on the body. Then the ways of delivering supplemental oxygen are described. Suctioning devices for keeping the airway clear of mucus or vomitus are discussed next. The last sections cover when to use oxygen, its possible hazards, its storage, and equipment for its delivery.

OBJECTIVES

The objectives of Chapter 9 are to

- define hypoxia and understand why patients sometimes need supplemental oxygen.
- learn how to use the various artificial ventilation devices.
- become familiar with suctioning devices and their use.
- recognize when supplemental oxygen is needed.
- identify the hazards of supplemental oxygen.
- learn how to handle oxygen in compressed gas cylinders, recognize the different types of regulators, and know when to replace a cylinder.
- become knowledgeable about the equipment available for oxygen delivery.

THE NEED FOR SUPPLEMENTAL OXYGEN

The atmosphere contains more oxygen than we need to maintain proper function of our vital organs: heart, lungs, and brain. Oxygen is present in the air at a concentration of about 20 percent. We inhale air containing 20 percent oxygen, extract about one-fourth of it, and exhale air containing 16 percent oxygen. Thus, during mouth-to-mouth ventilation, 16 percent oxygen is delivered from the EMT to the patient. This concentration is sufficient to sustain life. Because external chest compression produces at best an effective cardiac output of only 25 to 30 percent of normal, only a limited amount of oxygen is delivered to the body's vital organs. The combination of a low inspired oxygen concentration and a limited cardiac output leaves the patient grossly oxygen deficient (**hypoxic**) even with the best artificial ventilation and cardiac compression techniques.

Hypoxia rapidly damages vital organs; therefore, the use of supplemental oxygen as early as possible will increase the patient's chances for recovery. Oxygen should be delivered at 100 percent concentration to any patient who has sustained a cardiopulmonary arrest.

ARTIFICIAL VENTILATION EQUIPMENT

During cardiopulmonary arrest, circulation and ventilation are both absent. Artificial ventilation utilizing a high oxygen concentration must have an oxygen source and an effective method of delivery.

Pocket Mask with an Oxygen Inlet

A **pocket mask** with an oxygen inlet has been designed to provide supplemental oxygen during mouth-to-mouth ventilation (Figure 9.1). The use of this mask is strongly recommended for all EMTs performing basic life support. The mask allows the

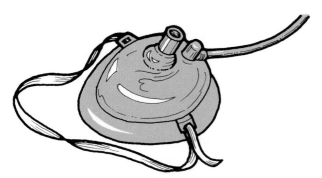

FIGURE 9.1 A pocket mask with a chimney can be used for mouth-to-mask ventilation. An inlet port for supplemental oxygen is shown.

EMT to ventilate the patient with air from his own lungs while at the same time supplying supplemental oxygen. The actual artificial breathing is done by the EMT, but significant oxygen enrichment of inspired air is possible. The major advantage of the mouth-to-mask system is that it frees both of the EMT's hands to keep the airway open and seal the mask to the face.

The mask, triangular in shape, has a narrow angle at the apex which is placed across the bridge of the nose. The base is placed in the groove between the lower lip and the chin. Rising from the center of the dome of the mask is a chimney with a 15 millimeter connector. The EMT should follow these steps when using the pocket mask during mouth-to-mask ventilation:

1. Stand or kneel at the patient's head and open the airway with a head-tilt maneuver.
2. Apply the mask to the face with the apex over the bridge of the nose and the base in the groove between the lower lip and chin.
3. Grasp the patient's mandible with the index, long, and ring fingers of each hand (the ring finger being on the ramus behind the angle) and place your thumbs on the dome of the mask. Maintain an airtight seal by applying firm pressure between the thumbs and the fingers (Figure 9.2a).
4. Keep the airway open by the upward and forward pull of the fingers on the mandible.
5. Take a deep breath and exhale through the open port of the chimney (Figure 9.2b).
6. Remove your mouth and observe the patient exhaling passively (Figure 9.2c). The timing of each breath is the same as that described

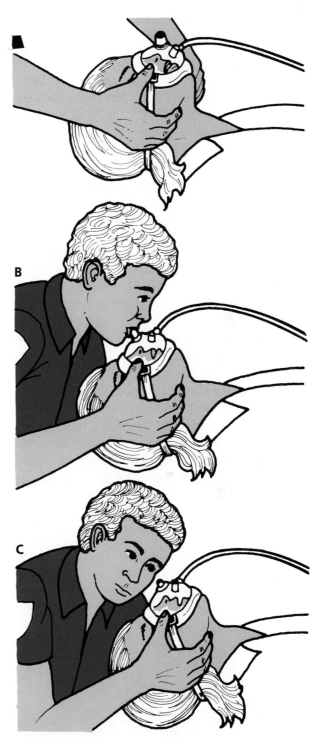

FIGURE 9.2 The steps in mouth-to-mask ventilation using a pocket mask: (a) The EMT seals the mask to the face using both hands. The apex of the mask is over the bridge of the nose, and the base is between the lips and chin. (b) The EMT exhales into the chimney of the mask. (c) During expiration, the EMT must see the chest fall and feel the motion of exhaled air on his cheek.

for the standard mouth-to-mouth technique of artificial ventilation (Chapter 6).

The oxygen concentration of air delivered to the patient can be increased by the addition of the gas through the oxygen inlet valve. Any oxygen delivered to the patient is diluted with the EMT's exhaled breath. For example, 10 liters of oxygen per minute running to the mask will provide the patient with inspired air at approximately 50 percent oxygen concentration; 15 liters per minute will provide inspired air at approximately 55 percent oxygen.

Provided that oxygen is being given and an airway can be maintained, this system also works well for the patient who is breathing spontaneously and does not require full ventilatory assistance but requires supplemental oxygen. The mask has an elastic strap for use with those patients who can breathe spontaneously.

The pocket mask may also be used for an infant. In this case the mask is turned around, and the apex is placed under the infant's chin while the base covers the bridge of the nose and the sides of the face (Figure 9.3). The EMT exhales small puffs of air into the open port of the chimney. The EMT must feel the resistance of the child's lung as air is breathed in and must hear and feel the exhaled air move out. Again, supplemental oxygen should be given as just described.

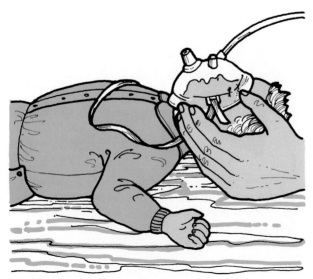

FIGURE 9.3 For an infant, the pocket mask is reversed, and the base is placed over the nose.

Artificial Airways

The primary function of an **artificial airway** is to prevent obstruction of the upper airway by the tongue and allow passage of air and oxygen to the lungs.

Oropharyngeal Airways

An **oropharyngeal airway** is positioned in the mouth with the curvature of the airway following the contour of the tongue. The flange should rest against the lips; the other end opens into the pharynx. This airway has an opening down the center or along either side to permit the free passage of air or oxygen and to allow easy access for suctioning. An oropharyngeal airway should be inserted only in an unconscious patient. If introduced into a conscious or semiconscious patient, it could cause vomiting or spasm of the vocal cords. If incorrectly placed, instead of maintaining the airway, the device can displace the tongue backward into the pharynx and actually produce airway obstruction. The technique for insertion of an oropharyngeal airway includes these steps:

1. Open the patient's mouth with one hand using the cross-finger technique described in Chapter 6.
2. Holding the airway upside down in the other hand, insert it into the patient's mouth, rotating it through 180 degrees until the flange comes to rest on the patient's lips or teeth. In this position, the airway will hold the tongue forward. Moistening the airway with a small amount of water will ease introduction (Figure 9.4).
3. Or, open the mouth, depress the tongue with a tongue blade, and slide the airway into place without rotating it as it passes.

The airway of an unconscious patient who is breathing spontaneously can be maintained with greater ease if an oropharyngeal airway is in place rather than with the constant use of the head-tilt or other maneuvers. The oropharyngeal airway should be used promptly for an unconscious patient who is breathing spontaneously. In the patient who is suspected of having a spinal injury, the oropharyngeal airway is a safe and effective means of keeping the airway open.

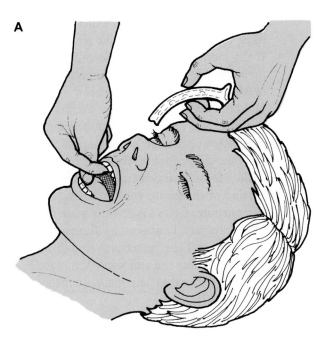

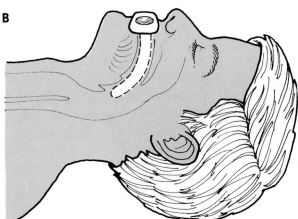

FIGURE 9.4 The oropharyngeal airway is rotated 180 degrees as it is inserted. (a) Using the cross-finger technique, the patient's mouth is opened. (b) The airway is then inserted until the flange rests on the lips or teeth.

Nasopharyngeal Airways

A conscious patient who is not able to maintain a natural airway may benefit from the use of a **nasopharyngeal airway.** This adjunct is usually well tolerated and is not as likely as the oropharyngeal airway to stimulate vomiting. It is not large enough in diameter, however, to accommodate a standard suction tip.

A nasopharyngeal airway is positioned in one nostril with its curvature following the curve of the

floor of the nose. The flange rests against the nostril while the other end opens into the pharynx. It must be well coated with a water-soluble lubricant before it is inserted. Care must be taken to select the patient's nostril large enough to accommodate the airway. In almost everyone, one nostril is larger than the other. Once the proper nostril is selected, the airway is inserted without force through the nostril until the flange rests against the skin (Figure 9.5).

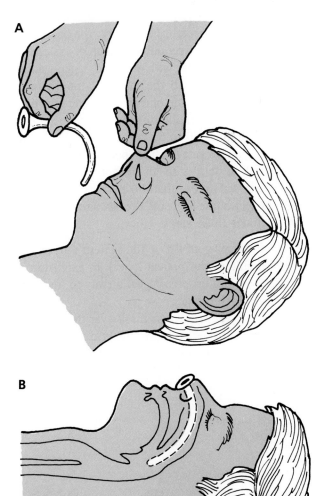

FIGURE 9.5 A nasopharyngeal airway can help to maintain an open airway in a conscious patient. (a) During insertion, its curvature should follow the curve of the floor of the nose. (b) Once in place, the flange should lie against the flare of the nostril so that the other end will lie in the pharynx.

If an obstruction is met as the airway is introduced, the airway should be removed and inserted into the other nostril.

The Bag-Valve-Mask System

The **bag-valve-mask system** should be used when it is desirable to deliver very high (greater than 50 percent) oxygen concentrations to the patient who is not breathing spontaneously (Figure 9.6). Both mouth-to-mouth and mouth-to-mask ventilation techniques can provide large volumes of inspired air — up to 4 liters per breath. In contrast, the bag-valve-mask system can deliver only as much gas as can be squeezed out of the bag with one hand, usually about 1 liter. However, with the mouth-to-mouth technique, the concentration of oxygen delivered is only 16 percent, and the mouth-to-mask technique at best will provide only 50 to 55 percent oxygen. At the same oxygen flow rate (10 liters per minute), the bag-valve-mask system with an oxygen reservoir will deliver air with more than 90 percent oxygen.

The technique for using the bag-valve-mask system includes these steps:

1. Position yourself at the patient's head and maintain the patient's neck in extension.
2. Insert an oropharyngeal airway to maintain an open airway.
3. Place the triangular mask over the patient's face with the apex over the bridge of the nose and the base in the groove between the lower lip and the chin. (To achieve this fitting, you must select the correct mask size.)
4. If the mask has an inflatable collar, blow it up before use to obtain a better and easier seal between the mask and the face.
5. Hold the mask in position by placing the little, ring, and long fingers on the mandible. The little finger is on the ramus, and the ring and long fingers are on the body of the mandible. Hold the index finger over the lower portion of the mask, while securing the upper portion of the mask with your thumb. Firm pressure between the fingers on the mandible and the finger and thumb on the mask maintains the seal while the mandible is pulled forward to help maintain the airway (Figure 9.7).
6. With the mask firmly applied to the patient's face and the neck maintained in extension with one hand, use your other hand to com-

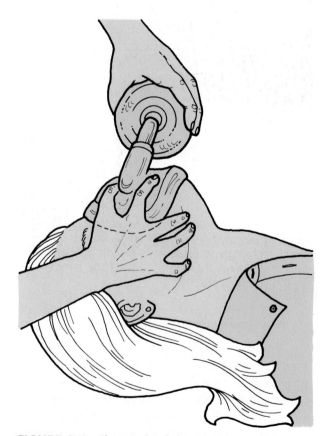

FIGURE 9.7 The mask of the bag-valve-mask system is held firmly against the patient's face. Three fingers are on the mandible, and the thumb holds the upper part of the mask.

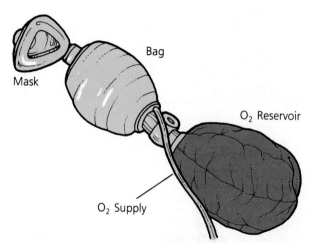

Bag

Mask

O₂ Reservoir

O₂ Supply

FIGURE 9.6 A bag-valve-mask system with all its component parts. Note the oxygen supply, oxygen reservoir, and resuscitation bag, in addition to the mask.

press the bag in a rhythmic manner once every 5 seconds (Figure 9.8). Proper ventilation must be evident by the rise and fall of the chest.

When this system is used with external chest compression, ventilation should be given during pauses in compression: one after every fifth or two after every fifteenth compression. At least 2 seconds should be allowed for each ventilation.

The EMT should adopt the following sequence in artificial ventilation when using a bag-valve-mask system with an airway.

1. Open the oxygen regulator and check that the pressure in the tank is adequate.
2. Connect the plastic oxygen line to the flowmeter nipple and connect the other end to the bag-valve-mask unit with the reservoir in place (Figure 9.9).
3. Turn on the flowmeter to deliver 10 liters of oxygen per minute.
4. Select the correct size of mask for the patient and attach the mask to the valve on the bag.
5. Open the patient's mouth using the cross-finger technique and insert an oropharyngeal airway.

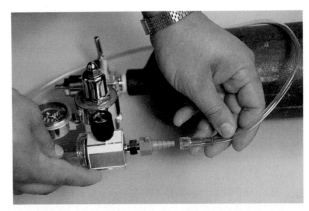

FIGURE 9.9 Connections of the bag-valve-mask with reservoir and oxygen tank flowmeter.

6. With one hand, maintain the face mask seal and neck extension.
7. With the other hand, ventilate the patient by squeezing the bag.
8. Check to be sure lung expansion is occurring.

SUCTIONING DEVICES

Portable and fixed suctioning equipment is essential for resuscitation. The portable unit must provide a vacuum pressure and flow adequate for effective pharyngeal suction. The unit should be fitted with wide bore, thick-walled, nonkinking tubing and rigid, plastic, **pharyngeal suction tips (tonsil tips)**. A nonbreakable collection bottle and a supply of water for rinsing the tips should be available. The fixed suction unit should generate an airflow of more than 30 liters per minute and a vacuum of more than 300 mm of mercury when the tubing is clamped. The suction yoke, collection bottle, water for rinsing, and the suction tube should be readily accessible to the EMT at the patient's head.

Plastic pharyngeal suction tips are best for suctioning the pharynx. They are large bore and do not collapse. A curved contour allows easy and rapid placement of the tip in the pharynx. They should be used with the greatest caution in conscious or semiconscious patients because of the hazard of inducing vomiting. Suction apparatus should be cleaned and decontaminated after each use.

When using suction, follow these steps:

1. Inspect the unit for proper assembly of all its parts; switch on the suction; clamp the

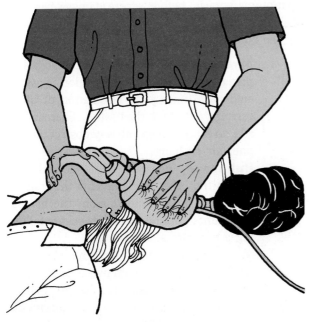

FIGURE 9.8 The bag-valve-mask system with an oxygen reservoir. Its limitations in terms of volume of oxygen delivered are apparent, since it can deliver only the volume that one hand can displace.

tubing and note if the pressure dial registers more than 300 mm of mercury.

2. Attach the pharyngeal suction tip to the tubing.

3. Open the patient's mouth with the cross-finger technique.

4. Insert the suction tip with it convex side along the roof of the mouth until the pharynx is reached (Figure 9.10).

5. After the tip is in place, release the clamp on the tube and suction.

6. Never suction for more than 15 seconds at one time, because suctioning removes oxygen from the airway very effectively.

7. Suctioning may be repeated only after the patient has been ventilated and reoxygenated.

WHEN TO USE SUPPLEMENTAL OXYGEN

Hypoxia, as noted earlier, is a condition in which there is a deficiency of oxygen reaching the tissues of the body. It is extremely dangerous, and if it persists, death will occur. Some tissues and organs, especially the heart, the central nervous system, lungs, adrenal glands, kidneys and liver, require a virtually constant supply of oxygen to function normally. Regardless of how well the mechanics of artificial ventilation are performed by the EMT, unless supplemental oxygen is used, recovery from hypoxia

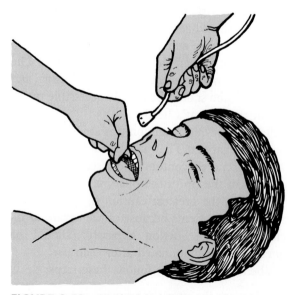

FIGURE 9.10 Suctioning of the oropharynx with a rigid plastic tonsil suction device.

will be slow and often incomplete. Therefore, it is essential that the EMT know the specific indications for the use of oxygen and the various modes of its storage and delivery.

Patients Requiring Oxygen Therapy

Oxygen should be given to two major groups of patients: those who are not breathing spontaneously and those who can breathe but who are unable to move a sufficient amount of air with each breath to ensure adequate oxygen delivery to the lungs. Those in the first group will rapidly develop hypoxia of the vital organs, especially the brain and heart. Death occurs within a matter of minutes if systemic hypoxia is not reversed. Patients in the second group will also be hypoxic. The onset and the degree of tissue damage will depend on the degree of respiratory inadequacy. These patients have poor air exchange and require oxygen and varying degrees of ventilatory support.

Conditions Causing Hypoxia

The early signs of hypoxia are **tachycardia** (abnormally fast heart rate), nervousness, and irritability. **Cyanosis** is a late finding. The ideal time for the correction of hypoxia is when the first signs and symptoms appear, before severe damage has been done to the essential organs. The following are some of the common conditions that cause hypoxia:

1. **Myocardial infarction** (heart attack). Hypoxia from myocardial infarction is associated with inadequate circulation of blood carrying oxygen to the tissues. There is usually no lung damage, airway obstruction, or poor air exchange.

2. **Pulmonary edema.** Fluid accumulates within the lungs and prevents the transfer of oxygen to the blood from the alveoli. Sometimes pulmonary edema occurs following a myocardial infarction.

3. Acute drug overdose. Respirations in patients who have taken an overdose of a drug may be very depressed. Infrequent, shallow breaths do not provide a sufficient amount of oxygen.

4. Pulmonary burns. Burns of the lungs result from inhalation of steam, hot fumes, and smoke. Such burns produce local pulmonary

edema and destroy lung tissue. In this situation, gas exchange in the lungs is impaired.

5. **Cerebrovascular accident** (stroke). The cause of hypoxia in a patient who has suffered a stroke is poor control of respiration by the brain. The rate and depth of breathing may both be severely decreased.

6. Chest injury. Hypoxia results because of pain and damage to the chest and underlying lung tissue.

7. **Shock.** Shock often occurs as a result of injuries in which much blood is lost. The capacity of blood to carry oxygen in the vascular system can be markedly reduced.

8. **Chronic obstructive pulmonary disease.** Long-standing chronic irritation of the lungs and air passages (smoking or inhaling toxic fumes) produces direct lung damage and increasingly poor gas exchange.

All patients who are hypoxic, from whatever cause, should be treated with supplemental oxygen. The method of oxygen delivery will vary, depending on the cause and the severity of the hypoxia.

HAZARDS OF SUPPLEMENTAL OXYGEN

Even though oxygen does not burn and does not explode, it does support combustion. A small spark can become a flame in an oxygen-enriched atmosphere. For example, a glowing cigarette can burst into flames. Therefore, any possible source of fire must be kept away from the area while oxygen is in use. This warning must be kept in mind at all times by the EMT.

With some chronic lung diseases such as emphysema, the normal carbon dioxide stimulus to respiration is no longer effective. In these conditions, a low blood oxygen level is the primary stimulus for the patient to breathe. Giving oxygen to patients with chronic lung disease may eliminate this stimulus to breathe and cause a decrease in ventilation to the point where breathing will cease altogether. Inspired oxygen concentrations greater than 25 to 30 percent must be given with great caution to these patients, and the EMT must be prepared at all times to provide artificial ventilation for patients with chronic lung disease.

However, keeping oxygen levels low should not be a consideration following a cardiopulmonary arrest. Patients experiencing cardiopulmonary arrest are dying. Nothing can be done to make the situation worse, since respiration is already as depressed as it can be. These patients need the maximal oxygen concentration that can be delivered until full resuscitation can be accomplished.

Oxygen given in high doses for prolonged periods of time can be toxic. In adults and children, **pulmonary fibrosis** (scarring of the lung) can develop, and in the newborn, **retrolental** (behind the optic lens) **fibroplasia** can occur and cause blindness. Pulmonary oxygen toxicity, however, in adults and children, only occurs after the lungs have been exposed for several days to an inspired oxygen concentration in excess of 50 percent, delivered at higher than normal pressures. The short-term delivery of high concentrations of oxygen does not cause such lung damage, and there is no valid reason to withhold it from a patient during and immediately after cardiopulmonary arrest. Similarly, the management of cardiac arrest in the newborn requires the use of high oxygen concentration for two reasons. First, the actual pumping capacity of the heart is reduced during the external chest compression. And second, most newborns who suffer arrest do so because of oxygen deficiency.

Oxygen deficiency in the very young is usually caused by a disease that impairs the passage of oxygen from the pulmonary alveoli to the lung capillaries. These two elements alone prevent large quantities of oxygen from being carried by the blood to the eyes. Again, retrolental fibroplasia is associated with long-term use (several days) of high oxygen concentrations and higher than normal inspiratory pressures. Therefore, during resuscitation the principles of oxygen administration are identical for adult, child, and neonate: All should be given oxygen in arrest situations.

SOURCES OF SUPPLEMENTAL OXYGEN

Compressed Gas Cylinders

In locations other than hospitals and similar facilities, oxygen is usually supplied as a compressed gas in seamless steel cylinders, available in various sizes. The two most frequently used in emergency medical care are the E and M cylinders (Figures 9.11 and 9.12). When filled with oxygen at a pressure between 2,000 and 2,300 pounds per square inch (PSI), the E size contains 650 liters, and the M size, 3,000 liters.

Cylinders of E size or smaller have outlet valves designed to accept pressure-reducing gauges of the yoke type (Figure 9.13). To prevent attachment of a pressure regulator for a different gas to an oxygen cylinder, the yoke contains a **pin-indexing safety attachment** (Figure 9.14). The system is comprised of a series of pins on the yoke that must be matched with the holes on the yoke attachment of the gas cylinder if a satisfactory connection is to be made. The arrangement of the pins and holes varies for different gases according to accepted national standards. Each cylinder of a specific gas has a given pattern and a given number of pins. When two or more different gases are being used, one cannot, for example, attach a cylinder of nitrous oxide to an oxygen

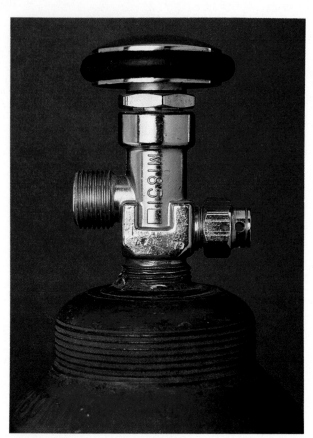

FIGURE 9.12   A size M oxygen cylinder has a valve with the threaded-connector gas outlet of the American Standard Safety System.

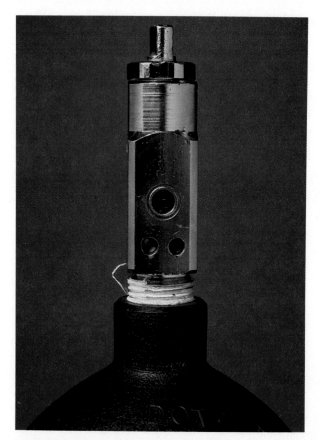

FIGURE 9.11   A size E cylinder with the pin-indexing safety system and gas outlet.

line by mistake because the nitrous oxide cylinder will not fit.

Cylinders larger than E size are equipped with threaded gas outlet valves (Figure 9.12). The inside and outside diameters of these threaded outlets vary according to the medical gas contained in the cylinder. Therefore, the gas cylinder will not accept a regulator valve unless it is properly threaded to fit that outlet. This safety system for large cylinders is known as the **American Standard System** (Figure 9.15). The purpose of these safety devices is to prevent the accidental attachment of a regulator to a wrong supply tank (for example, to nitrous oxide or carbon dioxide instead of to oxygen).

Regulators

Compressed gas cylinders must be handled carefully since their contents are under pressure. Regulators must be firmly attached to the cylinders before they are transported. A loose regulator or per-

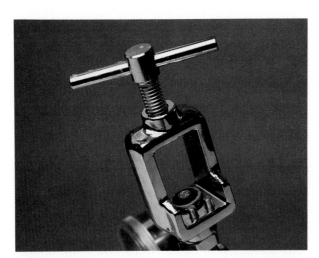

FIGURE 9.13 The yoke connector is used with small oxygen cylinders.

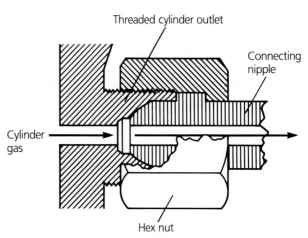

FIGURE 9.15 The typical American Standard connection is used to attach a reducing valve to a large high-pressure cylinder.

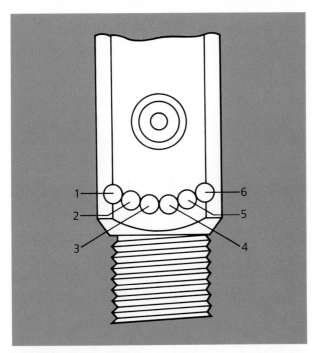

FIGURE 9.14 The locations of the pin-indexing safety system holes in a cylinder valve face. Various pairs constitute indexes for different gases.

foration of the tank can cause it to become a deadly missile.

Pressure Regulators

The pressure of gas in an oxygen cylinder is too high to be useful medically. **Pressure regulators** must be attached to medical gas cylinders to reduce the pressure to a level suitable for the operation of medical equipment, usually 40 to 70 pounds per square inch (PSI). Most pressure regulators in medical use today reduce the pressure in a single stage, although multistage regulators do exist. A two-stage regulator will initially reduce the pressure to 700 PSI and then to 40 to 70 PSI. After the cylinder pressure is reduced to a workable level, the final attachment for delivering the gas to the patient is usually through one of these two ways:

1. A quick-connect female fitting that will accept a quick-connect male plug from a pressure hose or ventilator or resuscitator.
2. A flowmeter that will permit the regulated release of gas measured in liters per minute.

Flowmeters

Flowmeters are usually permanently attached to pressure regulators on emergency medical equipment. The two types of flowmeters commonly in use are pressure-compensated flowmeters and Bourdon gauge flowmeters.

Pressure-Compensated Flowmeters. **Pressure-compensated flowmeters** have a float ball incorporated within a tapered calibrated tube. The float rises or falls according to the gas flow within the tube. The flow of gas is controlled by a needle valve located downstream from the float ball. Back pressure resulting from a restriction of gas (e.g., kinked tubing) will cause the float ball level to drop since the float will record only actual delivered flow. This type of flowmeter is affected by gravity and must always be maintained in an upright position (Figure 9.16).

Bourdon Gauge Flowmeters. The **Bourdon gauge flowmeter** is very common in emergency medical use because it is not affected by gravity and can be used in any position. It is actually a pressure gauge calibrated to record flow rate (Figure 9.17). The major disadvantage of this flowmeter is that it does not compensate for back pressure and will actually record a higher flow rate when any obstruction to gas flow is encountered downstream.

Humidification

Oxygen from a cylinder source is extremely dry. For all practical purposes, it is completely free from water vapor. Therefore, to prevent the drying of the patient's mucous membrane surfaces, **humidification** is an important component of oxygen administration (Figure 9.18). Excessive drying of the mucous membranes of the nose, mouth, and lungs can interfere with respiration. Humidification systems, because they contain water, can easily become contaminated and serve as a reservoir for infection. Therefore, if used on an ambulance, they must be kept clean and changed frequently.

Replacement of Oxygen Cylinders

Several methods are available for calculating how long an oxygen cylinder can be used before its con-

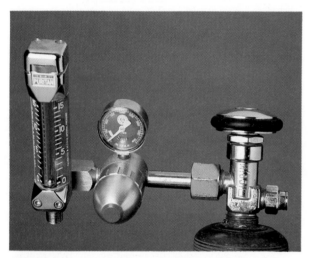

FIGURE 9.16 A pressure-compensated flowmeter attached to a large gas cylinder via a threaded connection allows a regulated flow from 0 to 15 liters of oxygen per minute.

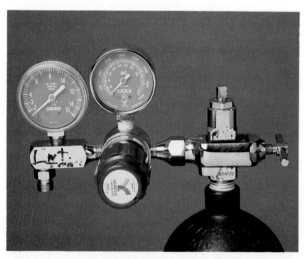

FIGURE 9.17 A Bourdon gauge flowmeter attached to a small gas cylinder via a yoke attachment allows a regulated flow from 0 to 15 liters of oxygen per minute.

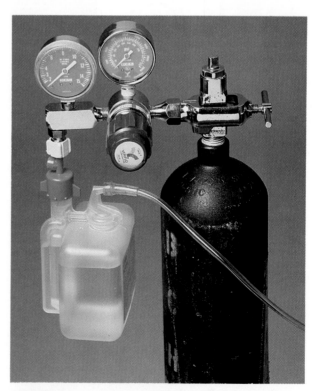

FIGURE 9.18 An evaporative oxygen humidifier is attached to a Bourdon gauge flowmeter/pressure regulator. Humidification prevents excessive drying of the mucous membranes of the nose, mouth, and lungs.

tents are depleted. It should be emphasized that one must always make arrangements to switch to a fresh cylinder before the one in use becomes completely empty. Normally, a cylinder is replaced at a certain level (usually 200 PSI) above the 0 PSI reading on the pressure gauge. This level may be called the **safe residual.** Knowing the current pressure reading, the current flow in liters per minute, and the safe residual, the EMT can calculate how much useful life remains in any cylinder. One way of calculating the remaining duration of flow in the cylinder after it has been used is shown in Table 9.1.

EQUIPMENT FOR OXYGEN DELIVERY

Nasal Cannula

With a **nasal cannula** (Figure 9.19), oxygen is administered to the patient through two small tubular prongs that fit into each nostril. If the flowmeter is set for 5 to 8 liters per minute, it is possible to obtain inspired oxygen concentrations ranging from 35 to 50 percent. Since the nasal cannula delivers dry gas directly into the nostrils, humidification is necessary if extensive drying or subsequent damage of the nasal mucosa is to be avoided with prolonged use. If prolonged oxygen administration by this method is anticipated, an air evaporative type of humidifier should be attached to the flowmeter. A patient who is a mouth breather or who has a nasal obstruction derives minimal benefit from this type of oxygen administration.

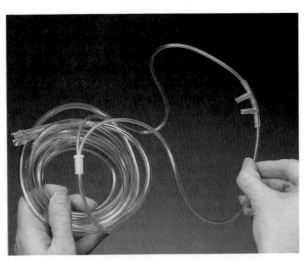

FIGURE 9.19 Nasal cannula used to administer oxygen in concentrations of 35 to 50 percent.

Simple Face Mask

Simple **face masks** (Figure 9.20) contain a small bore inlet port and an elastic strap for snug fit. Perforations on either side allow the escape of excess gases, especially during exhalation. Different sizes of face masks are available, including infant and pediatric. All types of masks are fitted to the face in the same manner — the apex across the bridge of the nose and the base between the lower lip and chin. With a flow rate of 6 to 10 liters per minute, inspired oxygen concentrations of 35 to 60 percent can be attained. Humidification is necessary in a manner similar to that described for the nasal cannula, when prolonged use is necessary.

TABLE 9.1   Calculating the Duration of Cylinder Flow (in Minutes)

Formula:	$\dfrac{\text{(Gauge pressure in psi} - \text{Safe residual)} \times \text{Factor}}{\text{Flowrate (liter flow per minute)}} = \text{Duration of flow (in minutes)}$
	Factors for various oxygen cylinders D 0.16 E 0.28 G 2.41 H & K 3.14 M 1.56
	Safe residual pressure is 200 psi
Example:	M cylinder, gauge pressure at 1,200 psi, safe residual is 200 psi, flowmeter set for 5 liters per minute. How long will the cylinder last?
Solution:	$\dfrac{(1,200 - 200) \times 1.56}{5} = \dfrac{1,560}{5} = 312$ minutes (or 5 hrs., 12 min.)

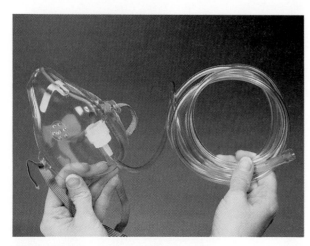

FIGURE 9.20   A simple face mask.

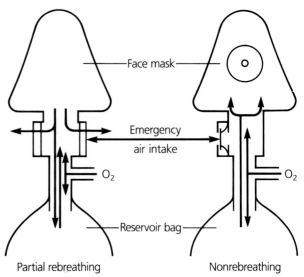

FIGURE 9.22   A nonbreathing and partial-rebreathing bag-valve-mask are compared.

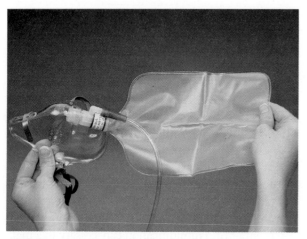

FIGURE 9.21   A simple face mask with attached bag connected by a one-way valve. If the valve is removed, a partial-rebreathing system is created.

Mask and Bag

In the **mask and bag system** (Figure 9.21), the mask is similar to the face mask just described. However, in this system, oxygen inflow fills the bag that is attached to the mask by a one-way valve. This system is occasionally called a non-rebreathing mask and bag. By removing the flapper valves on the mask, the system can be converted to a partial rebreathing mask and bag (Figure 9.22). Oxygen concentrations in excess of 60 percent in inspired air can be obtained with this system. There is no preset flow rate. Gas inflow must be set at whatever level will prevent the complete collapse of the bag during inhalation. With infants and children, obviously a smaller gas flow

bag will be needed since the volume inhaled each time will be less.

Flapper valves over the mask perforations serve as one-way ports of exhalation. This modification prevents taking in room air that could mix with and dilute the oxygen concentration. These exhalation valves may be removed if necessary. Humidification is necessary when prolonged administration is anticipated.

Venturi Masks

A **venturi mask** is a breathing unit that provides a specific concentration of oxygen through a delivery tube connected to a standard face mask (Figure 9.23a and b). Before the oxygen delivery tube reaches the mask, it passes through an air entrainment device that specifically regulates the concentration of delivered oxygen and also the volume of gas delivered to the patient per unit of time. Venturi masks are usually designed to deliver inspired oxygen concentrations of 24, 28, 35, or 40 percent. However, the stated concentrations are not entirely accurate, and some variations should be expected. Humidification is needed with prolonged use. The major advantage of this system is a high volume of inspired air with gradually increasing and controlled concentrations of oxygen. Venturi masks are especially useful for patients with chronic obstructive lung disease.

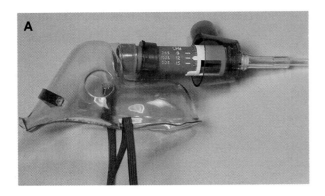

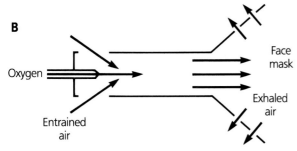

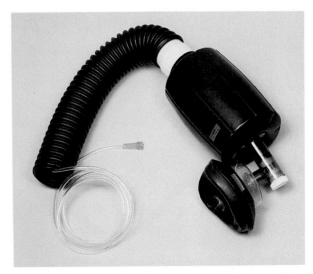

FIGURE 9.24 A bag-valve-mask resuscitator with modification for administration of a high concentration of oxygen.

FIGURE 9.23 (a) A typical venturi mask. (b) A diagrammatic representation of the functions of the venturi mask. As oxygen is delivered, a certain amount of room air is also entrained with each inhalation, providing a given oxygen concentration. The amount of room air taken in is dependent on the size of the ports through which the air passes.

Bag-Valve-Mask Resuscitators

All types of **bag-valve-mask resuscitators** have these common components (Figure 9.24):

1. An inflatable, deflatable bag
2. A valve that incorporates the exhalation port, the oxygen inflow, and a means of connection between the face mask and the bag
3. A face mask

The total amount of gas contained within the bag of an adult resuscitator is 1,200 to 1,600 cubic centimeters (cc). The pediatric bag contains approximately 500 to 700 cc, and the infant bag holds 150 to 240 cc. The majority of the bag-valve-mask resuscitators on the market today are available with modifications or accessories to permit the delivery of oxygen concentrations approaching 100 percent. Without these modifications, it is difficult to achieve concentrations above 50 percent.

The oxygen inlet of a bag-valve-mask resuscitator is attached to the flowmeter nipple of the oxygen cylinder by the small bore tube. These units may be used to assist the respiration of patients who are breathing spontaneously but are not receiving adequate air. The EMT using the unit for this purpose should deflate the bag simultaneously with the patient's inspiratory effort and ultimately attempt to achieve a more normal rate and depth of respiration. The function of the unit is under the manual control of the EMT.

Oxygen-Powered Mechanical Ventilation Devices

There are two basic types of oxygen-powered mechanical ventilation devices: automatic and manual. The most common of these devices are intermittent positive-pressure breathing (IPPB) resuscitators, demand-valve resuscitators (Figure 9.25), and resuscitator inhalators. Conventional, pressure-cycled, automatic resuscitators should not be used by EMTs for artificial ventilation, especially in conjunction with external chest compression. External chest compression prematurely triggers termination of the inflation cycle of these devices, and inadequate ventilation results.

Federal specifications require that resuscitators used in ambulances be manually controlled (timed cycle). Manually controlled resuscitators have high

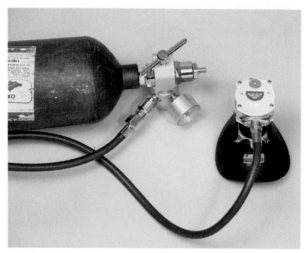

FIGURE 9.25 A demand-valve resuscitator with high-pressure hose and quick-connect fitting.

porting and tilting the patient's head and keeping the jaw elevated.

The amount of pressure necessary to ventilate a patient adequately will vary according to the size of the patient, the patient's lung volume, and the condition of the lungs. A patient with stiff, diseased lungs or chronic obstructive lung disease will require a greater pressure to receive a given volume than would be necessary for a patient with normal lungs.

The problem the EMT faces in using these resuscitators, just as with the bag-valve-mask units, is the airtight fit between the patient's face and mask. Practice and strict adherence to proper technique will minimize this problem.

Significant concern exists about the inherent danger in the use of these units, especially since they are widely available. Their usefulness makes it necessary to include them in this discussion, but the need for proper training must be emphasized if they are to be used by the EMT.

instantaneous flow rates that allow them to be used for artificial ventilation alone, as well as in conjunction with external chest compression. The majority of these units will function as inhalators for patients who are breathing spontaneously but require oxygen.

Manually controlled oxygen-powered resuscitators should do the following:

1. Provide flow rates of 40 liters per minute or more and an inspiratory pressure safety release valve that opens at approximately 50 cm of water. (The EMT must be alert for gastric distention as a result of such a high flow rate).
2. Provide 100 percent oxygen.
3. Operate satisfactorily under varying environmental conditions.
4. Have a position on the manual control so that both the EMT's hands can remain on the mask to provide an airtight seal while sup-

YOU ARE THE EMT...

1. What are the major advantages of mouth-to-mask ventilation over mouth-to-mouth ventilation?
2. The patient is unconscious and needs an artificial airway. Will you insert an oropharyngeal airway or a nasopharyngeal airway? Why?
3. What is hypoxia? What are the early signs of hypoxia? The late signs? How can it be reversed?
4. Why is it dangerous to give oxygen in concentrations greater than 25 to 30 percent to patients with chronic obstructive lung disease?

SECTION 4

BLEEDING AND SHOCK

10

The Control of Bleeding

OVERVIEW

Unquestionably, bleeding is one of the major emergency problems. The EMT must recognize its existence — obvious when it is external but not so obvious when it is internal — assess its seriousness, and know the limits of being able to control it effectively. Several methods exist for controlling obvious external bleeding, with varying degrees of risk associated with each. For internal bleeding, recognition of its existence and prompt transportation are paramount because the EMT has very limited means to control internal bleeding.

Chapter 10 first discusses the significance of bleeding. Then external bleeding and the six methods of controlling it are described. The last section of Chapter 10 discusses internal bleeding. The focus is on its seriousness because of the difficulty of controlling it in the field.

OBJECTIVES

The objectives of Chapter 10 are to

- understand the significance of bleeding, both external and internal.
- learn how to control external bleeding using direct pressure, pressure on a major artery, a tourniquet, a splint, an air pressure splint, or a pneumatic counterpressure device.
- recognize the signs and symptoms of internal bleeding and learn the principles of treating patients with suspected internal bleeding.

THE SIGNIFICANCE OF BLEEDING

Bleeding and **hemorrhage** mean the same thing, namely, that blood is escaping from arteries, capillary vessels, or veins. Bleeding may be external or internal. In either case it is dangerous. Hemorrhage initially causes weakness and, ultimately, if uncontrolled, shock and death. The average adult has 6 liters of blood. The acute loss of 10 percent of the circulatory blood volume (in an adult, 600 ml; in a child, 200 to 300 ml) is very dangerous. In an infant, the loss of 25 or 30 ml of blood can cause the signs of shock.

Blood is transported within the circulatory system through blood vessels. Injury and some diseases will disrupt vessels and result in bleeding. Characteristically, blood from an open artery is bright red and spurts under pressure, in time with the beat of the heart. Blood from an open vein is much darker and flows steadily without the spurt. Bleeding from damaged capillaries is a continuous, slow, steady ooze (Figure 10.1). The rapidity of bleeding is very important. The average adult may comfortably lose a unit (500 ml) of blood donated in a blood center over 15 to 20 minutes. While the blood is being withdrawn, the body can adapt to the decrease in blood

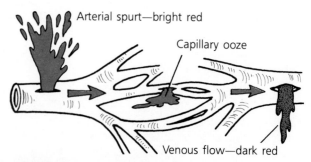

Arterial spurt—bright red

Capillary ooze

Venous flow—dark red

FIGURE 10.1 A capillary loop connecting an arteriole and a venule is shown in this schematic drawing. Bleeding on the arterial side is bright red and spurting; from the venous side it is dark red, or reddish-blue, with a steady flow. Bleeding from the capillaries themselves is a slow, steady ooze.

volume quite well. If larger amounts are lost, especially more suddenly, the patient may show the signs and symptoms of shock or may even die. In these circumstances, the blood loss has been so large or so fast that the body cannot compensate. In general, the body cannot compensate for acute blood losses greater than 10 percent of the total volume.

EXTERNAL BLEEDING

External bleeding is hemorrhage that can be seen coming from a wound. Some examples of external hemorrhage are bleeding from open fractures, bleeding from wounds, and nosebleeds. In most instances, bleeding stops naturally after 6 to 10 minutes because the body has many intrinsic mechanisms of defense, among them those that arrest bleeding. If a finger is cut, for example, blood will at first gush from the cut vessels. Then the cut vessel ends will constrict to diminish the hemorrhage. A clot then forms at the ends of the vessels, and bleeding stops as the clot increases in size and plugs the hole. Body tissues and tissue juice activate the clotting mechanisms within the blood. When exposed to these components, blood clots rapidly seal the injured portions of any vessel. Normally, blood within an artery or vein is protected from contact with body tissues or tissue juices by the vessel wall and therefore will not clot unless the vessel is injured.

In some patients who have undergone a severe injury, the damaged blood vessels may be so large that clots cannot occlude (block) them. Sometimes only a portion of the vessel wall may be cut; and, thus, the wall cannot retract or constrict. In these cases bleeding will continue unless stopped by external means. Blood loss may occasionally be so rapid that, if one waits for the bleeding to stop, the patient may bleed to death before normal protective processes can be activated. It is imperative that the EMT know how to control bleeding. In general, after securing an airway and being certain that the patient can breathe, the EMT must address the second matter for immediate concern — the control of hemorrhage.

Controlling External Bleeding

The control of external bleeding is often very simple. Almost all instances of external bleeding can be controlled by applying direct local pressure.

Pressure stops the physical flow of blood and permits normal blood coagulation to occur.

There are several ways to control bleeding when it is external, among them the following (Figure 10.2):

1. Direct pressure may be exerted over the wound by a finger or hand or by the application of a pressure dressing; this method is by far the most effective way to control local external hemorrhage.
2. Pressure on a major artery proximal to the wound may be applied to occlude blood flow in that artery. This method may diminish the rate of bleeding but will rarely stop it because all wounds receive blood flow from more than one artery.
3. A tourniquet may be applied proximal to the wound on an affected extremity.
4. A splint may be applied.
5. An air pressure splint may be used.
6. A pneumatic counterpressure device may be used.

Local Pressure

Bleeding is nearly always stopped when pressure is applied directly over the wound (Figure 10.2a). Initially, pressure may be applied with the finger or hand, but a sterile gauze pressure dressing is preferred; 4 × 4 or 4 × 8 sterile gauze pads should be used for small wounds and a sterile universal dressing for larger wounds. Once bleeding is controlled using local pressure, the compression can be maintained by wrapping the wound circumferentially and firmly with a sterile, roller, self-adhering bandage. The entire sterile dressing should be covered above and below the wound by the roller bandage, stretched sufficiently tight to control the hemorrhage. If sterile pads are not immediately available, a handkerchief, a sanitary napkin, a clean cloth, or a bare hand can be used to apply pressure.

A dressing should not be removed once it has been placed until the patient has been evaluated by the physician at the emergency department. Bleeding that continues after the dressing is in place usually means that not enough pressure has been applied to the wound. In such instances, additional manual pressure should be applied through the dressing, and then additional gauze pads should be applied over

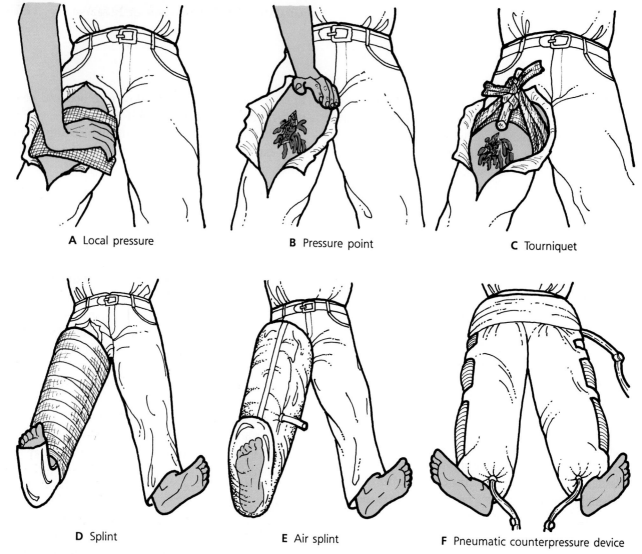

A Local pressure   **B** Pressure point   **C** Tourniquet

D Splint   **E** Air splint   **F** Pneumatic counterpressure device

FIGURE 10.2 The major means of controlling external bleeding: (a) local pressure; (b) pressure point; (c) tourniquet; (d) splint; (e) air splint; and (f) pneumatic counterpressure device.

the first dressing and secured with a second roller bandage.

Pressure Point Control

When pressure dressings are not available or when direct pressure with reinforced dressings does not control wound bleeding, proximal arterial pressure control can sometimes be used to slow bleeding (Figure 10.2b). Pulse points for the major arteries are described in Chapter 3. To use proximal arterial pressure well, the EMT must be thoroughly familiar with the location of these pulse points. Only rarely does compression of a major feeding artery completely arrest hemorrhage from a wound distal to that artery, because in most instances the wound is supplied by more than one major artery. Thus, this technique can aid temporarily in the control of severe

hemorrhage, but it should not be the primary or the sole method of bleeding control.

Tourniquet

The use of a tourniquet to stop bleeding is rarely if ever necessary. Tourniquets are not recommended because sometimes they can cause more damage to injured extremities than was caused by the injury itself. They can crush a considerable amount of tissue beneath them and cause permanent damage of nerves and blood vessels. If they are left on for a long time, all distal tissues will die. Their use is not indicated in wounds of the trunk, or for those distal to the elbow or knee. Thus, the range of injuries for which they may be effective is quite limited.

Nevertheless, a properly applied tourniquet may be lifesaving for a person whose bleeding from a major vessel cannot be controlled in any other way. Specifically, the tourniquet is useful in the patient who has severe bleeding from a traumatic amputation, either partial or complete, or in the patient for whom local pressure supplemented by proximal pressure point control has failed to arrest the hemorrhage. If a tourniquet must be used, it should be applied in the following manner (Figure 10.3):

1. Fold a triangular bandage until it is 3 to 4 inches wide and 6 to 8 layers thick.
2. Wrap this long, 4-inch-wide bandage twice around the extremity, at a point proximal to the bleeding but as far distal on the extremity as possible (Figure 10.3a).
3. Tie one knot in the bandage. Place a stick or rod on top of the knot and tie the ends of the bandage over the stick in a square knot (Figure 10.3b, c).
4. Use the stick as a handle and twist to tighten the tourniquet until the bleeding has stopped. Once the bleeding has ceased, make no more turns with the stick. Secure the stick in place and make the wrapping neat and smooth (Figure 10.3d). The technique of using a rod passed through a bandage to achieve pressure is called the "**Spanish Windlass.**" It is also occasionally used for the application of traction.

A blood pressure cuff can serve as an effective tourniquet (Figure 10.4). The cuff should be applied proximal to the bleeding point and inflated to a pressure just in excess of that required to arrest the bleeding.

The following precautions must be observed when using a tourniquet:

1. Use as wide a bandage as possible and be sure that it is tightened securely.
2. Never use wire or any other material that will cut into the skin.
3. Do not loosen the tourniquet. It will be loosened in the emergency department but not until measures have been taken to control the expected bleeding.
4. Never cover a tourniquet with a bandage. Leave it open and in full view. Always signify that the patient has had a tourniquet applied by writing "TK" and the time of tourniquet application on a piece of adhesive tape securely fastened to the patient's forehead (Figure 10.4). This important information must also be recorded on the ambulance run report form, and the emergency department personnel must be notified that a tourniquet is in place.
5. Never place a tourniquet below the knee or elbow. In these more distal areas in the extremity, nerves lie close to the skin and may be injured by the compression. Furthermore, rarely, if ever, does one encounter bleeding distal to the knee or elbow that will require tourniquet control.

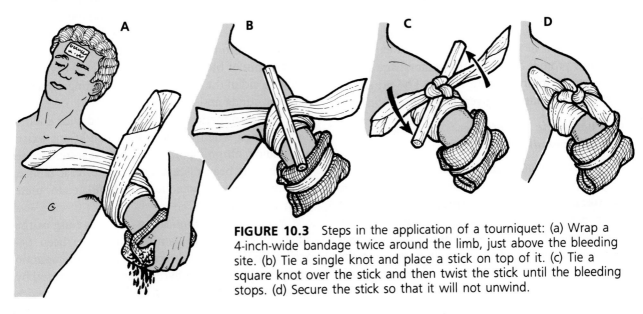

FIGURE 10.3 Steps in the application of a tourniquet: (a) Wrap a 4-inch-wide bandage twice around the limb, just above the bleeding site. (b) Tie a single knot and place a stick on top of it. (c) Tie a square knot over the stick and then twist the stick until the bleeding stops. (d) Secure the stick so that it will not unwind.

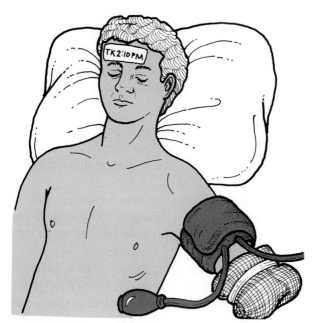

FIGURE 10.4 A blood pressure cuff can be used effectively as a tourniquet. With all tourniquets, a note must be made, usually taped to the patient's forehead, of the time of application.

6. If a blood pressure cuff is used, continuously monitor the gauge to be sure that the pressure is not being lost gradually.

Splints

Much bleeding from injured extremities occurs because muscles are lacerated by sharp ends of broken bones or because vessels lying near the fractured bone continue to bleed. As long as the fracture has not been stabilized, continued laceration and further damage of partially clotted vessels can occur. This continued irritation results in further bleeding. Often the application of a splint to a fractured extremity will allow prompt control of the hemorrhage associated with the injury (Figure 10.2d). The principles of applying splints are given in Chapter 15.

Pneumatic Counterpressure Devices and Pressure Splints

Many ambulances throughout the United States carry air pressure splints and some carry **pneumatic counterpressure devices** (Figure 10.2e, f). Air splints are used to control severe soft tissue hemorrhage when massive lacerations of soft tissue or fractures have occurred. The principle underlying the use of air splinting in the control of hemorrhage is that a pressure bandage may be applied to an entire

extremity rather than to a single laceration or a given area on the extremity. At the same time, effective splinting of the coexisting fracture can be accomplished. The use of such a splint for the pressure control of hemorrhage is entirely appropriate in the patient with only extensive soft tissue lacerations and no fracture (Figure 10.2e).

Frequently, hemorrhage is a severe or fatal complication of fractures of the pelvis or the proximal femur. Bleeding may not be observed externally in these patients because it occurs behind the peritoneum and into the tissues around both hips.

A pneumatic counterpressure device (**pneumatic trousers, air pressure pants,** or a **pneumatic antishock garment**) can be used in the treatment of hypovolemic shock from such injuries and from certain other causes. The device is effective in these specific instances:

1. For controlling significant bleeding into the tissues from a fractured pelvis or from fractures of the proximal femurs.
2. For helping to counteract significant intra-abdominal bleeding.
3. For stabilizing fractures of the pelvis and proximal femurs.
4. For supporting the systolic blood pressure when it falls below 100 mm Hg following trauma when a bleeding source is not evident.

The effectiveness of a pneumatic counterpressure device is based on the fact that the greatest portion of blood at any one time is in the capillary circulation. Compression of the abdomen and the lower extremities will force much of this blood from the capillaries into the central circulation and increase the amount of blood available to the vital organs. It will also aid in the local control of bleeding from soft tissue wounds and fractures.

The pneumatic counterpressure device should not be used when the following conditions exist: pregnancy, chronic pulmonary edema secondary to longstanding heart disease, and acute cardiac failure. Ideally, the device should not be left inflated for more than 2 hours.

Some major complications from the use of the pneumatic counterpressure device have been described in the medical literature. The most common complication is severe hypovolemic shock caused by unsupervised, or too rapid, deflation of the device in the emergency department. Once applied, and prior to deflation, emergency department personnel must be prepared to administer large volumes of intravenous fluids and blood to restore adequate blood volume before the device is deflated. Recently, there have been some reports of muscle tissue death caused by excess pressure within the garment when the garment was left inflated for prolonged periods of time. Finally, the medical literature reports some inappropriate uses of the pneumatic counterpressure device. It must be used only when indicated because of the potential for complications associated with its application.

There is general agreement that the garment can produce good stability for major pelvic and femoral fractures. It can also support the blood pressure in instances of hypovolemic shock quite well. The EMT must remember that emergency support of the blood pressure is achieved at the cost of unusual and sometimes lethal tissue pressures in the lower extremities and abdomen. A good result can be obtained by careful inflation in increments with constant monitoring of the blood pressure. As a general rule, pressure should be gradually increased in the leg portions of the garment before the abdominal portion is inflated. The pressures should not be increased beyond those that produce the return of an adequate (greater than 100 mm Hg) systolic blood pressure. In general, one should avoid extremity pressures above 40 mm Hg since these will damage the local tissue. Effectiveness of this mode of treatment is measured by the return of blood pressure toward normal and the stabilizing of vital signs.

While considerable work has been done to show that the use of pneumatic counterpressure devices increases carotid blood flow during cardiopulmonary resuscitation (CPR), there are no data demonstrating improved outcome from cardiac arrest with their use. Hence, these devices are not recommended for routine cardiopulmonary resuscitation in the treatment of cardiac arrest.

Whenever air pressure splints or pneumatic trousers are used, and it is necessary to transport the patient either in a helicopter or in areas where temperature changes may be marked, the EMT must remember that the volume of the air within the device will change in accordance with changes in external temperature and air pressure. In helicopters and in unpressurized airplanes, external pressure drops with increasing height, and the air in the splint expands. Accordingly, the splint will become much tighter than it was when applied. Similarly, cold makes air within the device contract. If an emergency requires the application of such a splint in cold areas, the pressure within it must be adjusted as the patient comes into a warm room or transporting vehicle. The air in the splint will then expand, and the splint will again tighten.

The EMT must inform the emergency department personnel about the patient's blood pressure, when the device was applied, and the results observed after its application. The EMT must also note and record the time the device was applied and inflated. Removal of a pneumatic counterpressure device is done only after gradual deflation, after the use of appropriate intravenous solutions, and with careful supervision. It is never done outside the emergency department. The technique of applying the pneumatic counterpressure device is illustrated in Figure 10.5.

Epistaxis

Nose bleed (**epistaxis**) is a common emergency. The amount of blood that a person can lose in a nose bleed may be enough to cause shock. The blood seen coming from the nose may represent only a small amount of the total loss, since much passes down the throat into the stomach as the patient swallows. A person who swallows a large amount of blood may become nauseated and may vomit. Bleeding from the nose can be caused by the following conditions:

1. A fractured skull
2. Facial injuries, including those caused by a direct blow with the fist
3. Sinusitis, infections, or other abnormalities of the inside of the nose
4. High blood pressure
5. Bleeding diseases

Bleeding from the nose or ears following a head injury may mean that a skull fracture is present. Such bleeding is difficult to control, and excessive pressure at the fracture site may increase pressure on the brain as the blood leaking out through the ear and the nose now collects within the head. Bleeding from the nose caused by a skull fracture should be treated with a dry sterile dressing with only moderate compression; excessive pressure should be avoided.

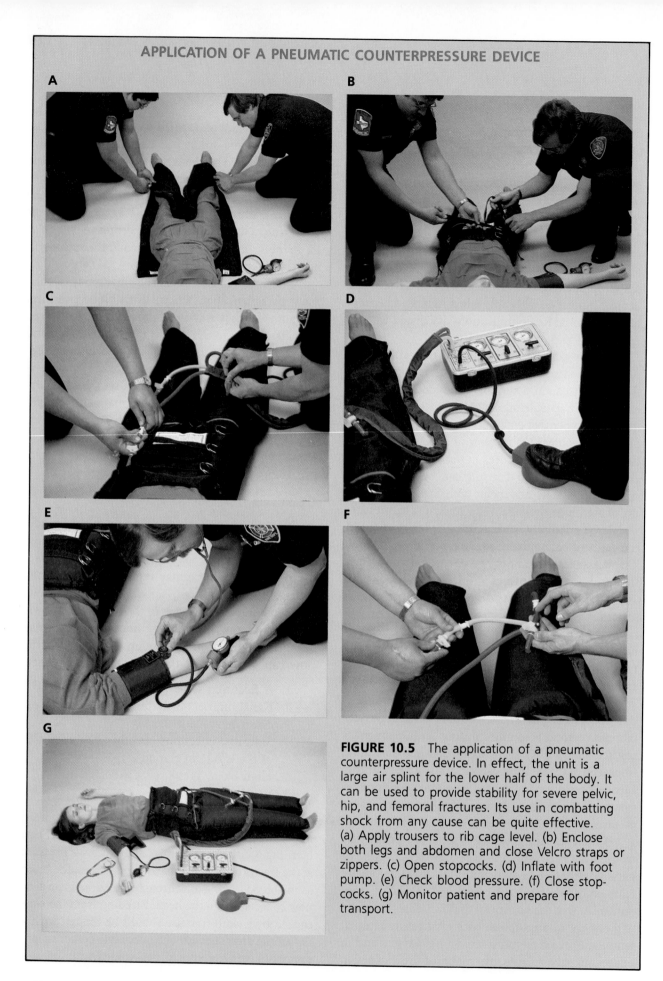

FIGURE 10.5 The application of a pneumatic counterpressure device. In effect, the unit is a large air splint for the lower half of the body. It can be used to provide stability for severe pelvic, hip, and femoral fractures. Its use in combatting shock from any cause can be quite effective.
(a) Apply trousers to rib cage level. (b) Enclose both legs and abdomen and close Velcro straps or zippers. (c) Open stopcocks. (d) Inflate with foot pump. (e) Check blood pressure. (f) Close stopcocks. (g) Monitor patient and prepare for transport.

Nose bleeds resulting from all other causes should be initially treated at the scene. The following techniques are successful in stopping most nose bleeds:

1. Apply pressure by pinching the nostrils together or by placing a rolled 4 × 4 gauze bandage between the upper lip and the gum and pressing against it with the fingers. The patient can sometimes apply enough pressure to stop the bleeding by stretching the upper lip tightly against the rolled bandage.

2. Keep the patient in a sitting position with the head tilted forward whenever possible so that the blood trickling down the back of the throat will not be aspirated into the lungs.

3. Keep the patient quiet. This rule is particularly important if the patient suffers from high blood pressure or is anxious. Anxiety will tend to increase the blood pressure, and the nose bleed will worsen.

4. Apply ice over the nose. Local cooling treatment is helpful in controlling hemorrhage.

The EMT must understand that the person with a prolonged nose bleed or one who is subject to frequent nose bleeds should be taken promptly to the hospital to be seen by a physician. Most nose bleeds arise from injury of the mucous membrane covering the nasal septum, which is anterior in the nose. Accordingly, the local measures listed above are frequently successful in stopping nose bleeds. A few nose bleeds, however, arise posteriorly, in the nasopharynx, and cannot be stopped by these normal emergency methods. This kind of nose bleed may require the application of a nasopharyngeal pack, which must be done in the hospital by the doctor. Therefore, any nose bleed that does not respond to the measures described above must be treated in the hospital to avoid the development of hypovolemic shock.

INTERNAL BLEEDING

Signs and Symptoms of Internal Hemorrhage

Although not usually visible, internal bleeding can be very serious, and the patient with severe internal hemorrhage may develop hypovolemic shock before the EMT realizes the extent of the blood loss. Bleeding, however slight, from any body orifice is serious, as it usually indicates an internal source of hemorrhage that may not be readily evident. Bleeding from the mouth or rectum or blood in the urine may indicate serious internal visceral injury or disease. Nonmenstrual bleeding from the vagina is always significant. Probably the most common evidence of internal bleeding is a bruise or contusion. It indicates hemorrhage into the soft tissues and may be seen after a slight or severe injury. Some other examples of internal hemorrhage are these:

1. Bleeding from a stomach ulcer
2. Bleeding from a closed fracture of any bone
3. Bleeding from a lacerated spleen

Signs that may point to internal bleeding and that are not evident at the body surface are those indicating the development of hypovolemic shock:

1. The pulse becomes weak and rapid ("thready").
2. The skin becomes cold and moist ("clammy").
3. The eyes are dull; the pupils may be dilated and slow to respond to light.
4. The blood pressure falls (late).
5. The patient is usually thirsty and almost invariably anxious, with a feeling of impending doom.
6. The patient may be nauseated and may vomit.

A person with a bleeding stomach ulcer may lose a large amount of blood internally very quickly. Fractured ribs may result in severe internal hemorrhage into the chest. Occasionally, with problems such as these, the patient may vomit blood or cough up bright red blood from an injured lung. Vomited blood may be bright red, dark red, or look like coffee grounds suspended in gastric juice (**coffee grounds vomitus**). A person who has suffered a severe blunt abdominal injury with a laceration of the liver or spleen may lose a considerable quantity of blood within the abdominal cavity. Ordinarily, in addition to the signs and symptoms of shock, this patient will have a tender abdomen which progressively distends.

A person with a fracture of the shaft of the femur can easily lose a liter of blood or more into the tissues of the thigh with little or no immediate external indication of such blood loss. Swelling is usually seen with closed fractures of major bones, largely as a result of an accumulation of blood around the ends of the fractured bone.

Control of Internal Bleeding

The control of internal bleeding depends on the site of the hemorrhage. There is nothing the EMT can do, in the field, to control internal hemorrhage within the body cavities or organs. The likelihood of this event must be suspected on the basis of injuries sustained and confirmed by observing the vital signs. Immediate transportation to the emergency department is required for the injured patient who has suspected internal bleeding. Usually, an operation or very complex equipment is needed to control the internal bleeding.

Some specific terms indicating acute internal bleeding from a variety of diseases and injuries are these:

1. **Hematemesis** (the vomiting of bright red blood)
2. **Hemoptysis** (the coughing up of bright red blood)
3. **Melena** (the passage of dark black stools with the consistency of tar)
4. **Hematochezia** (the passage of bright red blood from the rectum)
5. The vomiting of coffee-ground-like material from the stomach
6. **Hematuria** (the passage of blood in the urine)
7. **Ecchymosis** (a black and blue discoloration of the skin caused by bleeding)
8. **Hematoma** (a "blood tumor," a mass of blood accumulated in the soft tissues beneath the skin)

All patients with these findings are at high risk. They may continue to bleed or may bleed again massively at any moment. All patients suspected of having internal bleeding must be transported promptly to the hospital for evaluation and treatment. Diagnosis of the exact cause of bleeding is frequently facilitated if the doctor can see the patient while the bleeding is taking place.

Internal bleeding into the extremities can be managed quite well by the EMT on the scene in a number of ways. Splinting of an injured extremity may allow control. In most cases, single-extremity

air splints will effectively control the bleeding. Only on rare occasions will the use of a pneumatic counterpressure device be required. Tourniquets are not indicated for the control of closed, internal, soft tissue bleeding.

Internal bleeding in the abdomen and thorax cannot be controlled in the field. The most serious complication of internal bleeding in these areas, hypovolemic shock, can be stabilized by use of the pneumatic counterpressure device.

The principles of treating any patient with suspected internal bleeding in the field are these:

1. Monitor and record the vital signs at least every 10 minutes.
2. Treat obvious internal bleeding in an arm or leg by applying a splint.
3. Treat severe uncontrolled hypovolemic shock with a pneumatic counterpressure device.
4. Anticipate that the patient will vomit. Give nothing by mouth and keep the patient lying down, preferably on one side.
5. Elevate the patient's feet 6 to 12 inches to increase circulation to the vital organs.
6. Give oxygen. As blood is lost, the tissues of the body are deprived of their needed oxygen supplies. Inhalation of oxygen on the way to the hospital may be lifesaving.
7. Transport the patient as expeditiously as possible to the emergency department.

YOU ARE THE EMT...

1. One of the ways that external bleeding can be controlled is to apply direct pressure to the wound using a finger, hand, or pressure dressing. Describe three other ways you can control external hemorrhage.
2. Why aren't tourniquets used very often to control bleeding? Under what type of circumstances are they useful?
3. How do pneumatic counterpressure devices work to control bleeding? What must be done before these devices are deflated to prevent hypovolemic shock in the patient?
4. What is the difference between hematemesis and hemoptysis? Between ecchymosis and hematoma? What do these four terms have in common?

Shock

OVERVIEW

The term "shock" has a variety of meanings. For example, it is used to denote the receiving of any amount of electrical current by an individual; it is also used to describe the psychological reaction to bad news, fright, or other emotional stress. However, in this chapter shock describes a state of collapse and failure of the cardiovascular system. When that happens, blood circulation slows and eventually ceases. After even a few minutes without blood flow, the cells of certain organs die. If the conditions causing shock are not promptly treated, death soon follows.

Shock is caused by a number of different factors, including blood loss, dilation of blood vessels, and failure of the heart to pump effectively. It can also be brought on by respiratory failure and acute allergic reactions. Shock is frequently encountered by the EMT because it so often accompanies the events to which EMTs respond such as heart attacks and automobile accidents. Therefore, it is imperative that the EMT be able to recognize shock, treat it, and hopefully reverse it and save a life.

Chapter 11 begins with a description of the cardiovascular system and an explanation of perfusion, the absence of which brings on shock. Then eight different types of shock are described. The chapter next discusses the signs and symptoms of shock. The last section describes the general treatment for shock, including appropriate measures for treating each of the eight types of shock.

OBJECTIVES

The objectives of Chapter 11 are to

- understand the basic physiology of shock.
- identify the specific physiological process responsible for the eight types of shock.
- recognize the signs and symptoms common to all types of shock.
- learn the general treatment for shock and the specific treatment for particular types of shock.

THE PHYSIOLOGY OF SHOCK

The cardiovascular system circulates blood to all of the cells and tissues. Through this system, oxygen and nutrients are brought to each cell, and metabolic waste products are removed. Certain parts of the body such as the brain, the spinal cord, and the heart require a constant flow of blood to live. These organs cannot tolerate the arrest of blood flow for more than a few minutes or their cells will die. Furthermore, these tissues do not have the ability to generate new cells. Once the cells die they cannot be replaced, and permanent loss of function or death of the patient will result.

The cardiovascular system can be described as consisting of two parts: a container and its contents. The container consists of the heart and its system of blood vessels: arteries, veins, innumerable small arterioles and venules, and capillaries. They are the tubes that extend to every cell in the body. In the arteries, and at the arterial ends of the capillaries, the vessels have distinct muscular walls. They can open and close as directed by the nervous system. The size of the small capillaries that pass between individual cells to link arterioles with venules is controlled by these **sphincter muscles.** The opening (dilation) and the closing (constriction) of all of these vessels are entirely automatic and under the control of a specialized portion of the nervous system called the **autonomic nervous system.** The stimuli that cause the dilation and constriction of blood vessels include fright, heat, cold, the specific need of an organ or tissue for oxygen, and the specific need to dispose of metabolic waste. An individual does not exert any voluntary control over this system. Never are all the vessels fully dilated or fully constricted in a normal individual.

The second part of the cardiovascular system can be described as the contents in the container, or the blood. Normally there is just enough blood to fill the system entirely; in an average adult, this amount is 6 liters. The heart is a muscular pump that circulates the blood through the system. The heart pumps 6 liters of blood per minute through a system that can hold just 6 liters. Thus, every part of the system receives a regular supply of blood every minute. Any condition under which the system fails to provide sufficient circulation to every part of the body is called **shock.**

As mentioned previously, certain tissues cannot live without a constant, high level of blood flow. The heart, the central nervous system, the lungs, and the kidneys are tissues that must function continuously. Regardless of what happens, the functions of these organs must continue, and so they require a constant minimum blood supply. It is important to realize that not every part of the body, nor every part of every tissue, receives the same blood supply all the time. Certain tissues are used very heavily but on an intermittent basis. For example, muscles are at rest during sleep but require a large blood supply during exercise. The gastrointestinal tract requires a high flow of blood after eating; but it can be deprived of a good deal of this flow without significant problems after digestion is completed. Blood can be shunted automatically from such organs as the skeletal muscles and gastrointestinal tract in emergency situations to the heart, brain, lungs, and kidneys. This balance of blood supply to the various tissues and organs is regulated by the nervous system on a moment-to-moment basis in response to various stimuli. The vascular system is dynamic and constantly changing, depending on the needs of each of the body parts.

The term **perfusion** means the circulation of blood within an organ or tissue. An organ or an area of the body is perfused if blood is entering it through the arteries and leaving it through the veins. To reach the veins, the blood must pass through the arterioles, connecting capillaries, and venules. The blood gives up nutrients and oxygen and picks up the waste from the organ or tissue that is being perfused. Perfusion of the whole body by blood keeps the component cells of the body alive and healthy. The body depends on adequate, continuous perfusion of its organs and tissues by blood to bring food to them and to dispose of the metabolic waste products generated in the course of normal daily activities. In states of shock, perfusion of organs and tissues fails.

The EMT must know which organs of the body are more susceptible than others to the lack of adequate perfusion. The brain and the spinal cord (the central nervous system) cannot lack perfusion for more than 4 to 6 minutes without permanent damage to nerve cells. Permanent damage in the kidney results after inadequate perfusion for a period of 45 minutes. The heart requires constant perfusion or it will not function properly. Skeletal muscle, if subjected to the loss of perfusion for 2 hours, will be permanently damaged. The gastrointestinal tract can exist with limited (but not absent) perfusion for a number of hours. No part of the body can exist without adequate perfusion for an indefinite period of time. Permanent injury results when the organ system that is most sensitive to the lack of perfusion is damaged. In order, these organs are heart, central nervous system, lung, and kidney. Each of the figures included above for safe length of time without perfusion presumes a normal body temperature. An organ or tissue that is considerably below normal body temperature (98.6 degrees Fahrenheit or 37.0 degrees Centigrade) is much more resistant to damage from lack of perfusion.

It is important for the EMT to understand the concept of perfusion because it is the unifying element in shock. Of equal importance is understanding the varying susceptibility of tissues to the lack of perfusion. While shock has a number of separate causes, there are really only three ways in which each of the separate causes can induce shock. Whatever the cause of shock, the damage comes about because perfusion of organs and tissues is deficient. As soon as perfusion ceases or is impaired, tissues start to die. The three basic causes of shock are these (Figure 11.1):

1. The heart can be damaged so that it fails to act properly as a pump.
2. Blood can be lost so that the volume contained within the vascular system is insufficient for perfusion.
3. The blood vessels constituting the container can dilate so that the blood within them, even though it is of normal volume, is insufficient to fill the system and provide efficient perfusion.

In all instances, the results of shock are exactly the same. There is insufficient perfusion of blood through the tissues of the body to provide adequate food and oxygen and to carry away waste. All local

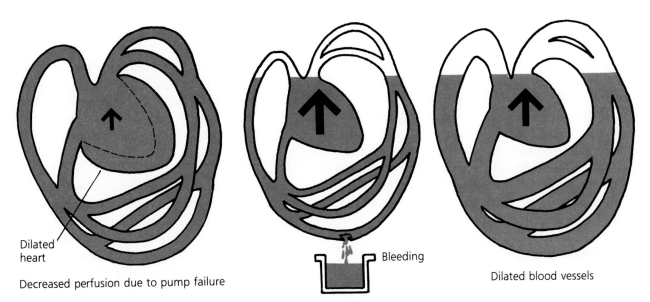

Dilated heart

Decreased perfusion due to pump failure

Bleeding

Dilated blood vessels

FIGURE 11.1   There are three basic causes of shock and impaired tissue perfusion: (a) pump failure due to heart disease; (b) decreased blood volume, usually a result of bleeding; and (c) dilation of blood vessels, making the container too large and decreasing the blood pressure.

body processes are affected. If the conditions causing shock are not promptly arrested and reversed, death soon follows.

The development of shock is a certain precursor of death unless it is treated and reversed. Shock itself, however, cannot be seen. It is a physiologic state with specific manifestations. Its signs and symptoms are a rise in pulse; pale, ashen, cool, moist skin; a poor urinary flow; agitation, anxiety, and a feeling of impending doom; air hunger; and ultimately a falling blood pressure. These signs must trigger a response in the EMT to treat imminent, severe cardiovascular collapse. In many critical situations the EMT should expect shock — for example, massive external or internal bleeding, multiple severe fractures, an acute abdomen, spinal injury, or severe infection could all bring on shock. Whatever the cause, the EMT must recognize the existence of shock promptly and institute definite measures to counteract it.

TYPES OF SHOCK

Shock may accompany many different emergency situations. Six types of shock are related to one of the three major vascular mechanisms described above:

1. Hypovolemic shock (blood loss)
2. Metabolic shock (loss of body fluid)
3. Neurogenic shock (loss of nervous control of the vascular system)
4. Psychogenic shock (the common faint)
5. Cardiogenic shock (inadequate functioning of the heart)
6. Septic shock (severe generalized infection with loss of blood volume and direct blood vessel damage)

In addition, there are two other kinds of shock that are nonvascular in nature: respiratory shock and anaphylactic shock.

Hypovolemic Shock

Following injury, shock is commonly a result of fluid or blood loss. This type of shock is called **hypovolemic (low volume) shock.** When due to blood loss, it is more specifically called **hemorrhagic shock.** External bleeding is common in patients who have suffered severe lacerations or fractures. Internal bleeding follows rupture of the liver, the spleen, or injury of the great vessels within the abdomen or the chest. Hypovolemic shock also results from severe thermal burns. In burns, a considerable amount of intravascular fluid, or plasma (the colorless part of blood), leaks from the circulatory system into the tissues that have been burned and that lie adjacent to the injury. Crushing injuries may also result in the loss of blood and plasma into the injured tissue from damaged blood vessels.

If **dehydration** (loss of body water) is present before the injury, the state of shock will be aggravated and will develop more rapidly. In all these circumstances, the common factor is an insufficient volume of blood within the vascular system (the container) to provide adequate circulation to all the organs of the body, resulting in hypovolemic shock.

Metabolic Shock

Occasionally, severe untreated illnesses may cause a state of **metabolic shock** because of profound fluid losses from vomiting, diarrhea, or excess urination. Severe disturbances of body fluid and chemical balance occur in uncontrolled diseases such as diabetes mellitus. These patients can become severely dehydrated and not have a sufficient volume of fluid within the vascular container to provide proper perfusion of tissues and organs. Patients who develop metabolic shock in the course of a chronic disease are desperately ill. They may have reached the end stage of their capacity to compensate for the problems of that particular disease. The EMT may be called to transport such a patient whose disease has been sorely neglected. During transport this patient will require all available support measures.

Neurogenic Shock

Damage of the spinal cord, particularly at the upper cervical levels, may cause significant injury to the part of the nervous system that controls the size and muscular tone of the blood vessels. **Neurogenic shock** is usually the result. In this condition, the muscles in the walls of the blood vessels are deprived of the nerve supply that causes them to contract. Thus, all the vessels below the level of spine injury dilate widely and increase the size and capacity of the vascular system. The available 6 liters of blood can no longer fill the enlarged vascular system and failure ensues. Even though no blood or fluid has been lost, perfusion of organs and tissues becomes inadequate and shock occurs. In this condition, a radical change in the size of the vascular system has caused shock.

It should be remembered that many other functions under the control of the nervous system are also lost in this situation. The most important of these, in an acute injury setting, is that the patient loses the ability to control body temperature. Body temperature in the patient with neurogenic shock can rapidly fall to match that of the environment.

Psychogenic Shock

Psychogenic shock, the common faint, is a sudden reaction of the nervous system that produces a temporary, generalized vascular dilation. The result is a temporary reduction of blood supply to the brain because the blood momentarily pools in dilated vessels in other parts of the body. When the blood supply to the brain is suddenly and sharply reduced, the brain ceases to function normally and a faint ensues. Fear, bad news, sometimes good news, the sight of an injury or blood, the prospect of medical treatment, severe pain, and anxiety are among the many precipitating causes of psychogenic shock. A person who is not feeling well, is tired or worried, or is obliged to stand quietly in a stuffy room may be susceptible to fainting.

Once fainting has occurred, the patient collapses and becomes supine; circulation to the brain is promptly restored and the episode passes quickly. In this type of shock, the major concern of the EMT is any injury sustained during the fainting spell, such as striking the head. The vascular cause of psychogenic shock is a sudden enlargement of the container so that perfusion, for the moment, becomes ineffective.

Cardiogenic Shock

Cardiogenic shock is caused by inadequate function of the heart. Circulation of blood throughout the vascular bed requires the constant pumping action of a normal and vigorous heart muscle. Many diseases can cause destruction or inflammation of this muscle. Within certain limits, the heart can adapt to these injuries. If too much muscular impairment occurs, however, as sometimes happens after a heart attack, the heart no longer functions well.

It is the muscular contraction of the heart that moves blood through the vessels at distinct pressures. A certain pressure is necessary to force the blood through the entire system. The heart must also beat enough times each minute so that the blood volume can be circulated throughout the system efficiently. Shock from cardiac origin develops when the heart muscle can no longer impart sufficient pressure to circulate the blood to all organs. It can also occur when the regularity of the heartbeat is so disrupted that the volume of blood within the system can no longer be efficiently handled. Direct pump failure is the cause of shock in this situation.

Septic Shock

In some patients who have severe bacterial infections, toxins (poisons) can be generated by the bacteria or by infected body tissues to produce a state called **septic shock.** In this condition, blood vessel walls are damaged and become leaky. They also lose the capacity to contract well. The shock state results from widespread dilation of vessels in addition to the loss of plasma through the injured vessel walls.

This type of shock is a complex problem. There is an insufficient volume of fluid in the container because much of the blood has leaked out of the vascular system (hypovolemia). At the same time, there is a larger than normal blood vessel bed to contain the smaller than normal volume of intravascular fluid. Septic shock almost always is seen as a complication of prolonged hospitalization or of some very serious illness, injury, or operation.

Respiratory Shock

A severe chest injury or obstruction of the airway may result in a patient's being unable to breathe adequately so that an insufficient amount of oxygen is inspired. These conditions can produce **respiratory shock.** Inadequate breathing capacity can produce shock as rapidly as the vascular causes. In these instances, shock is produced because an insufficient concentration of oxygen exists in the blood. The volume of blood, the volume of the vascular container, and the action of the heart are all normal. The supply of oxygen carried in the blood is not. Without oxygen the organs in the body cannot survive, and their functions promptly start to deteriorate.

Because this type of shock may develop in patients with airway obstruction or with diseased or injured lungs, the first step in adequate resuscitation is securing an airway and the second is restoring respiration. Circulation of nonoxygenated blood will have no benefit at all for the patient.

Anaphylactic Shock

Anaphylactic shock (anaphylaxis) occurs when an individual who has been sensitized to some substance by previous contact with it reacts violently to a subsequent dose or contact. It is the most severe form of an allergic reaction. Instances that most often cause allergic reactions may be grouped.

1. *Injection.* The injection of sera such as tetanus antitoxin or drugs such as penicillin may cause an immediate severe reaction.
2. *Ingestion.* The eating of certain foods such as shellfish or the use of some medications or drugs such as oral penicillin can cause slower but equally severe reactions in anyone sensitive to the agents.
3. *Sting.* The sting of a honeybee, wasp, yellow jacket, or hornet can cause very severe, immediate allergic reactions in those people who are allergic to the injected toxin.
4. *Inhalation.* The inhalation of dusts, pollens, or materials to which the patient is sensitive may similarly cause a rapid and severe reaction.

Anaphylactic shock is a very complex reaction. It is, however, encountered fairly commonly; therefore, the EMT should know its signs and treatment. Anaphylactic reactions occur in minutes or even seconds after contact with the substances to which the patient is allergic. Obvious reactions in the skin, respiratory system, and circulation result. The signs are not those usually associated with shock from other causes. The following evidences of an anaphylactic reaction are quite characteristic:

1. *Skin.* There is flushing, itching, or burning of the skin, especially in the face and upper chest. **Urticaria** (hives) may spread over large areas of the body. **Edema** (swelling), especially of the face and tongue, may occur. Specific marked swelling of the lips may be seen. Cyanosis may become marked about the lips.
2. *Respiratory system.* There is tightness or pain in the chest, with an irritating, persistent cough. Wheezing and **dyspnea** (difficulty in breathing) develop. Fluid pours into the bronchi in reaction to the sensitizing agent and the patient tries to cough up this fluid. The

smaller bronchi constrict, and the passage of air into the lungs becomes increasingly difficult. Expiration, normally the passive part of the breathing cycle, becomes forced. The fluid in the air passages and the constricted small bronchi cause the development of a characteristic wheeze as the patient works hard to exhale.

3. *Circulatory system.* Ultimately, there will be a perceptible drop in blood pressure, the development of a weak, barely palpable pulse, pallor, and dizziness. Fainting and coma may follow.

With anaphylactic shock, there is no loss of blood, no cardiac or vascular damage, and no vascular dilation. The body is, however, rapidly deprived of needed oxygen.

SIGNS AND SYMPTOMS OF SHOCK

Certain signs and symptoms are common to all types of shock, with the exception of anaphylactic shock, which presents certain additional special signs. These were described above for added emphasis. The following are common indicators for all the types of shock described earlier:

1. Restlessness and anxiety (may precede all other signs)
2. Weak and rapid pulse ("thready" or difficult to feel)
3. Cold and wet skin (commonly described as "clammy")
4. Profuse sweating
5. Paleness and maybe later cyanosis if oxygen delivery to tissues falls sufficiently
6. Shallow, labored, rapid, or possibly irregular or gasping respirations (especially if a chest injury is associated with the development of shock)
7. Dull and lusterless eyes with dilated pupils
8. Thirst
9. Nausea or vomiting
10. Gradual and steadily falling blood pressure. (In general, although some people normally have a systolic blood pressure of only 90 to 100 mm Hg, it is best to assume that shock is developing in any adult whose systolic

blood pressure is 100 millimeters of mercury or lower.)
11. Loss of consciousness in cases of rapidly developing or severe shock

The EMT must remember that although shock means failure of the cardiovascular system to perfuse blood through organs and tissues at proper pressures, the blood pressure is the last measurable parameter to change. Many mechanisms react automatically to help maintain the blood pressure. When a falling blood pressure is observed, shock is far along in development.

TREATMENT OF SHOCK

Any patient who exhibits any of the signs or symptoms of shock should be vigorously treated as soon as the diagnosis is made. Recognizing the probable cause of shock is important so that treatment can be adjusted accordingly. However, many specific principles of initial treatment can be applied to all patients in shock. These principles are listed as follows:

1. Secure and maintain a clear airway and give oxygen as needed. *Do this first before doing anything else.* Be certain the patient can breathe well. Assist or control respirations when appropriate.
2. Control all obvious bleeding by direct compression.
3. Elevate the lower extremities about 12 inches.
4. Splint fractures. Splinting will lessen bleeding and minimize pain and discomfort that can further aggravate shock.
5. Avoid rough and excessive handling.
6. Prevent the loss of body heat by putting blankets under and over the patient. Do not, however, overload the patient with covers or attempt to warm the person unduly.
7. In general, keep an injured patient supine; remember, however, that some patients in shock after a severe heart attack or with lung disease cannot breathe as well when supine as when sitting up or in a semi-sitting position. With such a patient use the most comfortable position.
8. Accurately record the patient's pulse, blood pressure, and other vital signs. Maintain a

record of them at 5-minute intervals until the patient is delivered to the emergency department.

9. Do not give the patient anything to eat or drink.

10. Plan the use of a pneumatic counterpressure device (also called a pneumatic antishock garment) if it is indicated. For those patients in shock from injuries of the pelvis, hips, or femurs or from intraabdominal bleeding, the use of the device may help. Occasionally, when the specific cause of shock is unknown, it may also help. The application, indications for its use, and hazards of this device are discussed in Chapter 10.

It is important for the EMT to observe the patient's breathing. Lack of oxygen may rapidly cause shock. Inadequate ventilation may be either the primary cause or a major contributing factor in shock. Respiratory difficulty may be the result of an easily removed obstruction in the throat or it may require full ventilatory support. The EMT should establish and maintain an open airway and be certain that breathing is adequate. Oxygen should be given to all patients in shock. A few assisted breaths using a ventilatory apparatus with added oxygen will substantially raise the patient's arterial blood oxygen concentration. If the cause of shock is hypovolemia, supplemental oxygen will permit the remaining blood to absorb and transmit a much higher than normal concentration of oxygen. This effect compensates to some degree for the actual loss of oxygen-carrying capacity with volume depletion.

All obvious external bleeding must be controlled. It is best done with sterile gauze compresses placed over the bleeding sites and secured with local circumferential pressure dressings. Sufficient pressure must be applied to stop any bleeding. The use of tourniquets is a last resort. Elevating the lower extremities of the patient allows the blood in the legs to be returned to the heart more rapidly. It is a simple way, after severe hemorrhage, of supplying as much blood to the heart as possible. It should not be attempted if the patient has fractures of the legs unless they are well splinted or the patient is on a spine board.

Fractures must be splinted. Splinting, at this point, is not a definitive treatment for the fracture.

It minimizes the amount of damage the broken ends of bone can do to adjacent soft tissues and thus decreases hemorrhage at the fracture site. In general, splinting makes it easier to move the patient and renders the patient much more comfortable. Some soft tissue injuries may very well be handled best by splinting and occasionally by the use of air splints for compression.

While the loss of body heat should be prevented, the EMT should not try to overwarm the patient. It is better that the patient be slightly cool than too hot. The use of external heat such as hot water bottles or heating pads may harm the person in shock.

Nor should any liquids be given by mouth to the patient in shock. The rule is specifically, *nothing by mouth,* under any circumstances, regardless of the patient's urgent requests. Nothing should be given orally until the patient has been seen in the emergency department by the doctor. Alcoholic drinks (depressants) are never given to treat shock; stimulants such as coffee have little or no value in the treatment of shock. The intense thirst that frequently accompanies shock may be alleviated by allowing the patient to chew or suck on a moistened piece of gauze.

Table 11.1 lists the general supportive measures for the major types of shock. Not every measure is used for every type of shock. The appropriate measures for each type of shock are explained in greater detail in the following sections.

Hypovolemic Shock

The emergency treatment of hypovolemic or hemorrhagic shock includes the control of obvious bleeding after the EMT is sure that the patient can breathe properly. The EMT must be aware that continued bleeding will result from (1) failure to apply sufficient pressure to obvious external bleeding points, (2) failure to splint fractures properly, or (3) failure to handle the injured patient gently. The lower extremities should be elevated by raising the legs from the hips and keeping the knees straight. This maneuver increases blood flow to the heart from the lower body and may combat shock using the patient's own blood to the best advantage. Remember that in a head-down position the entire weight of the abdominal organs falls on the diaphragm. The patient may be unable to breathe easily in this position and may require some assistance with ventilation. The legs should be elevated no more than 12 inches.

TABLE 11.1   General Supportive Measures for Major Causes of Shock

Type of shock	Give supplemental oxygen	Inject epinephrine	Elevate legs 12″	Apply antishock device	Look for other injuries	Transport supine
Hemorrhagic	Yes	No	Yes	Yes	Yes	Yes
Metabolic	Yes	No	Yes	Yes	No	Yes
Neurogenic	Yes	No	Yes	Maybe	Yes	Yes
Psychogenic	Maybe	No	No	No	Yes	Yes
Cardiogenic	Yes	No	No	No	No	No
Septic	Yes	No	Yes	Yes	No	Yes
Respiratory	Yes	No	Maybe	No	Yes	No
Anaphylactic	Yes	Yes	No	No	Maybe	No

The presence of internal hemorrhage is difficult to recognize. On occasion it can be identified when blood passes from the mouth or anus. Nothing can be done in the field to control internal bleeding. The EMT must recognize the existence and severity of internal bleeding and provide vigorous general support. That means being certain that the patient does not, in the instance of bleeding from the mouth, aspirate any vomitus into the lungs. Since so little can be done to control the bleeding itself, the patient must be transported as rapidly as possible to the emergency department.

In instances of hemorrhage about the pelvis, hips, or femurs, within the abdomen, or occasionally of obscure cause, a pneumatic counterpressure device may be very effective to control shock. Its use is described in Chapter 10.

Ventilatory support must be part of the treatment for hypovolemic shock. It may include only assisted ventilation and the use of supplemental oxygen while the patient is being transported to the hospital. It may require full ventilatory support. With too little circulating blood, additional oxygen may be lifesaving. The patient with hypovolemic shock must be taken as promptly as possible to the emergency department for definitive care.

Metabolic Shock

Metabolic shock is usually the result of an illness that has been present for a long time or has been extremely severe over a brief period. It is associated with unusual and excessive losses of fluid from vomiting, diarrhea, or urination. With inadequate food and fluid intake to cover the loss of body water, the patient will become severely dehydrated. This patient must be transported to the hospital as promptly as possible and again given all the support necessary, including oxygen during transport. The EMT should try to find out if any contributory illness such as diabetes or severe gastroenteritis might be present.

Neurogenic Shock

Shock that accompanies spinal cord injury is best treated by a combination of all known supportive measures. The patient who has suffered this kind of injury will ordinarily require hospitalization for a long time. Emergency treatment should be directed at obtaining and maintaining a proper airway, assisting impaired breathing as needed, conserving body heat with blankets, and providing the most effective circulation possible. The patient may not be losing blood, but the capacity of the vessels will become significantly larger than the volume of blood they contain. In this instance, the pneumatic antishock garment may be very useful. This patient will surely require supplemental oxygen so that the blood may carry a greater than normal concentration of this gas. The patient should be kept as warm as possible, since the normal control of body temperature may well be lost with the injury. Prompt transportation to the hospital is mandatory.

Psychogenic Shock

Usually, a common fainting spell will pass very quickly. If the attack has caused the patient to fall, the EMT must be alert for any injury sustained in the fall. The older patient is more likely to sustain such an injury. In the absence of any such injuries, the patient usually recovers promptly. As soon as the patient has fallen, collapsed, or become supine, the blood supply to the brain improves and consciousness returns quickly. If it does not, or if the patient is confused after such a mishap, the EMT must suspect a head injury, particularly if there has been a fall during the fainting spell. In such an instance, prompt transportation to the emergency department is necessary, with the recording of initial observations of vital signs and the level of consciousness, as well as the length of time that the patient was unconscious.

Cardiogenic Shock

The patient in shock as a result of a heart attack specifically *does not* require a transfusion of blood, intravenous fluids, elevation of the legs, or a pneumatic counterpressure device. In this condition, shock results from the heart's inability to handle the volume of blood that the patient already has. The heart muscle simply cannot generate the necessary power to pump the blood through the circulatory system. If chronic obstructive lung disease is associated with this condition, as is frequently the case, oxygenation of the blood passing through the lungs is further decreased. The chronic lung disease will aggravate the cardiogenic shock. This patient is often able to breathe better in a sitting position and may tell the EMT so. The patient should be permitted to sit up in this situation. Usually, these patients do not have any injury, but they have had and may still be having chest pain. The pulse commonly is irregular and may be weak. The blood pressure is low. Cyanosis is frequently present about the lips and underneath the fingernails. The patient may be anxious. Occasionally, patients who have had heart attacks vomit.

These patients should be treated by placing them in the position in which they can breathe most easily, by administering oxygen, by assisting ventilation when necessary, and by transporting them promptly

to the emergency department. Reassurance and a calm demeanor are required in treating them.

Septic Shock

The proper treatment of septic shock requires complex hospital management. If this condition is suspected, the patient must be transported to the hospital as promptly as possible while being given all the general support available. The use of oxygen during transportation is advisable. Ventilatory support may be necessary.

Respiratory Shock

The proper emergency management of shock as a result of inadequate respiration involves the immediate securing and maintaining of an airway. The mouth and throat down to the larynx must be cleared of mucus, vomitus, foreign material, or anything obstructing the air passages. Artificial ventilation, ventilatory aids, and mouth-to-mouth resuscitation may be necessary. Supplemental oxygen should be given. Prompt transportation to the emergency department is mandatory.

Anaphylactic Shock

The only really effective treatment for a severe, acute, allergic reaction is immediate, subcutaneous, intramuscular or intravenous injection of medication to combat the agent causing the reaction. In general, the injection of 0.5 to 1.0 ml of 1:1000 **epinephrine** will alleviate the immediate signs and symptoms of these reactions. Often the patient may know of a specific sensitivity and carry a kit containing epinephrine to combat the reaction. The patient should be assisted in using the epinephrine. The injection may need to be repeated as the signs and symptoms recur or worsen. Frequently, a drug that is a specific counteragent for the compound causing a reaction can be given. This specific treatment must be given by a doctor at a medical facility. Prompt transportation to the emergency department while giving all support possible is necessary. In general, the EMT will be principally concerned in supplying respiratory support and ventilatory assistance. The EMT should also attempt to discover what caused the reaction — was it a drug, an insect bite or sting, or food — and how the agent was received — was it by mouth, by inhalation, or by injection (needle or sting)?

The severity of such reactions can vary greatly. The symptoms may range from mild itching and burning of the skin to generalized edema, profound coma, and rapid death. Because it is often impossible to know at once how severe any reaction may become, the EMT must undertake the most prompt transportation to the emergency department possible and be prepared to give all available supportive measures en route.

YOU ARE THE EMT...

1. Which two organs of the body cannot lack perfusion for more than 4 to 6 minutes? Name three other organs that will be permanently damaged if they are not adequately perfused.
2. What are three basic causes of shock?
3. How does neurogenic shock differ from hypovolemic shock? What is septic shock?
4. What essential substance is the body deprived of in anaphylactic shock? Name four causes of anaphylactic shock.

SECTION 5

INJURIES

12 Injury

OVERVIEW

Injuries are the leading cause of death and disability in the United States among children and young adults. Each year, one person in three sustains an injury that requires medical treatment, and more than 140,000 people die from injuries. In fact, more Americans between the ages of 1 and 34 years die from injuires than from all other diseases combined. Trauma is the leading cause of death up to the age of 44 years, and it causes the loss of more working years of life than do cancer and heart disease combined. As can be seen from these statistics, the EMT will be exposed frequently to patients with injury. Indeed, one out of every eight hospital beds is occupied by a patient who has sustained an injury. Proper prehospital evaluation and care can do much to minimize suffering, long-term disability, and death from trauma.

Chapter 12 begins by defining the mechanisms of injury — that is, how the different forms of energy cause injury to the body. The chapter next describes various patterns of injury and how these injury patterns are related to the environment in which the EMT works. The last part of Chapter 12 discusses the principles of treatment of injuries — the primary survey, assessment of vital signs, stabilization of injuries prior to transport, and recognition of life-threatening symptoms that require immediate transport for treatment.

OBJECTIVES

The objectives of Chapter 12 are to

- define the mechanisms of injury.
- identify the patterns of injury.
- understand the basic principles of the treatment of injury.

MECHANISMS OF INJURY

Injury results from sudden exposure of the body to energy. The energy may be in the form of heat, electricity, or kinetic energy. **Kinetic energy** is energy in action that produces motion. The human body is frequently exposed to high levels of energy that cause permanent, sometimes fatal, damage to it. **Trauma,** another word for injury, is the term frequently used to describe the injury process.

The kinetic energy of an object in motion (such as a car) must be converted from speed into another form of energy when the motion stops. When the motion stops gradually (as when the brakes are applied), the kinetic energy is converted to heat (in the brakes). When the motion stops suddenly (as when the car strikes a wall), the energy of impact deforms the moving object, the object that is struck, or both (Figure 12.1). The human body's tolerance for sudden deformity is very limited. A gentle punch of the fist to the nose will cause the nose to deform temporarily and absorb the energy of impact without permanent damage. A violent punch, however, will cause greater deformity of the tissues of the nose and

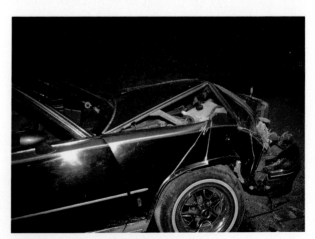

FIGURE 12.1 When the rapid motion of a vehicle suddenly stops, the kinetic energy is converted into deformity of the moving object.

result in permanent damage to them. The tissues will continue to deform until all of the kinetic energy is used up. Thus, tissue damage continues until all of the kinetic energy is spent. In high-energy injuries, several structures may be damaged at the same time.

The amount of kinetic energy that is present in a moving object is proportional to the mass (weight) of the object and to the square of its velocity. The formula

$$\text{Kinetic energy} = MV^2/2$$
$$(\text{where } M = \text{mass and } V = \text{velocity})$$

is used to calculate the kinetic energy of any object. It is this amount of energy that must be absorbed at the moment of impact. The more important factor in this formula is the velocity of the object because the amount of kinetic energy increases dramatically as the object's velocity increases.

The velocity factor is especially significant when considering the wounding potential of firearms. Although larger bullets cause more damage than smaller (less mass) ones, the more important variable is speed. As bullet speed increases, the amount of damage produced increases greatly. For this reason, gunshot wounds are separated into two basic categories: high velocity and low velocity. Bullets traveling at a muzzle velocity greater than 2,000 feet per second cause high-speed injury. The type and amount of tissue damage is much greater than that found in low-speed bullet injuries (Figure 12.2). Because the extent of injury is so different between these two types of gunshot wounds, the surgical treatment for each is different. Therefore, it is essential that the EMT identify the type of firearm used and report this information to the emergency department personnel.

The type of injury that occurs from the impact of kinetic energy also depends on the specific tissue that is being deformed. Soft tissue such as the skin can stretch or deform to some degree and sustain only minor damage. With further deformity, however, soft tissues will be torn apart and permanently damaged. Firmer tissues, such as bone and certain organs that are contained within a firm capsule — for example, the liver and spleen — can resist or absorb small forces. When a large amount of energy is applied, however, these tissues deform and ultimately break apart, causing fracture (bone) or rupture (liver and spleen).

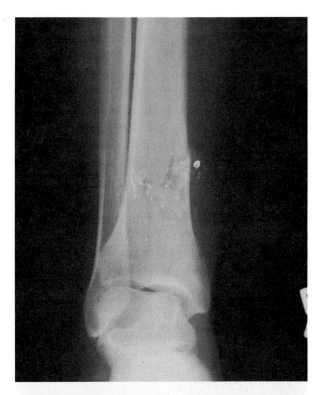

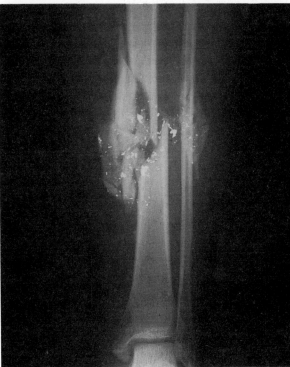

FIGURE 12.2 All gunshot wounds can inflict serious injury, but more injury is produced by high-velocity bullets. The x-ray (top) shows a simple fracture of the tibia produced by a low-velocity bullet wound. A high-velocity bullet (bottom) has caused the tibia to shatter.

Some structures of the body are more susceptible to injury than others. The brain and the spinal cord are especially fragile and vulnerable to injury. They are protected from injury by the surrounding skull, the spinal column, and several layers of soft tissues. The eye is another susceptible structure that lies recessed in the bony eye socket of the skull. The anterior portion of the eye is still vulnerable to injury, and even small forces may cause serious and permanent damage (Figure 12.3).

Forces applied to the body are generally separated into two broad categories: penetrating and blunt. In **penetrating injury,** there is usually a very small point of contact between the skin and the wounding implement. The force of impact is concentrated on this small point, and the wounding object is driven through the skin to produce a **laceration** or cut. When the skin is cut by a penetrating object, the wound produced is called an **open wound.** The penetrating object may only go through the skin or it may pass entirely through the body and exit at some distant site. All structures in its path are vulnerable to injury. Occasionally, the object remains in the body. Such objects are called **impaled foreign objects.** Blood loss from the open wound and the potential for infection resulting from the damage to the protective covering of the skin may create serious problems for the patient.

In **blunt trauma,** the area of contact between the object and the body is large enough so that skin penetration does not occur. However, the force of impact is transmitted through the skin, and the deeper tissues are damaged. Often blood vessels below the skin are sheared from their attachments, which produces bleeding under the skin and into the deeper body tissues. In addition, blunt trauma tends to cause hollow organs to rupture and solid organs to break apart (fracture or rupture).

Not all injury occurs as a result of the body's being struck by a moving object. Significant injury can also occur when the body is in motion and strikes a fixed object. Sudden deceleration or decreased speed occurs at the moment of impact, and both blunt and penetrating injury can result. In addition, specific deceleration injuries can occur because certain parts of the body come to a stop more rapidly than do others. For example, when the head strikes the dashboard in a car wreck, the skull quickly stops moving forward; however, the brain, which floats within the skull, continues to move forward until it strikes the inner surface of the skull. This "second impact" is often the cause of brain injury (Figure 12.4).

A similar phenomenon occurs with certain organs in the chest — the heart and aorta — and in the abdomen — the liver, small intestine, and spleen. Deceleration injury of the internal organs may be fatal, although the severity of such an injury may not be appreciated on initial examination because the

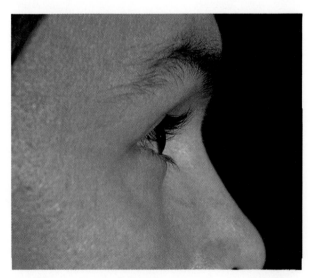

FIGURE 12.3 The eye is recessed in the skull to protect its fragile structures from injury; however, the front of the eye remains exposed and is quite vulnerable.

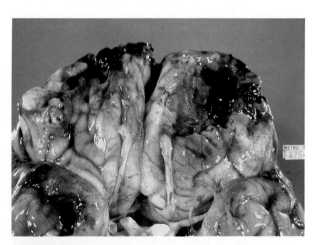

FIGURE 12.4 Sudden deceleration of the skull resulted in fatal brain injury when the brain continued its forward motion and struck the inside of the skull.

outward signs of injury, such as laceration or bruising, may not be great. The critical determinant of the degree of injury is the amount of kinetic energy that was absorbed at the moment of impact. The greater the force of impact, the greater the damage. The EMT must realize the potential for severe and multiple injuries with all high-energy (high-velocity) injuries. Car wrecks, gunshot wounds (especially high-velocity), and falls from heights are just a few examples of these high-energy injuries.

Other mechanisms of bodily injury exist as well. **Crushing injury** implies the application of force to body tissue over relatively long periods of time as opposed to the very short time of blunt and penetrating trauma. In addition to causing some direct soft tissue damage, continued compression of the soft tissues during the crushing will cut off their circulation and produce further tissue destruction. For example, a person whose legs are trapped under a collapsed pile of rocks will continue to suffer tissue damage until the compressing rocks are removed.

Another form of compression injury can result from the tissue damage itself. Whenever tissues are injured, swelling occurs. The cells that are injured leak watery fluid (**edema fluid**) into the spaces between the cells, which produces a local increase in size of the tissues. Swelling is the commonest response to injury. If the swelling is excessive or if it occurs in a confined space such as the skull, the tissue pressure will increase to dangerous levels. The pressure of the edema fluid may become great enough to compress the tissue and cause further damage, particularly if the blood vessels become compressed, cutting off the flow of blood to the tissue. Excessive swelling often follows injury of the brain, the spinal cord, and the extremities.

There are many different mechanisms of injury, and several factors determine the extent and severity of the injury produced. The amount of kinetic energy absorbed, the degree of tissue deformity and displacement, and the particular tissue injured are three important variables that the EMT must consider when evaluating an injured patient.

PATTERNS OF INJURY

The EMT will come in contact with a wide spectrum of injury and must be prepared to deal with many different types of trauma. However, the frequency of exposure to specific types of injury will be directly related to the environment in which the EMT works, because certain specific types of injury are more common in certain settings. For example, a great contrast is evident when comparing the types of injury commonly seen in urban and rural environments.

The EMT who works in a large city will respond to a great many injuries resulting from personal assaults with weapons such as knives and guns — injuries rarely seen in the rural environment. In addition, the urban EMT must be prepared to deal with patients injured in construction and industrial accidents. In contrast, in the rural setting the EMT will respond to a large number of agricultural accidents that are virtually unique to that environment. Such injuries may result from heavy farm machinery accidents, augers, corn pickers, combines, and many other specialized pieces of farm equipment (Figure 12.5). Silos and grain elevators present special dangers to both the injured patient and to rescue personnel, especially those unfamiliar with the potential for such hazards.

Other environments also present unique and unusual potentials for injury. EMTs who work near large bodies of water, particularly those used for recreational purposes, will respond to many different

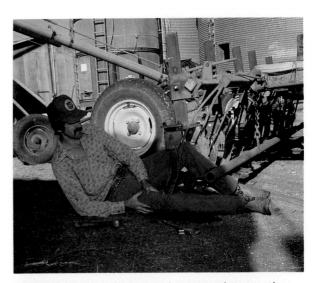

FIGURE 12.5 Certain injuries are unique to the environment in which they occur. For example, specialized farm equipment can cause unusual injuries and difficult extrication problems.

types of water-related injuries that range in severity from sunburn to drowning.

Because of the specialized nature of the injuries common to certain environments, it is essential that EMTs become familiar with the common patterns of injury seen in their particular locale. Furthermore, EMTs may have to develop specialized rescue and treatment skills to facilitate the management of environment-related injuries. For example, in rural areas, the EMT must become familiar with the unique injuries that farm machinery can cause and the specialized rescue and extrication techniques that these injury situations call for. Books, courses, and other instructional materials are available to prepare EMTs for this specialized type of work. As a general principle, all EMTs must become familiar with the injury patterns common in their area and be prepared to deal with them before training is completed.

PRINCIPLES OF TREATMENT OF INJURY

Because the EMT is so often called to evaluate and treat injuries, all EMTs must understand the basic principles of injury care. As with other emergencies, evaluating an injured person begins with the primary survey of airway, breathing, and circulation. One or more of these critical body functions is often impaired following injury. Prompt restoration of the airway, breathing, and circulation must therefore be the top priority in the care of any injured patient.

The second step in the general management of a patient who has been injured is to assess the vital signs. The injury frequently results in bleeding of the damaged tissues, and significant bleeding will result in tachycardia and hypotension. Injuries of the head, neck, and chest can interfere with the normal mechanisms of breathing. Many other injuries may also affect the vital functions and alter the vital signs. Thus, an initial assessment of the vital signs must be carried out in all injured patients. The vital signs must then be monitored at least every 15 minutes until the patient reaches the hospital. More frequent observations are needed in the seriously injured patient who has unstable vital signs.

Rapid deterioration of one or more of the vital signs is seen frequently in the severely injured patient. Initially, many patients are able to compensate for blood loss or moderate respiratory insuffi-

ciency. During this early phase, the vital signs are maintained near normal levels. However, with significant injury the compensatory mechanisms eventually fail, and the vital signs and vital functions deteriorate rapidly. That is why it is essential for the EMT to continue to monitor the vital signs in all injured patients in anticipation of the possibility of significant rapid deterioration. After evaluating the vital signs, a careful history of the injury, combined with a thorough secondary assessment, will help identify the areas of injury that need stabilization prior to transport.

Pain and loss of function usually accompany injury. Any patient who complains of pain should be considered as having a significant injury deserving a thorough evaluation. Because injury also frequently results in a loss of function of a specific organ or body part — for example, difficulty in breathing, double vision, or inability to bend the elbow — any complaint of loss of function should result in a complete, in-hospital evaluation.

The absence of these complaints does not mean that the patient has not sustained a significant injury. Obviously, the unconscious injured patient will not complain at all. In addition, sometimes the pain of a severe injury will be so great that the patient does not realize that he or she has sustained another equally serious, yet less painful, injury. Therefore, a secondary survey of all injured persons must be carried out to identify these common signs of injury:

1. Tenderness
2. Swelling
3. Ecchymosis
4. Deformity
5. Loss of function

Gentle palpation of the trunk and extremities is designed to identify areas of tenderness following injury. Frequently, more than one injury site may be present. A careful examination will reveal all points of injury and enable the EMT to set priorities for treatment.

Swelling, as described earlier, is a very common, nonspecific sign of injury. Damaged cells leak edema fluid very soon after injury. Massive swelling may occur as a result of damage to blood vessels and bleeding into the soft tissues. Thus, swelling is one of the earliest and most consistent signs of injury.

Ecchymosis (bruising or discoloration of the tissues) is caused by damage to blood vessels. Blood from the damaged vessels leaks into the area of injury and gives a blue or blue-black discoloration to the tissues.

When a force is applied to body tissues, they deform in an attempt to absorb the energy of impact. All tissues can deform to some degree without sustaining permanent damage. With excessive force, however, tissue damage and deformity occur. Deformity is readily seen in many fractured limbs as well as in soft tissues such as the skin that have been stretched or torn beyond their limits.

The patient often complains of a loss of function of a specific body part, and this loss may also be observed by the EMT. For example, impaired breathing following a chest injury can frequently be seen by the careful observer. Such observations are especially important in patients who for one reason or another are unable to express complaints about pain and loss of function.

With specific injuries, other specific symptoms and signs will be present. The subsequent chapters in this section detail these particular findings. A careful assessment of the patient's vital signs, symptoms, and physical signs will enable the EMT to evaluate the patient's condition and set priorities for treatment. In general, after the airway, breathing, and circulation have been secured, isolated injuries should be stabilized and the patient transported to the hospital for definitive treatment. In most cases, stabilizing the injury in the field will allow the patient to be transported in an efficient yet safe manner.

In rare circumstances, particularly with the multiply injured patient, it is not practical and sometimes not possible to achieve stable vital functions in the field. In this situation, delay in the field only serves to further decrease the patient's chances for survival. It has been said that with the severely injured patient there is a "golden hour" after the time of injury. It is during this hour that the patient must reach a trauma center where a team fully equipped and trained to treat severe injury can provide definitive care. Excessive delays in the field use up critical minutes for these severely injured patients. It should be emphasized, however, that most trauma patients can be stabilized in the field; less than 5 percent require immediate transport to the hospital with time only being taken to restore an airway, control obvious bleeding, stabilize the spine, and provide oxygen and ventilatory support en route.

Recently, several trauma scales have been developed to help the EMT in the field assess the severity of the injury and objectively identify those patients with injuries severe enough to require immediate and rapid transport to the hospital. The scales use the objective measurements of vital signs, level of consciousness, and specific sites of injury to give a severity of injury rating to the patient. The use of these trauma scales is discussed further in Chapter 45. In general, when treating a severely, multiply injured patient, the EMT should report all medical observations promptly to medical control for specific guidance regarding the extent of care to be provided in the field prior to transport.

The following chapters in this section describe the specific injuries that the EMT will encounter. The principles of evaluation and field stabilization are presented in detail for each of the areas of the body.

YOU ARE THE EMT...

1. You are responding to a gunshot injury. Why is it important for you to know the muzzle velocity of the weapon that inflicted the injury?
2. Explain how an accident or set of circumstances can simultaneously cause blunt injury and penetrating injury.
3. Your cousin works for a rural EMS, and you work for an urban EMS. You are having a "friendly argument" about who has the hardest job. What examples will you give of "difficult" city situations? What kind of situations do you think your cousin will describe? What problems do you both share?
4. What five common signs of injury should you look for during the secondary survey? Which of these signs can be detected in an unconscious person?

13

Soft Tissue Injury

ANATOMY AND PHYSIOLOGY OF THE SKIN

The skin, the largest single organ in the body, serves three major functions: (1) to protect the body in the environment, (2) to regulate the temperature of the body, and (3) to transmit information from the environment to the brain. The protective functions of the skin are numerous. Over 70 percent of the body is composed of water. The water contains a delicate balance of chemical substances in solution. The skin is watertight and serves to keep this balanced internal solution intact. The skin also protects the body from the invasion of infectious organisms — bacteria, viruses, and fungi. These organisms are everywhere and are routinely found lying on the skin surface and deep in its grooves and glands; they never, however, penetrate the skin. Germs cannot pass through the skin unless it is broken by injury; thus, the skin provides a constant protection against outside invaders.

The energy of the body is derived from chemical reactions (**metabolism**) that must take place within a very narrow temperature range. If the body temperature is too low, these reactions cannot proceed, metabolism ceases, and the body dies. If the temperature becomes too high, the rate of metabolism will increase. Dangerously high temperatures from too high a metabolic rate can result in permanent tissue damage and death.

The major organ for regulation of body temperature is the skin. Blood vessels in the skin constrict when the body is in a cold environment and dilate when the body is in a warm environment. In a cold environment, constriction of the blood vessels shunts the blood away from the skin to decrease the amount of heat radiated from the body surface. When the outside environment is hot, the vessels in the skin dilate, the skin becomes flushed or red, and heat radiates from the body surface. Also, in the hot environment, sweat is secreted to the skin surface from the sweat glands. Evaporation of the sweat requires energy. This energy, as body heat, is taken from the body during the evaporation process, which causes the body temperature to fall. Sweating alone will not reduce body temperature. Evaporation of the sweat must also occur.

Information from the environment is carried to the brain through a rich supply of sensory nerves that originate in the skin. Nerve endings that lie in the skin are adapted to perceive and transmit information about heat, cold, external pressure, pain, and the position of the body in space. The skin thus recognizes any changes in the environment. The skin also reacts to pressure on a portion of the body, pain, and pleasurable stimuli.

The skin is divided into two parts: the superficial epidermis, which is composed of several layers of cells, and the deeper dermis, which contains the specialized skin structures. Below the skin lies the subcutaneous layer of fat (Figure 13.1a). The cells of the **epidermis** are sealed to form a watertight protective covering for the body (Figure 13.1b).

The epidermis is actually composed of several layers of cells. At the base of the epidermis is the germinal layer, which continuously produces new cells that gradually rise to the surface. On the way to the surface these cells die and form the watertight covering. The epidermal cells are held together securely by an oily substance called **sebum,** which is secreted by the **sebaceous glands** of the dermis. The outermost cells of the epidermis are constantly rubbed away and then replaced by new cells produced by the germinal layer. The deeper cells in the germinal layer also contain pigment granules that (along with the blood vessels lying in the dermis) produce skin color.

The epidermis varies in thickness in different areas of the body. On the soles of the feet, the back, and the scalp it is quite thick, but in some areas of the body the epidermis is only 2 or 3 cell layers in thickness. The watertight seal provided by the epidermis prevents the invasion of bacteria and other organisms.

The deeper part of skin, the **dermis,** is separated from the epidermis by the layer of germinal cells. Within the dermis lie many of the special structures of the skin: sweat glands, sebaceous (oil) glands, hair follicles, blood vessels, and specialized nerve endings.

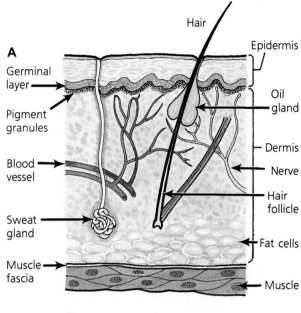

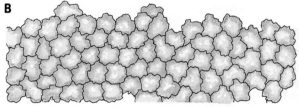

FIGURE 13.1 (a) The skin has two layers, the epidermis and the dermis. All of the major structures lie in the dermis. A layer of subcutaneous fat lies below the dermis. (b) Cells of the epidermis are fitted closely together on the skin surface to form a watertight protective layer.

Sweat glands produce sweat for cooling the body. The sweat is discharged onto the surface of the skin through small pores or ducts that pass through the epidermis onto the skin surface. The sebaceous glands produce sebum, the oily material that seals the surface epidermal cells. The sebaceous glands lie next to hair follicles and secrete sebum along the hair follicle to the skin surface. In addition to providing waterproofing for the skin, sebum keeps the skin supple so that it does not crack.

Hair follicles are the small organs that produce hair. There is one follicle for each hair connected with a sebaceous gland and also with a tiny muscle. The muscle serves to pull the hair into an erect position when the individual is cold or frightened. All hair grows continuously and is either cut off or worn away by clothing.

Blood vessels provide nutrients and oxygen to the skin. The blood vessels lie in the dermis. Small branches extend up to the germinal layer (there are no blood vessels in the epidermis). A complex array of nerve endings also lie in the dermis. These specialized nerve endings are sensitive to environmental stimuli: They respond to these stimuli and send impulses along the nerves to the brain.

Beneath the skin, immediately under the dermis and attached to it, lies the subcutaneous tissue. The **subcutaneous tissue** is largely composed of fat. The fat serves as an insulator for the body and as a reservoir for the storage of energy. The amount of subcutaneous tissue varies greatly from individual to individual. Beneath the subcutaneous tissue lie the muscles and the skeleton.

The skin covers all of the external surface of the body. The various openings to the body (mouth, nose, anus, and vagina) are not covered by skin. Called **orifices,** these openings are lined with mucous membranes (Figure 13.2). **Mucous membranes** are quite similar to skin in that they provide a protective barrier against bacterial invasion. Mucous membranes differ from skin in that they secrete **mucus,** a watery substance that lubricates the openings. Thus, mucous membranes are moist whereas the skin is dry. A mucous membrane lines the entire gastrointestinal tract from the mouth to the anus.

SOFT TISSUE INJURIES

Because the soft tissues are the first line of defense against most injuries, they are often damaged. Soft tissue injuries or wounds are divided into two types: closed and open. A **closed wound** is one in which soft tissue damage occurs beneath the skin or mucous membrane surface, but the surface remains intact. An **open wound** is one in which there is a break in the surface of the skin or the mucous membrane that lines the major body openings.

Closed Soft Tissue Injuries

Contusions and Hematomas

A blunt object that strikes the body will crush the tissue beneath the skin. This injury is called a **contusion,** or more commonly, a bruise. The epidermis remains intact. Damage beneath the epidermis will extend to varying depths, depending on the force of injury. In the dermis, cells are damaged and small blood vessels are usually torn. Varying amounts of edema fluid and blood leak into the damaged area. This leakage of edema fluid and blood produces swelling and pain. As blood accumulates in the damaged area, a characteristic discoloration occurs. Usually the discoloration is black or blue and is called an **ecchymosis** (Figure 13.3).

When large amounts of tissue are damaged beneath the outer layer of the skin, large blood vessels may tear and cause rapid bleeding. A pool of blood called a **hematoma** will collect within the damaged

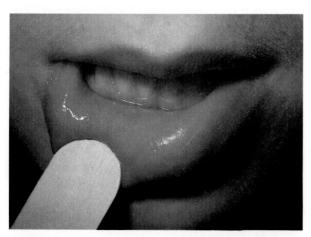

FIGURE 13.2 All body openings are lined with mucous membranes. Just like the skin, these membranes prevent the invasion of bacteria into the body. They secrete a watery mucus for lubrication and moisture.

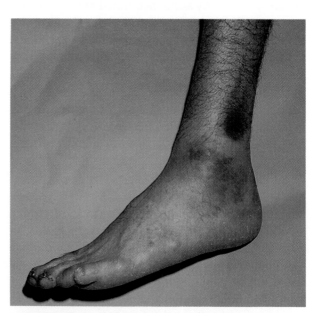

FIGURE 13.3 A closed soft tissue injury — a contusion — is characterized by swelling and ecchymosis.

tissue. Hematomas are literally blood tumors, and they will occur whenever large blood vessels are damaged. Their occurrence is not limited to soft tissue injuries; they can also occur following fractures or when blood vessels to any organ in the body are damaged. When a large bone such as the femur or pelvis fractures, the hematoma that forms may contain more than a liter of blood.

Closed soft tissue injuries are characterized by a history of injury, pain at the site of injury, swelling beneath the skin, and ecchymosis. They may be mild or quite extensive.

Management of Closed Soft Tissue Injuries

Small bruises require no special emergency medical care. With more extensive closed injuries, swelling and bleeding beneath the skin can be extensive and may even result in hypovolemic shock. The EMT can control bleeding and swelling in the deep soft tissues to some degree by applying ice and local compression immediately following the injury. Ice or cold packs will cause the blood vessels to constrict, which will slow the bleeding. Firm manual compression over the area of injury will compress the blood vessels and also decrease bleeding. Immobilizing the soft tissue injury with a splint is another way to decrease bleeding. In addition, application of cold packs and splinting decrease the patient's pain. Elevating the injured part to a level just above the level of the patient's heart decreases the amount of swelling in the region. Therefore, when treating a patient with a closed soft tissue injury, the EMT can think of ICES (ice, compression, elevation, and splinting) to remember the four steps in treatment.

Many closed soft tissue injuries are so severe that they cause fracture or injury to other important deeper structures. At times it is difficult to estimate the degree of injury to the deeper structures. Therefore, all closed soft tissue injuries should be treated with the immediate application of cold and then compression, elevation, and splinting as discussed in Chapter 15.

Open Soft Tissue Wounds

Open soft tissue wounds differ from closed wounds in that the protective skin layer is damaged. This damage can result in more extensive bleeding.

More importantly, however, once the protective skin layer has been violated, the wound becomes contaminated and may become infected. These two additional problems must be addressed in the treatment of open soft tissue wounds.

There are four types of open soft tissue wounds: abrasions, lacerations, avulsions, and puncture wounds (Figure 13.4).

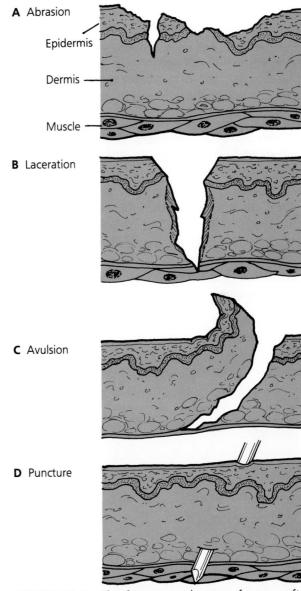

FIGURE 13.4 The four general types of open soft tissue injuries: (a) Abrasions involve variable depths of the dermis and epidermis. (b) Lacerations are cuts produced by sharp objects. (c) Avulsions raise flaps of tissue, usually along normal tissue planes. (d) Puncture wounds may penetrate to any depth.

Types of Open Soft Tissue Wounds

Abrasion. An **abrasion** is the loss of a portion of the epidermis and part of the dermis as a result of the skin being rubbed or scraped across a rough or hard surface. Blood may ooze from the injured capillary blood vessels in the dermis, but the abrasion usually does not penetrate completely through the dermis. Extremely painful, abrasions are known by a variety of common names: road burn, strawberry, and mat burn, to name a few (Figure 13.5).

Laceration. A **laceration** is a cut produced by a sharp object. The cutting object may leave a smooth or jagged wound through the skin and may penetrate into the subcutaneous tissue, the underlying muscles, and the associated nerves and blood vessels (Figure 13.6).

Avulsion. An **avulsion** is an injury in which a piece of skin is either torn completely loose from all of its attachments or is left hanging as a flap. Avulsed tissues ordinarily separate at normal anatomical planes, usually between the subcutaneous tissue and the muscle fascia. Usually there is significant bleeding from the bed of the wound. If the avulsed part remains attached only by a small pedicle of skin, the circulation to the flap may be in jeopardy (Figure 13.7).

Puncture Wound. A **puncture wound** results from a stab with a knife, ice pick, splinter, or any other pointed object or from a bullet. External bleeding from a puncture wound is usually not severe

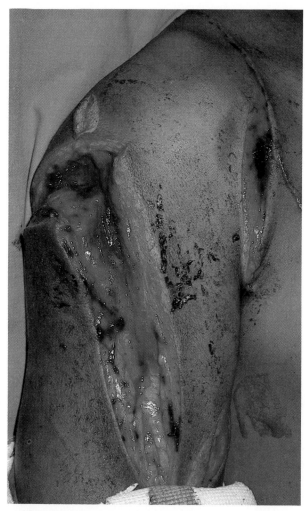

FIGURE 13.6 A laceration of the skin and subcutaneous tissue. The fascia covering the muscle is seen in the depths of the wounds.

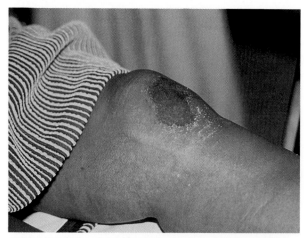

FIGURE 13.5 An abrasion of the skin. Blood is oozing from the damaged capillaries of the dermis.

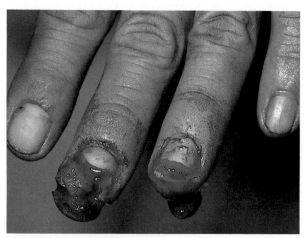

FIGURE 13.7 An avulsion attached only by a small pedicle of skin.

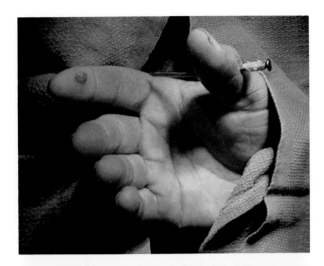

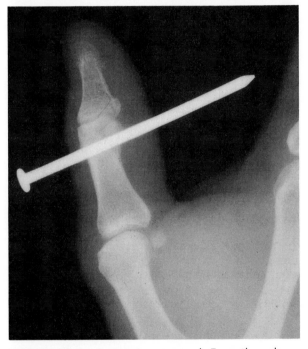

FIGURE 13.8 A puncture wound. Even though the entrance wound is small and the external bleeding is not severe, damage to the internal structures may be serious.

because the entrance wound is relatively small (Figure 13.8). However, the wounding object may injure structures deep within the body and cause rapid, fatal bleeding if the wound occurs in the chest or abdomen. Assessing the amount of damage sustained from a puncture wound is very difficult. Some puncture wounds, especially those in the extremities, may traverse the entire limb and exit on the opposite side. These are called **perforating (through**

and through) wounds. The EMT should always look for and note an exit wound, especially in the case of gunshot injury.

Management of Open Wounds

Initially, it is imperative to assess the extent and severity of the soft tissue wound. A complete assessment can be accomplished only by removing any clothing that is covering the wound. Usually it is better to tear or cut the clothing away from the wound rather than attempt to remove it in a normal manner because excessive motion of the injured part will cause pain and possibly additional tissue damage. Even when cutting or tearing the clothing, the EMT should remove it with as little movement of the patient as possible. What may seem an insignificant motion to the EMT may cause excruciating pain for the patient.

Once the wound is clear of any clothing, its severity can be assessed and treatment begun. Three general rules govern the management of open soft tissue wounds: (1) control bleeding, (2) prevent further contamination, and (3) immobilize the part.

With open wounds, the amount of bleeding may be extensive and severe. The first priority in the emergency management of an open wound is to control the bleeding by applying a dry sterile compression dressing to the entire wound. Initially, pressure is applied to the dressing by the hand of the EMT. Continued pressure is then maintained by firmly applying a roller bandage to the injured part. If bleeding continues or recurs, the original dressing should be left in place and a second dressing should be applied and secured with an additional roller bandage. Once the bleeding is controlled, the dressing is held in place with a splint (Figure 13.9).

All open wounds are contaminated. **Contamination** occurs as soon as the protective covering of the skin or mucous membrane is broken. Once contaminated, the wound is at risk for infection. It is impossible to sterilize a wound in the prehospital setting. The EMT, however, can prevent further contamination of an open wound by applying a dry, sterile dressing. This will help keep foreign matter such as hair, clothing, and dirt out of the wound and decrease the risk of secondary infection. However, in the initial management of open wounds, the EMT should not try to remove material in the wound no matter how dirty it may be. Rubbing, brushing, or

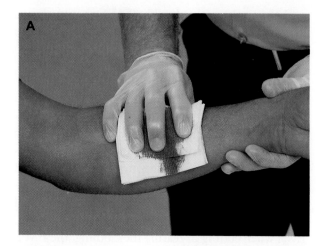

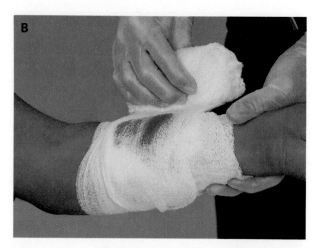

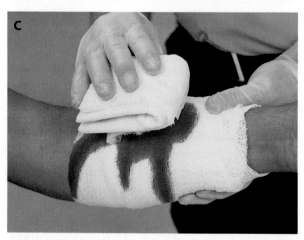

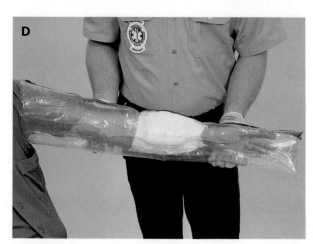

FIGURE 13.9 (a) Bleeding from an open wound is first controlled by manual pressure applied to a dry sterile dressing. (b) The dressing can be held in place by a circular pressure bandage. (c) If bleeding continues, an additional layer of compression dressing should be applied to the first dressing. (d) A splint is used to hold the dressing in place.

washing an open wound will only cause further bleeding. Cleansing of the wound is a procedure for the surgeon to carry out in the hospital.

Frequently, the control of bleeding from soft tissue wounds, whether or not they are associated with a fracture, is improved by splinting the extremity. Splinting will also help the patient feel more comfortable. In addition, splinting facilitates movement of the patient, thus minimizing further damage to an already injured arm or leg. Therefore, an initial step in the control of soft tissue bleeding is appropriate splinting to immobilize the injured part.

To summarize the treatment of open soft tissue injuries, the wound must be thoroughly inspected and then covered with a dry, sterile compression dressing to control bleeding and prevent further contamination. Once bleeding is controlled by compression, the limb should be splinted to further control bleeding, stabilize the injured part, minimize the patient's pain, and facilitate the patient's transport to the hospital. As with closed soft tissue injuries, the injured part should be elevated to just above the level of the patient's heart to minimize swelling.

Management of Avulsion Injuries

When a flap of skin has been partially avulsed, the circulation to the skin flap is jeopardized. The blood supply must come through the pedicle of the

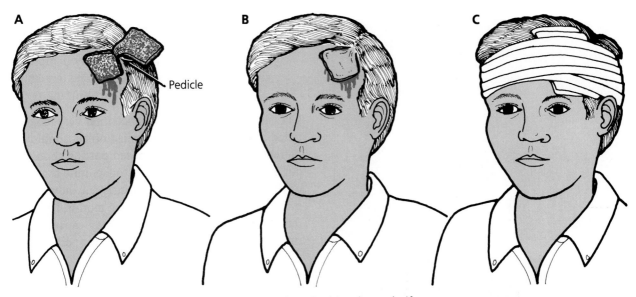

FIGURE 13.10 (a) An avulsed flap of skin may lose its blood supply if the pedicle attachment is kinked or twisted. (b) The flap should be carefully restored to a more normal position. (c) A compression dressing is then applied.

flap, which may be kinked if the flap is folded back on itself and not lying as it should. If compression is applied to the flap in this abnormal position, the blood vessels may be compressed and further diminish blood supply to the flap. Any partially avulsed flap of skin should be folded back onto the wound so that it is aligned normally. Once the flap has been replaced into its bed, a dry, sterile compression dressing should be placed over it (Figure 13.10).

If the avulsion is complete, meaning that it has produced an amputated piece of soft tissue, the avulsed or amputated part should be collected and taken to the emergency department along with the patient. The EMT may encounter persons who have had avulsion injuries of small or large pieces of skin or who have lost portions or all of an extremity. It is now often possible to replace or reimplant these totally avulsed tissues. Therefore, the avulsed part should be wrapped in sterile gauze and placed in a plastic bag. The bag should be placed in a cool container. The tissue, however, should not be allowed to freeze (Figure 13.11).

Management of Impaled Foreign Object

Occasionally, following a puncture wound the object (knife, splinter, or piece of glass) will remain in the wound (Figure 13.12). It is called an **impaled**

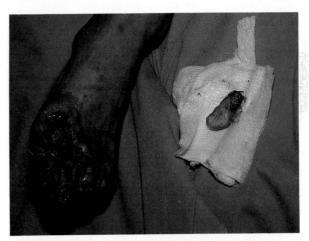

FIGURE 13.11 Amputated body parts should be saved, wrapped in a dry sterile gauze, placed in a plastic bag, kept cool, and transported with the patient to the hospital.

foreign object. In addition to controlling local bleeding, the EMT must follow three rules in treating a patient who has an impaled foreign object in a wound:

1. Do not move or remove the object. Any motion may cause damage to nerves, blood vessels, or muscles lying close to the object. Try to stop any bleeding from the entrance wound

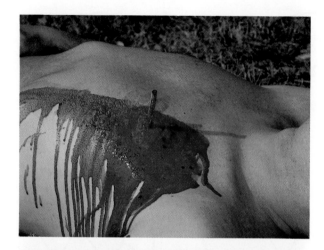

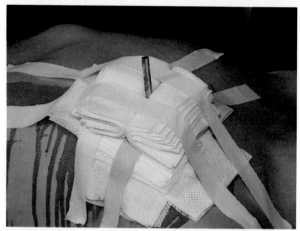

FIGURE 13.12 An impaled foreign object should be left in place and secured with a stabilizing dressing.

by applying direct pressure but avoid exerting any force on the impaled object or on any tissue directly adjacent to its cutting edge. The only time that an impaled object should be removed is when that object lies in the upper airway and causes obstruction of the airway. In this circumstance, the need to restore the airway should cause greater concern than the problems produced by removal of the foreign body.

2. Use a bulky dressing to stabilize the object. Any motion of the impaled object will cause further soft tissue damage. The impaled foreign body itself should be incorporated within the dressing so that its motion after the bandage is applied is minimized or eliminated.

3. Transport the patient promptly to the emergency department with the object still in place. Ordinarily, the patient will need an operation to remove the object and to examine the tissues immediately surrounding it.

Occasionally, the EMT will encounter very long impaled objects. Again, the impaled object should not be removed. Rather, the exposed portion should be cut off — that is, shortened — to facilitate transport of the patient. Before the object is cut, however, it must be secured to minimize any motion transmitted to the patient. Such motion may cause further internal damage and, most certainly, pain for the patient.

Management of Gunshot Wounds

Gunshot wounds are a form of puncture wound that have some unique characteristics that require special prehospital care. The degree of damage from a gunshot wound is directly proportional to the square of the velocity of the bullet. Thus, high-velocity gunshot wounds produce far more severe damage than low-velocity wounds. It is important for the EMT to try to find out what type of gun was used to inflict the wound. This information can be of great help to the physicians attending the patient who has sustained a gunshot wound.

Frequently, gunshot wounds are multiple. The EMT must inspect the patient carefully to identify the number and sites of the bullet wounds. Sometimes the patient or others at the scene will know how many rounds were fired, and careful inspection of the patient will reveal how many wounds are present. This information will also be of significant use to the emergency department physicians in their care of the patient.

Usually, the wound of entrance is smaller than the wound of exit when a through-and-through bullet wound occurs. Often the patient will have a small entrance wound on the anterior aspect of the body and a large exit wound on the opposite side. The EMT must look carefully for the exit wound. Because of its size, an exit wound may be bleeding excessively and yet not be as readily apparent as the entrance wound. In addition to being smaller in size, an entrance wound that is sustained at close range will have powder burns around its edges (Figure 13.13).

Careful recording of the circumstances of injury, the status of the patient, and the treatment given is most important with gunshot wounds because most will involve litigation at some future date. The EMT may be called by the court to testify regarding conditions at the scene and any treatment that was administered. Only a carefully written record will be of use to the EMT.

GENERAL PRINCIPLES OF THE APPLICATION OF DRESSINGS AND BANDAGES

All wounds require bandaging. In most instances splints will also be used to help control bleeding or provide firm support for the dressing. There are many different types of dressings and bandages, and the EMT should be familiar with their functions and their proper application. Dressings and bandages have three major functions: to control bleeding, to protect a wound from further damage, and to prevent further contamination of the open wound.

Sterile Dressings

All ambulances must carry sterile dressings. Universal dressings, conventional 4″ × 4″ and 4″ × 8″ gauze pads, an assortment of small adhesive-type dressings, and soft self-adherent roller dressings will provide coverage for most wounds (Figure

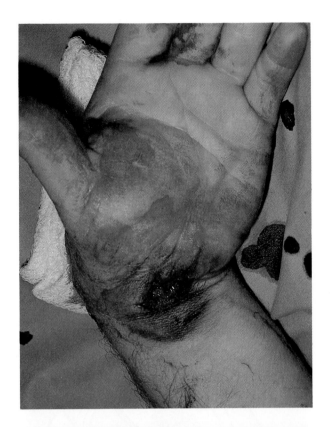

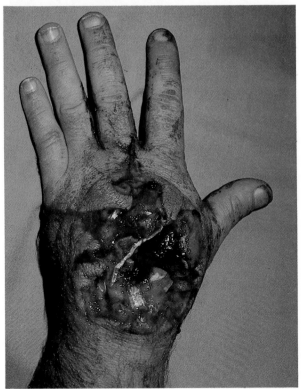

FIGURE 13.13 A close-range gunshot wound. Note the powder burns around the smaller entrance wound and the large wound of exit.

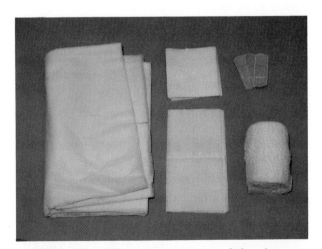

FIGURE 13.14 The standard types of dressings carried in an ambulance: universal dressings; conventional 4″ × 4″ and 4″ × 8″ gauze pads; small adhesive-type dressings; and soft self-adherent roller dressings.

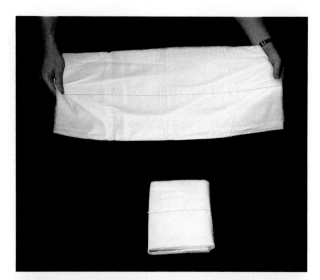

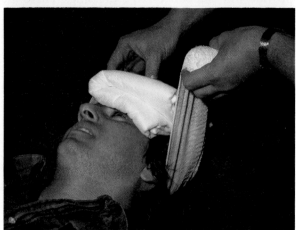

FIGURE 13.15 The universal dressing (top) can be folded to fit almost any large-size wound. It is held in place (bottom) by a self-adherent roller dressing.

13.14). A **universal dressing** is made of thick, absorbent material. It measures 9″ × 36″ and is packed folded into a compact size (Figure 13.15). These dressings are available commercially in sterilized packages. The universal dressing material can also be purchased in long 20-yard rolls that can be cut into 3-foot lengths, packaged, and sterilized for use. The universal dressing provides ideal coverage for large open wounds, and the smaller gauze pads should be utilized for less extensive wounds. The universal dressing is also an efficient pad for rigid splints.

Dressings must remain in place during transport. The stability of the dressing can be provided by soft roller bandages, rolls of gauze, triangular bandages,

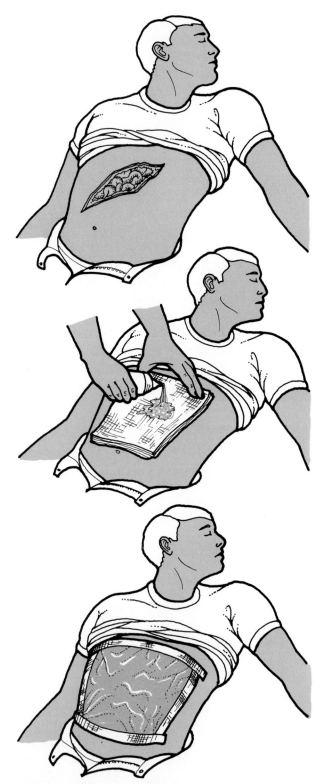

FIGURE 13.16 An abdominal evisceration is kept moist with a universal dressing soaked with sterile normal saline. The moistened dressing is sealed with aluminum foil securely taped on all sides to the skin of the abdomen.

or adhesive tape. The self-adherent soft roller bandages are probably easiest to use. They are slightly elastic, which makes them easy to apply. The layers adhere somewhat to one another, and the end of the roll can be tucked back into a deeper layer to secure it in place. Adhesive tape holds small bandages in place and helps secure larger dressings. Some people, however, are allergic to adhesive tape; paper or plastic tape should be used for these patients. Elastic bandages should not be used to secure dressings. With swelling, the elastic bandage may act as a tourniquet on an injured limb and cause further damage. Dressings should never interfere with circulation to the limb. The EMT should always check a limb distal to a dressing after it is applied for signs of impaired circulation or loss of skin sensation.

Occlusive Dressings

Occlusive dressings are used for **sucking chest wounds** and **abdominal eviscerations.** A sucking chest wound must be sealed so that air does not pass through it. The wound can be occluded by vaseline gauze, sterile aluminum foil, or other impermeable dressings that will block the passage of air. A large enough dressing must be used so that the dressing itself will not be sucked into the chest cavity. The dressing should be taped to the chest wall to keep it in place.

Abdominal eviscerations must be kept moist. Occlusive dressings serve this purpose best. Exposed abdominal organs should be covered with a moistened universal dressing. The universal dressing is then covered with sterile aluminum foil that is taped to the abdomen. This dressing will keep the exposed abdominal contents moist and prevent further contamination (Figure 13.16).

YOU ARE THE EMT...

1. Your patient has a closed soft tissue injury in her leg. Describe the four steps you will follow in treating it.
2. You know that lacerations and puncture wounds both may penetrate to any depth. What, then, is the difference between a laceration and a puncture wound?
3. Open soft tissue wounds are automatically contaminated and you should cover them to prevent further contamination. When do you use dry sterile dressings and when do you use occlusive dressings?
4. Is a gunshot wound considered an open soft tissue wound, a closed soft tissue wound, or both? Why? Why is it important that you find out what caliber of gun caused the injury?

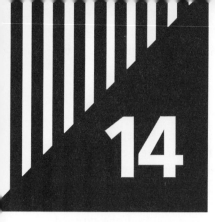

14

The Musculoskeletal System

OVERVIEW

The human body is a well-designed system whose form, upright posture, and movement are provided by the musculoskeletal system. As its combination form suggests, the term *musculoskeletal* refers to the bones and voluntary muscles of the body. The musculoskeletal system also protects the vital internal organs of the body. It is susceptible to external forces, however, that can cause injury. And more than muscles and bones are at risk. The tendons that attach muscles to bones, the joints that form whenever two bones come into contact, and the ligaments that hold the bone ends of a joint together all are susceptible to injury.

The EMT is expected to understand the basic anatomy of the body's skeletal system. Although muscles are technically soft tissue, they are considered in this chapter because of their close anatomic and functional relationship to the skeleton. Chapter 14 thus begins with a description of the three basic types of muscles. The rest of the chapter focuses on the anatomy of the skeleton.

OBJECTIVES

The objectives of Chapter 14 are to

- describe the three types of muscle found in the human body: skeletal muscle, smooth muscle, and cardiac muscle.
- be able to name and locate the major bones of the body.

MUSCLE

Muscles are a form of tissue that allows body movement. Although there are more than 600 muscles in the human body, they are generally divided into three types: skeletal, smooth, and cardiac.

Skeletal Muscle

Skeletal muscle forms the major muscle mass of the body. It is called skeletal muscle because it attaches to the bones of the skeleton. It is also called **voluntary muscle** because all skeletal muscle is under direct voluntary control of the brain and can be stimulated to contract or relax at will. Skeletal muscle is also called **striated muscle** because it has characteristic stripes (striations) when viewed under the microscope. All bodily movement results from skeletal muscle contraction or relaxation. Usually, a specific motion is the result of several muscles contracting and relaxing simultaneously.

All skeletal muscles are supplied with arteries, veins, and nerves (Figure 14.1). Arterial blood brings oxygen and nutrients to the muscle, and the veins carry away the waste products of muscular contraction (carbon dioxide and water). Muscles cannot function without this ongoing supply of oxygen and nutrients and removal of waste products. Muscle cramps result when insufficient oxygen or food is carried to the muscle or when acidic waste products accumulate and are not carried away.

Skeletal muscle is under the direct control of the nervous system and responds to a command from the brain to move a specific body part. Specific nerves pass directly from the brain to the spinal cord. There they connect with other nerves that exit from the spinal cord and pass to each skeletal muscle. Electrical impulses are carried from the cells in the brain and spinal cord along the **peripheral nerves** to each muscle, signaling it to contract. When this normal nerve supply is lost through brain injury, spinal cord injury, or peripheral nerve injury, the voluntary con-

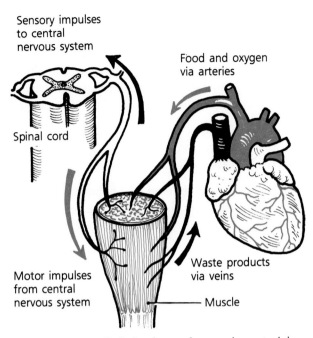

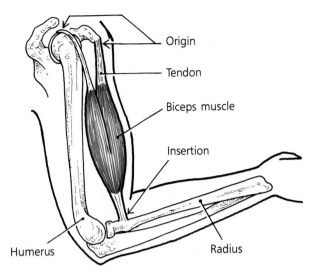

FIGURE 14.1 All skeletal muscles receive arterial blood carrying oxygen and nutrients. Waste products of muscle activity are removed by veins. Peripheral nerves, which extend from the spinal cord to each skeletal muscle, transmit electrical signals from the brain that cause the muscle to relax or contract.

FIGURE 14.2 The biceps muscle causes the elbow to bend (flex) when it contracts. Note the points of tendon origin and insertion. As the muscle fibers contract and shorten, the origin and insertion are pulled closer together with motion occurring at the elbow joint.

trol of the muscle is lost and the muscle becomes paralyzed.

Most skeletal muscles attach directly to bone by tough, ropelike cords of fibrous tissue called **tendons.** A tendon is a continuation of the fascia that covers all skeletal muscles. The **fascia** is much like the skin of a sausage in that it encases the muscle tissue. At either end of the muscle the fascia extends beyond the muscle to attach to a bone. This **musculotendinous unit** crosses a joint and is responsible for the motion of that joint. The proximal point of attachment of the musculotendinous unit is called its *origin,* and the distal bony attachment is called the *insertion* of the muscle (Figure 14.2). When a muscle contracts, a line of force is created between the origin and the insertion, which pulls the points of origin and insertion closer together. This motion occurs at the joint between the two bones.

Smooth Muscle

Smooth muscle carries out much of the automatic work of the body; therefore, it is also called

involuntary muscle. Under the microscope, it does not have the striations that are found in skeletal muscle; thus it is called smooth muscle. Smooth muscle is found in the walls of most tubular structures of the body, such as the gastrointestinal tract, the urinary system, the blood vessels, and the bronchi of the lungs. Contraction and relaxation of smooth muscle propels or controls the flow of the contents of these structures along their course. For example, the rhythmic contraction and relaxation of the smooth muscles of the wall of the intestine propel ingested food along its course, and smooth muscle in the walls of a blood vessel can alter the diameter of the vessel to control the amount of blood flow through it (Figure 14.3). Smooth muscle responds only to primitive stimuli such as stretching, heat, or the need to relieve waste. An individual cannot exert any voluntary control over this type of muscle. A more extensive description of smooth muscle function can be found in Chapter 24.

The Diaphragm

The **diaphragm** is unique because it has characteristics of both voluntary and involuntary muscle. Under the microscope it has striations like skeletal muscle. Also, it is attached to the costal arch and the lumbar vertebrae like other skeletal muscles.

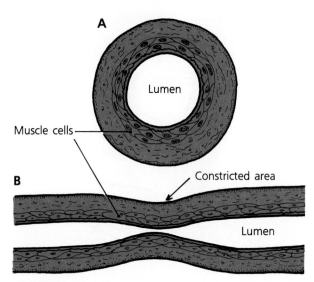

FIGURE 14.3 (a) Smooth muscle lines the walls of the tubular structures of the body. (b) Contraction of the muscles narrows the diameter of the structure, and relaxation allows the diameter to increase in size.

Thus, in many ways it looks like a voluntary muscle; however, we do not have complete voluntary control over its function. When we take a deep breath, the diaphragm flattens and its central part moves downward. This movement increases the volume of the chest cavity, allowing us to inhale air. When the diaphragm relaxes, its central part rises and air is expired. For the most part, breathing is an automatic function that continues all the time, and thus the diaphragm muscle should be thought of as an involuntary muscle. Automatic control of breathing can be overridden by the conscious person, and one can breathe faster or slower or hold one's breath for short periods of time. However, this voluntary control cannot continue indefinitely, and in the end automatic control resumes. Hence, although the diaphragm looks like voluntary skeletal muscle and is attached to the skeleton, it behaves like involuntary muscle most of the time.

Cardiac Muscle

The heart is a large muscle comprised of a pair of pumps of unequal force — one of lower and one of higher pressure. The heart must function continuously from birth to death. It is an especially adapted involuntary muscle with a very rich blood supply and its own intrinsic regulatory system. Microscopi-

cally, it looks different from both skeletal and smooth muscle. Cardiac muscle can tolerate an interruption of its blood supply for only a few seconds. It requires a continuous supply of oxygen and glucose for normal function. Because of its special structure and function, cardiac muscle is placed in a separate category.

SKELETON

The skeleton is composed of 206 bones. The functions performed by the skeleton are to:

1. Give form to the body.
2. Allow bodily movement.
3. Provide protection of vital, internal organs.
4. Produce red blood cells.
5. Serve as a reservoir for calcium, phosphorus, and other important body chemicals (Figure 14.4).

The skeleton is a framework for the attachment of muscles; it allows an erect posture against the pull of gravity and gives a constant and recognizable form to the body. Yet it is designed to allow motion of the body as well. The bones come in contact with one another at joints where controlled motion is accomplished by muscle action.

The skeleton also affords protection of vital internal organs. The brain lies within the skull. The heart, lungs, and great vessels are protected by the thorax. Much of the liver and spleen are protected by the lowermost ribs. The spinal cord is contained within and protected by the bony spinal canal formed by the vertebrae.

The central portion of all bones is composed of bone marrow. **Bone marrow** produces red blood cells. These red blood cells have a short life span of about 120 days. Thus, the bone must continuously supply new red blood cells to the circulation to assure adequate transport of oxygen and carbon dioxide.

Each bone is composed of a protein framework that allows for its growth and remodeling. Calcium and phosphorus are deposited into this framework to make the bone hard and strong. Throughout the lifetime of the individual, calcium and phosphorus are constantly being deposited in bone and withdrawn from it under the control of a very complex, metabolic system. Calcium must be maintained at a very specific concentration in the circulation for

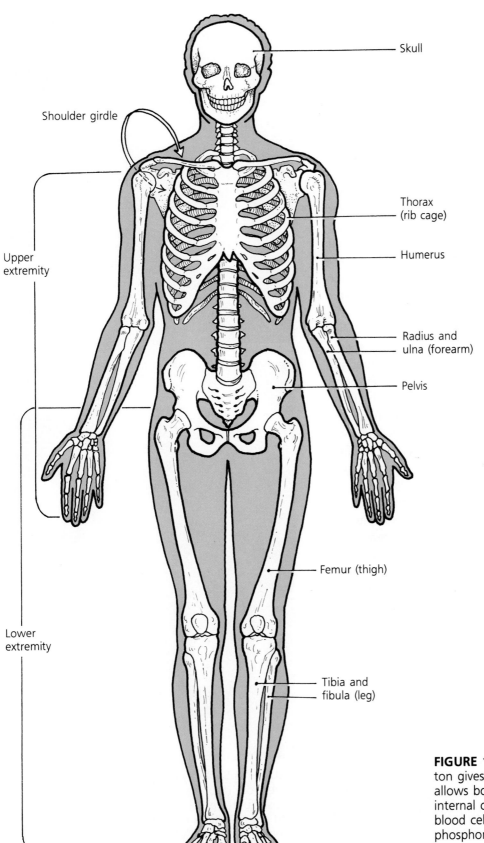

Skull

Shoulder girdle

Thorax
(rib cage)

Humerus

Upper
extremity

Radius and
ulna (forearm)

Pelvis

Femur (thigh)

Lower
extremity

Tibia and
fibula (leg)

FIGURE 14.4 The human skeleton gives form to the body, allows bodily movement, protects internal organs, produces red blood cells, and stores calcium, phosphorus, and other body chemicals.

skeletal muscles to contract normally and for proper function of cardiac muscle.

Bone is just as much a living tissue as are muscle, skin, and other tissues. A rich blood supply constantly provides the oxygen and nutrients required by the bones. Each bone also has an extensive nerve supply. Thus, a fracture of bone will produce severe pain from irritation of the nerves as well as significant bleeding from damage to the bone's blood vessels.

Although bones form the skeleton, not every bone is fully developed at birth. Bones must be rigid and unyielding to fulfill their structural support function, but they must also grow and adapt as the human being grows. As a rule, bone growth ends when a person reaches the late teens. Unless some abnormality is present, there is usually little outward skeletal change after this period.

Bones in young children are more flexible than in the adult and therefore are less likely to fracture. However, since children are so active, fractures still occur frequently. Bone heals by forming new bone. It is the only tissue in the body that heals by forming more of itself. Other tissues in the body heal by forming scar tissue. Scar tissue, however, is not strong enough to function as bone should; therefore, bone has retained the ability to heal by forming more of itself.

As humans age, bone gradually becomes weaker. This condition of gradual, progressive weakening of the bone is called **osteoporosis.** Osteoporosis is particularly common in women and is especially severe after menopause. Thus, elderly people, and in particular postmenopausal women, are more susceptible to fracture because of the weakened condition of the bone. Even trivial injuries may produce significant fractures in patients with osteoporosis (Figure 14.5).

Anatomy of a Bone

The various parts of a bone are designated by specific names depending on their shape and function. Many bones have a rounded end that allows joint rotation. This part is called the head. The region below the head is called the neck. The shaft is the long, straight cylindrical midportion of a bone. The **condyles** (called **malleoli** at the ankle and **styloid processes** at the wrist) are prominences at one or both ends of the bone that usually serve as points

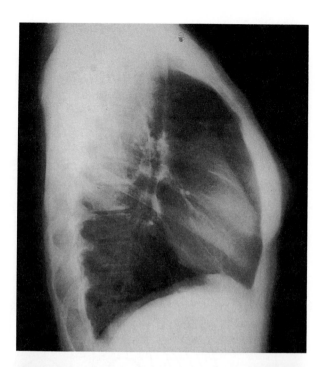

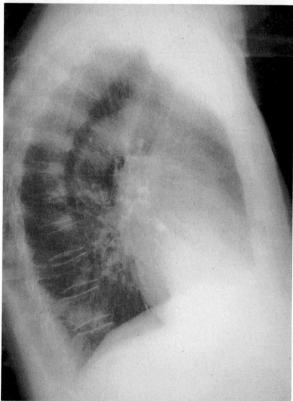

FIGURE 14.5 X-ray of the spine of healthy 25-year-old (top) and a 79-year-old with osteoporosis (bottom). Note the loss of bone density with age. Multiple fractures of the vertebrae have resulted in collapse of the spine and a "humpback" deformity.

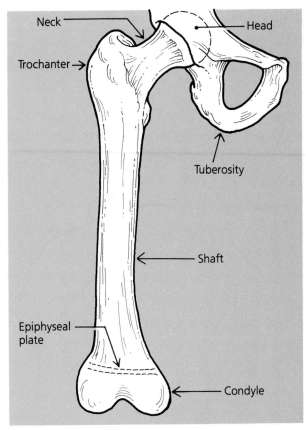

FIGURE 14.6 Specific regions of many bones have special names as indicated by the labels on this "typical bone."

of ligament attachment. **Tuberosities** and **trochanters** are prominences of the bone where tendons insert (Figure 14.6).

The **epiphyseal plate** is a transverse cartilage plate near the end of a long bone of a child. It is responsible for the growth in length of the bone. Because it is made of cartilage, it can be seen on an x-ray as a clear transverse line near the end of the child's bone.

Joints

Wherever two bones come in contact, a **joint (articulation)** is formed. Most joints allow motion — for example, the knee, hip, or elbow — whereas some bones fuse with one another at joints so that a solid, immobile, bony structure results. For instance, the skull is composed of several bones that fuse as the child grows. The infant, whose skull bones are not yet fused, has "soft spots" called **fontanelles** between the bones. The fontanelles close as the bones fuse together when the child's skull reaches the adult size. Some joints have slight limited motion. The bone ends are held together by fibrous tissue. Such a joint is called a **symphysis.**

A joint consists of the ends of the bones that make up the joint and the surrounding, connecting, and supporting tissue (Figure 14.7). Most joints in

FIGURE 14.7 (a) The knee joint is stripped of the soft tissues that surround it to demonstrate its capsule and ligaments. (b) The knee is cut longitudinally to show the interior of the joint.

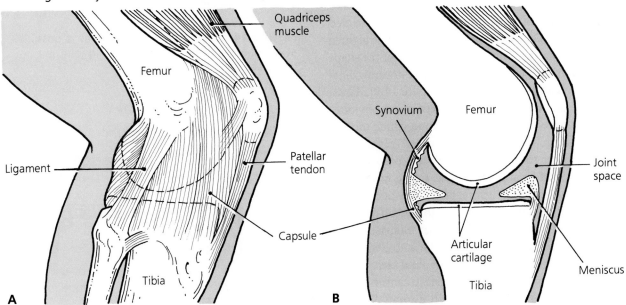

the body are named by combining the names of the two bones that form that joint. For example, the sternoclavicular joint is the articulation between the sternum and the clavicle.

In joints where motion occurs, the ends of bones that articulate with each other are covered with a smooth, shiny surface called **articular cartilage.** Inside some joints, most notably the knee, cushions made of cartilage fill up spaces between the bone and aid in the gliding motion of the joint. Such a cushion is called a **meniscus,** or sometimes simply a **cartilage.** If injured and torn from its attachments, the meniscus can produce symptoms of locking or catching in the joint.

The bone ends of a joint are held together by a fibrous tissue **joint capsule.** At certain points around the circumference of the joint, the capsule is lax and thin so that motion can occur. In other areas it is quite thick and resists stretching or bending. These bands of tough, thick capsule are called **ligaments.** A joint such as the sacroiliac joint that is virtually surrounded by tough, thick ligaments will have little motion, whereas a joint such as the shoulder, with few ligaments, will be free to move in almost any direction (and will, as a result, be more prone to dislocation).

The degree of freedom of motion of a joint is determined by the extent to which the ligaments hold the bone ends together and also by the configuration of the bone ends themselves. The hip joint is a **ball-and-socket joint,** which allows rotation as well as bending (Figure 14.8). The finger joints and the knee are **hinge joints,** with motion restricted to one plane. They can only bend (flex) and straighten (extend). Rotation is not possible because of the shape of the joint surfaces and the strong restraining ligaments on both sides of the joint (Figure 14.9). Thus, while the amount of motion varies from joint to joint, all joints have a definite limit beyond which motion cannot occur. When a joint is forced beyond this limit, damage to some structure must occur: either the bones that form the joint will break, or the supporting capsule and ligaments will be disrupted.

The inner surface of the joint capsule (the **synovium**) produces a fluid that nourishes and lubricates the articular cartilage. It is called **synovial fluid.** It is thick, almost oily, and clear yellow in color. Normally, only a few cubic centimeters of synovial fluid are present within a joint. With in-

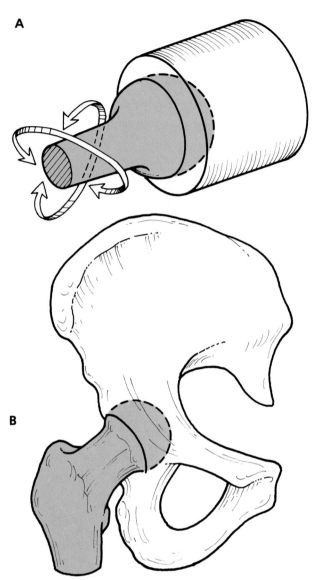

FIGURE 14.8 (a) Motion in all planes is possible at a ball-and-socket joint. (b) The hip joint is a typical ball-and-socket joint.

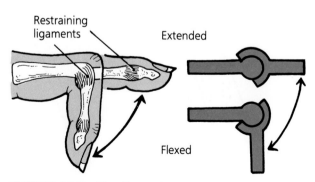

FIGURE 14.9 The finger joints are hinge joints, which allow motion in only one plane.

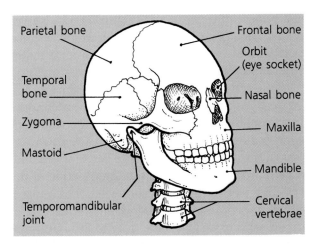

FIGURE 14.10 The skull includes the bones of the cranium, which are fused, and the facial bones. The mandible (lower jaw) is freely movable.

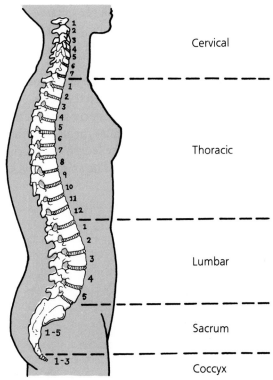

FIGURE 14.11 The spinal column consists of 33 vertebrae in 5 definite sections. The vertebrae protect the spinal cord.

jury or disease, however, more fluid is produced to protect the joint, resulting in swelling inside the capsule — for example, the so-called "water on the knee."

The Skull

The skull has two major divisions: the cranium (brain case) and the face (Figure 14.10). The **cranium** is composed of a number of thick bones that fuse together to form a shell that protects the brain. The face is also composed mostly of bones fused together to provide protection for important structures. For example, the **orbit** (eye socket) is composed of two facial bones, the maxilla and the zygoma, as well as the frontal bone of the cranium, to form a solid bony rim that protrudes around the eye to protect it. The **maxilla** contains the upper teeth and forms the **hard palate,** or roof of the mouth. The **mandible,** or lower jaw, is the only movable facial bone having a joint (the **temporomandibular**) with the cranium just in front of the ear. The nasal bone is very short, as the majority of the nose is composed of flexible cartilage. The **mastoid process** of the cranium is a bony prominence behind the ear.

The Spinal Column

The **spinal column** is the central supporting structure of the body (Figure 14.11). It is composed of 33 bones, each called a **vertebra.** The spine is divided into these five sections:

1. Cervical (neck)
2. Thoracic or dorsal (upper part of the back)
3. Lumbar (lower part of the back)
4. Sacral (part of the pelvis)
5. Coccygeal (coccyx or tailbone)

The vertebrae are named according to the section of the spine in which they lie and are numbered from top to bottom. The first seven vertebrae form the **cervical spine** (C1 through C7). The next 12 vertebrae make up the **thoracic** or **dorsal spine.** One pair of ribs articulates with each of these thoracic vertebrae. The next five vertebrae form the **lumbar spine,** or the lower back. The five sacral vertebrae are fused together to form one bone called the **sacrum.** The sacrum is joined to the iliac bones of the pelvis with strong ligaments at the sacroiliac joints to form the **pelvic girdle.** The last three or four vertebrae form the **coccyx,** or tailbone.

The skull rests on the first cervical vertebra and articulates with it. The **spinal cord** is an extension of the brain. It is composed of virtually all the nerves that carry messages between the brain and the rest of the body. It exits through a large hole (the **foramen magnum**) in the base of the skull and is contained within and protected by the vertebrae of the spinal column.

The front part of each vertebra consists of a round, solid block of bone called the **body.** The back part of each vertebra forms a **bony arch.** This series of arches from one vertebra to the next forms a tunnel that runs throughout the length of the spine and is called the **spinal canal.** The spinal canal encases

and protects the spinal cord (Figure 14.12). Nerves branch from the spinal cord and exit from the spinal canal between each two vertebrae to form the motor and sensory nerves of the body (Figure 14.13).

The vertebrae are connected by ligaments, and between each two vertebral bodies is a cushion, the **intervertebral disc.** These ligaments and discs allow some motion to occur between every two vertebrae, thus allowing the trunk to bend forward and back; however, they also act to limit motion of the vertebrae so that the spinal cord will not be injured. When a fracture of the spine occurs, protection of the spinal cord and its nerves may be lost. Until the fracture is stabilized, the EMT must guard, above all, against injury to the spinal cord.

The spinal column itself is virtually surrounded by muscles; however, the **posterior spinous process** of each vertebra can be palpated, as it lies just under the skin in the midline of the back (Figure

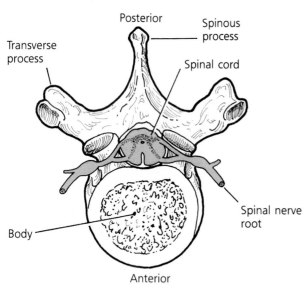

FIGURE 14.12 The top view of a thoracic vertebra showing the spinal canal protecting the spinal cord.

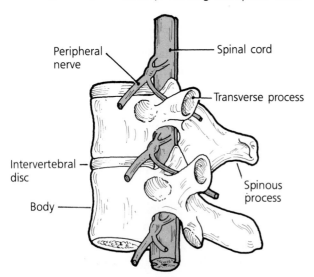

FIGURE 14.13 Between each two adjacent vertebrae, peripheral nerves exit the spinal canal. These nerves transmit information between the brain and specific parts of the body.

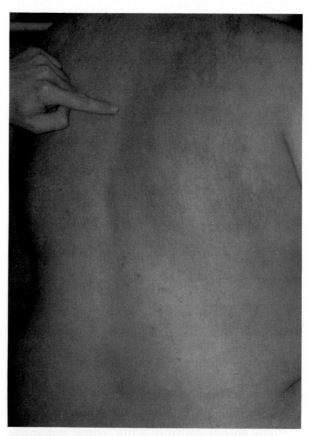

FIGURE 14.14 Even in the obese patient, it is usually possible to palpate the posterior spinous processes in the midline. The spine of C7 is usually the most prominent.

14.14). The most prominent and most easily palpable spinous process is that of the seventh cervical vertebrae at the base of the neck.

The Thorax

The **thorax** (the rib cage) is made up of the ribs, the 12 thoracic vertebrae, and the **sternum** (breast bone) (Figure 14.15). There are 12 pairs of **ribs,** which are long, slender, curved bones. Each rib forms a joint with its respective thoracic vertebra and then curves around to form the rib cage. At the front of the rib cage, ribs 1 through 10 connect with the sternum through a bridge of cartilage. For the lower five ribs, this cartilaginous bridge is called the **costal arch.**

The sternum forms the middle part of the front of the thoracic cage. This bone is approximately 7 inches long and 2 inches wide. The sternum has three parts: the **manubrium,** the **body,** and the **xiphoid process.** The junction of the manubrium (upper part) and the body of the sternum is located at the level of the second ribs. Here there is a consistent bony prominence that can be palpated on all patients. This bony prominence is called the **angle of Louis.** The xiphoid process of the sternum projects from the lower part of the body. It is made of cartilage and is very tender to palpation.

The Upper Extremity

The proximal portion of the upper extremity is called the **shoulder girdle** (Figure 14.16). It consists of three bones: the clavicle, the scapula, and the humerus. The shoulder girdle serves as a base of attachment for the upper extremity to the trunk. The upper extremity can be moved through a wide range of motion, allowing the hand to be placed in almost any position. This motion occurs at three joints within the shoulder girdle: the **sternoclavicular joint,** the **acromioclavicular joint,** and the **glenohumeral joint.** Only slight motion occurs normally at the sternoclavicular and acromioclavicular joints. On the other hand, the ball-and-socket arrangement of the glenohumeral joint (the true shoulder joint) allows great freedom of motion in almost any direction.

The **clavicle** (collar bone) is a long, slender bone that lies just under the skin and serves as a support or prop for the upper extremity. Its medial end is attached by very strong ligaments to the manubrium of the sternum to form the sternoclavicular joint. Its

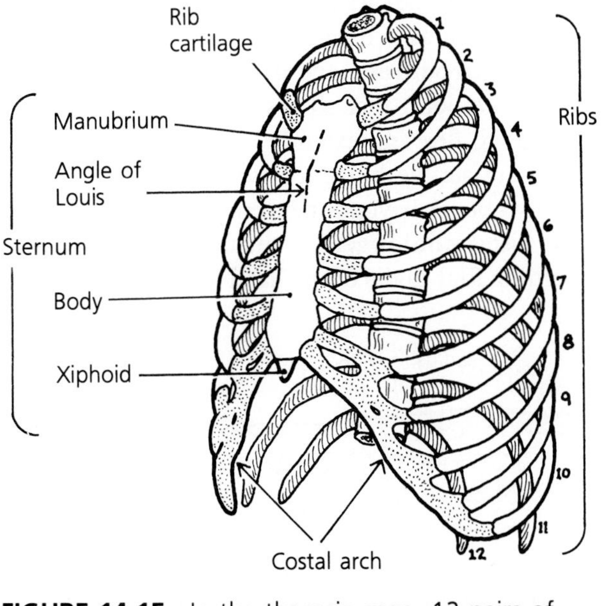

FIGURE 14.15 In the thoracic cage, 12 pairs of ribs articulate with the vertebrae in the spinal column through small joints. The first 10 pairs also articulate with the sternum or the costal arch in front, through a cartilaginous bridge.

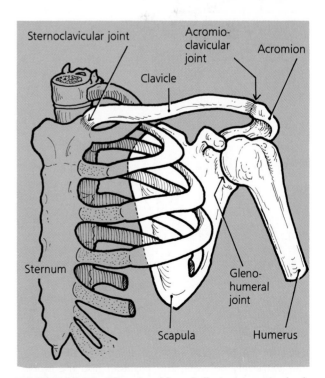

FIGURE 14.16 The shoulder girdle is composed of the clavicle, scapula, and proximal humerus.

lateral end forms a joint with the acromion process of the scapula to create the acromioclavicular joint.

The **scapula** (shoulder blade) is a large, flat, triangular bone interposed between the clavicle and the humerus and held against the back of the thorax by large muscles. It has two specially named regions that form joints with the clavicle and the humerus. The **acromion process,** anteriorly, forms part of the acromioclavicular joint, and the **glenoid fossa** is the recess for the articulation of the humeral head, forming the glenohumeral joint. The spine and medial border of the scapula can be seen and palpated posteriorly. The acromion process forms the rounded edge of the shoulder girdle and can be felt anteriorly as one walks a finger along the clavicle and across the acromioclavicular joint.

The head of the **humerus** is covered by muscles that form the rounded prominence of the shoulder girdle laterally. The humerus extends from the shoulder to form the supporting structure for the arm, and the distal end articulates with both the radius and ulna at the **elbow joint** (Figure 14.17).

The humerus, with its long, straight shaft, serves as an effective lever for heavy lifting. The section of the upper extremity containing the humerus is called the arm.

The humerus articulates with the two bones of the forearm, the **radius** and **ulna,** to form a relatively simple hinge joint, the elbow. On the back of the elbow three prominences can be seen and easily palpated. They are the medial and lateral condyles of the humerus and the **olecranon process** of the ulna (Figure 14.17).

The forearm is composed of many muscles that are supported by the underlying radius and ulna. At the elbow, the ulna is larger than the radius, but at the wrist, the radius is the larger bone. The radius rotates about the ulna, which allows the palm to be turned up or down. At the wrist, the ends of the radius and ulna (the styloid processes) lie directly under the skin and can be easily palpated. The radial styloid is slightly longer than the ulnar styloid. The radius lies on the lateral, or thumb, side of the forearm, and the ulna is on the medial or little-finger side (Figure 14.18).

The wrist joint is a modified ball-and-socket articulation formed by the ends of the radius and ulna and several small wrist bones. There are eight bones in the wrist. They are called the **carpal bones.** Extending from the carpal bones are five **metacarpals,** which serve as a base for each of the digits. The thumb (**carpometacarpal**) joint is a modified ball-and-socket joint that allows the thumb to rotate as well as to flex and extend. The other joints in the hand are simple hinge joints. In the thumb, there are two bones beyond the metacarpal: the proximal and distal **phalanges** (singular, *phalanx*). The remaining four digits of the hand are named in order:

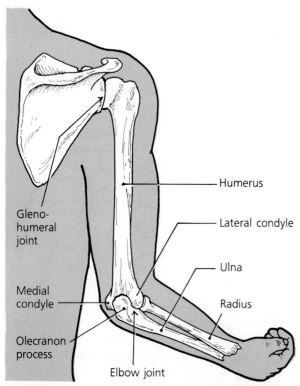

FIGURE 14.17   The arm is that portion of the upper extremity between the shoulder and the elbow joint. Three bony prominences can be seen at the elbow joint.

Glenohumeral joint
Humerus
Lateral condyle
Ulna
Medial condyle
Radius
Olecranon process
Elbow joint

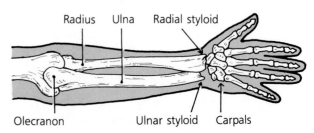

Radius   Ulna   Radial styloid
Olecranon   Ulnar styloid   Carpals

FIGURE 14.18   The forearm is made up of two bones, the radius and the ulna. The radius is larger distally and lies on the thumb side of the forearm. The ulna is larger proximally and lies on the little-finger side.

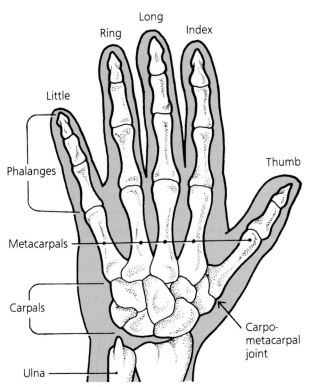

FIGURE 14.19 The bones of the wrist and hand. Note the proper name of each digit.

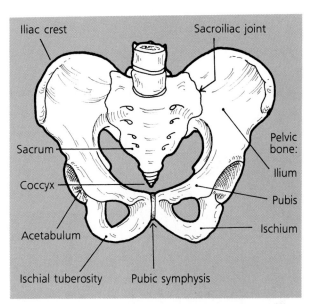

FIGURE 14.20 The pelvis is comprised of three bones: the sacrum and the two pelvic bones. The sacrum firmly articulates with the two pelvic bones posteriorly, and anteriorly the symphysis pubis joins the two pelvic bones.

the index, the long, the ring, and the little finger. Each of these contains three phalanges (Figure 14.19).

The Pelvis and Lower Extremity

The **pelvis** (Figure 14.20) is a bony ring that is formed posteriorly by the sacrum and anterolaterally by the large winglike pelvic bones. Each pelvic bone is formed by the fusion of three separate bones, much as the skull is composed of several bones fused together. The three bones are the **ilium,** with its iliac crest laterally; the **ischium,** with its ischial tuberosity palpable in the buttocks; and the **pubis,** palpable anteriorly.

The sacrum and the two pelvic bones articulate at three joints: the two posterior **sacroiliac joints** and the anterior, midline **symphysis pubis.** All three joints allow very little motion, as they are firmly held together by strong ligaments. Thus, the pelvic ring is strong and stable, for it is designed to support the body weight and protect the structures within the pelvic cavity (the bladder, the rectum, and the female reproductive organs). On the lateral side of each pelvic bone where the three component bones

join is the socket for the hip joint. This depression in which the femoral head fits very snugly is called the **acetabulum.**

The lower extremity consists of the thigh, the leg, and the foot (Figure 14.21). The **femur** (thigh bone) is the longest and one of the strongest bones in the body. The femoral head forms the hip joint with the acetabulum of the pelvis. This ball-and-socket joint allows flexion, extension, **adduction** (motion of the limb toward the midline), and **abduction** (motion of the limb away from the midline), as well as internal and external rotation of the entire lower extremity.

In the proximal lateral thigh, the prominence of the **greater trochanter** of the femur can be easily palpated. This prominence is sometimes called the "hip bone." The shaft of the femur is surrounded by large muscles (the quadriceps anteriorly and the hamstrings posteriorly). Just above the knee, the medial and lateral femoral condyles can be palpated.

Between the thigh and the leg is the **knee joint,** the articulation between the distal femur and the proximal tibia. The knee is the largest joint in the body and is essentially a hinge joint, allowing only flexion and extension. Adduction, abduction, and rotation of the knee joint are resisted by complex ligaments that are quite susceptible to injury.

Anterior to the knee joint is the **patella** (kneecap). It lies within the tendon of the quadriceps muscle and protects the front of the knee joint from injury.

The leg is that portion of the lower extremity between the knee and the ankle joint (Figure 14.22). It contains two bones: the tibia and the fibula. The **tibia** (shin bone), the larger bone, lies in the anterior aspect of the leg. Its edge is just under the skin and is easily palpable from the tibial tuberosity (the insertion of the patellar tendon) to the medial malleolus at the ankle. The **fibula** lies laterally. Its head can be palpated on the lateral aspect of the knee joint, and its distal end forms the lateral malleolus of the ankle joint.

The **ankle joint** is a hinge joint that allows flexion and extension of the foot on the leg. The end of the tibia provides a smooth articular surface for

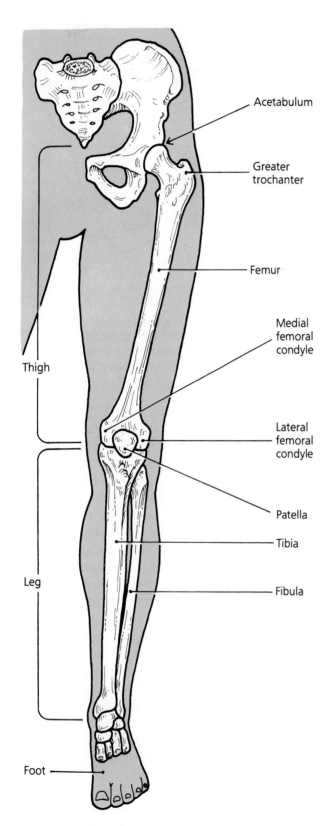

FIGURE 14.21 The femur is the single bone of the thigh. The leg is formed by the fibula and the tibia. The foot contains seven tarsal bones.

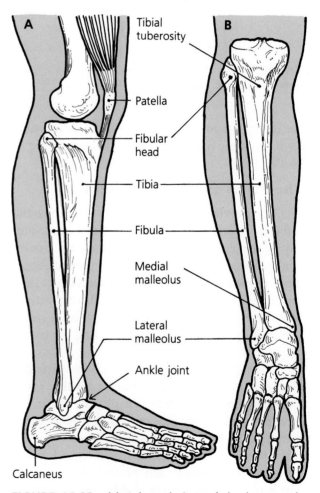

FIGURE 14.22 (a) A lateral view of the knee and leg showing the patella in the tendon of the quadriceps muscle. (b) An anterior view of the leg.

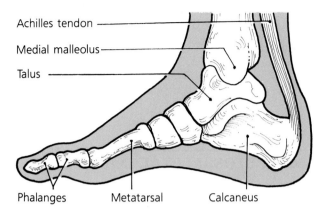

Achilles tendon
Medial malleolus
Talus

Phalanges   Metatarsal   Calcaneus

FIGURE 14.23 This view of the ankle and foot shows the articulation of the talus with the distal tibia. The talus and calcaneus are both tarsal bones.

the **talus** (ankle bone) (Figure 14.23). The talus is one of seven **tarsal bones.** The **calcaneus (os calcis,** or heel bone) is the other large tarsal bone. It forms the prominence of the heel. The **Achilles tendon** inserts into the back of the calcaneus. There are five **metatarsals** that articulate with the tarsal

bones, and, as in the hand, each gives rise to its respective digit. The great toe has two phalanges, and the lesser four toes have three phalanges each, similar to the arrangement of the bones in the fingers.

YOU ARE THE EMT...

1. Would you describe the biceps muscle as smooth or skeletal muscle? Why? Which muscle looks like skeletal muscle but behaves like involuntary muscle?
2. You know that bones heal by forming new bone. Can this process still occur in an elderly person? Describe the condition called osteoporosis.
3. Your patient has "water on the knee." What is the medical explanation for this phenomenon?
4. What is the difference between hinge joints and ball-and-socket joints? Name two hinge joints and two ball-and-socket joints.

15 Fractures, Dislocations, and Sprains

OVERVIEW

Musculoskeletal injuries are among the most common problems seen in emergency care work. The EMT must check each injured patient for the possibility of fracture, dislocation, or sprain and be prepared to manage that injury properly. Effective emergency care of musculoskeletal injuries not only decreases immediate pain and reduces the possibility of shock and further nerve or vessel injury; it also improves the patient's chances for a rapid recovery and early return to normal activity.

Chapter 15 begins with a description of the types and causes of musculoskeletal injuries. It then discusses fractures, dislocations, and sprains. The chapter next describes the steps in the examination of musculoskeletal injuries. The last part of Chapter 15 focuses on the treatment of musculoskeletal injuries — specifically, the methods of splinting and transporting the injured patient.

OBJECTIVES

The objectives of Chapter 15 are to

- describe the types and causes of musculoskeletal injuries.
- recognize the various types of fractures.
- recognize a dislocation.
- recognize a sprain.
- learn how to carry out an examination of an injured limb.
- learn how to treat a musculoskeletal injury, including the various methods of splinting and the proper way to transport a patient with an injured limb.

TYPES AND CAUSES OF MUSCULOSKELETAL INJURY

A **fracture** is any break in the continuity of a bone. The break may range in severity from a simple crack to severe shattering that produces multiple fracture fragments. The break can occur anywhere on the surface of the bone, even across the articular surface (Figure 15.1). There is no difference between a fractured and a broken bone; both terms have the same meaning.

Dislocation means disruption of a joint so that the bone ends are no longer in contact. Such a disruption of the joint can happen only if the supporting ligaments and capsule of the joint tear, allowing the bone ends to separate completely from each other (Figure 15.2).

A **fracture-dislocation** is a twofold injury in which the joint is dislocated and a part of the bone near the joint also fractures (Figure 15.3).

A **sprain** is a joint injury in which the joint is partially, temporarily dislocated and some of the supporting ligaments are either stretched or torn. Following the injury, the joint surfaces fall back into alignment so that immediately after the injury persistent displacement of the joint surfaces does not occur (Figure 15.4). Sprains vary in severity from mild to severe, depending on the amount of damage that has occurred to the supporting ligaments. A severe sprain often causes as much damage to the supporting ligaments and the joint capsule as a complete dislocation.

A **strain,** sometimes called a **muscle pull,** is a stretching or tearing of a muscle. Unlike the sprain, no ligament or joint damage occurs. A strain is a muscle injury. The muscle fibers are partially pulled apart and produce pain and occasional swelling and ecchymosis of the local soft tissues.

Because musculoskeletal injuries occur so frequently, the EMT must be able to evaluate them properly. Injury to the bones and joints is often

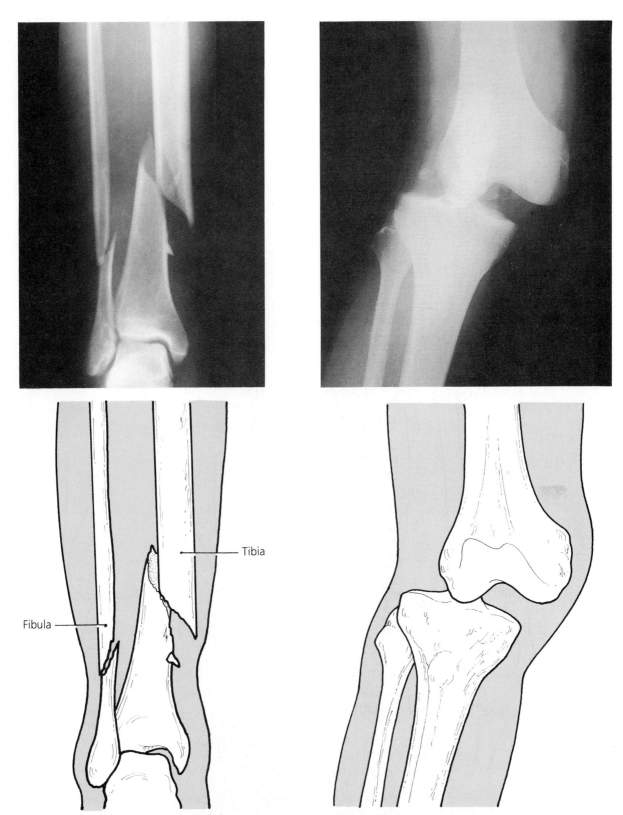

FIGURE 15.1 Fracture of the tibia and fibula. (top) X-ray appearance of fracture fragments; (bottom) line drawing of the fracture.

FIGURE 15.2 Dislocation of the knee joint. (top) X-ray appearance of the dislocated joint; (bottom) line drawing of the dislocation.

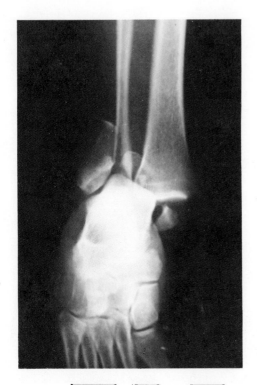

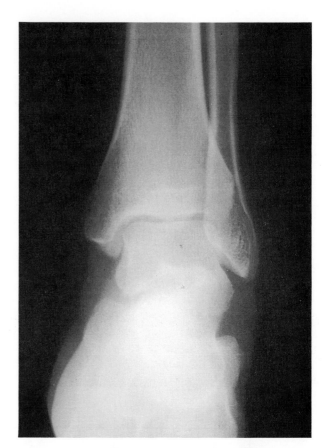

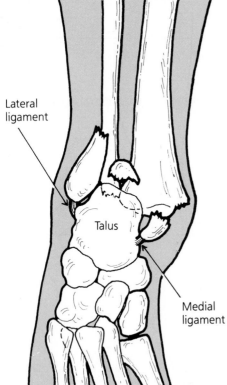

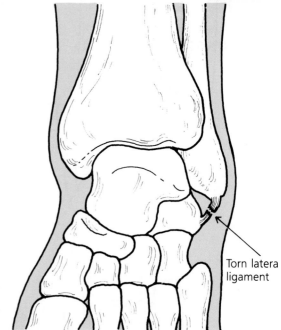

FIGURE 15.3 Fracture-dislocation of the ankle joint. (top) X-ray appearance of the talus dislocated from the distal tibia with fracture of both the medial and lateral malleoli; (bottom) line drawing of the fracture-dislocation.

FIGURE 15.4 An ankle sprain. (top) X-ray of the injured ankle appears normal because there is no injury of the bones. (bottom) The line drawing, however, shows that the supporting ligament on the lateral side of the ankle has been torn.

associated with injury to the surrounding soft tissue (especially the adjacent nerves and arteries). In addition, other areas of the body at a distance from the fracture may sustain injury as well. Therefore, the EMT should not focus exclusively on a patient's obviously deformed arm or leg without first completing a primary assessment to be certain that associated and perhaps even more serious injuries are not overlooked.

Significant force is usually required to cause fractures or dislocations. The force may be applied to the limb in a variety of ways. Direct blows, indirect forces, twisting forces, or high-energy injury all may cause significant musculoskeletal injury (Figure 15.5). A direct blow is a common cause of fracture. The fracture from a direct blow occurs at the point of impact. For example, the patella may be fractured if it strikes the dashboard in an automobile accident.

Indirect forces can also result in fracture or dislocation. In such instances, the force is applied to one part of the limb, and the site of injury is some distance away from the point of impact, usually proximal to it. The best example of an indirect force that causes a fracture is the wide range of fractures that occur when an individual falls and lands on an outstretched hand. The patient may fracture the bones of the wrist, the forearm bones, the humerus, or even the clavicle. Indeed, this is the most common mechanism of fracture of the clavicle.

Twisting forces can also result in musculoskeletal injury. Such a force is a common cause of tibial fractures as well as knee and ankle ligament injuries. With this mechanism of injury, the foot is usually fixed to a point on the ground as the patient falls. Skiing injuries frequently occur this way when the ski becomes caught and the skier falls, applying a twisting force to the lower extremity.

High-energy injury, as in automobile accidents, falls from heights, gunshot wounds, and injuries from other extreme forces, will produce severe damage to the skeleton, its surrounding soft tissues, and the vital internal organs it is designed to protect. More than one bone in a limb may be fractured or dislocated, and multiple injuries to many parts of the body will commonly occur following high-energy injury.

Not all fractures result from the application of a violent force, however. Some people have a localized destructive lesion of bone, such as a bone tumor, that will weaken the bone so that only a slight force

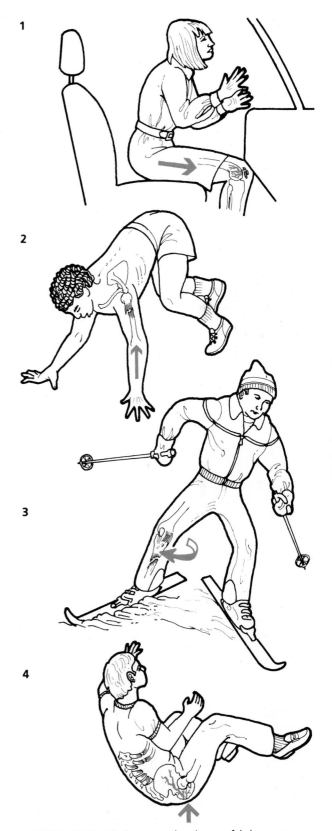

FIGURE 15.5 Various mechanisms of injury may produce fractures and dislocations.

will cause it to break. A very common generalized bone disease, **osteoporosis,** weakens the bone and causes it to be very susceptible to fracture with minimal force. Osteoporosis is very common in elderly patients, particularly postmenopausal females. Minor falls, simple twisting injuries, or even contraction of the muscles can cause a bone to fracture in people who have osteoporosis. Thus, the EMT must be very suspicious of a fracture in any older patient who has sustained even a mild injury.

FRACTURES

Fracture Classification

The most important factor to identify in the initial evaluation of a fracture, or any extremity injury, is the integrity of the overlying skin and soft tissues. Just as with soft tissue injuries, fractures are classified as open (compound) or closed.

An **open,** or **compound, fracture** is any fracture in which the overlying skin has been damaged (Figure 15.6). Laceration of the skin can occur from

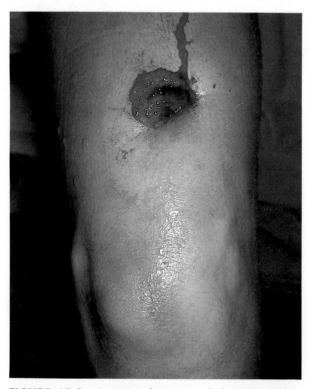

FIGURE 15.6 An open (compound) fracture with exposed bone. The fracture does not have to be visible to be classified as open.

sharp bone ends protruding through it or by a direct blow that lacerates the skin at the time of the fracture. The wound may vary in size from a small puncture wound to a gaping hole with much exposed bone and soft tissue. The bone may or may not be visible in the wound. Regardless of the extent and severity of the injury to the skin, any fracture in which the protective covering of skin has been damaged is considered to be an open fracture. In contrast, a **closed fracture** is one in which the skin has not been penetrated by the bone ends and no wound exists anywhere near the fracture site.

It is extremely important for the EMT to determine whether the fracture is open or closed. Open fractures are much more serious than closed fractures for two reasons. First, greater blood loss will occur with open fractures than with closed fractures. Second, and more important, the bone is contaminated by being exposed to the outside environment and the fracture site may become infected. An infected fracture sometimes causes serious life-long problems for the patient. For these reasons, all fractures should be described to emergency department personnel as either open or closed so that the proper treatment can be undertaken upon arrival at the hospital.

Fractures are also described by the degree of displacement of the fracture fragments. A **displaced fracture** produces deformity of the limb. The deformity will be slight if the displacement is minimal, or it may be extreme if gross displacement of the fracture fragments has occurred. Many different deformities may occur. Angulation at the fracture site and rotation of the limb distal to the fracture site are common displacements. In addition, the limb may be shortened if the fracture fragments are displaced and their ends overlap (Figure 15.7).

The deformity associated with displaced fractures makes their diagnosis easy. It is much more difficult to diagnose **nondisplaced fractures** without the aid of x-rays. Because there is no deformity, these fractures may be missed or thought to be only a bruise or a sprain. A high index of suspicion is necessary when evaluating an injured person who complains of pain in the extremity. A patient exhibiting any one of the signs of fracture described later in this chapter must be considered to have a fracture and treated as such, even if there is no deformity of the limb.

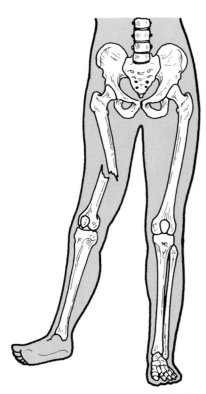

FIGURE 15.7 Fracture of the shaft of the right femur with angulation, shortening, and rotation of the limb below the fracture site.

On occasion, special terms are used to describe particular types of fractures. Because these terms are used commonly by medical personnel, the EMT should be familiar with their meaning:

Greenstick fracture: Occurs only in children and is an incomplete fracture that passes only part-way through the shaft of a bone (Figure 15.8).

Comminuted fracture: One in which the bone is broken into more than two fragments (Figure 15.9).

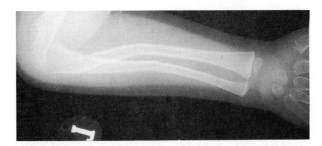

FIGURE 15.8 X-ray of a greenstick fracture of the radius and ulna. These incomplete fractures occur only in children.

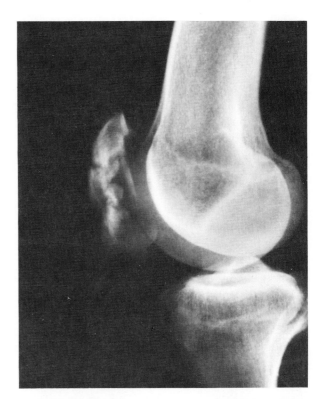

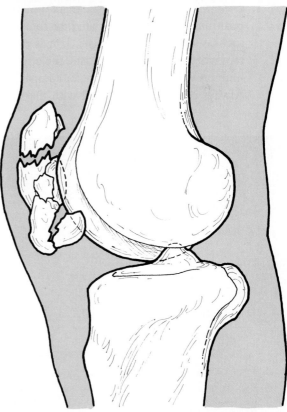

FIGURE 15.9 A comminuted fracture of the patella. (top) X-ray appearance of the patella; (bottom) line drawing of the comminuted fracture.

Pathologic fracture: Occurs through weak or diseased bone and can be produced by a minimal force (Figure 15.10).

Epiphyseal fracture: Occurs in growing children. It is an injury to the growth plate of a long bone that may lead to an arrest of bone growth if not properly treated (Figure 15.11).

Signs and Symptoms of Fractures

Any patient with a history of injury who complains of musculoskeletal pain must be suspected of having sustained a fracture. While bone ends protruding through the skin or gross deformity of a limb make fracture recognition easy, many fractures, particularly nondisplaced fractures, are less obvious. The EMT must know the following seven signs of fractures. All seven signs do not need to be present to make the diagnosis. The presence of any one of these signs should arouse suspicion of a fracture, and the proper emergency treatment should then be instituted.

1. *Deformity.* The limb may lie in an unnatural position, shortened, angulated, or rotated at a point where no joint exists. If it is uncertain whether a deformity exists, the opposite limb provides a mirror image for comparison. Always compare the injured with the unin-

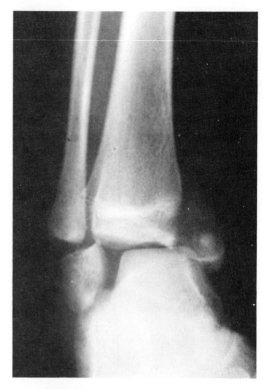

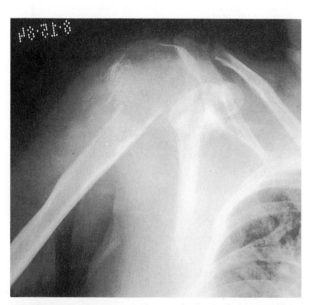

FIGURE 15.10 X-ray of a pathologic fracture that has occurred through the upper end of the humerus weakened by a tumor.

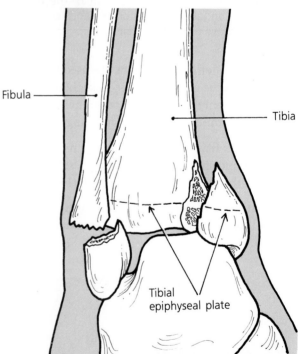

FIGURE 15.11 Epiphyseal (growth) plates are present in children near the ends of all long bones. (top) X-ray appearance of a displaced fracture completely along the epiphysis of the distal fibula and a vertical fracture perpendicular to the epiphyseal plate of the distal tibia near the medial malleolus; (bottom) line drawing of these epiphyseal fractures.

jured opposite limb when checking for deformity (Figure 15.12).

2. *Tenderness.* Tenderness is usually sharply localized at the site of the injury. This sensitive spot can be located by gently palpating along the bone with the tip of one finger. This sign is called **point tenderness** and is the most reliable indication of an underlying fracture (Figure 15.13).

3. *Inability to use the extremity* (**guarding**). A patient who has sustained a fracture or serious injury usually guards the injured part and will

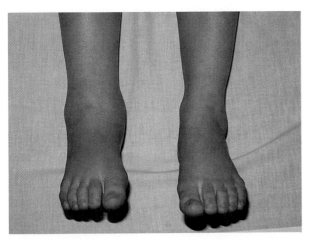

FIGURE 15.12 The EMT should always compare the injured limb with the uninjured opposite limb when checking for deformity.

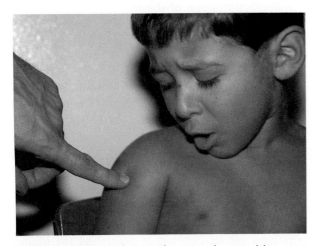

FIGURE 15.13 Point tenderness, the sensitive spot at the site of injury that can be located by gentle palpation along the bone with the tip of the EMT's finger, is the most reliable sign of an underlying fracture.

refuse to use it because motion causes increased pain. It is the patient's way of "splinting" the injured limb to minimize motion and pain. While the *inability* to use a limb is a reliable sign of a significant injury, the EMT must realize that the reverse is *not* true. The *ability* to use an extremity does not mean that a fracture does not exist. Occasionally, nondisplaced fractures are not very painful, and some patients may continue to use an injured limb even though a fracture is present. Such is the case particularly with multiple fractures where one injury is very painful and masks the pain of other fractures.

4. *Swelling and ecchymosis.* Fractures are virtually always associated with swelling and bruising of the surrounding soft tissues. These signs are also present following almost any injury and are not specific for fractures. However, rapid swelling occurring immediately after an injury usually indicates bleeding from the fracture site into the soft tissues from damaged blood vessels. Indeed, the swelling may be so severe as to mask the deformity of a limb produced by the broken bones. Generalized swelling of the limb will also occur as a result of fracture several hours after the injury.

5. *Exposed fragments.* An open fracture's bone ends may protrude through the skin or be seen in the depths of the wound itself, an obvious sign of fracture.

6. *Crepitus* (grating). A grating or grinding sensation called **crepitus** can be felt and even sometimes heard when the raw bone ends rub together.

7. *False motion.* Motion at a point in the limb where it usually does not occur is a positive indication of fracture. This is called **false motion.**

The first five signs listed are the only ones that need to be evaluated to diagnose a fracture in the field. The last two signs only appear when a limb is moved or manipulated. Crepitus and false motion, however, are extremely painful to the patient, and the limb should not be manipulated to elicit these signs. Inspection of the limb with the clothing removed will allow the EMT to see any deformity, swelling, ecchymosis, or exposed bone fragments. An unwillingness of the patient to use the injured limb indicates guarding and loss of function. Finally, palpation with one finger over the injured bone will elicit point tenderness. Any one of these signs is sufficient grounds to assume that a fracture is present.

DISLOCATIONS

With dislocation of a joint, injury to the supporting ligaments and capsule is so severe that the joint surfaces are completely displaced from one another. The bone ends lock in the displaced position, making any attempt at motion of the joint very difficult as well as very painful. Among the joints most susceptible to dislocation are the small joints of the fingers, the shoulder, the elbow, the hip, and the ankle. The following signs and symptoms are seen with a dislocated joint:

1. Marked deformity of the joint
2. Swelling in the region of the joint
3. Pain at the joint which is aggravated by any attempt at movement
4. Virtually complete loss of normal joint motion (a "locked" joint)
5. Tenderness to palpation about the joint

SPRAINS

A joint sprain is produced when a joint is twisted or stretched beyond its normal range of motion. As a result, some of the supporting capsule and ligaments are stretched or torn. Since it is an injury to a joint, a sprain should be considered to be a partial dislocation. Because the bone ends are not completely displaced from one another by the force of injury, they can fall back into alignment when the force is released. Therefore, the severe deformity seen with a dislocated joint is not present with a sprain. Sprains vary in severity from a very slight injury to severe disruption of the supporting ligaments and capsule. Although sprains most often occur in the knee and ankle, any joint may be sprained. The following are signs of sprain:

1. *Tenderness.* Point tenderness can be elicited over the injured ligaments just as point tenderness is found over a fracture site.

2. *Swelling and ecchymosis.* A sprain will usually result in tearing of blood vessels, producing swelling and ecchymosis at the point of ligament injury.
3. *Inability to use the extremity.* Because of the pain of injury, the patient is often unable to use the limb normally.

The perceptive student will realize that the signs of a sprain are the same as some of those for a fracture. Indeed, it is impossible at times to differentiate between a nondisplaced fracture and a sprain. The important point to remember is that while an injury may appear to be just a sprain, a fracture may be present as well. In the field, the working diagnosis whenever any one of the signs of fracture, dislocation, or sprain is present should be "injury to the limb." Even though the EMT will often be able to make a more specific diagnosis of fracture, dislocation, or sprain, all extremity injuries require evaluation in the emergency department. The basic principles of field management are the same for all three types of limb injury.

EXAMINATION OF MUSCULOSKELETAL INJURIES

There are three essential steps in the examination of all patients with musculoskeletal injuries:

1. General assessment of the patient
2. Examination of the injured part
3. Evaluation of the distal neurovascular function

A general, primary assessment of the injured patient must be carried out before attention is focused on an injured limb. As pointed out earlier, multiple injuries occur frequently, and the patient's general condition must be assessed and stabilized first. Bleeding from an extremity should be controlled as part of the primary stabilization, but further treatment of the extremities should await full stabilization of the patient's vital functions.

Once the patient's general condition is stabilized, attention can be directed at evaluating the injured limb. Inspection and palpation are used to identify musculoskeletal injuries. The EMT should look at the injured limb and compare it with the opposite, uninjured side. The clothing should be gently and carefully removed so that a thorough inspection will reveal any of the following: (1) open fracture or dislocation (and its accompanying risk of contamination and infection), (2) deformity, (3) swelling, and/or (4) ecchymosis. Then the EMT should gently palpate the extremities and the spine to identify any areas of point tenderness — the best indicator of an underlying fracture, dislocation, or sprain.

Following inspection and palpation, the presence of a significant limb injury will have been identified in most instances. It is not important to differentiate fractures, dislocations, sprains, or just simple contusions. The working diagnosis in most instances will be "injury to the limb." All limb injuries are treated in the same manner and therefore it is not critical to differentiate between the various types of extremity injuries.

If the patient has no signs of injury following inspection and palpation, the EMT should ask the patient to move each limb carefully. With any significant musculoskeletal injury, movement of an injured part will be painful for the patient. The patient can usually localize the point of maximal discomfort. If even the slightest motion by the patient produces pain, no further motion should be attempted. This step should not be attempted when evaluating an injured person who complains of neck or back pain, because even the slightest motion may cause permanent damage to the spinal cord.

Once an injury to the limb has been diagnosed, it is essential to perform an evaluation of the distal neurovascular function. Many important vessels and nerves lie close to the bone, especially around the major joints. Therefore, any fracture or dislocation may have associated vessel or nerve injury. A neurovascular examination must be carried out initially and repeated every 15 minutes until the patient is hospitalized.

It is also imperative to recheck the neurovascular status after any manipulation of the limb (such as splinting). This reevaluation after a splint is applied is most important because manipulations during splinting might have caused a bone fragment to press against or impale an important nerve or vessel. A pulseless limb will die if circulation is not restored, and priority must be given to such patients in the emergency care system. The following neurovascular examination should be carried out and recorded for each injured limb:

1. *Pulse.* Palpate the pulse distal to the point of injury. Palpate the radial pulse in the upper extremity and the posterior tibial pulse in the lower extremity (Figure 15.14).
2. *Capillary refill.* Note and record skin color, identifying any pallor or cyanosis. The capillary bed is best seen in the finger or toe underneath the nail. Firm pressure on the tip of the nail will cause the nailbed to blanch

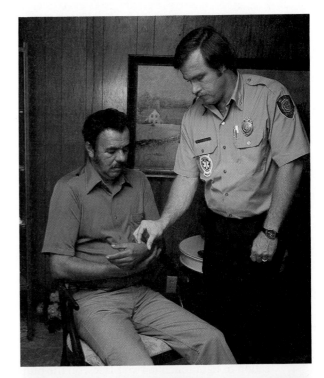

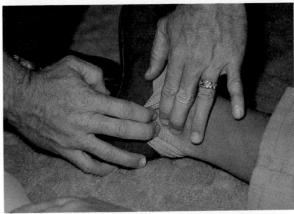

FIGURE 15.14 The first step in a neurovascular examination following a limb injury is to palpate the pulse distal to the injury: (top) palpation of the radial pulse; (bottom) palpation of the posterior tibial pulse.

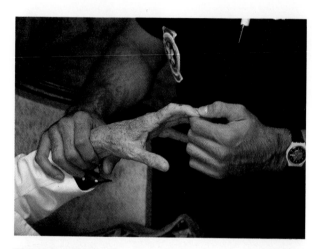

FIGURE 15.15 The second step in a neurovascular examination following a limb injury is to note and record skin color. Capillary refill (best seen in the nailbed) should be pink and brisk.

(turn white). Upon release of the pressure, the normal pink color should return to the nailbed by the time it takes to say "capillary filling." If a pink color does not return in this 2-second interval, it is considered delayed and indicates impairment of circulation. The capillary refill should be pink and brisk (Figure 15.15).

3. *Sensation.* The patient's ability to sense light touch in the fingers or toes distal to a fracture site is a good indication that the nerve supply remains intact. In the hand, check sensation to light touch in two places: on the pulp of the index and the little fingers. In the foot, feeling on the pulp of the big toe and on the dorsum of the foot laterally should be checked (Figure 15.16).

4. *Motor Function.* When injury is proximal to the hand or foot, make an estimate of muscular activity. If the injury involves the hand or foot itself, do not perform this test because it will cause pain for the patient. The test can be done simply by having the patient open and close the hand for an upper extremity injury and wiggle the toes or move the foot up and down to test the motor function of the lower extremity (Figure 15.17). Sometimes, attempt at motion will produce pain at an injury site. If pain occurs, do not persist with this part of the examination.

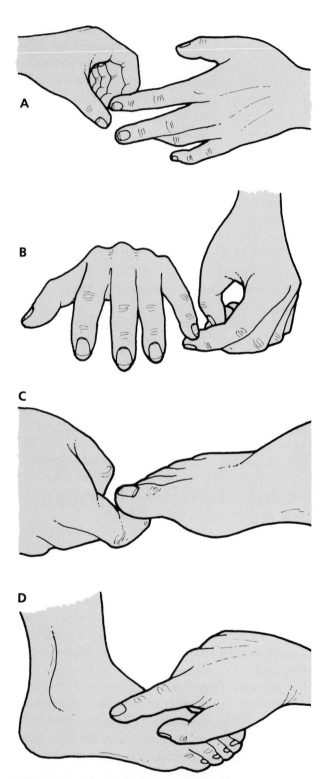

FIGURE 15.16 The third step in a neurovascular examination following a limb injury is to check sensation in four critical areas: (a) the pulp of the index fingertip; (b) the pulp of the little fingertip; (c) the pulp of the big toe; and (d) the dorsolateral aspect of the foot.

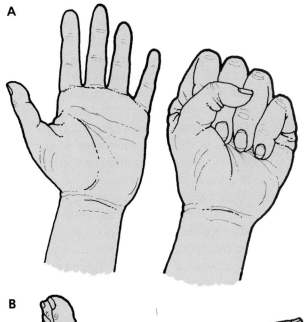

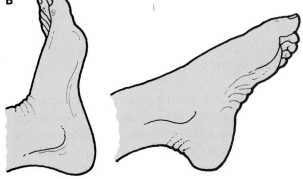

FIGURE 15.17 The fourth step in a neurovascular examination following a limb injury is to check motor function: (top) upper extremity motor function is tested by having the patient open and close the hand; (bottom) lower extremity motor function is tested by wiggling the toes or moving the entire foot up and down.

In the unconscious patient, many of the steps just listed cannot be carried out because they require patient cooperation. After the primary assessment is completed and vital functions are stabilized, *any* limb deformity, swelling, ecchymosis, or false motion should be considered evidence of a limb injury and treated as such. Monitoring the distal pulses and capillary filling can be done in the unconscious patient, but assessing sensation and motor function cannot be done without the cooperation of the patient. In addition, the EMT must always assume that *any unconscious, injured patient has a spinal fracture that will require spinal immobilization.*

TREATMENT OF MUSCULOSKELETAL INJURIES

The emergency management of fractures, dislocations, and sprains takes place after the injured patient's vital functions have been assessed and stabilized. Then, and only then, should attention be directed to the musculoskeletal injury.

All open wounds are managed initially by covering the entire wound with a dry, sterile dressing and applying local pressure to control bleeding (Figure 15.18). Once a sterile compression dressing has been applied to an open fracture, it can be managed in the same way as a closed fracture by applying an appropriate splint. Emergency department personnel must be notified of all wounds that have been dressed and splinted.

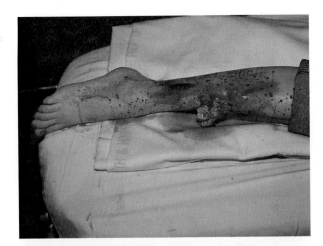

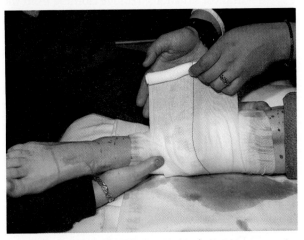

FIGURE 15.18 The first step in the management of any open extremity wound is the application of a dry sterile compression dressing.

Splinting

All fractures, dislocations, and sprains should be splinted before the patient is moved unless the patient's life is in immediate danger. Splinting prevents the motion of fracture fragments, a dislocated joint, or damaged soft tissues, thus reducing pain. Splinting also facilitates the transfer and transportation of the patient. In addition, splinting will help prevent the following:

1. Further damage of muscles, the spinal cord, peripheral nerves, and blood vessels from broken bone ends.
2. Laceration of the skin by broken bone ends. One of the primary indications for splinting is to prevent the conversion of a closed fracture to an open fracture.
3. Restriction of distal blood flow resulting from pressure of the bone ends on blood vessels.
4. Excessive bleeding of the tissues at the injury site.

Because splinting has so many advantages, all extremity injuries, regardless of their severity, should be splinted prior to transport.

A splint can be fashioned from any material. It is simply a device to prevent motion of the injured part. However, the EMT should have an adequate supply of standard commercial splints and only occasionally should have to improvise. The following are general principles of splinting that all EMTs should know how to carry out:

1. In most situations, remove clothing from the area of any suspected fracture or dislocation to allow inspection of the limb for open wounds, deformity, swelling, and ecchymosis.
2. Note and record the circulatory (pulse and capillary refill) and neurological (sensation and movement) status distal to the site of injury. Continue to monitor the neurovascular status until the patient reaches the hospital.
3. Cover all wounds with a dry sterile dressing before applying a splint. Notify the receiving hospital of all open wounds.
4. Do not move the patient before splinting extremity injuries unless there is an immediate hazard to the patient or the EMT.

5. In a suspected fracture of the shaft of any bone, make sure the splint immobilizes the joint above and the joint below the fracture.
6. With injuries in and around the joint, make sure the splint immobilizes the bone above and the bone below the injured joint.
7. Pad all splints to prevent local pressure.
8. During application of the splint, use your hands to minimize movement of the limb and to support the injury site until the limb is completely splinted.
9. Align a limb severely deformed from a fracture of the shaft of a long bone with constant gentle manual traction so that it can be incorporated into a splint.
10. If resistance to limb alignment is encountered when traction is applied, splint the limb in the position of deformity.
11. In all suspected spine injuries, only correct the deformity enough to obtain an effective airway and allow application of a splint.
12. When in doubt, *splint*.

Principles 9 and 10 refer to the use of traction in managing musculoskeletal injury. **Traction** is defined as the action of drawing or pulling on an object. Traction is the most effective way to realign fractures of the shaft of the long bones so that the limb can be splinted more effectively. Excessive traction can be very harmful to an injured limb. When applied correctly, however, traction will stabilize the bone fragments and improve the overall alignment of the limb. The EMT should not attempt to reduce the fracture or force all the bone fragments back into anatomic alignment. This is the physician's responsibility. In the field the goals of traction are (1) to stabilize the fracture fragments to prevent excessive movement, and (2) to align the limb sufficiently to allow it to be placed in a splint.

The amount of pull required to accomplish these objectives will vary but rarely will exceed 15 pounds. The least amount of force necessary to achieve alignment of the limb is the amount that should be employed. When applying traction, the EMT must grasp the foot or hand firmly so that once the traction pull is applied it will not be released until the limb is fully splinted. Discomfort to the patient will be minimized by having a second person support the injured limb under the site of the fracture.

The direction of traction pull is always along the long axis of the limb. The EMT should imagine where the normal, injured limb would lie and pull along the line of that normal, imaginary limb. The alignment of the deformed, injured limb will then approximate this posture as gentle traction is applied (Figure 15.19). Grasping the foot or hand and the initial pull of traction will usually cause slight discomfort as the fragments move. This initial discomfort will quickly subside and further gentle traction may then be applied. If the patient strongly resists the traction or if it causes more pain that persists, it must be stopped and the limb must be splinted in the deformed position.

The EMT must remember that many different materials can be used as splints if necessary. Even when no splinting materials are available, the arm can be bound to the chest wall and an injured leg can be splinted to the patient's uninjured leg to provide at least temporary stability. While splints can be fabricated from many different materials, there are three basic types: rigid, soft, and traction splints.

Rigid Splints

Rigid splints are made from firm material and are applied to the sides, front, and/or back of an injured extremity to prevent motion at the injury site.

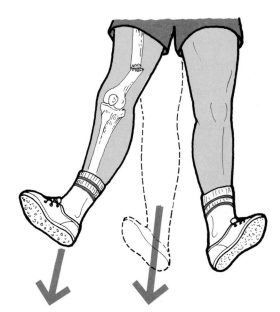

FIGURE 15.19 Gentle traction should be applied to the limb in a line parallel to the normal axis of the injured, deformed limb.

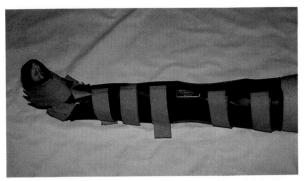

FIGURE 15.20 A rigid splint. Two EMTs are needed to apply a rigid splint.

Common examples of rigid splints include padded board splints, molded plastic and metal splints, padded wire ladder splints, and folded cardboard splints (Figure 15.20). Two EMTs following these steps are needed to apply rigid splints:

1. First EMT: Gently support the limb at the site of injury and apply gentle steady traction if necessary. Maintain this support until the splint is completely applied.
2. Second EMT: Place the rigid splint under or alongside the limb.
3. Place padding to assure even pressure and even contact between the limb and the splint, paying particular attention to bony prominences.
4. Apply bindings to hold the splint securely to the limb.
5. Check and record the distal neurovascular function.

When severe limb deformities are present — as is the case with many dislocations — or when resistance or pain is encountered upon application of gentle traction to the fracture of a shaft of a long bone, the deformed limb must be splinted in the position of deformity. In this situation, splinting is accomplished by appling padded board splints to each side of the limb and securing them with soft roller bandages (Figure 16.15 and 17.12).

Soft Splints

The most commonly used **soft splint** is the precontoured, inflatable, clear plastic **air splint.** These splints are available in a variety of sizes and shapes, with or without a zipper that runs the length of the splint. After application, the splint is inflated by mouth — never with a pump. The air splint is comfortable for the patient, provides uniform contact, and has the added advantage of applying firm pressure to a bleeding wound.

The air splint has some disadvantages, particularly in cold weather areas. The zipper can stick, clog with dirt, or freeze. With significant temperature changes, the pressure of the air in the splint will vary, decreasing with cold and increasing in warm environments. Changes in pressure will also occur with changes in altitude — sometimes becoming a problem with helicopter transport of patients.

The method of applying an air splint depends on whether or not it has a zipper. With either type, all wounds are first covered with a dry, sterile dressing. If the splint has a zipper, the injured limb is held slightly off the ground with gentle traction and

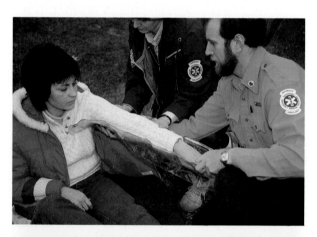

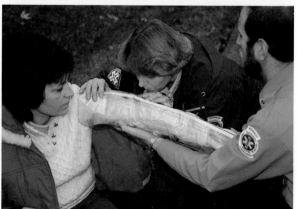

FIGURE 15.21 A zippered air splint. (top) The deflated splint is first placed under the limb and zipped up. (bottom) Then the EMT inflates the air splint by mouth.

support under the site of injury; the open, deflated splint is then placed around the limb, zipped up, and inflated by mouth (Figure 15.21).

If a nonzippered or partially zippered type of air splint is used, two EMTs should follow these steps:

1. First EMT: Place your arm through the splint. Once your hand is extended beyond the splint, grasp the hand or foot of the injured limb (Figure 15.22a).
2. Second EMT: Support the patient's injured limb until splinting is accomplished.
3. First EMT: Apply gentle traction to the hand or foot while sliding the splint onto the injured limb (Figure 15.22b). The hand or foot of the injured limb should always be included in the splint.
4. Inflate the splint by mouth (Figure 15.22c).
5. With either type of air splint, test the pressure in the splint after application. With proper inflation, you should be just able to compress the walls of the splint together with a firm pinch between the thumb and index finger near the edge of the splint (Figure 15.22d).
6. As with any other splint, check and record the distal neurovascular function after application and monitor it periodically until the patient reaches the hospital.

Other soft splints such as pillow splints and a sling and swathe are used extensively and will be discussed in Chapters 16 and 17.

Traction Splints

A **traction splint** holds a lower extremity fracture in alignment through a constant, steady longitudinal pull on the extremity. The famous orthopedic surgeon, Sir Hugh Owen Thomas, invented this splint, and it is frequently called the **Thomas splint.** When traction is applied to the foot through the ankle hitch, a force is exerted by the upper end of the splint against the ischial tuberosity of the patient's pelvis. This force is called **countertraction.** The splint must be seated well on the ischial tuberosity for effective countertraction. Because countertraction is essential to proper function of the splint, it is not suitable for use in the upper extremity because countertraction forces cannot be tolerated by the major nerves and blood vessels in the patient's axilla.

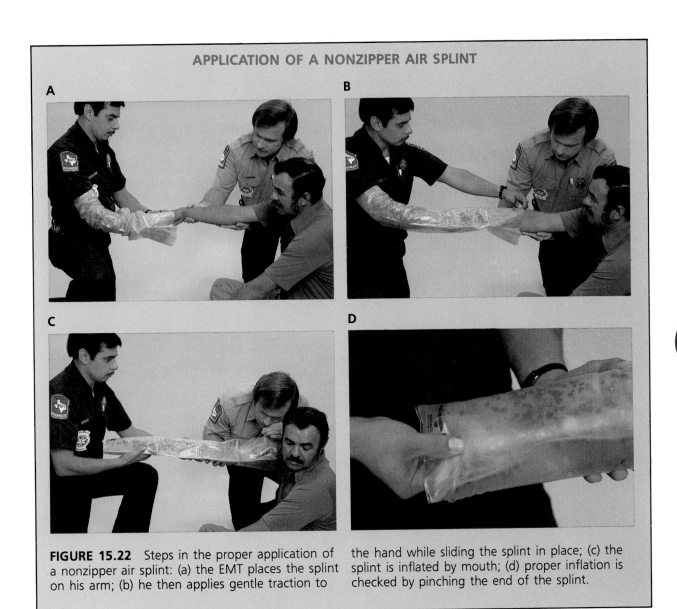

APPLICATION OF A NONZIPPER AIR SPLINT

A

B

C

D

FIGURE 15.22 Steps in the proper application of a nonzipper air splint: (a) the EMT places the splint on his arm; (b) he then applies gentle traction to the hand while sliding the splint in place; (c) the splint is inflated by mouth; (d) proper inflation is checked by pinching the end of the splint.

Proper application of a traction splint requires two well trained EMTs working together. It is impossible for one person to apply this splint. Knowledge of the precise technique of application of the traction splint is extremely important. The EMTs should practice the steps over and over until the sequence and necessary teamwork have become routine. Seven steps must be followed (Figure 15.23):

1. Cut open the patient's trouser leg or otherwise expose the injured lower extremity so that it is possible to see exactly what is being done.

2. Place the splint beside the patient's uninjured leg and adjust it to the proper length (the ring at the ischial tuberosity and the splint extending 12 inches beyond the foot) (Figure 15.23a). Open and adjust the four Velcro support straps that should be positioned at the mid-thigh, above the knee, below the knee, and above the ankle.

3. First EMT: Manually support and stabilize the injured limb so that no motion will occur at the fracture site while the second EMT fastens the appropriately sized ankle hitch about the patient's ankle and foot (Figure

A

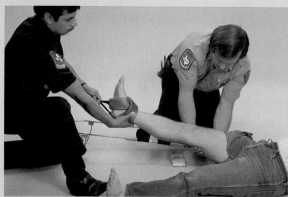

B

C

D

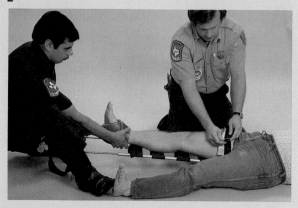
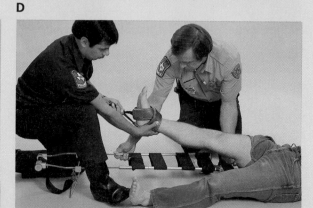

E

F

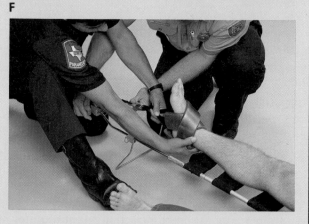

G

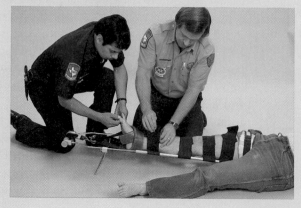

FIGURE 15.23 Proper sequence of steps used in the application of a traction splint to an injured lower extremity: (a) the EMT positions the splint against the patient's uninjured leg and adjusts it to the proper length; (b) the ankle hitch is fastened around the patient's ankle and foot; (c) the leg is supported at the site of suspected injury; (d) the EMT slides the splint into position under the patient's leg; (e) the groin area is padded, and the ischial strap is fastened; (f) the loops of the ankle hitch are connected to the end of the splint; (g) the support straps are fastened.

15.23b). The shoe is customarily removed from the foot.

4. First EMT: Support the leg at the site of the suspected injury (Figure 15.23c), while the second EMT simultaneously applies gentle longitudinal traction manually to the ankle hitch and foot. Only enough traction is applied to align the limb so that it will fit into the splint. Do not attempt to align the fracture fragments anatomically.

5. First EMT: Slide the splint into position under the patient's limb (Figure 15.23d), making certain that the ring is seated well on the ischial tuberosity. Pad the groin and gently apply the ischial strap (Figure 15.23e).

6. First EMT: While the traction is maintained, connect the loops of the ankle hitch to the end of the splint (Figure 15.23f). Then apply gentle traction to the connecting strap between the ankle hitch and the splint, just strongly enough to maintain limb alignment. Some splints come with a ratchet mechanism to tighten the strap. This mechanism can generate an excessive amount of force, which can overstretch the limb and cause further injury to the patient.

7. Once proper traction has been applied, fasten the support straps so that the limb is securely held in the splint (Figure 15.23g).

Traction splints are used primarily to secure fractures of the shaft of the femur or the tibia. Several different types of lower extremity traction splints are commercially available. Each brand has its own unique method of application. The EMT must be thoroughly familiar with and practiced in the technique of applying the particular splint being used.

Because traction splints immobilize the limb by producing countertraction on the ischium and in the groin, care must be used to pad these areas well and especially to avoid excessive pressure on the external genitalia. Commercial padded ankle hitches are readily available and must be used rather than pieces of rope, cord, or tape. Such improvised hitches are painful and can obstruct circulation in the foot.

Transportation

Once an injured limb is adequately splinted, the patient is ready to be transferred to a litter and transported. The exact position of the patient will vary somewhat, depending on the type of injury. With most isolated upper extremity injuries, the patient will be most comfortable in a semiseated position rather than lying flat. Either position is acceptable. With lower extremity injuries, the patient should lie supine, with the limb elevated slightly, about 6 inches, to minimize swelling. In all cases, the injured part should be positioned slightly above the level of the heart (Figure 15.24). The injured limb

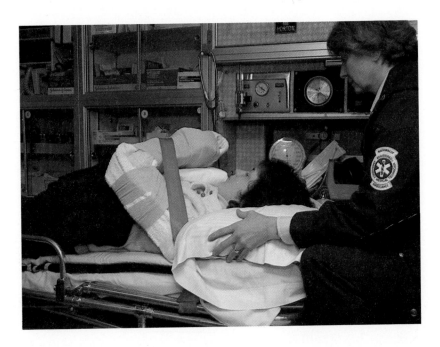

FIGURE 15.24 The patient should always be transported with the injured part positioned slightly above the level of the heart.

should never be allowed to flop about or dangle off the edge of the litter.

Swelling can also be minimized to some degree by applying cold packs to the splinted injury site. Care must be taken to avoid placing the cold packs directly on the skin or other exposed tissues. Placing a cold pack on top of an air splint or other thick, insulating material, however, will not be of any benefit.

Very few, if any, musculoskeletal injuries require excessively rapid ambulance transportation. Once dressed and splinted, the limb is stable and orderly transportation can be undertaken. With the pulseless limb, a sense of urgency develops, and the patient must be given a higher priority in the transportation system. If the hospital is only a few minutes away, reckless speeding to the emergency department will make little or no difference to the patient's eventual outcome. If the treatment facility is an hour or more away, however, evacuation of the patient by helicopter or rapid ground transportation should be given high priority. In every instance of impaired circulation to the distal limb, medical control should be notified of the patient's problem so that proper steps can be taken once the patient arrives in the emergency department.

YOU ARE THE EMT...

1. Your patient has a compound fracture of the tibia. Is this an open or closed fracture? Which is more serious? Why?
2. A young boy has fallen out of a tree and is guarding his arm. What does that mean? What is guarding a sign of?
3. A strain is a muscle injury. What kind of injury is a sprain? What are three signs of a sprain?
4. You are not sure if your patient's ankle is sprained, dislocated, or broken. Why should you splint it? What kind of splint will you use?

Shoulder and Upper Extremity Fractures and Dislocations

16

INJURIES TO THE CLAVICLE AND SCAPULA

The clavicle (collarbone) is one of the most frequently fractured bones in the body. Fracture of the clavicle most commonly occurs in children, usually from a fall on the outstretched hand. Clavicle fractures are also seen in association with crushing injuries of the chest. A patient with a fracture of the clavicle will complain of pain in the shoulder girdle and will usually hold the injured arm against the chest wall, supporting the elbow or forearm with the opposite hand to "splint" the site of injury (Figure 16.1). Frequently, a younger child will complain of pain throughout the limb and express unwillingness to use any part of that limb. These complaints make it difficult to localize the point of injury. Generally, there is swelling and point tenderness over the clavicle. Occasionally the skin is tented over a fracture fragment because the clavicle lies just beneath the skin. The clavicle lies directly over the major arteries, veins, and nerves that supply the upper extremity. Thus,

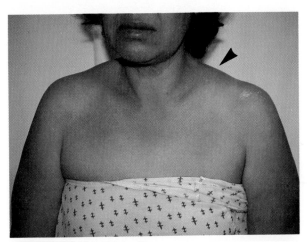

FIGURE 16.1 The clavicle is one of the most frequently fractured bones, especially among children. The patient will usually "splint" the injured limb by holding the arm against the chest wall to prevent motion of the fracture fragments.

fractures of the clavicle may damage these important neurovascular structures.

Fractures of the scapula occur much less frequently because this bone is well protected by many large muscles. Scapular fractures almost always occur following a violent blow to the back, directly over the scapula. Because the force required to break the scapula is so great and because the thoracic cage lies just beneath it, a patient suspected of having a scapular fracture must be evaluated very carefully. Respiratory insufficiency secondary to rib fractures or other chest injury may exist. The signs of scapular fracture include abrasions, contusions, swelling, and tenderness about the scapula, as well as signs of respiratory difficulty (Figure 16.2). The patient will limit use of the arm because of pain at the fracture site.

The joint between the outer end of the clavicle and the acromion process of the scapula is called the **acromioclavicular joint** (Figure 16.3). This joint

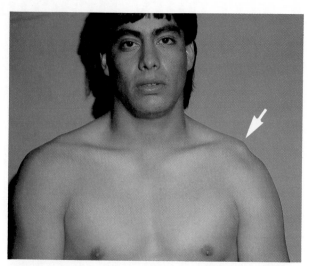

FIGURE 16.3   Acromioclavicular separation. Note the prominence of the dislocated outer end of the clavicle.

is frequently dislocated, especially in football players. The injury is often called a **shoulder separation** or simply an **A/C separation.** Dislocations occur when the individual falls and lands on the point of the shoulder, driving the scapula distally away from the outer end of the clavicle. Pain, including point tenderness over the acromioclavicular joint, is usually accompanied by prominence of the distal end of the clavicle.

Fractures of the clavicle and scapula and acromioclavicular separations can all be splinted effectively with a sling and swathe. The principal effect of the **sling** is to support the weight of the upper extremity and relieve the downward pull of gravity on the injury site. The triangular sling must apply gentle upward support to the olecranon process of the ulna to be effective. The knot of the sling should be tied to one side of the neck so that it does not press uncomfortably on the cervical spinous processes (Figure 16.4).

A sling alone, however, will not provide full immobilization of the shoulder region. A **swathe** must be added to bind the arm to the chest wall for adequate immobilization. The swathe should be tight enough to secure the limb to the chest wall to prevent it from swinging freely. However, it should not be so tight as to compress the chest and compromise breathing. The hand should remain exposed so that neurovascular evaluation can be performed periodically after the splint has been applied.

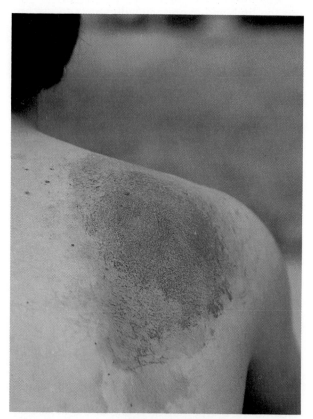

FIGURE 16.2   Contusions or abrasions over the scapular region may indicate a fracture. The EMT must be aware of the high likelihood of respiratory problems found frequently with this injury.

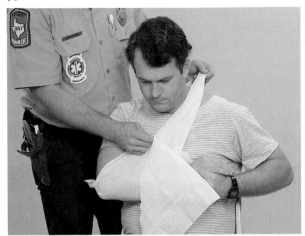

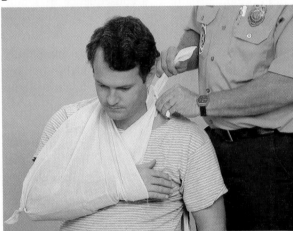

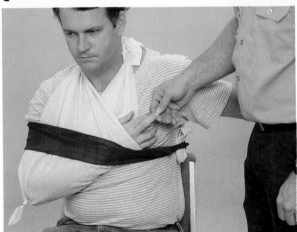

FIGURE 16.4 Splinting with a sling and swathe: (a) The sling should be applied so that the knot is tied to one side of the neck; (b) the sling should support the weight of the arm; (c) a swathe is used to bind the arm to the chest wall to prevent it from swinging freely.

DISLOCATION OF THE SHOULDER

The shoulder joint, the articulation between the humeral head and the glenoid fossa of the scapula (the **glenohumeral joint**), is the most commonly dislocated large joint in the body. Almost always, the humeral head dislocates anteriorly, coming to lie in front of the scapula. This anterior dislocation of the humeral head is caused by forceful abduction and external rotation of the arm. Shoulder dislocation is extremely painful, and the patient will resist any motion of the locked joint. The patient will try to protect the injured shoulder by holding the dislocated arm with the opposite hand to "splint" it. On careful inspection from the front, the EMT will see that the normal rounded contour of the shoulder is not present when compared with the opposite side (Figure 16.5). Instead, the shoulder is squared off — flattened laterally. The humeral head can be seen protruding anteriorly, lying underneath the pectoralis muscle on the anterior chest wall. Frequently there is numbness in the upper extremity because the head

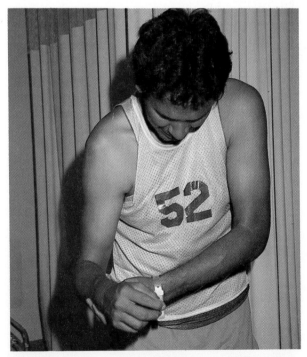

FIGURE 16.5 Anterior dislocation of the shoulder. The normal rounded contour of the shoulder is not present when compared with the opposite side, and there is a space between the elbow and the patient's chest wall.

of the humerus is pressing on the major nerves in the axilla (armpit).

Dislocation of the shoulder disrupts many of the supporting ligaments on the anterior aspect of the shoulder joint. Often these ligaments do not heal well after the shoulder dislocation is reduced (put back in place). Therefore, some patients will have frequent, recurrent dislocations of this joint that will eventually require surgical repair. Much less force is required to dislocate a shoulder that previously has been dislocated, and many patients will have recurrent dislocations of the shoulder with trivial trauma. Simply raising one's hand to put on a T-shirt is all that may be necessary to allow the humeral head to slip out of place. The EMT will care for many patients who have primary or recurrent dislocations of the shoulder joint. Never, however, should the EMT attempt to reduce a dislocated shoulder. This maneuver should only be done in the hospital after x-rays have been taken.

Immobilizing a shoulder dislocation is difficult because the patient will hold his or her arm in a fixed position away from the chest wall. Any attempt to bring the arm in toward the chest will produce pain. The joint must be splinted in the position that is most comfortable for the patient. The EMT can overcome the difficulty that this fixed position of the arm causes by gently placing a pillow or rolled blanket between the arm and chest wall to fill up the space between them (Figure 16.6). Once the arm is stabilized against the pillow, the elbow can usually be flexed to 90

degrees without causing further pain for the patient. A sling can then be applied to the forearm and wrist to support its weight. The arm in the sling is secured to the pillow and chest with a swathe. The patient should be transported in a sitting or semiseated position.

FRACTURE OF THE SHAFT OF THE HUMERUS

The shaft of the humerus is frequently broken. Two regions of this bone are prone to fracture. In the elderly, the proximal portion near the shoulder joint is frequently fractured as a result of a fall. Fracture near the midshaft occurs more frequently in the young adult, usually as a consequence of a more violent injury.

The proximal shaft fracture causes mild to moderate deformity of the upper arm. Frequently, deformity is masked by swelling and by the large muscles that surround this part of the arm (Figure

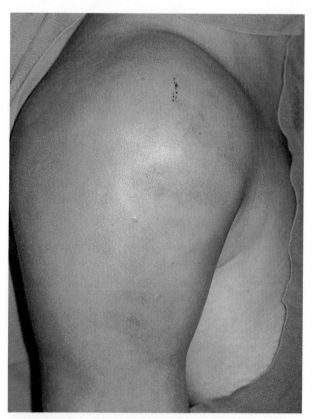

FIGURE 16.7 Fracture of the proximal end of the humerus is usually associated with significant soft tissue swelling at the fracture site.

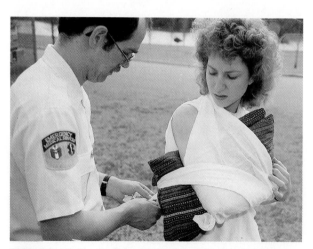

FIGURE 16.6 A dislocated shoulder must be splinted in the position of deformity with a pillow, sling, and swathe.

16.7). With fractures of the midshaft of this bone, there is usually gross angulation at the fracture site and marked instability of the fracture fragments (Figure 16.8).

Occasionally, because of the close proximity of the radial nerve to the humeral shaft (Figure 16.9), this nerve is lacerated, compressed, or trapped at the

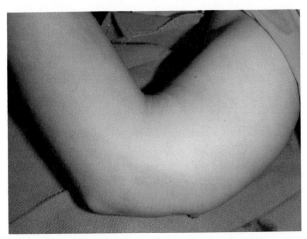

FIGURE 16.8 Fractures in the midshaft of the humerus are usually displaced, producing significant deformity of the arm.

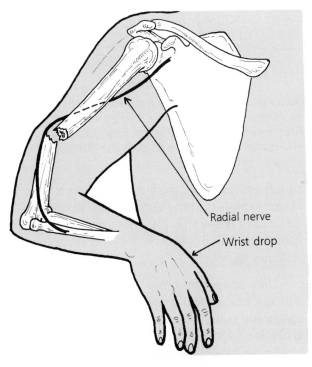

Radial nerve

Wrist drop

FIGURE 16.9 The radial nerve lies right against the shaft of the humerus and may be damaged or trapped in the fracture site.

midshaft fracture site. When this nerve is injured, the patient will be unable to extend (**dorsiflex**) the wrist or fingers. The patient may also experience numbness on the dorsum of the hand. The weakness produces the characteristic "**wrist drop**" of a radial nerve palsy.

Fractures of the proximal humerus and all minimally displaced fractures of the shaft of this bone can be immobilized with a sling and swathe. The chest wall is used as a splint, and the injured arm is secured to the chest wall, as with injuries about the shoulder girdle. A short padded board splint may be placed on the lateral side of the arm under the sling and swathe to provide additional lateral support (Figure 16.10).

With a severely angulated fracture of the shaft of the humerus, traction should be applied to realign the fracture fragments prior to splinting. With one hand the EMT should support the site of the fracture and with the other hand grasp the two humeral condyles just above the elbow. Pulling gently in line with the normal axis of the limb will align the arm so that splinting can be accomplished more effectively (Figure 16.11). Once gross alignment of the limb is achieved, the arm is splinted with a sling and swathe, supplemented by a padded board splint on the lateral aspect of the arm. If significant pain or resistance to gentle traction is encountered, the fracture should be splinted in the deformed position with a padded wire ladder splint or a padded board splint and pillows to support the injured limb.

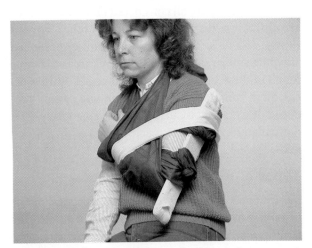

FIGURE 16.10 A sling and swathe, supplemented with a lateral padded board splint, provides good immobilization for humeral shaft fractures.

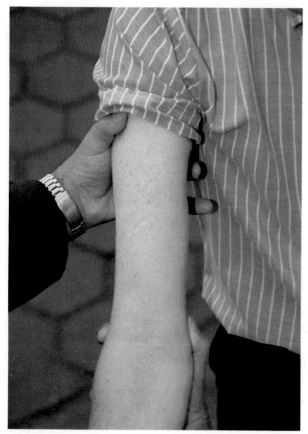

FIGURE 16.11 To align the severely deformed arm with a humeral fracture, gentle traction is applied to the humeral condyles.

INJURIES ABOUT THE ELBOW

Fractures and dislocations occur commonly around the elbow. They are all considered here because they are difficult to distinguish from each other without the use of x-rays. The clinical deformities produced are quite similar, and the emergency care is the same for all of these injuries. Nerve and vessel injuries occur quite commonly in this region and can be produced or worsened by inappropriate emergency care, particularly by excessive manipulation of the injured joint.

Types of Elbow Injuries

Fracture of the Distal Humerus. Fracture of the distal end of the humerus is called a **supracondylar fracture** because the fracture line lies just across the humerus above the level of the condyles (Figure 16.12). These fractures are commonly seen in children. Frequently a significant rotation of the frac-

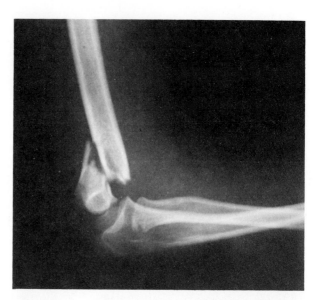

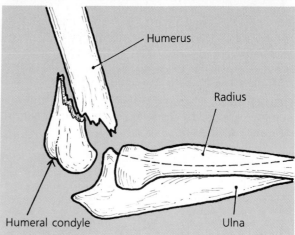

FIGURE 16.12 Supracondylar fracture of the humerus: (top) X-ray of the injured elbow; (bottom) line drawing showing fracture line lying just across the humerus above the level of the condyles.

ture fragments takes place and produces a deformity and exposes the bone surfaces to the nearby vessels and nerves (Figure 16.13). Nerve and vessel injury is common with this fracture. Swelling occurs rapidly and may be severe.

Dislocation of the Elbow. This injury usually occurs in teenagers and young adults and is frequently an athletic injury. The ulna and radius, which both articulate with the distal humerus, are most commonly displaced posteriorly, making the olecranon process of the ulna much more prominent (Figure 16.14). The joint is locked with the forearm moderately flexed on the arm. Any attempt at motion of

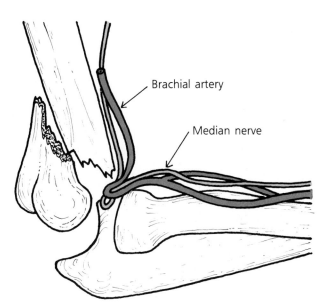

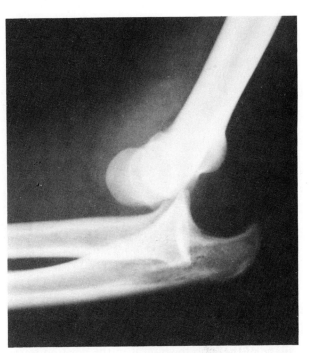

FIGURE 16.13 Note the close proximity of the brachial artery and median nerve to the fracture fragments in a supracondylar fracture.

the elbow is very painful. As with a supracondylar fracture, there is swelling and the potential for significant vessel or nerve injury.

Elbow Joint Sprain. Sprains of the elbow joint occur only rarely. It is not uncommon to see a child who has sustained a mild or moderate elbow injury that could readily be dismissed as a simple sprain. Very frequently the "sprain" turns out to be a nondisplaced or minimally displaced fracture or a partial dislocation of this joint that requires prompt treatment to avoid problems later as the child grows. Thus, all elbow injuries, regardless of their apparent severity, require x-ray evaluation in the emergency department.

Olecranon Fracture. Fracture of the olecranon process of the ulna is usually the result of a direct blow. Thus, abrasions or lacerations are commonly present over this fracture site.

Care of Elbow Injuries

All elbow injuries must be taken seriously, and caution must be exercised in their emergency management. A very careful distal, neurovascular evaluation must be performed on all patients with elbow injuries.

If strong pulses and good capillary filling are present when the patient is first evaluated, the frac-

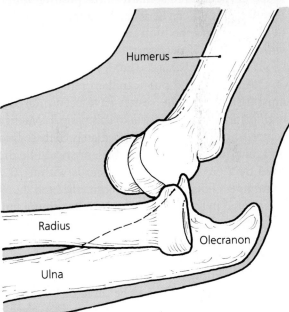

FIGURE 16.14 Dislocation of the elbow: (top) X-ray of the elbow; (bottom) line drawing showing prominence of the olecranon process.

ture or dislocation should be splinted in the position in which it is found. Two padded board splints, applied to each side of the limb and secured with soft roller bandages, will usually provide adequate stability. The boards should extend from the shoulder joint to the wrist joint, immobilizing the entire bone above and below the injured joint (Figure 16.15). A

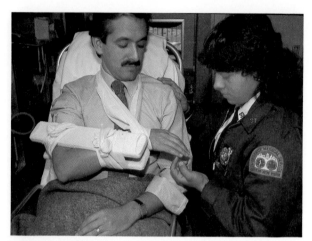

FIGURE 16.15 Two padded board splints adequately stabilize the injured elbow. A collar and cuff further support the weight of the arm.

padded wire ladder splint can also be molded to the shape of the limb to splint it in the position found. A collar and cuff can be added to support the weight of the arm, and the limb can be further supported with a pillow, if necessary.

If the patient's hand is cold, pale, or has a weak or absent pulse and poor capillary refill, the EMT must assume that the vessels have been injured; a high priority must be given to this patient. Medical control should be notified immediately of these findings, and further care of this patient should be dictated by a physician. If the patient is within 10 to 15 minutes of definitive medical care, the limb should be splinted in the position in which it is found, and the patient should be transported promptly to the hospital.

If the circumstances are such that there will be a prolonged time before definitive medical care can be reached, the EMT may be directed by medical control to try to realign the limb to improve circulation to the hand. If the pulseless limb is significantly deformed at the elbow, gentle manual traction in line with the long axis of the limb should be applied to decrease the deformity. This maneuver may restore the pulse. Excessive manipulation should never be attempted, however, as it will only worsen the vascular problem. If the pulse can be restored by gentle longitudinal traction, the limb should be splinted in the position that allows the strongest pulse. If no pulse returns after one manipulation, the limb should be splinted in the most comfortable position for the

patient. Prompt transfer to the emergency department is required for all patients with impaired distal circulation.

FRACTURES OF THE FOREARM

Fractures of the shaft of the radius and the ulna are common in persons of all age groups but are seen particularly often in children. Usually both bones break at the same time when the injury is the result of a fall on the outstretched hand, although the fractures may be at different levels in the forearm (Figure 16.16). An isolated fracture of the shaft of the ulna may occur as the result of a direct blow to it.

Fracture of the distal radius is especially common in the elderly, osteoporotic patient. In fact it is so common that it has a special name, **Colles' fracture.** It results from a fall on the outstretched hand that usually produces a characteristic **silver fork deformity,** because the injured wrist assumes a curvature similar to the profile of a dinner fork

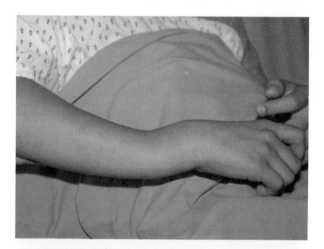

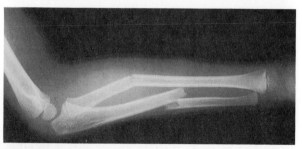

FIGURE 16.16 (top) Fractures of both bones of the forearm occur in children as a result of a fall on the outstretched hand. (bottom) X-ray showing fractures of the shafts of the radius and the ulna.

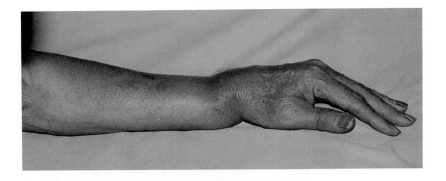

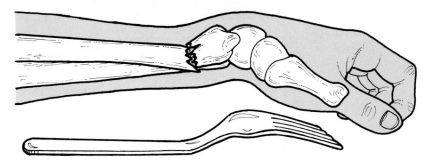

FIGURE 16.17 Fracture of the distal radius, also called a Colles' fracture, produces a characteristic silver fork deformity.

(Figure 16.17). In children a fracture similar in appearance passes through the epiphyseal plate.

A variety of splints can be used to immobilize fractures of the forearm bones. A padded board, air, or pillow splint are all effective. Immobilization of fractures of the shaft of these bones must include the elbow joint. Elbow joint splinting is not essential with fractures near the wrist, but the patient will be more comfortable if a sling or supporting pillow is added to the immobilization.

INJURIES TO THE WRIST AND HAND

Dislocation of the wrist is uncommon. It is usually associated with fracture of one or more of the carpal bones, producing a fracture-dislocation. Wrist sprains frequently occur. Another common injury is an isolated, nondisplaced fracture of one of the carpal bones. As with other joint injuries, these wrist bone fractures cannot be diagnosed without x-rays. Thus, all apparent wrist sprains must be splinted until they can be evaluated in the emergency department.

The EMT will respond to a great variety of hand injuries. All can be potentially serious for the patient. Industrial, recreational, and home accidents commonly result in lacerations (with frequent underlying nerve, tendon, or vessel injury), burns, amputations, fractures, or dislocations. The very intricate

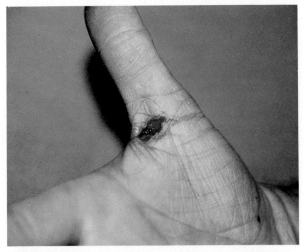

FIGURE 16.18 A small laceration to the base of the thumb that, upon surgical exploration, was found to have produced laceration of two tendons and two nerves.

function of the fingers and hand is so important that any injury, if inadequately or belatedly treated, may result in permanent deformity and disability. All injuries to the hand must be evaluated promptly by a physician so that proper care can be instituted. Even simple lacerations should be treated with respect (Figure 16.18). Dislocated finger joints should not be "popped" back into place. Any amputated parts should be brought with the patient to the hospital.

All hand and wrist injuries can be effectively splinted with a **bulky hand dressing.** All wounds are first covered with a dry, sterile dressing. The injured hand is then formed into what is called the "position of function": The wrist is slightly dorsiflexed and all finger joints are flexed moderately (Figure 16.19). This is the position in which one would most comfortably hold a baseball. A soft roller bandage is then placed into the palm of the hand. A padded board splint is applied to the palmar side of the hand and wrist and secured with a soft roller bandage throughout the length of the splint. The splinted hand and wrist should then be propped on a pillow or on the patient's chest during transportation to the hospital.

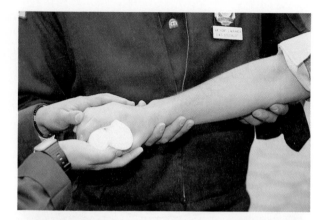

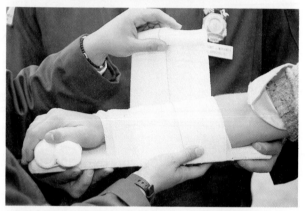

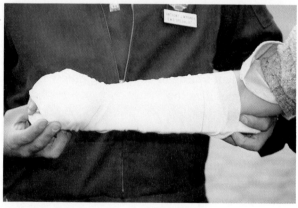

FIGURE 16.19   The injured hand is splinted in the "position of function" — the position that one would most comfortably hold a baseball.

YOU ARE THE EMT...

1. What is the difference between a shoulder separation and dislocation of the shoulder? How would you treat each injury?
2. You suspect your patient has a humeral shaft fracture. After performing a careful neurovascular evaluation, you decide the limb does not need to be realigned before splinting. What findings contributed to this decision? What signs would have made you decide realignment was necessary?
3. What bone is involved in a Colles fracture and produces a silver fork deformity? These fractures are more common in elderly people who suffer from what disease? How would you treat this injury?
4. Your patient is a young girl who fell off a deck about 12 feet off the ground. She has pain in her arm and is holding it to her chest with her other arm. What other injury should you suspect and what will you look for to confirm your suspicions?

Injuries of the Pelvis and Lower Extremity

OVERVIEW

The bones of the pelvis and lower extremity are large and strong because they are designed for weight bearing. Injuries to these structures usually result from severe trauma such as from falls and automobile accidents. These injuries can range in severity from a simple contusion to severe multiple fractures that often result in permanent deformity and loss of function.

The general principles of splinting as outlined in Chapter 15 should be followed with injuries to the lower extremity, after, of course, the EMT performs a general primary assessment of the patient. Serious problems identified in the primary survey must be stabilized before the limb injury is evaluated and splinted. The EMT must also evaluate and monitor the distal neurovascular function frequently until the patient is delivered to the hospital.

Chapter 17 examines pelvic fractures, dislocation of the hip joint, fractures of the proximal femur, femoral shaft fractures, knee injuries, tibia and fibula fractures, ankle injuries, and foot injuries. The discusssion of each of these injuries includes their signs and symptoms, how to evaluate them, and the best way to stabilize them.

OBJECTIVES

The objectives of Chapter 17 are to

- identify and know how to stabilize injuries of the pelvis, including fractures of the pelvis and dislocation of the hip joint.
- learn how to evaluate and splint fractures of the proximal femur and the femoral shaft.
- become familiar with injuries about the knee, including injuries of the knee ligaments, dislocation of the knee, fractures about the knee, and dislocation of the patella.
- know the techniques of splinting fractures of the tibia, fibula, ankle, and foot.

INJURIES TO THE PELVIS

Fractures of the Pelvis

Closed fracture of the pelvis is commonly a result of direct compression in which the pelvis is literally crushed by a heavy impact. This injury is often seen after a fall from a height or a direct crushing blow to the pelvic region. Indirect forces can also produce injury of the pelvis — for example, in a car wreck, the knee can strike the dashboard of the car, whereupon the impact of the force is transmitted along the femur, driving the femoral head into the pelvis and causing it to fracture (Figure 17.1). Not all pelvic fractures result from violent trauma. Even a simple fall can produce a closed fracture of the pelvis, especially among elderly people who have osteoporosis.

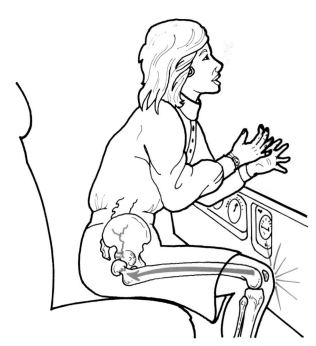

FIGURE 17.1 When the knee strikes the dashboard forcefully, the energy of impact can be transmitted to the hip, fracturing the pelvis or even dislocating the hip.

Fractures of the pelvis may be accompanied by severe blood loss. Very large blood vessels lie adjacent to the pelvis and are easily torn or lacerated at the time of the fracture. A large amount of blood can drain from these lacerated vessels into the **retroperitoneal space,** an area that can hold several liters of blood. As a result, the patient may develop hypovolemic shock and even die from blood loss following a fracture of the pelvis. Keeping in mind the possibility of shock associated with this fracture, the EMT must take immediate steps to combat it, even if there is only minimal swelling or other external signs of bleeding. The extent of blood loss in a closed fracture of the pelvis may not be apparent because the bleeding occurs within the pelvic cavity into the retroperitoneal space. The patient's vital signs must be monitored carefully during stabilization and transport.

Open fractures of the pelvis are quite rare because the pelvis is surrounded by heavy muscles. Occasionally, pelvic fracture fragments will lacerate the rectum or vagina and create an open fracture.

The urinary bladder is especially susceptible to injury following a fracture of the pelvis. Pelvic bone fragments may lacerate the bladder, or the force of impact at injury may cause the bladder to rupture. Thus, the important structures that the pelvis is designed to protect (the blood vessels, the bladder, the vagina, and the rectum) are all susceptible to injury once the protective pelvic ring has been broken.

Fracture of the pelvis should be suspected in any patient who has sustained a high-velocity injury. The patient will frequently complain of pain in the pelvic region or the lower abdomen. Because the area is covered by heavy muscles and other soft tissues, deformity of the pelvis or swelling in the pelvic region is difficult to see. The best sign of fracture of the pelvis is tenderness on firm compression and palpation. Because of its ring-like structure, firm inward compression on the two iliac crests will produce pain at a fracture site at any point around the pelvic ring (Figure 17.2). In addition, firm palpation with the palm of the hand over the symphysis pubis will elicit tenderness if there is injury to the anterior portion of the pelvic ring. If there has been injury to the bladder or the urethra, the patient will have lower abdominal tenderness and may have **hematuria** (blood in the urine) or a bloody discharge from the urethral opening.

Once the diagnosis of a pelvic fracture is suspected, the patient's vital signs must be monitored closely because of the high likelihood of developing hypovolemic shock. Isolated fractures of the pelvis can be immobilized with a long spine board or a scoop stretcher. A pneumatic antishock garment should be placed on the spine board or stretcher underneath the patient (Figure 17.3). During transport, the foot of the immobilization device should be elevated 6 to 12 inches. If the patient develops signs of hypovolemic shock due to a severe pelvic

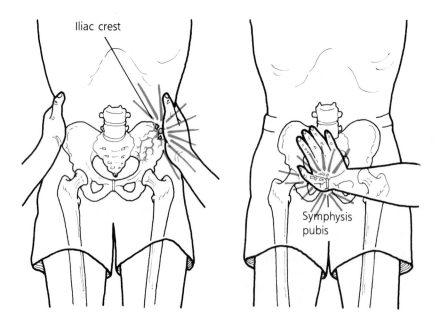

Iliac crest

Symphysis pubis

FIGURE 17.2 Fracture of the pelvis. Tenderness over the iliac crests or pubic symphysis is a sign of pelvic fracture.

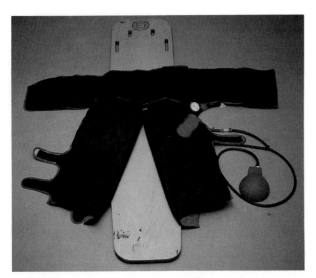

FIGURE 17.3 Any patient suspected of having a pelvic fracture should be placed on a spine board or stretcher with a pneumatic antishock garment in place. The garment can then be applied and inflated promptly should the patient develop signs of hypovolemic shock.

fracture, immobilization should be supplemented with a pneumatic antishock garment (Chapter 10). The device will provide adequate immobilization of the fracture and will also decrease the severity of the hypovolemic shock. Once the pneumatic antishock garment is applied, all of the rules governing its use (particularly the method of deflation and removal) must be followed.

Dislocation of the Hip Joint

The hip joint is a very stable ball-and-socket joint that dislocates only following significant injury. Virtually all dislocations of the hip are posterior. The femoral head is displaced posteriorly, coming to lie in the muscles of the buttock. Posterior dislocation of the hip most commonly occurs during automobile accidents, when an indirect force is applied to the knee and the entire femur is driven posteriorly, dislocating the joint. Thus, hip dislocations should be suspected in any patient in a car wreck in which a contusion, laceration, or obvious fracture is present in the knee region.

Very rarely does the femoral head dislocate anteriorly. In this circumstance, the legs are suddenly and forcefully spread wide apart.

Posterior dislocation of the hip is frequently complicated by injury to the **sciatic nerve.** Located di-

rectly behind the joint, the sciatic nerve is the most important nerve in the lower extremity. It controls the activity of some of the muscles in the thigh and all of the muscles below the knee as well as all the sensation in the leg and foot. When the head of the femur is forced out of the acetabulum, it damages the sciatic nerve by pressing on it or stretching it (Figure 17.4). Partial or complete paralysis of this nerve can result from posterior dislocation of the hip. The patient with paralysis of the sciatic nerve will have decreased sensation in the leg and foot. In addition, there will frequently be weakness of the foot muscles, particularly those muscles that **dorsiflex,** or raise, the toes or the foot. This muscular weakness is commonly called a "**foot drop**" and is characteristic of damage to the sciatic nerve.

A characteristic deformity occurs with posterior dislocation of the hip. The patient lies with the hip joint flexed (the knee drawn up toward the chest), and the thigh rotated inward and adducted across the midline of the body (Figure 17.5). The flexed thigh on the dislocated side lies across the midline of the body over the top of the thigh of the normal leg. With the rare anterior dislocation of the hip, the limb is in the opposite position — extended straight out, rotated outward, and pointing away from the midline of the body. Because of the unique deformities associated with dislocation of the hip, inspection of the patient will usually lead the EMT to the

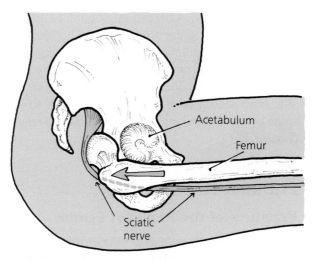

FIGURE 17.4 Posterior dislocation of the hip joint allows the head of the femur to press against the sciatic nerve, causing partial or complete paralysis of this nerve.

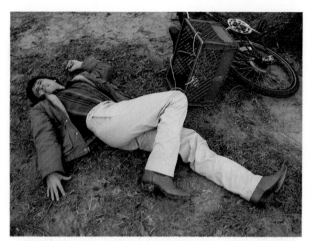

FIGURE 17.5   The usual position of a patient with a posterior dislocation of the hip: The hip joint is flexed and the thigh is rotated inward and adducted across the midline of the body.

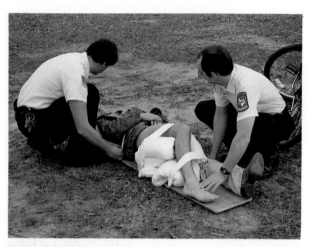

FIGURE 17.6   Posterior dislocation of the hip is splinted with the limb in the deformed position, supported with pillows and secured to the long spine board with straps.

correct diagnosis. The patient will have severe pain in the hip, and any attempted motion of the joint will be met with great resistance. Palpation of the lateral and posterior aspects of the hip region will elicit tenderness, and in some thin individuals the femoral head can be palpated lying below the muscles of the buttock. Careful examination of sensation and motor function in the lower extremity will identify sciatic nerve injury.

As with any other dislocated joint, no attempt should be made to reduce the dislocated hip in the field. The dislocation must be splinted in the position of deformity. The patient should be placed supine on a long spine board. The limb should be supported with pillows and rolled blankets, particularly under the flexed knee. Then the entire limb should be secured to the spine board with long straps. The limb should be stabilized well enough to the spine board to eliminate all motion in the hip region (Figure 17.6).

INJURIES TO THE FEMUR

Fractures of the Proximal Femur

Some of the most common fractures are those of the upper (proximal) end of the femur. Over the years these fractures have been called "**hip fractures**," even though the hip joint is rarely involved. The break goes through the neck of the femur, the

intertrochanteric area, or across the proximal shaft of this bone. The fractures are then respectively called femoral neck, intertrochanteric, or subtrochanteric fractures. Fractures of the upper end of the femur occur in two distinctly different groups of patients — the elderly and young adults. Fractures of the hip most commonly occur in elderly persons (particularly women) with osteoporosis. Because of the brittleness of the osteoporotic bone, a simple fall sustained while standing or walking may result in fracture. On rare occasions fracture of the proximal end of the femur occurs in a younger individual with normal bone who sustains more severe trauma.

All patients with displaced fractures of the proximal femur have a very characteristic deformity. They lie with the leg externally rotated, and the injured leg is usually shorter than the opposite uninjured limb (Figure 17.7). If the fracture is not displaced, this deformity will not be present. Most patients with a fracture of the hip will be unable to walk or move the leg because of pain. Usually the pain is in the hip region or along the inner aspect of the thigh. On occasion, however, the pain is referred to the knee, and it is not uncommon for an elderly person with a fracture of the hip to complain of knee pain after a fall. Because fractures of the proximal femur are so common, any elderly individual who has fallen and complains of pain in the hip or knee, even though there is no deformity, should be splinted and transported to the emergency department for x-rays.

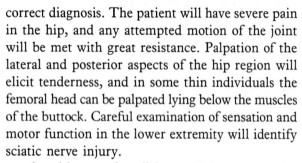

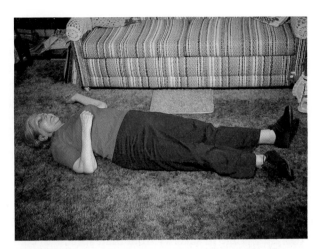

FIGURE 17.7 The patient with a displaced "fractured hip" will have shortening and external rotation of the injured limb.

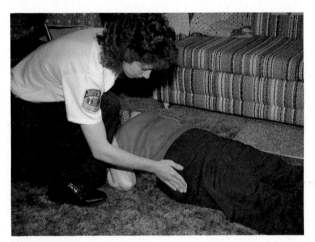

FIGURE 17.8 Palpation of the greater trochanter is usually painful in the patient with a "hip fracture."

Palpation about the hip region will usually elicit tenderness in a patient with a fracture of the hip. The EMT should apply gentle, manual pressure to the greater trochanter to elicit this tenderness (Figure 17.8).

The method of splinting the fractured hip will be determined by the age of the patient and the severity of the injury. Fractures of the hip that occur as a result of violent injury in young people are best immobilized with a traction splint or the combination of a pneumatic antishock garment and a spine board. The traction splint is applied in the same manner as for femoral shaft fractures (see Chapter

15). Special care should be taken to protect the injured region about the hip from excessive pressure from the ring of the traction splint. In the seriously or multiply injured patient, the pneumatic antishock garment will provide effective immobilization of the pelvis and hip region when combined with a spine board. In addition, the pneumatic antishock garment will help control hemorrhage in the region.

In contrast to the multiply injured patient, the elderly individual with an isolated hip fracture does not require a traction splint for adequate immobilization. Effective immobilization can be obtained by placing the patient on a long spine board or a scoop stretcher using pillows or rolled blankets to support the injured limb. The EMT should carefully secure the injured limb to the stretcher with long straps or cravats (Figure 17.9).

All patients with hip fractures may lose significant amounts of blood. The EMT should therefore watch for shock in these patients and monitor the vital signs carefully.

Femoral Shaft Fractures

Fractures of the femur can occur in any part of the shaft, from the hip region to the femoral condyles just above the knee joint. Following fracture, the large muscles of the thigh go into spasm to "splint" the unstable limb. The muscle spasm frequently produces significant deformity of the limb, with severe angulation or rotation at the fracture site.

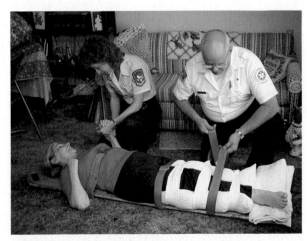

FIGURE 17.9 Splinting of most patients with a "hip fracture" can be accomplished with a spine board and pillows.

Usually the limb shortens significantly as well. Often, fractures of the femoral shaft are open, and fragments of bone may protrude through the skin.

There is always a significant amount of blood loss following a fracture of the shaft of the femur. As much as 500 to 1,000 ml of blood can be lost with this fracture. With open fractures, the amount of blood loss may be even greater. Thus, it is not unusual for a patient with a fracture of the femur to develop hypovolemic shock. The EMT must be extremely careful in handling these patients, since any extra movement or fracture manipulation will increase the blood loss.

Because of the severe deformity that occurs with these fractures, bone fragments may penetrate or press on important nerves and vessels and produce significant damage to them. Careful evaluation of the distal neurovascular function is imperative in patients who have sustained a fracture of the shaft of the femur.

Clothing must be removed from the limb of a patient suspected of having a fracture of the shaft of the femur so the injury site can be adequately inspected for any open wounds. The patient's vital signs must be monitored closely and continually to identify the onset of hypovolemic shock. The EMT must be prepared to combat shock should it occur.

If a wound is present, it should be covered with a dry, sterile compression dressing. If the foot or leg below the level of the fracture shows signs of impaired circulation (pale, cold, or pulseless), gentle longitudinal traction should be applied to the deformed limb. The traction is applied in line with the long axis of the limb, and the leg is gradually turned from the deformed position to restore the limb's overall alignment. Frequently, restoring the limb to a more normal position will restore or improve circulation to the foot. If there are no signs of the return of circulation after traction has been applied and realignment achieved, a serious vascular injury may have occurred, and the patient will require prompt medical treatment.

A fracture of the femoral shaft is best immobilized with a traction splint. In addition to knowing the precise sequence of steps to apply the splint properly, the EMT must practice the splinting technique frequently to maintain the necessary skills. The technique for applying a traction splint is described in Chapter 15.

INJURIES ABOUT THE KNEE

Many different types of injuries can occur about the knee. Ligament injuries, for example, will range from mild sprains to complete dislocation of the joint. The patella can also dislocate. In addition, all of the bony elements of the knee (the distal femur, the upper tibia, and the patella) can fracture. The knee is very vulnerable to injury, and injuries frequently occur in this region.

Injuries of the Knee Ligaments

The knee is especially prone to ligament injuries that may range in severity from mild sprains to complete disruption of one or more of the stabilizing ligaments. These injuries occur when abnormal bending or twisting forces are applied to the joint. They are commonly seen in both recreational and competitive athletes. The ligaments on the medial side of the knee are the ones most frequently injured. This injury usually results when the foot is fixed to the ground and the lateral aspect of the knee is struck by a heavy object such as when a football player is clipped or tackled from the side (Figure 17.10).

Usually the patient with a knee ligament injury will complain of pain in the joint and is unable to use the extremity normally. Examination will show swelling and occasionally ecchymosis, as well as point tenderness at the area of ligament injury.

All suspected knee ligament injuries must be splinted. The splint must extend from the hip joint to the foot, thus immobilizing the bone above the

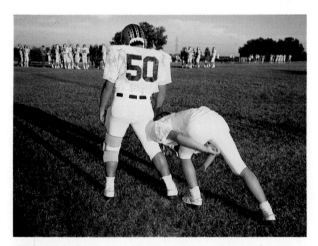

FIGURE 17.10 The knee joint is especially vulnerable to injury, particularly during athletics.

injured joint (the femur) and the bone below (the tibia). A variety of splints can be used: a padded rigid long leg splint, two padded board splints securely applied to the medial and lateral aspects of the limb, or a long leg air splint. A long spine board, a pillow splint, and simply binding the injured limb to the opposite uninjured limb are also acceptable but less effective splinting techniques.

Usually the patient will be able to straighten the knee to allow the splint to be applied. If resistance or pain is encountered when the EMT attempts to straighten the knee, it should be splinted in the flexed position. Following the application of the splint, the distal neurovascular function must be assessed and monitored until the patient reaches the hospital.

Dislocation of the Knee

Complete disruption of the ligaments supporting the knee may result in dislocation of the joint. When this happens, the proximal end of the tibia completely displaces from its articulation with the lower end of the femur, usually producing a significant deformity. While substantial ligament damage always occurs with a knee dislocation, the seriousness of this injury is not related to the ligament damage but to injury to the popliteal artery. Frequently the popliteal artery is lacerated or compressed by the displaced tibia (Figure 17.11). When a dislocation of the knee is suspected because of gross deformity, severe pain, and an inability to move the joint, the EMT must always check the distal circulation carefully before

any other step is taken. If the distal pulses are absent, medical control should be notified immediately because further steps in field stabilization must be directed by medical control.

If adequate distal pulses are present, a dislocated knee should be splinted in the position in which it is found, and the patient should be transported promptly to the hospital. No attempt should be made to manipulate or straighten any severe knee injury when strong distal pulses are present. If the limb with good pulses is straight, standard long leg splints should be applied to at least two sides of the limb to provide adequate immobilization (Figure 17.12). If the knee is bent and the foot has a good pulse, the joint should be splinted in this position. Parallel padded board splints secured at the hip and ankle joint will provide a stable A-frame splinting configuration. The limb should be further supported with pillows and straps to a spine board or stretcher to eliminate any motion of the limb during transport (Figure 17.13).

On rare occasions the medical control physician may request that the EMT realign a deformed, pulseless limb in order to restore distal circulation. The EMT should only make one attempt to realign the limb and thus reduce compression of the popliteal artery. The limb should be gently straightened by applying gentle longitudinal traction in the axis of the limb. The distal pulse points should be monitored during the application of traction to determine if the pulse returns. The limb should be splinted in the

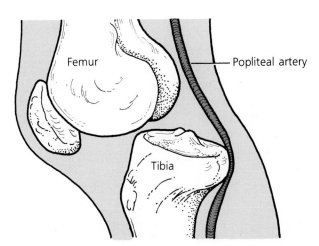

FIGURE 17.11 Dislocation of the knee frequently results in serious injury to the popliteal artery in the back of the knee.

Femur — Popliteal artery

Tibia

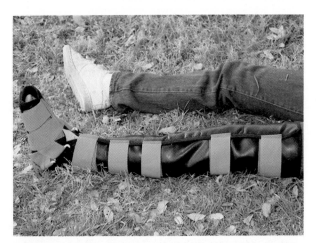

FIGURE 17.12 When the injured knee is straight, it should be splinted with two padded board splints extending from the hip to the ankle.

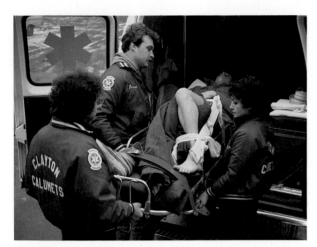

FIGURE 17.13 The flexed knee can be immobilized adequately by padded board splints applied securely to each side of the limb.

position in which the strongest pulse is felt. If traction significantly increases the patient's pain, no further attempts should be made to realign the limb. Once manual traction is applied, it must be maintained until the limb is fully splinted; otherwise the limb will return to its deformed position.

If the EMT is unable to restore the distal pulse, the limb should be splinted in the position most comfortable for the patient; then the patient must be transported rapidly to the hospital. Medical control should be notified of the status of the distal pulse so that arrangements can be made in advance to receive the patient.

Fractures about the Knee

Fractures about the knee may occur at the distal end of the femur, at the proximal end of the tibia, or in the patella. Nondisplaced or minimally displaced fractures are sometimes confused with ligament injury because of their local tenderness and swelling. On the other hand, displaced fractures about the knee may produce significant deformity and be confused with a knee dislocation. When fractures about the knee are suspected, they should be managed in a manner similar to the knee injuries just described. If there is an adequate distal pulse and no significant deformity, the limb should be splinted with the knee straight. If there is significant deformity and an adequate pulse, the joint should be splinted in the position of deformity. If the pulse is absent below the level of the injury, medical control should

be notified immediately, and the EMT should follow the instructions from medical control with regard to further management of this injury.

Dislocation of the Patella

The patella may be dislocated from its articulation with the front of the distal femur. This injury usually occurs in teenagers and young adults engaged in athletic activities. Some patients will have recurrent dislocations of the patella in which only a minor twisting of the knee will produce the dislocation, just as occurs with recurrent dislocation of the shoulder. Usually the dislocated patella displaces to the lateral side, and the knee is held in a partially flexed position. The displacement of the patella produces a significant deformity (Figure 17.14).

This injury should be splinted in the position in which it is found, usually with the knee flexed to a moderate degree. Padded board splints applied to the medial and lateral aspects of the joint extending from the hip to the ankle will provide adequate immobilization when combined with pillows to support the limb on the stretcher.

Occasionally, as the splint is being applied, the patella will return to its normal position, spontaneously. If the patella does return to its normal position, the limb should be immobilized as for a knee ligament injury in a padded long leg splint or a long leg air splint. Even if the patella does return to its normal position, the patient will need to be evaluated in the emergency department. Any time a joint

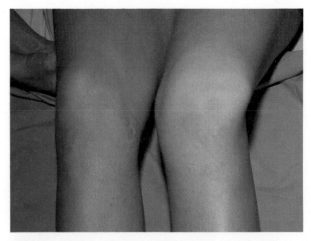

FIGURE 17.14 The typical appearance of a dislocated patella, with the patella displaced laterally and the knee moderately flexed.

reduces spontaneously, the EMT should report this occurrence to emergency department personnel so that they will know the severity of the injury.

INJURIES TO THE TIBIA AND FIBULA

Fracture of the shaft of the tibia or the fibula may occur at any place between the knee joint and the ankle joint. Usually both bones fracture simultaneously. Because the tibia is located just beneath the skin, open fractures of this bone are quite common. These fractures may result in severe deformity, with significant angulation or rotation (Figure 17.15).

Fractures of the tibia and fibula should be immobilized with a padded, rigid long leg splint or an air splint that extends from the foot to the upper thigh. Alternatively, a traction splint may be used; however, constant traction is not usually necessary to maintain limb alignment with tibial fractures. As with most other fractures of the shaft of long bones, severe deformity should be corrected prior to splinting by applying gentle longitudinal traction. The goal

of applying traction is to achieve adequate alignment of the limb so that a standard splint can be applied. It is not necessary to replace the fracture fragments in their anatomic position.

Vascular injury is not uncommon with fractures of the tibia and fibula and is frequently due to the distorted position of the limb following injury. Realignment of the limb will frequently correct the impaired blood supply to the foot. If adequate circulation is not present or is not restored when the limb is realigned, the patient must be transported promptly to a hospital and the emergency department notified en route.

INJURIES TO THE ANKLE AND FOOT

Ankle Injuries

The ankle is one of the most commonly injured joints. Injuries occur in people of all ages and range in severity from a simple sprain that heals after a few days' rest to severe fracture-dislocations. As is true with other joints, it is sometimes difficult to distinguish nondisplaced ankle fractures from a simple sprain by clinical examination (Figure 17.16). Therefore, any ankle injury that produces pain, swelling, localized tenderness, or the inability to bear weight must be evaluated by a physician. The most frequent mechanism of ankle injury is twisting, with stretching or tearing of the supporting ligaments. A more extensive twisting force may produce fracture of one or both malleoli (Figure 17.17). When dislocation of the ankle occurs, it is usually associated with fractures of both malleoli.

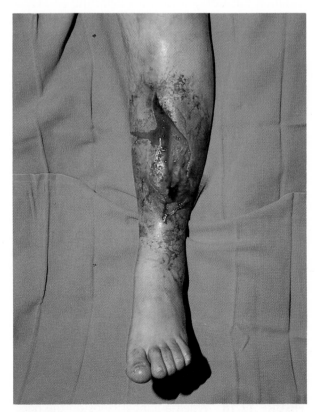

FIGURE 17.15 The typical appearance of an open fracture of the tibia and fibula.

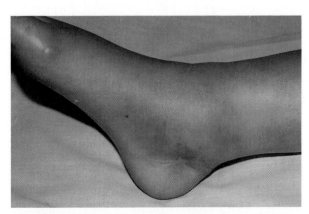

FIGURE 17.16 Swelling about the ankle is characteristic of both sprains and fractures.

The wide spectrum of injuries to the ankle should all be managed in the same way. All open wounds should be dressed, distal neurovascular function should be evaluated, any gross malalignment should be corrected by applying gentle longitudinal traction to the heel, and a splint should be applied before the traction is released. Splinting can be accomplished with a padded rigid splint, an air splint, or a pillow splint. The splint should include the en-

tire foot and extend up the leg to the level of the knee joint.

Foot Injuries

Injuries of the foot can result in the fracture of one of the several tarsals, metatarsals, or phalanges of the toes. Toe fractures are especially common.

Of the tarsal bones, the calcaneus is the most frequently fractured. Fracture of this bone usually occurs when the patient falls or jumps from a height and lands directly on the heel(s). The force of injury causes the calcaneus to be compressed and produces immediate swelling and ecchymosis about the heel. If the force of impact is great enough, as from a fall from a roof or tree, additional fractures may occur as well. Frequently, the force of injury is transmitted up the legs to the spine, producing a fracture of the lumbar spine (Figure 17.18). When a patient who has jumped or fallen from a height complains of heel pain, the EMT must question the patient about back pain and check the spine for tenderness or deformity.

Injuries of the foot are associated with significant swelling but rarely with gross deformity. Vascular injuries are uncommon. As in the hand, lacerations

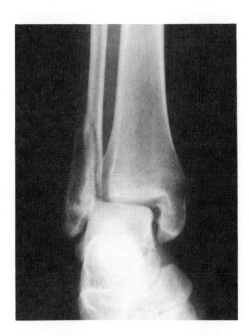

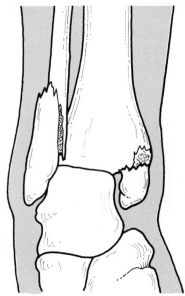

FIGURE 17.17   (top) X-ray of an ankle fracture. (bottom) Line drawing showing that both malleoli are broken.

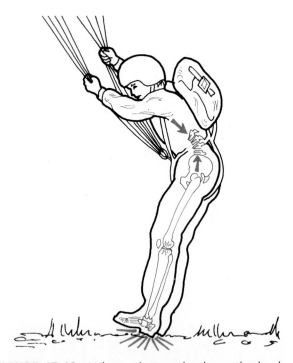

FIGURE 17.18   When a jumper lands on the heels, the energy is transmitted to the spine, producing spine injury as well as injury to the foot and ankle.

about the ankle and foot may damage important underlying nerves and tendons. Puncture wounds of the foot occur frequently and may cause serious infection if not treated early. All of these injuries must be evaluated and treated by a physician.

Splinting of the foot is accomplished with a rigid padded board splint, an air splint, or a pillow splint, all of which must immobilize the ankle joint as well as the foot (Figure 17.19). The toes should remain exposed for periodic neurovascular checks.

Slight elevation of the foot after splinting will minimize swelling. When the patient is lying on the stretcher, the foot should be propped up approximately 6 inches. All patients with lower extremity injuries should be transported supine so that adequate elevation of the limb can be accomplished. The foot and leg should never be allowed to dangle off the stretcher on the floor or ground.

Any patient who has fallen from a height and complains of heel pain should, in addition to having the foot splinted, be transported on a long spine board to immobilize any possible spinal injury (Figure 17.20).

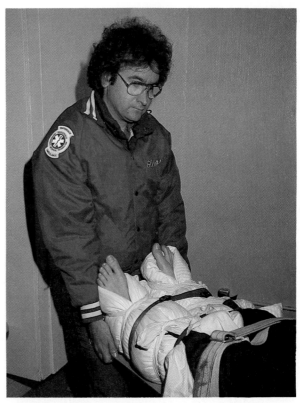

FIGURE 17.20 Any patient who has fallen from a height should be transported on a long spine board to immobilize any possible spine injury.

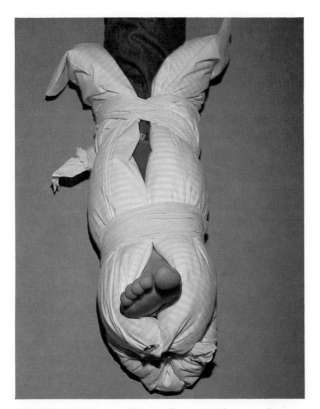

FIGURE 17.19 A pillow splint provides excellent immobilization of the foot with suspected fractures.

YOU ARE THE EMT...

1. Your patient has a closed pelvic fracture. What internal organs could be injured? What are some of the signs of such injuries?
2. Why is hypovolemic shock likely to occur with pelvic and femoral injuries? How should you combat it once you determine the patient is in shock?
3. Your patient has a serious knee injury, but you are not sure if his knee is dislocated or fractured. What are the signs of each? How should you prepare this patient for transport?
4. You have identified posterior dislocation of the hip in a patient injured in an automobile accident. What signs led you to this diagnosis? What would anterior dislocation of the hip look like?

18

The Nervous System

OVERVIEW

The nervous system is a complex system of nerve cells that enables all parts of the human body to function. It is basically composed of the brain, the spinal cord, and several billion nerve fibers that carry information to and from all parts of the body. Because the nervous system is so vital, it is well protected. The brain lies beneath the skull, and the spinal cord lies inside the bony spinal canal. Despite its being well protected, the nervous system can be injured from serious impacts and blows. In order to make an accurate assessment of nervous system injuries, the EMT must understand the anatomy of the nervous system and how it functions.

Chapter 18 first describes the anatomic and functional components of the nervous system. It then discusses its two basic anatomic divisions: the central nervous system and the peripheral nervous system. The chapter next presents the nervous system's two functional divisions: the somatic nervous system and the autonomic nervous system. The last part of the chapter describes how the nervous system is protected within the body.

OBJECTIVES

The objectives of Chapter 18 are to

- understand the anatomic and functional components of the nervous system.
- describe the central and peripheral nervous systems.
- describe the somatic and autonomic nervous systems.
- identify the protective coverings of the nervous system.

ANATOMIC AND FUNCTIONAL COMPONENTS OF THE NERVOUS SYSTEM

Anatomically, the nervous system is divided into two parts: the central nervous system and the peripheral nervous system. The **central nervous system (CNS)** is made up of the brain and the spinal cord. From a practical point of view, the central nervous system can be considered the part of the nervous system that is covered and protected by bones. The brain is covered by the skull, and the spinal cord is covered by the spinal column. The major parts of most nerve cells (the nucleus and the cell body) lie within the central nervous system. Many of the nerve cells in the central nervous system have long fibers that extend from the cell out of the central nervous system through openings in the bony covering to form a cable of nerve fibers that link the central nervous system to the various organs of the body. These cables of nerve fibers make up the **peripheral nervous system.** The two major types of nerve fibers are sensory and motor nerve fibers. The **sensory nerves** carry information from the body to the central nervous system, while the **motor nerves** carry information from the central nervous system to the muscles of the body.

The nervous system controls virtually all activities of the body. Body activities can be separated into two broad categories: those over which one has voluntary control (voluntary) and those over which one has no voluntary control (involuntary). The part of the nervous system that regulates activities over which there is voluntary control is called the **somatic nervous system.** Such activities include walking, talking, and writing. Many body functions occur without voluntary control. These activities are under the control of the **autonomic, or involuntary, nervous system.** The autonomic nervous system controls automatic body functions such as digestion, dilation and constriction of blood vessels, sweating, and all other involuntary actions necessary for basic bodily functions. Some of the cells that form the autonomic nervous system are inside the central nervous system, while others lie alongside the spinal cord in the cervical and lumbar regions.

Thus, the nervous system as a whole can be divided *anatomically* into the central and peripheral nervous system, and *functionally* into somatic (voluntary) and autonomic (involuntary) components.

CENTRAL AND PERIPHERAL NERVOUS SYSTEMS

Central Nervous System

The central nervous system is composed of the brain and the spinal cord.

The Brain

The **brain** is the controlling organ of the body. It is the center of consciousness. It is responsible for all our voluntary body activities, the perception of our surroundings, and the control of our reactions to the environment. In addition, it enables us to experience all the fine shadings of thought and feeling that make us individuals. The brain is subdivided into several areas, all of which have specific functions. Three major subdivisions of the brain are the cerebrum, the cerebellum, and the brain stem.

The largest part of the brain is the **cerebrum.** The cerebrum is sometimes called the "gray matter." It makes up about three-fourths of the volume of the brain and is itself composed of several lobes — frontal, parietal, temporal, and occipital (Figure 18.1). The cerebrum on one side of the brain controls activities on the opposite side of the body. Each lobe of the cerebrum is responsible for a specific function. For example, one group of brain cells in the frontal lobe is responsible for the activity of all the voluntary muscles of the body. Brain cells in this area generate impulses which are sent along nerve fibers that extend from each cell into the spinal cord. Another area in the parietal lobe has cells that receive sensory impulses from the peripheral nerves of the body. Other parts of the cerebrum are responsible for other body functions. For instance, the occipital region, on the back of the cerebrum, receives visual impulses for the eyes, and areas deep within the brain control hearing, balance, and speech. Still other parts

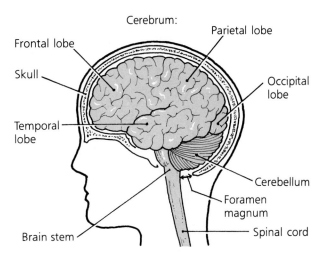

FIGURE 18.1 The brain lies well protected within the skull. Its major subdivisions are the cerebrum, cerebellum, and brain stem.

of the cerebrum are responsible for emotions and other characteristics of an individual's personality.

Underneath the great mass of cerebral tissue lies the **cerebellum,** sometimes called the "little brain" (Figure 18.1). The major function of this area is to coordinate the various activities of the brain, particularly body movements. Without the cerebellum, very specialized muscular activities such as writing or sewing would be impossible.

The **brain stem** is so called because the brain appears to be sitting on this portion of the central nervous system as a plant sits on its stem. The brain stem is the most primitive part of the central nervous system. It lies deep within the cranium and is the best protected part of the central nervous system (Figure 18.1). The brain stem is the controlling center for virtually all those body functions that are absolutely necessary for life. Cells in this part of the brain control cardiac, respiratory, and other basic body functions.

The brain has many other anatomic areas, all of which have specific and important functions. The brain receives a vast amount of information from the environment, sorts it all out, and directs the body to respond appropriately. Many of the responses involve voluntary muscle action, while others are automatic and involuntary.

The Spinal Cord

The **spinal cord** is the other major portion of the central nervous system (Figure 18.2). Like the

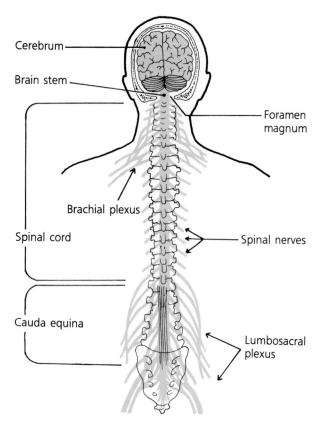

FIGURE 18.2 The spinal cord is the continuation of the brain stem. It exits the skull at the foramen magnum and extends down to the level of the second lumbar vertebra.

brain, the spinal cord contains nerve cell bodies, but the major portion of the spinal cord is made up of nerve fibers that extend from the cells of the brain. These nerve fibers transmit information to and from the brain. All the fibers join together just below the brain stem to form the spinal cord. The spinal cord exits through a large opening at the base of the skull called the **foramen magnum.** It is encased within the spinal canal down to the level of the second lumbar vertebra. The **spinal canal** is created by the vertebrae, stacked one on the other. Each vertebra surrounds the cord to form the bony spinal canal (see Figures 14.12 and 14.13, page 170).

The major function of the spinal cord is to transmit messages between the brain and the body. These messages are passed along the nerve fibers as electrical impulses, just as messages are passed along a telephone cable. The nerve fibers are arranged in specific bundles within the spinal cord to carry the messages from one specific area of the body to the brain and back.

The Peripheral Nervous System

The peripheral nervous system is composed of 31 pairs of **peripheral nerves** called **spinal nerves** and 12 pairs called **cranial nerves.** At each vertebral level from the first cervical to the fifth sacral on each side of the spinal cord, a spinal nerve root exits the spinal cord and passes through an opening in the bony canal (Figure 18.3). This spinal nerve is composed of nerve fibers from nerve cells that originate within the spinal cord. The nerve fibers conduct sensory impulses from the skin and other organs to the spinal cord. They also conduct motor impulses from the spinal cord to the muscles that are present in that segment of the body. For example, between the seventh and eighth ribs the spinal nerve carries sensory fibers from the skin between those two ribs and also has motor nerve fibers to innervate the intercostal muscle between the seventh and eighth ribs (Figure 18.4). This specific arrangement of nerve fibers becomes more complex and confusing in both the cervical and lumbar regions because of the large number of muscles in the arms and legs that must be supplied with nerve fibers. The spinal nerve roots combine to form complex nerve networks (**plexuses**)

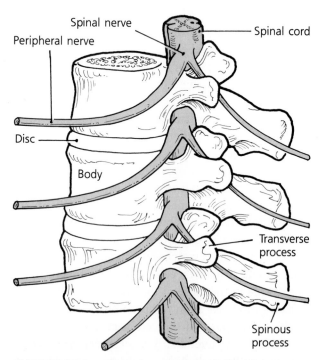

FIGURE 18.3 At each vertebral level spinal nerves containing both motor and sensory fibers exit the spinal canal between each pair of vertebrae.

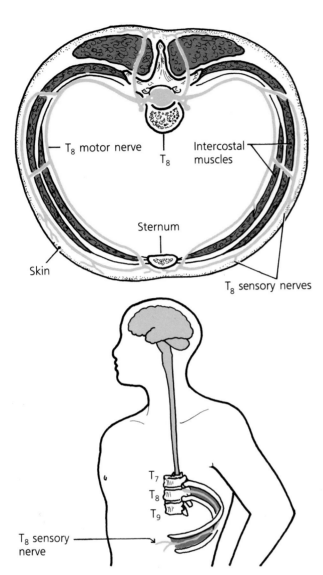

FIGURE 18.4 The T$_8$ peripheral nerve supplies motor nerve fibers to the intercostal muscles between the seventh and eighth ribs and sensory nerve fibers to the skin in this interspace.

in these two areas — the **brachial plexus** for the upper extremity and the **lumbosacral plexus** for the lower extremity (Figure 18.2).

Twelve pairs of peripheral nerves called cranial nerves exit the brain through holes in the skull. For the most part, they are very specialized nerves designed to provide specific functions in the head and face. For example the facial nerves (seventh cranial) send motor impulses to many of the facial muscles.

There are three major categories of peripheral nerves: sensory nerves, motor nerves, and connecting nerves.

Sensory Nerves

Sensory nerves of the body are quite complex. There are many different types of sensory cells in the nervous system. One type forms the retina of the eye; others are responsible for the hearing and balancing mechanisms in the ear. Other sensory cells are located within the skin, muscles, joints, lungs, and other organs of the body. When a sensory cell is stimulated, it transmits its own special message to the brain. There are special sensory nerves to detect heat, cold, position, motion, pressure, pain, balance, light, taste, and smell, as well as other sensations. Specialized nerve endings are adapted for each cell so that it perceives only one type of sensation and it transmits only that message.

The sensory impulses constantly provide information to the brain about what the different parts of our body are doing in relation to our surroundings. Thus, the brain is continuously made aware of its surroundings. The cranial nerves supply sensations directly to the brain. Visual sensations (what we see) reach the brain directly by way of the **optic nerve** (second cranial nerve) in each eye. The nerve endings for the optic nerve lie in the retina of the eye. The nerve endings are stimulated by light, and the impulses are carried along the nerve which passes through a hole in the back of the eye socket and carries impulses to the occipital portion of the brain.

When sensory nerve endings in the extremities are stimulated, the impulses are transmitted along a peripheral nerve to the spinal cord. The cell body of the peripheral nerve lies in the spinal cord. The impulses are then transmitted from that cell body to another nerve ending in the spinal cord. The impulse is then transmitted up the spinal cord to the sensory area in the parietal lobe of the brain where the sensory information can be interpreted and acted upon by the brain (Figure 18.5).

Motor Nerves

Each muscle in the body has its own motor nerve. The cell body for each motor nerve lies in the spinal cord, and a fiber from the cell body extends out as part of the peripheral nerve to its specific muscle. Electrical impulses produced by the cell body in the spinal cord are transmitted along the motor nerve to the muscle and cause it to contract. The cell body in the spinal cord is stimulated by an im-

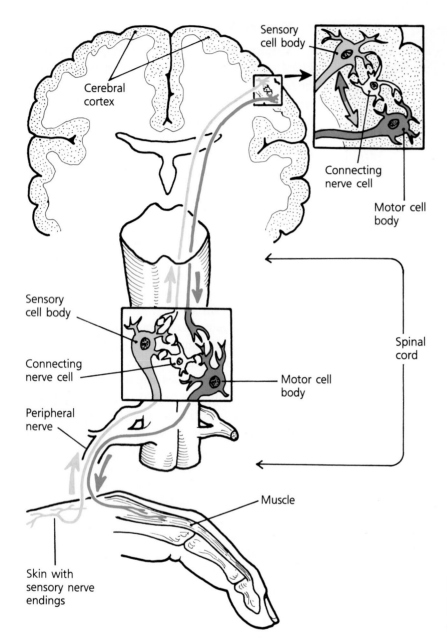

FIGURE 18.5 A simplified schematic representation of the nerves in the central and peripheral nervous systems.

pulse produced in the motor strip of the cerebral cortex. This impulse is transmitted along the spinal cord to the cell body of the motor nerve.

Connecting Nerves

Within the brain and the spinal cord are cells with short fibers that connect the sensory nerves with the motor nerves. In the spinal cord they connect the sensory and motor nerves directly, bypassing the brain. These **connecting nerves** allow sensory and motor impulses to be transmitted from one nerve to another within the central nervous system.

FUNCTIONAL DIVISIONS OF THE NERVOUS SYSTEMS

The Somatic Nervous System

The somatic nervous system controls the voluntary activities of the body. Sensory information from the peripheral nerves is interpreted by the cerebral cortex of the brain. The brain then sends signals to voluntary muscles in response to these sensory stimuli. The somatic nervous system is responsible for almost all of the body's coordinated muscular activities such as walking, eating, and driving a car.

The Autonomic Nervous System

The autonomic nervous system is involuntary — the brain has no voluntary control over its activity. It is a very primitive system that controls the function of many of the body's vital organs. The autonomic nervous system is composed of two counterbalancing parts: the sympathetic nervous system and the parasympathetic nervous system. These two divisions have equal and opposite effects on the body's vital organs, increasing or decreasing their activity depending on basic bodily needs.

The Sympathetic Nervous System

The cells of the **sympathetic nervous system** lie outside of the spinal canal in clusters on either side of the cervical and lumbar spine near the points where the spinal nerve roots exit the canal. The sympathetic nerves respond to stress and prepare the body to respond to threatening situations (the "fight or flight" phenomenon). Thus, the sympathetic nervous system causes blood vessels to constrict, stimulates sweating, increases the heart rate, causes the sphincter muscles to constrict, and prepares the body to respond to stress.

The Parasympathetic Nervous System

In contrast, the **parasympathetic nervous system** acts in the opposite manner. The cells of the parasympathetic nervous system are found in the brain stem and also in the sacral area of the spinal cord. Its functions are opposite those of the sympathetic nervous system. The parasympathetic nervous system causes blood vessels to dilate, slows the heart rate, and relaxes muscle sphincters, among other effects.

Both divisions of the autonomic nervous system are equally effective. They tend to counterbalance one another so that stable and effective basic body functions can be maintained.

Activities of the Somatic and Autonomic Nervous Systems

The combined actions of the somatic and the autonomic nervous systems control all the body activities. The body responds either voluntarily or involuntarily to external stimuli. There are three basic categories of nervous system activity: voluntary, involuntary, and reflex.

Voluntary Activity

The skeletal muscles are under voluntary control. A person can decide to move his arm or leg to accomplish a specific task. A conscious decision is made to perform this task. Sensory input will be used to determine the specific muscular activity. Driving a car is an example of voluntary activity of the nervous system. Sensory input from the eyes and ears and the general sensation of road bumps and vehicle speed are synthesized in the brain. This information dictates the specific muscular activity necessary to drive the car toward a specific objective, avoiding danger. This action is a series of willed or voluntary acts, each resulting from a separate conscious decision to act.

Involuntary Activity

Both the central nervous system and the autonomic nervous system control basic bodily functions independent of the thought process. Breathing, for example, is done automatically. Although, to a certain extent, we can breathe rapidly or hold our breath by conscious will, neither can be done indefinitely. A complex system of chemical controls takes over when a person approaches danger from excessive voluntary breathing control. The respiratory rate is controlled involuntarily until normal levels of oxygen and carbon dioxide are restored. This response is one of the most primitive functions of the brain and is present at every level of animal development. Similarly, heart rate, dilation and constriction of blood vessels, and the function of many other organs are controlled by involuntary activity of the central and autonomic nervous systems.

Reflex Activity

The connecting nerves in the spinal cord complete a **reflex arc** between the sensory and motor nerves of the limbs. An irritating stimulus to the sensory nerve (such as heat) will be transmitted from the sensory nerve along the connecting nerve directly to the motor nerve, causing it to be stimulated (Figure 18.6). The muscle responds promptly, withdrawing the limb from the irritating stimulus even before this information can be transmitted to the brain. The doctor who taps on the patellar tendon with a rubber hammer is testing to see if the patient's reflex arcs are intact.

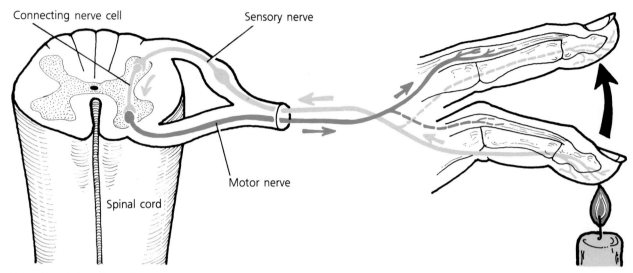

FIGURE 18.6 The reflex arc is a primitive response to irritating stimuli that allows prompt stimulation of the muscles to withdraw from the source of irritation.

PROTECTIVE COVERINGS OF THE NERVOUS SYSTEM

The cells of the brain and spinal cord are soft and easily injured. Once damaged, cells in the central nervous system cannot be regenerated or reproduced. Therefore, the body has developed an extensive protective covering for the central nervous system (Figure 18.7). The entire central nervous system is contained within this bony protective framework. The skull is covered by a thick layer of skin (the **scalp**) and underneath the skin by a layer of muscle fascia. The spinal canal is also surrounded by a thick layer of skin and muscles.

The skull and spinal canal are thick and withstand injury very well. The skull, in fact, has two layers — an inner table and an outer table — doubling the amount of bone protecting the brain. In addition to these layers of protective covering, the central nervous system is further protected by a set of special coverings called the **meninges.** The meninges are three layers of tissue that suspend the brain and the spinal cord within the skull and the spinal canal. These layers are distinct. The outer one is a tough fibrous layer, much like leather, called the

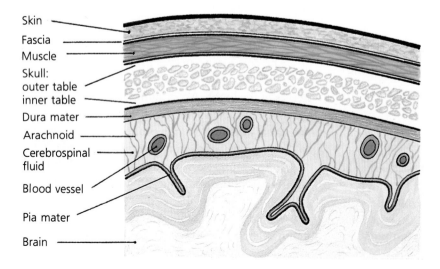

FIGURE 18.7 The central nervous system has several layers of protective covering: the skin, muscles and their fascia, bone, and the meninges.

dura mater. The dura mater forms a sac to contain the central nervous system. The peripheral nerves exit through small openings in the dura.

The inner two layers of the meninges are much thinner than the dura mater. They are called the **arachnoid** and the **pia mater.** Blood vessels that nourish the brain and spinal cord lie in these layers. **Cerebrospinal fluid** fills the spaces between the arachnoid and the pia mater. The brain and spinal cord essentially float in this cerebrospinal fluid. The fluid is an excellent shock absorber that buffers the central nervous system from injury. All of these protective layers combine to isolate the central nervous system and protect it from injury. That is why closed head injuries can result in serious problems caused by these firm protective coverings. Severe injury may cause bleeding of the vessels under the dura. The hematoma that develops (a **subdural hematoma**) will compress the softer brain tissue. The increased pressure inside the confined space of the skull will require prompt surgical decompression to avoid permanent brain damage. If the outer protective layers are damaged (the skin, fascia, skull, and dura), cerebrospinal fluid may leak to the body surface.

Such cerebrospinal fluid leaks most frequently occur from the nose and the ears. Cerebrospinal fluid is clear and watery. If a head injury patient has a "runny nose" or watery fluid draining from the ear or from an open skull fracture, the EMT must assume that the watery fluid is cerebrospinal fluid.

YOU ARE THE EMT...

1. The nervous system can be divided *anatomically* into what two divisions? Into what two parts is it divided *functionally*?
2. What are the three categories of peripheral nerves? Describe the function of each.
3. Which part of the nervous system causes blood vessels to constrict? Which part causes them to dilate? Are constriction and dilation voluntary or involuntary activities? Why?
4. How is the central nervous system protected from injury? What kinds of injuries do you think might endanger the central nervous system?

19 Head Injuries

OVERVIEW

Over 70 percent of the injuries sustained in automobile accidents involve the head. The degree of damage can range from a trivial scalp laceration to a severe brain injury that rapidly causes death. All head injuries are potentially life-threatening. To ensure full recovery and satisfactory return to normal function, proper emergency treatment is vital.

In spite of the seriousness of brain injuries, a very large percentage of patients survive and return to normal function if proper initial treatment is given promptly. Effective emergency care, combined with prompt transportation to the hospital, will minimize many of the long-term problems associated with head injury and increase the patient's chances for survival. The fact that a patient has sustained a severe head injury does not mean that the injury is fatal; however, the patient's chances for survival and resumption of normal existence depend a great deal on the quality of the initial care.

Chapter 19 first presents the three general principles of treatment for head injuries: maintaining an airway, immobilizing the cervical spine, and assessing the level of consciousness. The chapter next describes the treatment for specific head injuries. Then certain other areas of prehospital care of head injuries are discussed. The last section of Chapter 19 describes how the EMT assesses the severity of a head injury once the airway and cervical spine have been stabilized.

OBJECTIVES

The objectives of Chapter 19 are to

- understand the general principles of treatment for head injuries.
- know how to treat specific head injuries.
- become familiar with other aspects of prehospital care of head injuries.
- learn how to assess the severity of a head injury after initial treatment.

GENERAL PRINCIPLES OF TREATMENT FOR HEAD INJURIES

The treatment of head injury patients must be guided by these three general principles, which are designed to protect and maintain the critical function of the central nervous system:

1. Maintain an adequate airway and adequate ventilation with supplemental oxygen.
2. Protect the cervical spine from injury.
3. Assess the patient's level of consciousness and continue to monitor it.

In addition, the EMT must look for other injuries, control bleeding, be prepared for convulsions, and transport the patient with extreme care.

Airway Maintenance

The most important step in the treatment of patients with head injury, regardless of severity, is the establishment of an adequate airway with supportive ventilation and the administration of oxygen. More than any other part of the body, the brain requires a constant, rich supply of oxygen. Inadequate ventilation will result in death within a few minutes unless oxygen is supplied artificially. Unconsciousness produced by a head injury will cause the patient to lose voluntary airway control and may produce severe **hypoxia.** Direct injury to the brain may damage the respiratory control center and bring about a change in the rate and depth of breathing. Most importantly, the injured brain is even more sensitive to low blood levels of oxygen than is the normal brain, and an injured brain cannot tolerate hypoxia as well as the normal brain.

One of the major problems associated with brain injury is swelling of the brain. Just as any other injured tissue, the brain swells when it has been injured. Swelling is aggravated by low oxygen levels in the blood and is decreased or minimized by high oxygen levels. For these many reasons, it is of primary importance in the head injury patient (particularly the unconscious patient) to secure an adequate airway, assure adequate ventilation, and provide supplemental oxygen. Supplemental oxygen should always be administered because there is strong evidence that oxygen decreases swelling in the acutely injured brain. The EMT should not wait for the appearance of cyanosis to diagnose low arterial oxygen levels. Cyanosis is a very late finding in head injury patients, and many patients will need ventilatory support before cyanosis appears.

Altered breathing patterns are very common following head injury. Indeed, some patients may breathe more deeply or more rapidly than normal following a head injury. Altered breathing patterns in a head injury patient should alert the EMT to the possibility of brain injury, particularly brain stem injury.

Although it is imperative to restore the airway, the high incidence of associated cervical spine injuries requires that secondary maneuvers be used to open the airway. The standard head-tilt/chin-lift maneuver that is used in cardiopulmonary resuscitation may cause significant further damage to an already injured cervical spine. The airway in the unconscious head injury patient should be restored using the jaw-thrust maneuver described in Chapter 6.

Once the airway is established, the rate and depth of respirations should be assessed to be certain that they are of good quality. Patients who have sustained a head injury frequently have abnormal respiratory patterns and do not ventilate sufficiently on their own. There are several causes of inadequate ventilation, among them the following:

1. Brain damage itself may impair the stimulus to breathe or cause irregular and/or shallow respirations.
2. In association with a spinal injury, paralysis of some of the muscles of respiration may limit the patient's ability to ventilate adequately.
3. Patients with head injuries may have associated injuries of the chest that also may limit ventilation.

Cervical Spine Immobilization

Approximately 10 percent of patients with head injuries who are unconscious after a fall or auto-mobile accident will also have suffered a neck injury with spinal cord damage. Determining which patient has sustained a spinal injury is often difficult, particularly when the patient is semiconscious or unconscious.

Any manipulation of the injured cervical spine may cause permanent and irreversible damage to the spinal cord. Because this risk is so great, the EMT must assume that all unconscious head injury patients have sustained a cervical spine injury. The spine must be protected from any further damage with prompt and secure splinting. The specific techniques of cervical spine immobilization are outlined in Chapter 20.

Certain clues on physical examination of the unconscious patient can be used to identify the presence of a spinal cord injury. For example, the EMT should observe the chest and abdomen as the patient breathes. Distention of the abdomen with little or no movement of the chest indicates that the diaphragm is performing the principal breathing function and that the chest muscles are paralyzed. The diaphragm can continue to function because it is controlled by nerves that arise high in the neck, usually above the area of a cervical spine injury. The chest muscles are under the control of peripheral nerves that originate in the thoracic spine. Therefore, with a cervical spine injury the diaphragm may continue to function and the muscles of the thorax will be paralyzed.

Another clue to spinal cord injury is hypotension because of dilation of the blood vessels below the level of the spinal injury. Thus, the head injury patient may be hypotensive with a systolic blood pressure below 100 millimeters of mercury, even though there may be no signs of external bleeding.

The semiconscious patient can be checked for loss of sensation — a third clue to spinal cord injury. The skin over the legs, abdomen, thorax, and face should be pinched gently. The patient will grimace or withdraw from the irritating pinch only in the areas in which sensation is present.

Assessment of the Level of Consciousness

The single most important step in evaluating a patient with a head injury is assessing the level of consciousness. The EMT should determine the level of consciousness immediately after completing the primary survey of the patient. The **AVPU scale** described in Chapter 4 should be used to assess the patient's level of consciousness. The initial level of consciousness should be determined, and the time at which that observation is made must be recorded. The level of consciousness should then be checked every 10 minutes and recorded on the ambulance street form, along with the time of the observation.

Any change in the level of consciousness (either improvement or deterioration) is the most important measurement any medical person can make in the head injury patient. Frequently the level of consciousness will fluctuate — improving, deteriorating, and then improving again with time. On other occasions there will be a gradual progressive deterioration in the patient's response to stimuli. Such deterioration usually indicates serious brain damage that may require prompt and vigorous surgical treatment. Attending physicians must know when loss of consciousness occurred. The baseline neurological evaluation that the EMT performed in the field will be compared with the neurological evaluations obtained once the patient reaches the emergency department. The sooner this baseline evaluation can be obtained, the more information physicians will have for planning an appropriate course of treatment. It cannot be stated too often that the state of consciousness of a patient or any change in it is the single most important observation the EMT can make to assess the severity of brain damage.

TREATMENT FOR SPECIFIC HEAD INJURIES

Scalp Laceration

Scalp lacerations may be minor or very extensive. Because the face and scalp both possess an unusually rich blood supply, significant amounts of blood may be quickly lost, even from very small lacerations. On rare occasions, blood loss from a scalp laceration may be severe enough to cause hypovolemic shock. In the multiply injured patient, bleeding from scalp or facial lacerations will contribute to hypovolemia. Bleeding from scalp lacerations can almost always be controlled by local manual pressure with a dry sterile dressing directly over the wound. The EMT will have to apply firm compression for several minutes in some instances in order to control the bleeding from scalp lacerations. Some-

times triangular or square flap types of lacerations of the scalp will occur. The flap of skin should be folded back down onto its bed before the compression dressing is applied. As with bleeding from other areas, the dressing should not be removed, even if it becomes saturated with blood. A second dressing should be applied over the first one to reinforce it. Manual pressure should be continued until the bleeding is controlled. Once the bleeding is under control, the compression dressing can be secured in place with a soft, self-adhering circumferential roller bandage (Figure 19.1).

Concussion

A blow to the head or face may cause concussion of the brain. There is no universal agreement on the definition of concussion except that it involves a temporary loss of some or all of the ability of the brain to function. No permanent physical damage occurs to the brain tissue. The concussion may result in a temporary abnormal function of any part of the brain. For example, the person who "sees stars" after being struck in the head has suffered a concussion that affects the occipital portion of the brain. Concussion may result in unconsciousness and even the inability to breathe for short periods of time. The patient may be confused or have a loss of memory (**amnesia**). Occasionally the patient cannot remember events that occurred prior to the injury (**retrograde amnesia**).

Usually the concussive state is of short duration. In fact, it is often over by the time the EMT arrives. Nevertheless, any patient who has sustained a head injury should be questioned for symptoms of a concussion. In addition to having a clear memory of the accident, the patient should not complain of dizziness, weakness, visual changes, or any other symptoms that would indicate temporary loss of part or all of the brain's function. If the patient has any complaints consistent with a concussion, regardless of the patient's degree of recovery, the level of consciousness should be observed and recorded. The patient should then be monitored closely over the next several hours to assure that progressive neurological symptoms do not develop.

Contusion

Just as with any other soft tissue in the body, the brain may sustain a contusion, or bruise, when

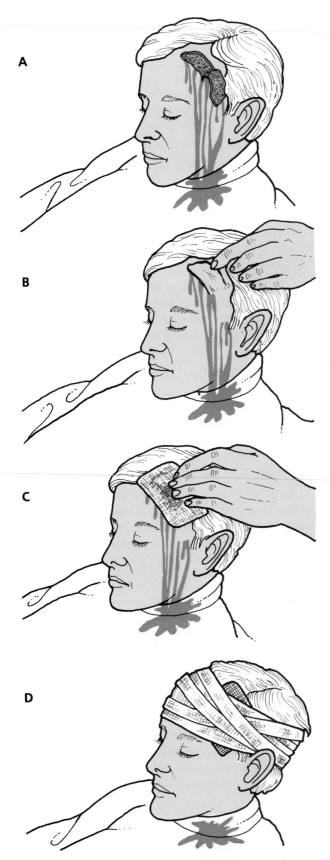

FIGURE 19.1 Scalp laceration. (a) Bleeding from a scalp laceration may be extensive; often, flap-type lacerations occur. (b) The flap should be replaced in its bed before (c) compression is applied with a dry, sterile bandage. (d) Once bleeding is controlled, the dressing can be secured with a soft roller bandage.

an object hits the skull. Contusion is a far more serious condition than concussion because physical injury to the brain tissue has occurred. As with other soft tissue contusions, there is associated bleeding and swelling from injured blood vessels. Contusion produces more long lasting and perhaps permanent damage to brain tissue. A patient who has sustained a brain contusion may exhibit any or all of the signs of brain damage (altered vital signs, numbness or weakness, loss of consciousness, or dilation of the pupils).

The brain tissue itself is easily damaged by extensive bleeding and swelling of the tissues into the confined space of the skull. The increased intracranial pressure itself causes damage to the brain that may result in progressive deterioration of the level of consciousness and even death.

The importance of adequate ventilation and the administration of oxygen cannot be overemphasized in the treatment of patients with this condition. High blood oxygen levels will decrease the amount of brain swelling and thus minimize the amount of brain damage that may occur. The patient's level of consciousness must be monitored closely, and the patient must be transported promptly to the hospital for expert neurological evaluation and care.

Intracranial Bleeding

The brain occupies nearly the entire space inside the skull. There is very little room for a hematoma resulting from laceration or rupture of a blood vessel within the skull. Severe injury that causes laceration of a blood vessel inside the brain or laceration of the meninges that cover the brain produces an **intracranial hematoma**. These hematomas are found in three areas:

1. Outside the dura and under the skull: **epidural hematomas.**
2. Beneath the dura but outside of the brain: **subdural hematomas.**
3. Within the substance of the brain tissue itself: **intracerebral hematomas.**

The signs and symptoms produced by intracranial bleeding are the result of pressure on the brain from the expanding hematoma within the skull (Figure 19.2). Usually the signs and symptoms develop promptly after a closed head injury but sometimes — particularly with the subdural hematoma

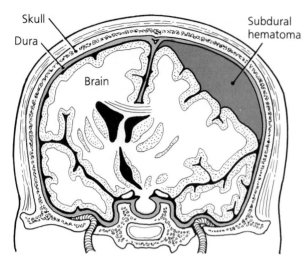

FIGURE 19.2 Bleeding from damaged blood vessels under the dura produces a subdural hematoma that compresses brain tissue, causing permanent brain injury.

— the bleeding may occur slowly over several days, and the patient develops progressive neurological problems. The patient with an expanding hematoma inside the skull requires prompt surgical treatment to avoid permanent brain damage. When the bleeding occurs rapidly within the brain, the patient's neurological status may deteriorate quite rapidly, within a matter of minutes. Any patient who develops rapidly progressive deterioration of neurological signs following a head injury should be considered to have an intracranial hematoma that will require rapid evaluation and probably surgical treatment.

Skull Fractures

The main function of the skull is to protect the brain from mechanical injury. A fracture of the skull is an indication that a significant force has been exerted on the head. Of course, very serious brain injury can occur even without fracture of the skull. As with any other fracture, skull fractures may be open or closed, depending on the integrity of the overlying scalp. The diagnosis of a skull fracture is usually made at the hospital by x-ray examination, but the EMT may conclude that a fracture is present if the patient's head appears deformed. If the scalp has been lacerated, there may be a visible crack in the skull. Injuries from bullets or other penetrating weapons almost always result in fracture of the skull. Another sign of skull fracture is ecchymosis that develops under the eyes (**"raccoon eyes"**) or be-

hind the ear over the mastoid process (**"Battle's sign"**) (Figure 19.3).

An indirect indication of fracture of the skull is the appearance of clear or pink, watery fluid dripping from the nose, from the ear, or from an open scalp wound. This watery fluid is **cerebrospinal fluid,** and it can leak to the outside only if the dura and the skull have both been penetrated. When cerebrospinal fluid is seen draining from the skull, no attempt should be made to pack the wound, the ear, or the nose. Firm packing of the draining site will block the escape of cerebrospinal fluid and may cause additional pressure on an already damaged brain. A scalp wound that is draining cerebrospinal fluid should be covered with sterile gauze to prevent further contamination, but it should not be bandaged tightly.

The treatment of skull fractures is directed primarily at the underlying brain injury, with attention being directed to the airway for adequate ventilation and close monitoring of the patient's level of consciousness. Any open wound should be covered with a dry sterile dressing. Splinting of skull fractures is not necessary, although the skull should be protected from any further injury. All patients with skull fractures must have the cervical spine totally immobilized because of the risk of associated spinal injury.

ADDITIONAL PREHOSPITAL CARE OF HEAD INJURIES

Care of Additional Injuries

A head injury may be isolated or it may be part of massive multiple trauma. Therefore, the patient who has a severe head injury must also be evaluated for other injuries. Many patients who sustain a head injury have been involved in high-velocity accidents and may have sustained injury to other body systems. A thorough secondary survey should be done to identify these other injuries, and appropriate emergency care should be provided prior to transport.

Control of Bleeding

All open wounds should be treated with a dry sterile compression dressing to control bleeding. Open skull fractures should also be treated with a dry sterile dressing. If cerebral spinal fluid is leaking from the fracture site or from the ear or nose,

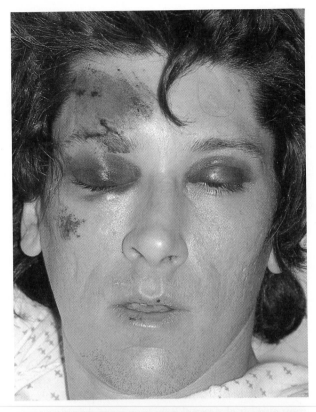

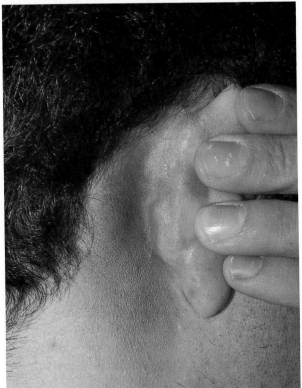

FIGURE 19.3 Signs of skull fracture: (top) bruising around the eyes; (bottom) bruising behind the ear over the mastoid process, or "Battle's sign."

a dry sterile dressing should be applied lightly to the draining area.

Management of Convulsion

It is not uncommon for the head injury patient to have a convulsion or seizure as a result of the injury. Immobilization of the cervical spine and maintenance of an adequate airway are difficult to achieve during a convulsion. During the convulsion, the patient must be protected from further injury. A bite block or padded tongue blade should be easily accessible to the EMT to help maintain the airway if the head injury patient starts to convulse.

Positioning the Patient

The ideal position for a patient with an isolated head injury is with the head of the stretcher elevated about 6 inches to promote the drainage of blood from the brain. This position will minimize swelling of the brain. Once the spine is adequately immobilized, the head should be elevated to minimize brain swelling.

Bleeding in the mouth or throat, vomiting, or excessive mucus may obstruct the upper airway. Suctioning should be used to clear any fluids that accumulate in the upper airway. The patient should be immobilized well enough that he can be turned on his side to facilitate clearing of the airway if necessary (Figure 19.4).

ASSESSING THE SEVERITY OF A HEAD INJURY

When assessing the head injury patient, the EMT should carefully evaluate the following:

1. Vital signs
2. Level of consciousness
3. Patient's ability to communicate and perceive the surroundings
4. Pupils' reaction to light
5. Sensation and motor function in the extremities

The EMT must observe and record the head injury patient's vital signs after completing the primary survey and stabilizing the airway and cervical spine. Unusual and unexpected vital signs may be seen in the head injury patient. Bleeding from the scalp may

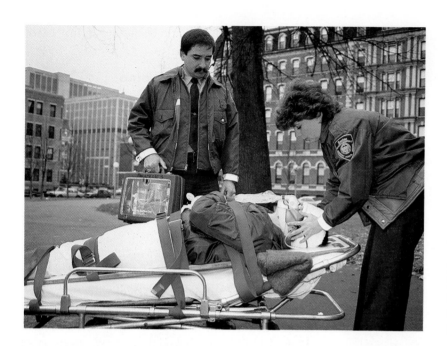

FIGURE 19.4 The patient with a head injury should be securely immobilized on a spine board. The head of the stretcher should be elevated 6 inches. The airway must be maintained and oxygen given.

be excessive, but bleeding within the skull usually is of a relatively small volume because of the confined space. Thus, low blood pressure and hypovolemic shock are almost never the result of bleeding into the brain alone. Hypotension in a head injury patient almost always indicates the presence of a spinal cord injury or serious blood loss from another injury in some other part of the body.

Intracranial hemorrhage frequently produces a slowing of the pulse rate and a rise in the blood pressure. The presence of these signs should alert the EMT to the possibility of intracranial bleeding, which may be life-threatening if not treated promptly.

As has been said several times already, an initial assessment of the patient's level of consciousness is the single most important evaluation the EMT can make to assess the presence of severe or progressive brain damage. Using the AVPU scale, the patient's level of consciousness must be evaluated and recorded every 10 minutes until the patient reaches the emergency department.

Following a head injury of any severity, a patient who exhibits any abnormal behavior must be considered to have sustained at least a concussion. It is imperative that this patient be observed very closely over the ensuing 24 hours to be certain that progressive neurological signs and symptoms do not develop. Because a patient may develop the symptoms of a subdural hematoma several days, or even

weeks, after injury, the EMT must suspect head injury as the cause of any abnormal behavior or loss of normal brain function. For example, alcoholics may exhibit abnormal behavior from drinking to excess, but alcoholics are also prone to falling and sustaining head injury. The abnormal behavior of someone who appears to be intoxicated may be the result of a head injury sustained several days earlier. Thus, any patient who exhibits the least bit of abnormal behavior, who is disoriented regarding time, place, or person, or who exhibits amnesia or any other sign of concussion should be transferred to the hospital for full evaluation and continued observation.

The size of a patient's pupils and their reaction to light should also be evaluated periodically. The muscles that control dilation and constriction of the pupils are very sensitive to changes in pressure within the brain. An early sign of increased intracranial pressure is a change in the pupils' response to light. As soon as the patient's level of consciousness has been assessed, the reaction of each pupil to light should be determined. The pupil should constrict promptly when light is shined into the eye. A dilated pupil that does not respond to light is an indication of significantly increased intracranial pressure and impending permanent brain damage. The size of the pupil of the eye and its ability to constrict in reaction to a bright light beamed into it are important clinical signs. The EMT should make a sketch of the pupil on the ambulance street form to indicate any difference in size. Any change in pupil reaction is an extremely important observation to record since it is an indicator of progressive brain damage.

Finally, the EMT should try to estimate the strength of the upper and lower extremities and assess sensation in all four limbs. As with the other signs, progressive loss of strength or sensation is an important indicator of progressive brain damage. Any complaints of numbness or weakness by the patient should be recorded, along with the time of onset of these symptoms.

Close observation and careful recording of the patient's vital signs, level of consciousness, pupillary reaction, sensation, and motor function will provide an effective means of assessing the degree of severity of the head injury. The baseline measurements established in the field will serve as a useful point of reference when similar evaluations are carried out in the emergency department. This baseline should be established as soon as possible so that any critical changes in the patient's condition can be identified promptly and proper medical care can be provided.

YOU ARE THE EMT...

1. Why is a brain contusion more serious than a brain concussion?
2. If the patient has "raccoon eyes" or "Battle's sign," what kind of injury would you suspect? How would you treat this injury?
3. Why do you have to immobilize a patient with a head injury? Why do you elevate the head of the stretcher during transport?
4. You have been called to treat a young man who is confused about where he is and who is not making any sense when he talks. His mother tells you that he "walked away," apparently unhurt, from an automobile accident five days ago. What kind of injury do you suspect? How serious could this problem be? How will you evaluate this patient?

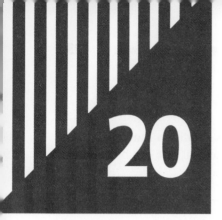

20 Injury to the Spine

OVERVIEW

Injury to the spine that disrupts the protection of the spinal cord can produce permanent paralysis. Over the past 10 to 15 years, since the advent of effective emergency medical services in the United States, there has been a gradual decrease in the incidence of paralysis from spinal injury. Most authorities agree that this decrease is a direct result of effective prehospital care of patients with spinal injury.

EMTs have learned how to recognize spinal injury even when the symptoms are not obvious. They have also learned how to clear and maintain airways without endangering the spinal cord, how to remove helmets (and when *not* to remove them) after sports and motorcycle accidents, and most important, how to splint spine injury patients. These techniques, when employed properly, will significantly minimize the risk of paralysis in the injured patient.

Chapter 20 first discusses fractures and dislocations of the spine. Next it describes the symptoms and signs of spinal injury. Then the chapter explains how the EMT decides if spinal injury is present and how, once diagnosed, spinal injuries are treated. The last section of Chapter 20 discusses the complications of spinal cord injury.

OBJECTIVES

The objectives of Chapter 20 are to

- describe fractures and dislocations of the spine.
- identify the symptoms and signs of spinal injury.
- know how to diagnose spinal injury.
- learn the emergency treatment of spine injury patients.
- become familiar with the complications of spinal cord injury.

FRACTURES AND DISLOCATIONS OF THE SPINE

The **spine** is a segmented column of 33 **vertebrae,** stacked one on the next and extending from the base of the skull to the tip of the coccyx (Figure 20.1). Lying between each of the cervical, thoracic, and lumbar vertebrae are the **intervertebral discs.** The vertebrae are tied together by strong ligaments that allow a small amount of bending motion to occur

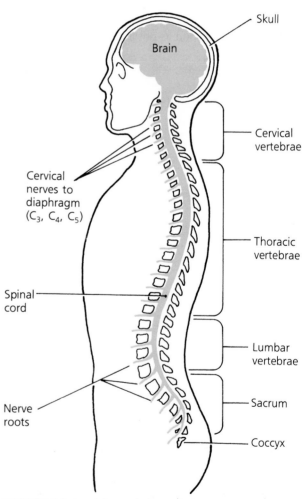

FIGURE 20.1 A lateral view of the spine shows the spinal cord lying inside the spinal canal.

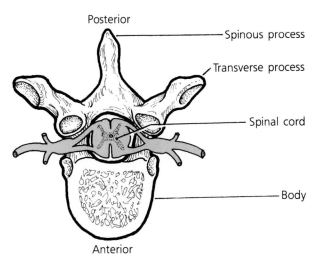

FIGURE 20.2   Top view of a typical thoracic vertebra showing how the spinal cord lies protected inside the bony spinal canal.

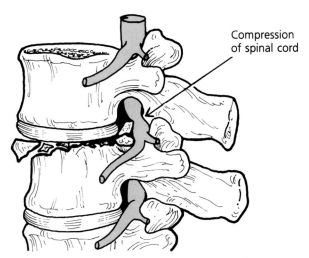

FIGURE 20.3   If the spine is unstable, even a small shift of one vertebra on the next may damage or even crush the spinal cord.

between adjacent vertebrae. The ligaments, however, prevent any shifting of one vertebra onto the adjacent ones. Posteriorly, each vertebra has a tunnel that extends from top to bottom (Figure 20.2). When stacked one upon another in the spinal column, the vertebrae create a bony **spinal canal** in which the **spinal cord** lies and is protected.

Most injuries to the spine produce ligament sprains or nondisplaced fractures that heal well and have an excellent long-term prognosis. Sometimes, however, displaced fractures or dislocations of the spine will damage the spinal cord or the nerve roots and cause permanent paralysis or even death. Distinguishing between those injuries that are not dangerous and those that may jeopardize the spinal cord is difficult and often requires special x-ray studies. The EMT at the scene of an accident can never be certain that the suspected spine injury is safe or dangerous, so it is best to consider all spine injuries as potentially dangerous and treat them as such.

If injury to the spinal column has made it unstable, it can no longer protect the spinal cord. The spinal cord fills most of the spinal canal. Even slight displacement of one vertebra on the next will pinch or shear the spinal cord. With an unstable fracture or dislocation, displacement of one millimeter may be enough to compress, pinch, or shear the spinal cord (Figure 20.3). This damage may make the difference between normal function and perma-

nent paralysis. Therefore, it is imperative that no further motion occur in an unstable spine and that rigid splinting be achieved.

Recognizing a possible spinal injury is one of the EMT's major responsibilities. The EMT should be suspicious of spinal injury when called to see any patient who has received a high-velocity injury. The types of trauma most likely to produce a spinal fracture are automobile and motorcycle accidents, diving injuries, falls from a height, and cave-ins. In addition, any unconscious injured patient and any patient who has sustained a facial or scalp laceration or contusion must be assumed to have a spinal injury. Thus, when dispatched to an accident scene and when sizing up any of these injury situations, the EMT must *"think spinal injury."*

SIGNS AND SYMPTOMS OF SPINAL INJURY

The EMT must be able to recognize those complaints of the patient (**symptoms**) and those physical findings (**signs**) that indicate the possibility of spinal injury.

Symptoms

Pain. A conscious patient will be aware of pain in the spine and be able to direct the EMT's attention to the area of injury in the back or neck. However, with an unconscious patient, this most important and reliable symptom will not be present. Occasionally, a conscious patient with a spinal fracture will not complain of pain. This will sometimes happen because the patient is lying very still ("splinting" his injury) or perhaps because other, more painful injuries are distracting the patient's attention from the spinal fracture.

Numbness, Tingling, or Weakness. If the conscious patient complains of tingling, loss of feeling, or weakness in one or more of the extremities, spinal cord damage probably exists.

Pain with Movement. If the patient attempts to move the injured area of the spine, pain may occur or increase significantly. The EMT should *never* try to test this increase in pain by moving the patient. Do not encourage anyone with neck or back pain to move. Proceed immediately with splinting.

Signs

Deformity. Deformity of the spine is a certain indication that significant injury has occurred. However, most patients with spinal fractures and spinal cord injury do not have an obvious deformity. It only occurs with severe injury with marked displacement of the bony fragments. Absence of a deformity in no way eliminates the possibility of a fracture or dislocation of the spine. When it is present, deformity is most often seen in the cervical spine with the head twisted or cocked to one side.

Tenderness. **Point tenderness** over any portion of the spine is sufficient reason to suspect spinal injury. The spinous processes of all cervical, thoracic, and lumbar vertebrae can be palpated in the midline posteriorly. The spine of C7 is especially prominent at the base of the neck. Point tenderness anywhere along the spinous processes is a strong indication of a significant spinal injury.

Lacerations or Contusions. Cuts and bruises are reliable signs that strong forces have been applied to the body. Almost all cervical spine fractures or dislocations result from a blow to the head. Therefore, any cut or bruise on the head or face is a very reliable indication of spinal injury (Figure 20.4). Patients with serious injuries in other areas of the spine are likely to have bruises over the shoulders, the back, or the abdomen.

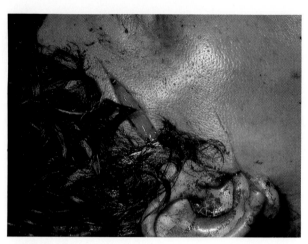

FIGURE 20.4 Lacerations of the head should make the EMT suspect a spinal injury.

Paralysis or Anesthesia. Any weakness or loss of sensation (**anesthesia**) that can be demonstrated on physical examination should be considered a sign of spinal injury. The EMT should touch the patient's fingers, toes, arms, and legs to assess feeling in these regions. Muscle function can be tested by judging the strength of the grip by asking the patient to squeeze the EMT's fingers. The EMT can test lower extremity strength by asking the patient to move his feet up and down. Any patient who has loss of sensation or weakness must be assumed to have a spinal cord injury.

Spinal cord injuries in the neck may cause paralysis of all four extremities as well as impairment of breathing. Spinal fractures at the level of the waist will cause numbness and/or paralysis below that level, but breathing and strength and sensation in upper extremities will not be affected (Figure 20.5).

DIAGNOSIS OF SPINAL INJURY

EMTs will suspect spinal injury whenever they arrive at an accident caused by any of the mechanisms described earlier. All patients so injured must be evaluated for the possibility of a spinal injury. In the conscious patient, the following four steps can be taken to determine the presence of a possible spinal injury.

1. Ask the patient or witnesses about the nature of the accident, and question the patient carefully about areas of pain, numbness, or weakness.

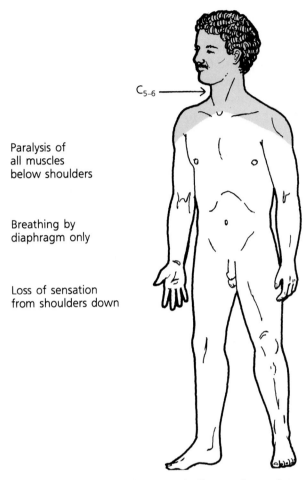

C$_{5-6}$

Paralysis of
all muscles
below shoulders

Breathing by
diaphragm only

Loss of sensation
from shoulders down

FIGURE 20.5 The white area indicates the region of numbness and paralysis from a spinal cord injury at the level of the fifth and sixth cervical vertebrae.

2. Look for contusions, lacerations, and abrasions about the face, head, or trunk and look for any deformity of the spine.
3. Feel for any irregularity, deformity, or point tenderness along the spinous processes posteriorly. Check the arms and legs for decreased sensation.
4. Check for weakness or paralysis by asking the patient to wiggle fingers and toes, unassisted.

If any one of these four signs or symptoms is present, injury of the spine must be assumed and appropriate splinting undertaken. No further manipulation of the spine by either the patient or the EMT should be performed. The patient should not be allowed to move until spinal immobilization is complete.

Sometimes the EMT will suspect a spinal injury in a patient who has been involved in a car wreck, fallen from a great height, or experienced some other high-velocity accident. Yet the patient does not complain of pain, numbness, or weakness, and no soft tissue injury or deformity is evident. No point tenderness can be elicited on palpation of the spine, and no numbness or weakness exists in the extremities. When this situation exists and the EMT is still suspicious that a spinal injury may be present because of the mechanism of injury, the patient should be instructed to slowly and carefully move the spine to see if motion produces pain at a specific location. The patient should be instructed to bend his head forward, backward, and to each side gently and carefully and then slowly bend forward from the waist. If any of these motions causes pain in this otherwise symptom-free patient, spinal injury must be considered a possibility. Of course, this step should *never* be performed if any of the other signs or symptoms described earlier are present.

The unconscious patient presents a more difficult problem. This person will not be able to cooperate with the full evaluation, and thus many of the signs and symptoms present in the conscious patient cannot be identified. Whenever unconsciousness has resulted from an accident that is known to cause spinal injury, the EMT must assume that the patient has an associated spinal fracture until proven otherwise. All patients who have been injured and are unconscious must be assumed to have sustained a spinal injury.

EMERGENCY TREATMENT OF SPINAL INJURY

Proper emergency care of a spinal fracture may prevent the need for weeks of medical care and years of permanent disability. The EMT has the opportunity to prevent paralysis and death. On the other hand, failure to diagnose a possible spinal injury or ineffective splinting of the unstable spine might cause significant, long-term problems for the patient.

The emergency care of spinal injury follows the same rules as emergency care for all other major injuries: Restore the airway and assure adequate ventilation, control serious bleeding using local pressure dressings, and most importantly, splint the patient before moving.

Restoring the Airway

The EMT must always be aware of the danger of causing permanent paralysis through improper handling of the patient with a cervical spine injury. However, this possibility should not interfere with providing an open airway for the patient, because the inability to breathe will result in death. In the spine injury patient with an obstructed airway, the EMT should restore an adequate airway by using the jaw-thrust maneuver described in Chapter 6. The head-tilt/chin-lift maneuver should not be used because it may cause further damage to the cervical spine. In the unconscious patient, the tongue can be pulled forward out of the pharynx using the jaw thrust to avoid any manipulation of the neck. If this maneuver is successful, the airway can be maintained with an oropharyngeal airway, but it must be closely monitored. Suctioning equipment must be available, as the airway will frequently need to be cleared of blood, saliva, or vomitus. Oxygen should be given to any patient with marginally effective respirations.

If the jaw-thrust maneuver does not relieve airway obstruction, the alignment of the neck must be improved to open the airway. Two EMTs will be needed. The first EMT should firmly grasp the patient's head with both hands and simultaneously pull the head gently and firmly away from the trunk and turn it to the front, bringing the head to the "eyes

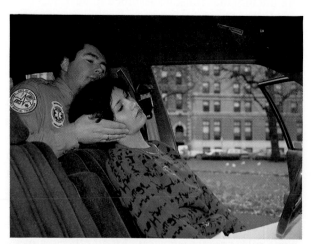

FIGURE 20.6 When alignment of the neck must be improved to establish an open airway, the EMT grasps the head firmly with two hands and applies gentle traction, bringing the head back to the "eyes-forward" position.

forward" position (Figure 20.6). A force of approximately 10 pounds will be required. The realignment of the head on the trunk is accomplished gradually in a step-wise fashion. After partial realignment is achieved, the first EMT maintains the head in the new position while the second EMT repeats the jaw-thrust maneuver to open the airway. The head is realigned only enough to open the airway. Extreme hyperextension and hyperflexion of the head on the trunk are always avoided because these are the positions in which spinal cord damage is most likely to occur. Once the airway is open, the head has to be held in the new position until it can be fully splinted.

Helmet Removal

Many patients with neck injuries are motorcyclists or football players who may be wearing protective helmets. In the vast majority of instances, the helmet does not need to be removed. Indeed, it is frequently fitted so snugly to the head that it can be secured directly to the spinal immobilization device. There are only two circumstances in which part or all of the helmet should be removed: (1) when the face mask or visor interferes with adequate ventilation or with the EMT's ability to restore an adequate airway, or (2) when the helmet is so loose that securing it to the spinal immobilization device will not provide adequate immobilization of the head.

When part of the helmet is interfering with ventilation, the visor of a motorcycle helmet should be lifted away from the face, or the face guard of a football helmet should be removed. Most football face guards are fastened to the helmet by four rubber clips. These clips can be cut easily with a sharp knife or scissors and the face guard removed (Figure 20.7). The chin strap should also be loosened to facilitate the chin-lift or jaw-thrust maneuvers. In most instances, exposing the face and jaw will allow the EMT access to the airway to secure adequate ventilation. Only if these steps do not allow adequate access to the airway should the entire helmet be removed.

The second indication for helmet removal is a loose helmet that cannot be adequately incorporated into the spinal immobilization device. Such a loose helmet can be removed quite easily. Sometimes, however, for some unusual reason, a snugly fitting football or motorcycle helmet might have to be re-

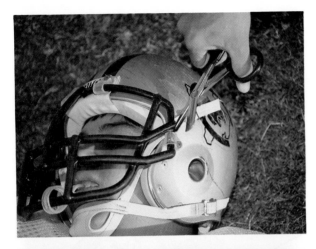

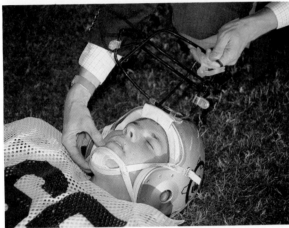

FIGURE 20.7 When airway access must be achieved in an injured football player, the face guard can be removed by (top) cutting the clips that attach it to the helmet and (bottom) lifting it out of the way.

moved to secure an adequate airway. In such circumstances, the following specific protocol should be carried out. Note that this procedure requires two EMTs.

1. First EMT: Stand or kneel above the patient's head and support the head by placing a hand on each side of the helmet with your fingers on the patient's mandible (Figure 20.8a).

2. Second EMT: Cut or loosen the chin strap while the first EMT maintains head support (Figure 20.8b).

3. Second EMT: Place one of your hands on the patient's mandible with your thumb on one side and the long and index fingers on the opposite side. Place your other hand behind

the patient's neck and apply firm pressure to the occipital region. This maneuver transfers the head support from the first to the second EMT (Figure 20.8c).

4. First EMT: Remove the helmet, remembering that it is usually egg-shaped and therefore must be expanded laterally to clear the ears. (Many football helmets have jaw pads that will be caught on the ears if they are not first removed.) If the helmet provides full facial coverage, it must be tilted backward to avoid striking the nose (Figure 20.8d).

5. Second EMT: Throughout the removal process maintain in-line support from below to prevent tilting of the head (Figure 20.8e).

6. First EMT: After removing the helmet, place your hands on either side of the patient's head, firmly grasping the mandible and base of the skull, to provide stable support until the patient is adequately splinted (Figure 20.8f).

The EMT should keep in mind that helmet removal is usually not necessary. If adequate access to the airway can be obtained and maintained and if the head is secure inside the helmet, the helmet can be left in place and secured to the spinal immobilization device to provide adequate splinting of the spinal injury.

Splinting of Spinal Injuries

Once the EMT suspects a spinal injury, all efforts must be made to avoid damage to the spinal cord. Once the airway is secure, it is imperative that the head and trunk be stabilized so that any displaced bone fragments will not impinge upon the spinal cord. Further abnormal motion — even as little as 1 or 2 millimeters — may cause significant spinal cord injury. One EMT must immediately begin stabilization by holding the head firmly with two hands. Whenever possible, the EMT should be behind the patient, placing each hand around the base of the skull, supporting the mandible with the index and long fingers and the occiput with the thumbs and palms (Figure 20.9, top). Gentle traction to lift the head to the position where the patient's eyes are looking straight ahead may be necessary on occasion to facilitate splinting. *At no time* should the head or neck be twisted or excessively flexed or extended.

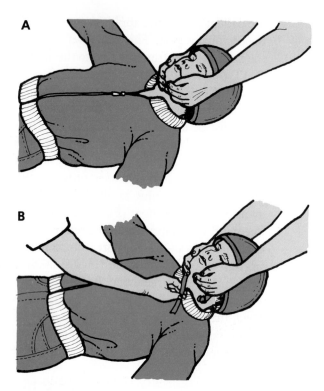

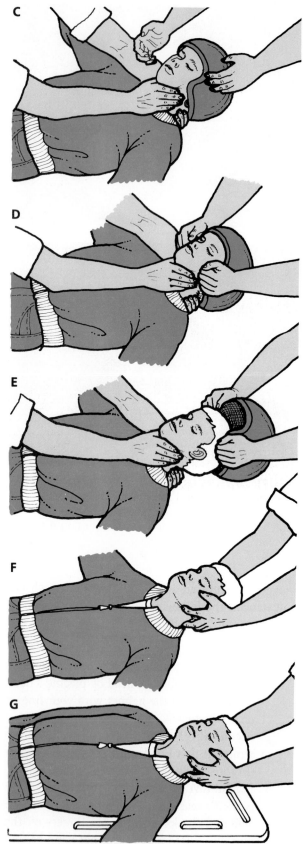

FIGURE 20.8 The proper steps of helmet removal are illustrated: (a) One EMT supports the head by placing a hand on each side of the patient's mandible. (b) The chin strap is loosened. (c) The second EMT places one hand on the mandible, the thumb on one angle, and the long and index fingers at the other angle. With the other hand, the second EMT supports the occipital region of the head. (d) The first EMT removes the helmet with as little motion of the head as is possible. The helmet must be expanded to clear the ears and rotated to clear the nose. (e) The second EMT provides continued support of the head. (f) After helmet removal, the first EMT resumes support of the head with hands on both sides of the patient's head, the palms over the ears, and the mandible supported by the fingers. (g) Head support is maintained until the patient is fully splinted.

If resistance or increased pain is encountered when the head is being stabilized manually, further traction should not be applied, and the neck must be splinted in the deformed position.

While one EMT continuously supports the head with manual traction, the second EMT places a firm extrication collar around the neck to provide some stability (Figure 20.9, bottom). While the extrication collar provides some support, it will not replace the support given by the EMT's hands. Manual sup-

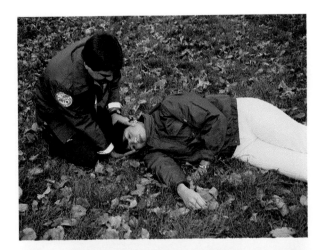

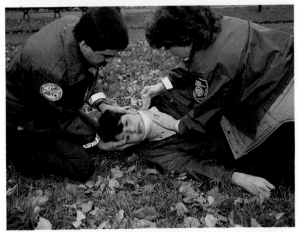

FIGURE 20.9 (top) Initial stability of the head is provided by manual support. (bottom) Additional support is achieved with the use of a firm extrication collar.

port of the head must be maintained until the patient is fully secured to the spine board.

The patient who is lying down is next placed supine on a long spine board or other spinal immobilization device. If found lying prone, the patient is turned as a unit, with one EMT supporting the head to be certain that the entire head/spine complex moves in unison. Then, using the **four-person log roll** (or the **straddle slide** if necessary) as described in Chapter 45, the patient is transferred as a unit to the board, avoiding any rotation of the head, shoulders, or pelvis. Bystanders can be recruited to assist if necessary, but an EMT must instruct them fully before the patient is moved.

Specially designed head supports are next positioned against either side of the head (Figure 20.10a).

The head and the supports are then firmly secured to the spine immobilization device with adhesive tape, Velcro straps, or with several turns of a soft roller bandage applied at the forehead level (20.10b). No chin strap is used.

Empty spaces under the knees, lower back, or neck can be filled with a pillow or a rolled blanket. The patient's chest and arms, pelvis, and lower extremities are secured to the device with straps or cravats (Figure 20.10c). The patient's hands should be loosely tied together to prevent the arms from flopping during transfer. The wrists should be crossed and a cravat or soft roller bandage loosely tied around the wrists to hold them secure (Figure 20.10d).

The patient should be so well secured to the device that the entire unit can be turned to the side to facilitate airway management if necessary (Figure 20.11, left). When vertical rescue or other complex extrication is necessary, two 9-foot straps will further secure the trunk to the device as illustrated (Figure 20.11, right).

When a spine injury patient is found in a sitting position, the short spine board or other short spinal extrication devices are used to splint the cervical and thoracic spine. The EMT must first stabilize the head with two hands and secure the airway. Gentle traction may be used to bring the head to the "eyes-forward" position if pain or resistance is not encountered. The firm extrication collar is then applied while manual support of the head continues (Figure 20.12a). The spinal extrication device is then wedged between the patient's buttocks and the seat (Figure 20.12b). The upper end of the device is tilted toward the head, and then the EMT, while supporting the head gently, brings the occiput up against it (Figure 20.12c). With the head supported manually, the trunk is secured to the extrication device with straps (Figure 20.12d). Any space between the neck and the device should be filled with soft padding. The head is then firmly secured to the device with Velcro straps applied only at the forehead level (Figure 20.12e).

The next step is to place the partially immobilized patient on the long spine board. The long board is placed next to the patient's buttocks, perpendicular to the trunk (Figure 20.13, top). The patient is turned to a parallel position with the long board and then slowly lowered onto it (Figure 20.13, middle). Then the patient is lifted as a unit, and the long board

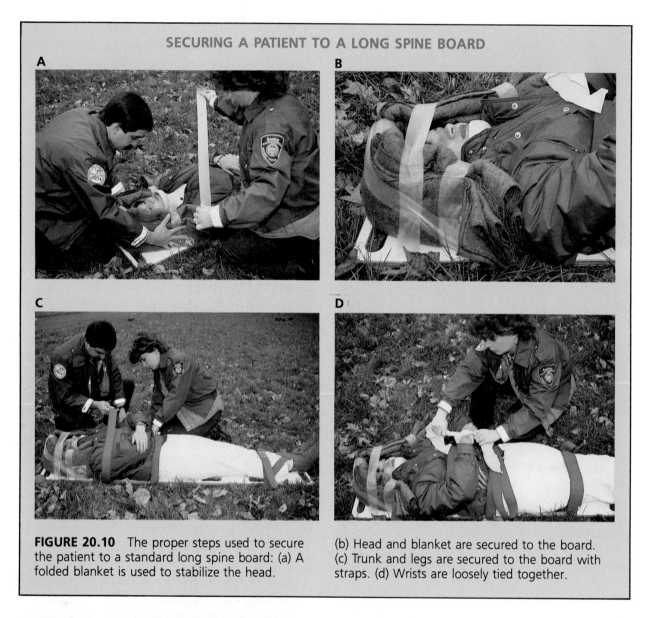

SECURING A PATIENT TO A LONG SPINE BOARD

A

B

C

D

FIGURE 20.10 The proper steps used to secure the patient to a standard long spine board: (a) A folded blanket is used to stabilize the head.

(b) Head and blanket are secured to the board. (c) Trunk and legs are secured to the board with straps. (d) Wrists are loosely tied together.

FIGURE 20.11 (left) The patient may be safely turned on one side, or (right) lifted vertically when properly secured to the board.

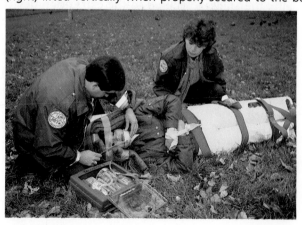

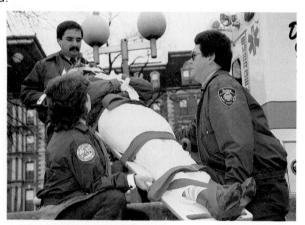

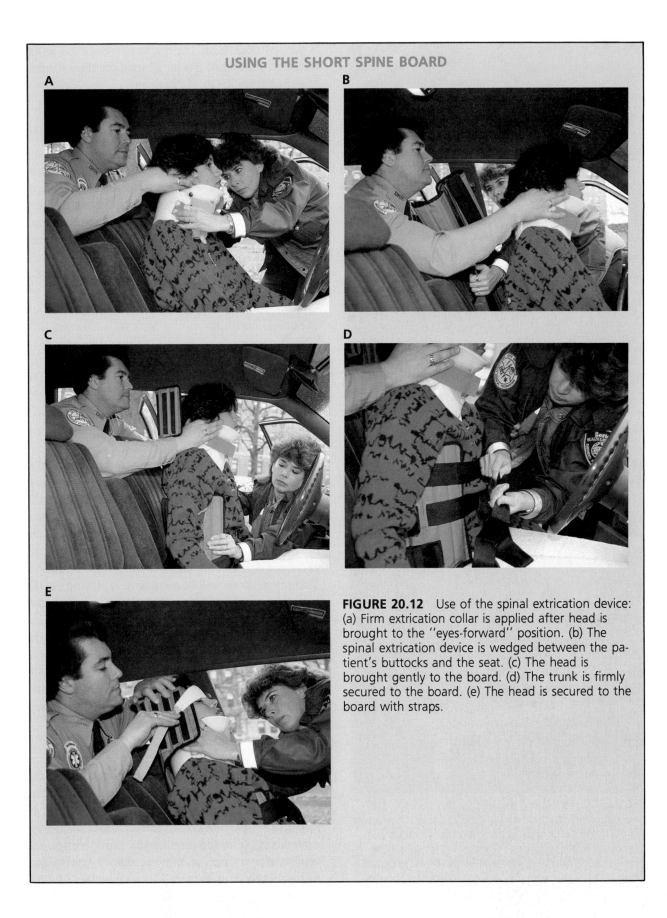

USING THE SHORT SPINE BOARD

FIGURE 20.12 Use of the spinal extrication device: (a) Firm extrication collar is applied after head is brought to the "eyes-forward" position. (b) The spinal extrication device is wedged between the patient's buttocks and the seat. (c) The head is brought gently to the board. (d) The trunk is firmly secured to the board. (e) The head is secured to the board with straps.

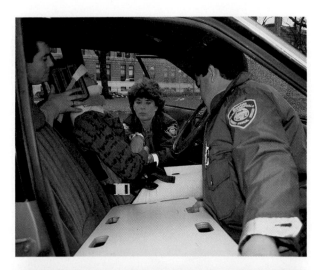

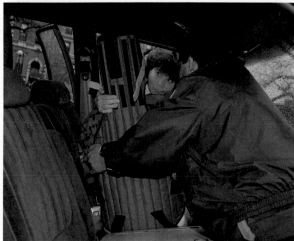

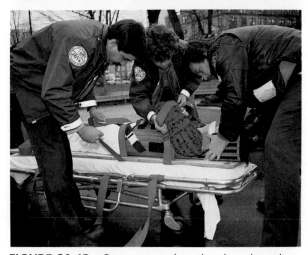

FIGURE 20.13 Once secured to the short board, the patient is placed on the long board for transport to the hospital. (top) The long board is placed perpendicular to the patient's buttocks. (middle) The patient is turned and lowered onto the long board. (bottom) The two boards are then secured together.

is slipped underneath the extrication device. The extrication device and the long board are then secured together (Figure 20.13, bottom).

COMPLICATIONS OF SPINAL CORD INJURY

In addition to paralysis and numbness, the patient with a cervical spine fracture and spinal cord injury may develop two specific problems before reaching the hospital: impaired breathing because of paralyzed chest muscles or neurogenic shock.

Impaired Breathing

The motor nerves to the diaphragm branch off the spinal cord high in the neck (C3, C4, and C5), and are rarely injured by fractures or dislocations of the cervical spine (see Figure 20.5). However, the nerves that control the chest wall muscles leave the spinal cord below the neck region. If the spinal cord is damaged at the mid-cervical level, these nerves will be paralyzed, along with the muscles of the abdomen, arms, and legs.

A patient with a spinal cord injury whose chest wall muscles and abdominal muscles have been paralyzed can breathe only with the diaphragm. As the EMT observes the pattern of breathing in this patient, the chest wall will move only slightly. In contrast, because of the motion of the diaphragm, the abdomen will move in and out with each respiration. The respirations will be weak and rapid so that the patient may seem to be panting. These signs indicate the diaphragm is the only muscle supporting respiration. When the diaphragm is unable to substitute adequately for the paralyzed chest and abdominal muscles, the person with spinal cord damage will have respiratory insufficiency. The EMT should monitor the patient's breathing, suction as necessary, and provide oxygen-enriched air if necessary.

Neurogenic Shock

Neurogenic shock results from paralysis of the nerves that control the size of the blood vessels. The arteries and veins of a paralyzed person increase in size (dilate), particularly in the abdomen and lower extremities. This dilation of the blood vessels increases the volume of the circulatory system and consequently decreases the blood pressure. The circulatory system may fail because not enough blood can be returned to the heart.

The treatment for neurogenic shock is to splint the spine and put the patient in the shock (**Trendelenburg**) position by elevating the foot of the long spine board. This position will help blood to drain from the enlarged vessels in the abdomen and lower extremities and return to the heart for active circulation. The foot of the spine board should be elevated about 12 inches. Excessive elevation should be avoided because it may cause the bowels and other abdominal viscera to fall against the underside of the diaphragm and compromise the patient's principal remaining breathing mechanism. Twelve inches of elevation is sufficient to assist blood in its return to the heart and will not significantly impair the work of the diaphragm.

YOU ARE THE EMT...

1. How can you determine whether a spinal injury is minor or serious? What are the major signs and symptoms of possible spinal injury?
2. You restored the airway and carefully splinted a spine injury patient. During transport she develops impaired breathing. What could be causing this problem and how will you treat it?
3. You are "on duty" at the local football game. One of the players is down and you are evaluating him. He does not have any numbness, tingling, or weakness in his fingers or toes. He says he just had the wind knocked out of him and is OK now. He wants to get up and walk back to the bench. What will you do?
4. What is neurogenic shock? How should you treat it?

21 Injuries of the Eye

OVERVIEW

The eye is an organ of special sense, developed for vision. It has a lens system that is similar to that of a camera. This system focuses an image, which special sensory cells in the retina change into an electrical message that is carried by the optic nerves to the occiput of the brain. The brain receives the sensory message and interprets it. This entire process is what is called "seeing."

Life revolves around our eyes, and early on children are warned about protecting their eyes. But accidents happen — car accidents, industrial accidents, household accidents, environmental accidents. Whatever the cause, eye injury is serious and painful. Correct initial emergency treatment by the EMT will minimize pain and may very well help prevent permanent loss of vision.

The first part of Chapter 21 examines the anatomy of the eye. The major part of the chapter is devoted to injuries of the eye, including injuries from foreign bodies, burns, lacerations, and blunt trauma. Eye abnormalities that alert the EMT to suspect underlying head injury are discussed next. The last section of Chapter 21 briefly discusses contact lenses and eye prostheses.

OBJECTIVES

The objectives of Chapter 21 are to

- become familiar with the anatomy of the eye.
- recognize various types of eye injury and learn how to apply correct emergency treatment for each.
- be alert for abnormalities of the eyes that may indicate underlying head injury.
- know how to manage patients with contact lenses and artificial eyes.

ANATOMY OF THE EYE

Like a fine camera, the eye has many intricate parts; all are important if the eye is to function properly (Figure 21.1). The eye is globe-shaped and approximately 1 inch in diameter. The shape of the **globe** is maintained by fluid contained within it. The fluid behind the lens is clear and jellylike and is called the **vitreous humor;** the fluid in front of the lens is more watery and is called the **aqueous humor.** When the globe is lacerated, one of these fluids may leak out.

The surface covering the front part of the globe is clear and transparent so that light may enter the eye. It is called the **cornea.** The rest of the surface of the globe is made of a tough tissue called the **sclera,** or the white part, of the eye. In the visible portion of the eye, the sclera is covered by a layer of smooth mucous membrane called the **conjunctiva.** This layer of conjunctiva also covers the undersurface of the eyelids. Thus, when the lids move, the two smooth surfaces covered with conjunctiva slide over one another. Inflammation of the conjunctiva gives the eye a characteristic red color (**"pink eye"**) and is called **conjunctivitis.**

A circular muscle lies just behind the cornea with an opening in its center. Like a camera, this muscle

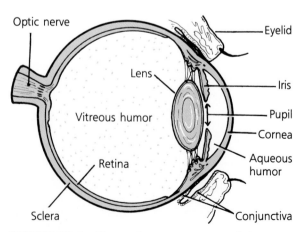

FIGURE 21.1 The major components of the eye.

adjusts the size of the opening to regulate the amount of light that enters the eye. The circular muscle is called the **iris,** and the color of the cells coating the muscle gives the eye its characteristic brown, green, or blue color. The circular opening in the middle of the muscle is called the **pupil.** Behind the iris is the **lens,** which focuses an image on the light-sensitive layer at the back of the eye, the retina. The **retina** is a layer of cells at the back of the eye that changes the light image into electrical impulses that can be carried by the optic nerve to the brain. Between the retina and the sclera on the back of the globe is a layer of blood vessels that nourish the eye, especially the retina. This layer is called the **choroid.** The retina and choroid are held against the sclera by the pressure of the vitreous humor.

The **lacrimal system** consists of lacrimal (tear) glands and ducts (Figure 21.2). This system is important for protection of the eye. Lacrimal glands produce tears that act as a lubricating substance to prevent the conjunctiva covering the front of the eye from drying. Tears also serve to flush foreign material from the surface of the eye. Small **tear glands** are located in the conjunctiva, and a large gland is located beneath the upper eyelid. **Tear ducts** are located on the inner side of the eye along the upper and lower lids. They drain the tears into the nose.

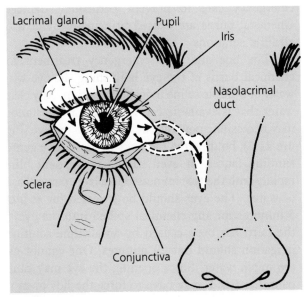

FIGURE 21.2 The lacrimal system (shown in white) consists of tear glands and ducts. Tears act as lubricants and keep the front of the eye from drying out.

The upper and lower eyelids protect the eyes. The inside of the eyelids is covered with the very smooth conjunctiva, which is continuously moistened by tears. The upper eyelid covers most of the surface of the eye and is shaped by a tough internal fibrous plate (the **tarsal plate**). It has a separate muscle (the **levator palpebrae**) to lift it. The eyelids are closed by the contraction of a circular muscle around the orbit called the **orbicularis oculi.**

The pupil of the eye becomes smaller in bright light and larger in dim light, just as the aperture of a camera is adjusted. The pupil also becomes smaller when an individual is viewing near objects. These adjustments are automatic and occur almost instantaneously.

INJURIES OF THE EYE

Proper emergency care of the injured eye first requires a thorough examination to determine the extent and nature of any damage. The examination should be performed with great care so as not to aggravate existing injury. Correct initial emergency treatment will minimize pain and may very well help prevent permanent loss of vision.

Following an injury to the eye region, the EMT should look for the following specific abnormalities or conditions: swollen or lacerated eyelids from blunt or penetrating injury. The conjunctiva frequently becomes bright red soon after irritation or injury. The cornea readily loses its smooth, wet appearance after injury. In a normal, uninjured eye, the entire circle of the iris is visible, the pupils are round and equal in size, both eyes move together in the same direction when following the EMT's moving finger, and each pupil reacts equally with the other when exposed to light.

Foreign Bodies in the Eye

Although large objects may be prevented from penetrating the eye by the bony orbit that surrounds it, moderate-sized and smaller foreign bodies of many different types can enter the eye and cause significant damage. Even a very small foreign body such as a grain of sand lying on the surface of the conjunctiva of the eye will cause severe irritation. The conjunctiva will become inflamed and red almost immediately (Figure 21.3). The eye will begin to produce tears in an attempt to flush out the irritating

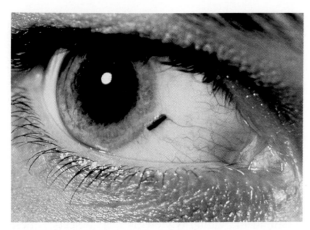

FIGURE 21.3 Small foreign bodies on the cornea of the eye will cause severe irritation, with redness and tearing.

object. Intense pain is produced by irritation of the conjunctiva, and the patient has difficulty keeping the eyelids open because the irritation is further aggravated by bright light.

If a small foreign body is lying on the anterior surface of the patient's eye, the eye should be irrigated gently with normal saline solution. Irrigation with 500 to 1,000 cc of saline will frequently flush away loose, small particles. After it is flushed away, a foreign body will often leave a small scratch on the surface of the conjunctiva that will cause the patient to continue to complain of irritation even after the particle has been removed.

Foreign bodies stuck to the cornea or lying under the upper eyelid usually will not wash out with a gentle irrigation. The EMT should never attempt to remove a foreign body that is stuck to the cornea. The undersurface of the upper eyelid may be examined for the presence of a foreign body. The lid should be *everted* or pulled forward and upward away from the eyeball. If a foreign body is found on the undersurface of the lid, it can be removed with a moist, sterile, cotton-tipped applicator (Figure 21.4).

Large foreign bodies may be impaled in the eye. They must be removed by a physician. The EMT should support the object with a dry, sterile dressing to prevent further contamination and to minimize motion of the object. Then the injured eye should be covered with a paper cup or cardboard cone to prevent the object from being driven farther into the eye. Cover the other eye, too, even though only the one eye is injured. Because the eyes move to-

gether, covering both eyes will keep both quiet and will prevent undue motion on the injured side (Figure 21.5).

A person with both eyes covered obviously cannot see and may become frightened easily. This is especially true in children. Covering both eyes without a warning may be unwise as the patient may become uncooperative and struggle, causing more damage to the eye. Calm reassurance and a quiet matter-of-fact explanation of why both eyes are being covered temporarily are essential before the EMT covers the eyes. Once both eyes are covered, the patient will need assistance and continuous reassurance when being moved from one place to another. The EMT should keep the patient informed verbally about what is happening. A gesture as simple as holding the patient's hand will often provide the support and reassurance that is needed.

Burns of the Eye

The eye can be burned by chemicals, heat, and light rays. The delicate tissues of the eye may be permanently damaged, and prompt emergency care must be directed at stopping the burning process and preventing further damage to the eye.

Chemical Burns

Injuries from chemical burns require immediate emergency care to prevent permanent damage. Chemical burns are caused principally by acid or alkaline solutions.

The one and only emergency treatment for chemical burns of the eye is flushing the eye with water or a sterile saline irrigation solution. Any clean water that is available can be used. Circumstances may necessitate pouring the water into the eye (Figure 21.6), holding the patient's head under a gently running faucet, or even having the patient blink rapidly with the face immersed in a large pan or basin of water. The eyes should be irrigated for at least 5 minutes for any chemical spilled into the eye; if the burn has been caused by an alkaline solution, irrigation should last 20 minutes. One cannot use too much water. Since opening the eye may cause pain, the EMT may have to force the lids open so the eye can be irrigated adequately. During irrigation it is especially important to protect the uninjured eye. The irrigation fluid should not be allowed to run into the good eye from the injured eye and possibly burn

REMOVAL OF A FOREIGN BODY FROM UNDER THE UPPER EYELID

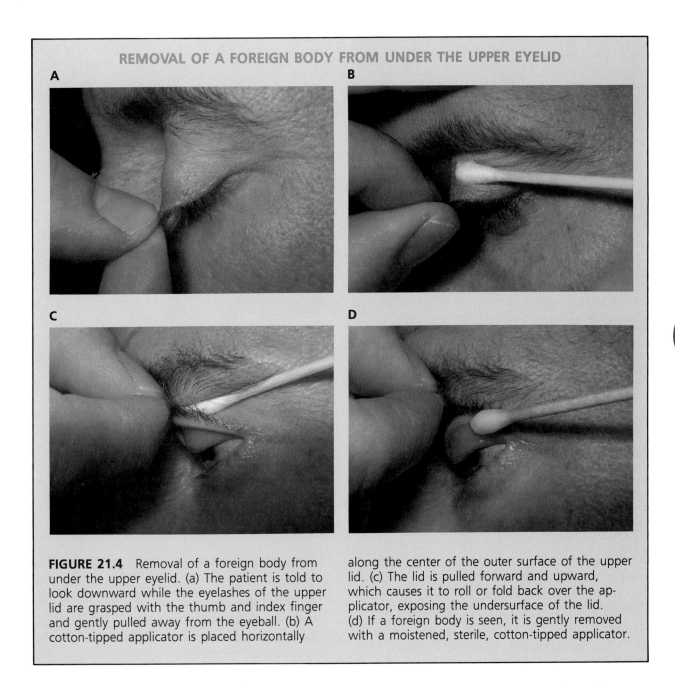

FIGURE 21.4 Removal of a foreign body from under the upper eyelid. (a) The patient is told to look downward while the eyelashes of the upper lid are grasped with the thumb and index finger and gently pulled away from the eyeball. (b) A cotton-tipped applicator is placed horizontally along the center of the outer surface of the upper lid. (c) The lid is pulled forward and upward, which causes it to roll or fold back over the applicator, exposing the undersurface of the lid. (d) If a foreign body is seen, it is gently removed with a moistened, sterile, cotton-tipped applicator.

it. After irrigation is completed, a clean dressing should be applied to cover the eye and the patient taken promptly to the hospital for further care. If the eye irrigation can be carried out satisfactorily in the ambulance, it should be done en route.

Thermal Burns

When a patient suffers burns of the face from a fire, the eyes usually close rapidly because of the heat. This reaction is a natural reflex to protect the eye from further injury. However, the eyelids remain exposed and are frequently burned. Burns of the eyelids require very specialized care. It is best to transport the patient who has burned eyelids promptly to the hospital without further examination. Both eyes should be covered with a sterile dressing moistened with sterile saline prior to transport.

Light Burns

Exposure to extremes of light can cause significant damage to the eye. The rays of light will be focused on the retina, and the sensory cells can be

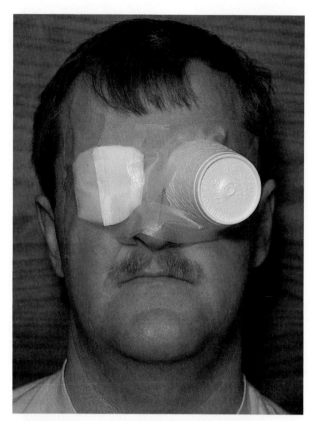

FIGURE 21.5 A large foreign body in the eye should be left in place, secured with a dressing, and prevented from moving. The uninjured eye should be covered in order to prevent motion of the injured eye.

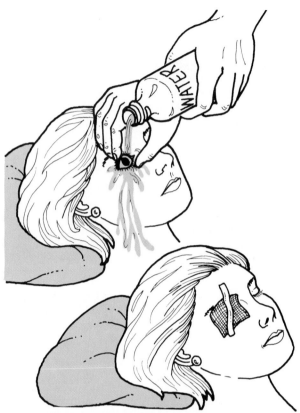

FIGURE 21.6 The emergency treatment of a chemical burn of the eye is copious irrigation of the eye with water or sterile saline. After irrigating for at least 5 minutes, a sterile patch dressing should be applied lightly to the eye.

damaged significantly. Infrared rays, eclipse light (if the patient has looked directly at the sun), and laser burns cause injuries to the retina that are generally not painful but may result in permanent vision damage.

Ultraviolet rays from an arc welding unit, from prolonged exposure to a sun lamp, or to a bright snow-laden area (snow blindness) can cause a superficial burn of the eyes. This kind of burn often is not painful at first, but extreme pain may be experienced 3 to 5 hours later as the damaged cornea responds to the injury. The patient develops a severe conjunctivitis with redness, swelling, and excessive tear production. The pain from these corneal burns may be diminished by covering each eye with a sterile, moist pad and having the patient lie down during transport to the hospital. The patient should be protected from exposure to bright lights and should be seen by a physician as soon as possible.

Lacerations and Blunt Trauma to the Eye

Lacerations

Lacerations of the eyelids require very careful repair to restore both appearance and function. Bleeding from a lacerated eyelid may be profuse, but it usually can be controlled by gentle manual pressure. If there is a laceration in the globe itself, no pressure should be applied to the eye; compression can interfere with the blood supply at the back of the eye and result in loss of vision from damage to the retina. Furthermore, the pressure may squeeze the vitreous humor out of the eye and cause irreparable damage. Penetrating injuries of the eye should be treated following these four important principles:

1. Never exert pressure on or manipulate the injured eye in any way.
2. If part of the eyeball is exposed, gently apply a moist, sterile dressing to prevent drying.

3. Cover the injured eye with a protective cup or metal eye shield.

4. Cover the opposite eye with a bandage to decrease movement on the injured side.

On rare occasions following a serious injury, the eyeball may be displaced out of its socket. No attempt should be made to reposition it. It should be covered and stabilized with a moist, sterile dressing. The patient should be transported to the hospital lying in the supine position.

Blunt Trauma to the Eye

Blunt trauma can cause a number of serious injuries of the eye, even though the lids and eyeball itself may appear to be intact. One injury that is seen frequently is a **hyphema,** which is bleeding into the anterior chamber of the eye that obscures part or all of the iris (Figure 21.7). Blunt trauma can also cause fracture of the orbit or of the bones that support the floor of the orbit (a **blowout fracture**). These frac-

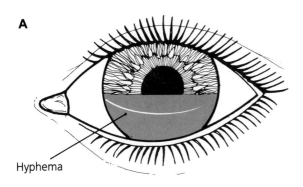

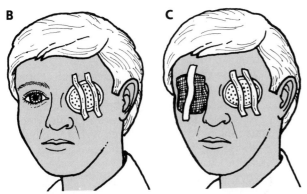

FIGURE 21.7 (a) Blunt trauma to the eye often produces a hyphema with blood accumulating in the anterior chamber overlying the iris. (b) Patients with blunt trauma to the eye should have an eye shield applied. (c) The opposite eye should be patched to minimize motion.

tures can entrap some of the muscles that control eye movement. Because of the limited motion secondary to the muscle entrapment, the patient may experience double vision.

Any patient who complains of pain, double vision, or decreased vision following a blunt injury to the eye region should be placed on a stretcher and transported promptly to the emergency department. The eye should be protected from further injury with a metal shield, and the uninjured eye should be patched to minimize movement on the injured side.

UNDERLYING HEAD INJURY

Abnormalities in the appearance or function of the eyes often occur following a closed head injury, and careful examination of the eyes may lead the EMT to suspect a head injury. Any of the following findings should alert the EMT to the possibility of an underlying head injury:

1. One pupil larger than the other.
2. The eyes not working together or pointing in different directions.
3. Failure of the eyes to follow the movement of the EMT's finger upon command.
4. Bleeding into the sclera (white portion) of the eye.
5. Protrusion or bulging of one eye.

Any of these observations must be recorded, along with the time they are made. In addition, in an unconscious patient the EMT should remember to keep the eyelids closed, as drying of the tissues can cause permanent injury and may result in blindness. The lids can be covered with a moist gauze or gently held closed with clear tape. Normal tears will then keep the tissues moist.

CONTACT LENSES AND EYE PROSTHESES

Many people wear contact lenses. They can be the small, hard plastic lenses that are usually tinted or large clear soft ones that are very difficult to see. The EMT should never attempt to remove a contact lens if there is any question of injury to the eye, since manipulation of the lens can aggravate the damage. The only time that contact lenses should be removed immediately in the field is with a chemical burn of the eye. The lens can trap the chemical and make dilution with an irrigation solution difficult. Unconscious patients who are wearing hard contact

lenses should have them removed, because prolonged wearing with the eyes closed can damage the cornea. In these patients, contact lens removal will usually be done by the emergency department personnel.

If it is necessary to remove a hard contact lens, a suction cup, the end moistened with saline, can be used. Soft contact lenses are removed by placing a couple of drops of saline onto the lens and gently pinching the lens between the thumb and index fingers; it can then be lifted from the surface of the eye (Figure 21.8).

In general, and particularly following trauma to the eye, the EMT should not attempt to remove contact lenses. Emergency department personnel should always be advised of the presence of contact lenses so that proper care can be provided in the hospital.

The patient may be wearing an artificial eye (an eye prosthesis). The EMT should suspect the presence of an artificial eye when it does not respond to light, move synchronously with the opposite eye, or appear quite the same as its mate. Sometimes it is quite difficult to distinguish an artificial eye from a natural one. If the EMT suspects the patient has an artificial eye, the patient should be asked about this possibility so that there is no misleading or incorrect information about the patient's eye function. With regard to the emergency care, no harm will be done if an artificial eye is given the same care as a normal eye.

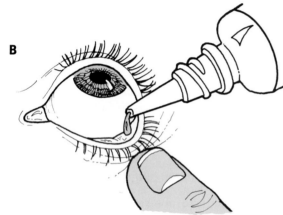

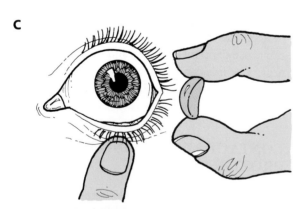

FIGURE 21.8 (a) A special suction cup, moistened with saline, is convenient for removing a small hard contact lens. (b) To remove a soft contact lens, one or two drops of saline or irrigating solution are applied, and (c) the lens is pinched off with the thumb and index finger.

YOU ARE THE EMT...

1. How does an injured eye differ in appearance from a normal, uninjured eye?
2. What part of the eye can foreign objects be flushed from? How are small foreign objects removed? Large foreign objects?
3. Eye injuries sometimes mean an underlying head injury has also occurred. What findings would make you suspect underlying head injury?
4. Why must you be careful not to exert any pressure when treating penetrating eye injuries? What other treatment principles should you follow with lacerations and blunt trauma to the eye?

Injuries of the Face and Throat

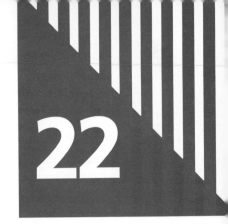

22

OVERVIEW

The face contains many specialized and important structures. Because of their prominence, these structures are vulnerable to injury and damage that may lead to permanent loss of many critical functions. The eyes are the most important of the facial structures. Their basic anatomy and the various categories of eye injuries are covered in Chapter 21. While perhaps less vital than the eyes, the other structures of the face present special problems when they sustain injury. The most serious problem is partial or complete upper airway obstruction. They are also often linked to cervical spine injuries. The EMT must understand that the emergency treatment of injuries of the face and throat are often related to the management of respiratory problems and spinal injuries.

The first section of Chapter 22 focuses on injuries of the face, including soft tissue wounds, injuries of the nose, and facial fractures. The second section discusses injuries of the throat and neck.

OBJECTIVES

The objectives of Chapter 22 are to

• understand how facial injuries can lead to upper airway obstruction and learn how to treat soft tissue wounds of the face, injuries of the nose, and facial fractures.
• learn how to treat patients with injuries of the neck and throat, including fractures of the larynx and/or trachea.

INJURIES OF THE FACE

The face and neck are vulnerable to injury because of their relatively unprotected position. Soft tissue injuries and fractures of the bones of the face occur commonly. These injuries will vary greatly in severity. Some may be potentially life-threatening and many will leave disfiguring scars if not treated properly. When treating a person with a facial injury, it is most important to remember that a cervical fracture may also have been sustained in the same accident. Care must be taken to protect and adequately immobilize the potential spine injury.

Injuries about the face frequently lead to partial or complete obstruction of the upper airway. Several factors may contribute to upper airway obstruction:

1. Bleeding from facial injuries can be profuse with large blood clots in the upper airway.
2. Loosened teeth or dentures may be dislodged into the throat.
3. Injuries of the mouth and nose may produce significant deformity of the airway.
4. Soft tissue injury may produce severe swelling of the tissues that encroach upon the airway.
5. In the semiconscious or unconscious patient, the head often is turned or twisted to one side.
6. Direct injury to the larynx or trachea will result in bleeding and swelling.
7. Associated brain injury may interfere with the control of breathing.

Soft Tissue Wounds

Soft tissue injuries of the face and scalp are common. Contusions usually cause local swelling. Some contusions of the scalp and forehead will produce a fairly large hematoma that forms a definite lump under the skin. Abrasions of the facial skin sometimes lead to significant disfiguring scar formation. Lacerations and avulsion injuries are especially common. Frequently, a flap of skin is peeled back from the underlying muscle fascia. Because they are well supplied with arteries and veins, the face and scalp usually bleed copiously from even trivial soft tissue wounds.

Emergency care of soft tissue injuries of the face and scalp is identical to the treatment of soft tissue injuries elsewhere. The local application of ice will aid in controlling the swelling of contused soft tissues. Bleeding is controlled by applying direct pressure with a dry sterile dressing. A circumferential wrap of elasticized roller gauze applied around the head will hold the pressure dressing in place. Excessive pressure should not be applied to a scalp laceration if a skull fracture is suspected. When penetrating injury exposes brain tissue, the eye, or other important structures, the EMT should cover the exposed parts with a sterile dressing to protect them from further damage.

When a laceration extends through the cheek directly into the mouth, it may be necessary to apply pressure with a sterile dressing against both the inside and the outside of the cheek in order to control the bleeding (Figure 22.1). Objects penetrating the cheek usually must be removed before the bleeding can be controlled.

The EMT should always check for bleeding inside the mouth. Broken teeth and lacerations of the tongue may cause profuse bleeding in the mouth. If enough blood is swallowed, this hemorrhage may not be apparent outside the mouth. All persons who have sustained facial trauma should have the inside of the mouth inspected for such bleeding.

Blood draining into the throat can produce vomiting and airway difficulties. The airway should be opened and cleared with suction. Because the head injury patient may have sustained a cervical spine injury, care must be taken to avoid all airway maneuvers that may cause damage to the spinal cord. The spine should be stabilized and then the patient should be turned on his side so that any blood or vomitus can drain out of the mouth rather than pool in the pharynx and obstruct the airway.

With a facial injury, the EMT should always check to see if any tissue is missing. Frequently, pieces of skin will be avulsed and can be found lying near the patient. Any free piece of tissue should be recovered, wrapped in a sterile dressing, placed in a plastic bag, kept cool, and transported to the

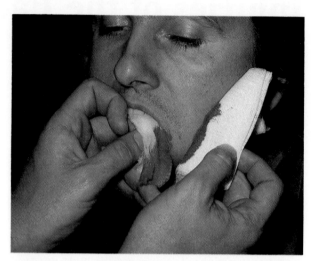

FIGURE 22.1 A penetrating laceration "through and through" the cheek will require a pressure dressing over both wounds to control bleeding.

emergency department with the patient. These pieces of skin often can be replaced surgically.

Flap-type injuries of the skin occur frequently on the face and scalp. As with flap injuries in other parts of the body, the flap of tissue should be folded back to its normal position before a dry, sterile dressing is applied to it. If the flap is left in its twisted or kinked position, a compression dressing applied to it will compress the blood vessels entering the flap through its pedicle and cut off the blood supply to the flap. Therefore, the flap should be folded back into the bed from which it was avulsed. A dry sterile compression dressing can then be applied in a standard manner to hold it in place and control bleeding (see Figure 19.1, page 225).

Injuries of the Nose

Soft tissue injuries of the nose usually result from blunt trauma and produce bleeding. An ice pack applied over the bridge of the nose or pinching the nostrils together, when it can be tolerated, may control the bleeding. A roll of gauze packed between the upper teeth and upper lip will sometimes help exert pressure on the blood vessels that supply the nose to help control the nosebleed (Figure 22.2).

Objects inhaled or stuffed into the nose may cause severe pain and occasionally bleeding. Generally, they do not cause complete airway obstruction. Such foreign bodies should be removed only by a physician at the emergency department. Attempting

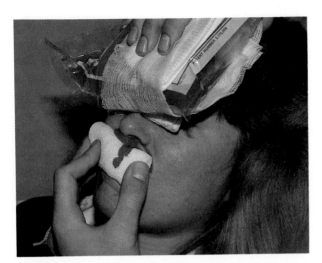

FIGURE 22.2 Bleeding from the nose following injury can be controlled by applying ice and placing a roll of gauze snugly under the upper lip.

to remove them in the field will often result in their being pushed farther back into the nose, and make later removal more difficult.

Facial Fractures

Fractures of the facial bones commonly result from blunt impact — for example, collision of the patient with a steering wheel or windshield. The fracture may involve the nose, the orbit, the maxilla, or the mandible. Fractures about the nose and mouth produce deformity, loose bone fragments, swelling, and bleeding that may combine to cause airway obstruction. Any patient who has sustained a direct blow to the mouth or nose should be considered to have a facial fracture. Many times these fractures are not evident on the first examination, as the patient may only have some swelling and local pain. Other clues to the possibility of a fracture are irregularity of the bite, absent or loose teeth, the inability to swallow or talk, increased salivation, bleeding in the mouth, and, obviously, loose or mobile bone fragments. In all of these injuries, extreme care must be taken that the airway does not become obstructed. The patient with a significant facial fracture is at continuous risk for developing airway obstruction as further bleeding and swelling occur. The upper respiratory passages should be cleared of any obstructing material and the airway should be maintained and ventilation assisted during transport to the hospital.

INJURIES OF THE THROAT

Soft tissue wounds of the neck may also produce severe bleeding and swelling that may result in upper airway obstruction. The primary consideration in patients with injuries to the throat is the adequacy of the upper airway. It must be established and maintained. Bleeding should be controlled with direct manual pressure with a dry sterile dressing. The cervical spine must be stabilized and protected from further injury.

Occasionally, the EMT will be required to treat a patient with an impaled foreign object in the neck or throat. The object should be stabilized and bandaged in place. Impaled foreign objects in the neck should never be removed except on the operating table.

The larynx and/or trachea may be fractured in any crushing injury to the anterior aspect of the neck. Impact against a steering wheel, attempt at suicide by hanging, or a clothesline injury sustained while riding a bicycle all are ways that the trachea could fracture. When this injury occurs, loss of voice, severe and sometimes fatal airway obstruction, and even occasionally air leakage into the soft tissues of the neck may result. The presence of air in the soft tissues produces a very characteristic crackling sensation on palpation called **subcutaneous emphysema** (Figure 22.3). Fracture of the cervical spine is often present with these injuries.

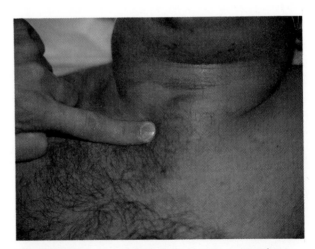

FIGURE 22.3 Fractures of the larynx or trachea can cause air to leak from the airway into the subcutaneous tissue. Subcutaneous emphysema has a characteristic crackling sensation upon palpation.

Emergency care of injuries of the larynx and trachea consists of securing the upper airway, administering supplemental oxygen by face mask, and splinting the cervical spine. Keeping the patient calm and breathing slowly may be lifesaving, as rapid breathing usually makes the situation worse. Oxygen inhalation should be used whenever this injury is suspected; however, positive pressure ventilation (with a bag-valve-mask) should be avoided whenever possible because air may be forced out of the injured trachea into the soft tissues and produce subcutaneous emphysema, compounding the problem. These are very serious, life-threatening injuries, and the patient must be transported promptly to the hospital for treatment.

YOU ARE THE EMT...

1. Why do you have to be concerned about possible spinal injuries when you see facial injuries?
2. The patient has hit the windshield in an automobile accident. He is not bleeding. What types of injuries should you be looking for? What symptoms should you be looking for?
3. How will you treat an avulsion injury which begins in the forehead area and extends into a portion of the scalp?
4. Identify five causes of upper airway obstruction from injuries about the face.

Injuries of the Chest

23

OVERVIEW

Injuries of the chest are of major importance because of the high likelihood of direct injury to the heart or lungs. Any injury to the chest is serious. Unless properly treated, chest injury may be rapidly fatal. Since the body has no capacity to store oxygen, any injury that interferes with normal breathing must be treated without delay to prevent permanent damage to those tissues that depend on a continuous supply of oxygen.

Another problem with chest injuries is internal bleeding. Blood from lacerations of the chest organs and major blood vessels can collect in the chest cavity, compressing the lungs. Or, air can enter the chest cavity and prevent expansion of the lungs — a function vital to the breathing process. All of these injuries are life-threatening and require fast action by the EMT. A few minutes is often all that separates life and death in these emergencies.

Chapter 23 first describes the signs and symptoms of chest injury. It then covers the general principles of treatment for all chest injuries. The chapter next discusses specific types of chest injury and their emergency care. The last section of Chapter 23 describes common complications that can occur following chest injury. The student should carefully review Chapter 5 on the normal anatomy and function of the respiratory system before reading this chapter.

OBJECTIVES

The objectives of Chapter 23 are to

- identify the signs and symptoms of chest injury.
- review the general principles of the care of chest injuries.
- recognize specific chest injuries and learn their emergency care.
- become familiar with the complications that can accompany chest injuries.

SIGNS AND SYMPTOMS OF CHEST INJURY

Chest injuries are divided into two categories: open or closed. **Open chest injuries** are those in which the chest wall has been penetrated by some object such as a knife or bullet. Open chest injury may also be caused by severe rib fractures in which the broken end of the rib lacerates the chest wall and the skin.

In **closed chest injuries** the skin is not broken. These injuries are generally caused by blunt trauma, as when the chest strikes the steering wheel or an object falls on the chest. Lacerations of the contents of the chest may still occur from broken ribs or when vital structures are torn from their attachments to the chest cavity, but the skin and chest wall are not penetrated.

The important signs of chest injury, either open or closed, are the following:

1. Pain at the site of the injury
2. Pain localized around the site of an injury that is aggravated by or occurs with breathing (pleuritic pain)
3. Dyspnea (difficulty breathing, shortness of breath)
4. Failure of one or both sides of the chest to expand normally with inspiration
5. Hemoptysis (the coughing up of blood)
6. A rapid, weak pulse and low blood pressure
7. Cyanosis

Following an injury to the chest, any change in the normal pattern of breathing is a particularly important sign. A healthy, uninjured person breathes from 6 to 20 times per minute without difficulty and without pain. Respiratory rates in excess of 24 breaths per minute usually indicate respiratory distress. The patient with injury to the chest will have an increased respiratory rate and will breathe more shallowly because it hurts to take a deep breath. Pain commonly occurs following injury to the chest. As with any other injury, pain and tenderness will be present at the point of impact as the result of a bruise or fracture. In addition, the pain is aggravated by the normal process of breathing. Irritation or damage to the pleural surfaces causes pain with each breath when these normally smooth surfaces move. This sharp pain with each respiration is called **pleuritic pain** or **pleurisy.**

Difficulty in breathing is called **dyspnea.** In the injured patient dyspnea has many different causes. It may occur because the patient's chest is not expanding properly due to the loss of normal nervous control of breathing, because the airway is obstructed, or because the lung itself is being compressed from within the chest by accumulated blood or air. Dyspnea in the injured patient indicates significant compromise of the function of the lung(s) that may require prompt, vigorous support and treatment.

The EMT should carefully observe the chest wall in patients who have sustained an injury. Failure of the chest wall to expand when the patient inhales is an extremely important sign. It indicates that the muscles of the chest have lost their ability to work appropriately. This loss of muscle function may be a result of direct injury to the chest wall, or it may be related to an injury of the nerves that control those muscles.

Hemoptysis (coughing up of blood) usually indicates that the lung has been lacerated. With injury of the lung, blood can enter the bronchial passages and is coughed up as the patient tries to clear the airway.

A rapid, weak pulse and low blood pressure are signs of hypovolemic shock. Shock following chest injury may result from insufficient oxygenation by the poorly functioning lung. It can also result from extensive bleeding from lacerated structures within the chest cavity.

Cyanosis — a bluish discoloration seen most readily around the lips and fingernails — indicates that blood is not being oxygenated sufficiently. Cyanosis in the patient with a chest injury indicates inadequate ventilation: The patient is unable to provide a sufficient supply of oxygen to the blood through the lung.

Many of these signs and symptoms occur simultaneously. When any one of them follows an injury to the chest, the EMT must realize that the patient requires hospital care.

GENERAL PRINCIPLES OF THE CARE OF CHEST INJURIES

Despite the many different types of chest injuries, all, almost uniformly, require the same initial care. For this reason this section reviews the general principles of the emergency treatment of chest injuries regardless of their cause.

The effectiveness of emergency medical care is directly related to the ability of the patient to breathe; therefore, initial attention must be given to the airway and respiration. The upper airway must be cleared and maintained. Ventilatory support and oxygen should be administered whenever respiratory distress exists. The overriding first consideration is to achieve normal respiratory function to provide adequate oxygenation to those tissues, particularly the brain and heart, that need a continuous supply of oxygen.

Open chest wounds must be covered with a dry, sterile dressing. Bleeding from the chest wall must be controlled by direct manual pressure. Embedded or protruding foreign objects — knives and the like — should be bandaged in place to stabilize them and to minimize movement. These impaled foreign objects should not be removed in the field.

If rib fracture is suspected, the patient should be made comfortable and kept quiet so that the possibility of further damage to the lungs, heart, or chest wall from the broken ribs is minimized. Fractured ribs may be splinted using several types of external support. The most commonly used device is a sling and swathe (Figure 23.1). Applying adhesive tape or other strapping to the chest wall is unnecessary. Furthermore, tight strapping limits the ability of the chest to expand and interferes with the normal respiratory effort.

The patient's vital signs should be observed and recorded frequently. They are the only means the EMT has to diagnose and follow the course of internal bleeding and to monitor the patient's respiratory function.

All patients with significant chest injury should be transported promptly to the hospital. Sometimes the patient will be in such extreme distress that immediate transport is necessary. In this situation, the patient's airway should be maintained, oxygen should be administered, and attempts to control bleeding should be carried out en route to the hospital.

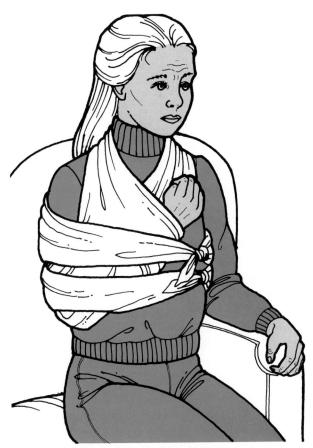

FIGURE 23.1 A sling and swathe will provide support for most fractured ribs. The humerus is used as a splint to support the injured ribs and decrease motion. Full immobilization of the ribs is difficult to achieve and may be harmful to the patient.

In sequence, the following steps should be used to handle patients with chest injuries:

1. Be certain the airway is clear and maintain it.
2. Use supplemental oxygen and be prepared to give respiratory support with mechanical aids or mouth-to-mouth ventilation, if necessary.
3. Observe, record, and monitor the vital signs.
4. Control all sites of obvious external bleeding.
5. Cover penetrating wounds into the chest cavity promptly.
6. Carefully monitor the effect of treatment and be ready to transport the patient rapidly because the patient's status may deteriorate quite rapidly following injury to the chest.
7. Transport all patients promptly to the emergency department and notify the hospital in advance of the type and severity of the injury sustained.

SPECIFIC CHEST INJURIES AND THEIR EMERGENCY CARE

Rib Fractures

Fracture of the ribs is seen very frequently. These fractures are usually caused by direct blows or compression injuries of the chest. Violent force is not always required to cause rib fracture, particularly in the elderly. The upper four ribs are rarely fractured since they are protected by the shoulder girdle. The fifth through tenth ribs are those most commonly fractured. Only rarely are the eleventh and twelfth ribs fractured, because they are small and have greater freedom of movement (floating ribs).

A common finding in all patients with a single or multiple rib fractures is pain localized at the site of the fracture. By asking the patient to place one finger on the exact area of the pain, the EMT can often determine the location of the injury. There may or may not be a rib deformity, a chest wall contusion, or a laceration in the area. Deep breathing, coughing, or movement is usually quite painful. The patient generally tries to remain still and will take shallow breaths. Often the patient will lean toward the injured side and place a hand over the fractured area to "splint" the fractures and ease the local pain.

The EMT should be sure that the patient is ventilating adequately by assessing the patient's respiration rate and other vital functions. Isolated simple rib fractures usually do not require any external support or splinting. The patient should be placed in a comfortable position on the litter and transported promptly to the hospital. A patient with multiple rib fractures will be made more comfortable and find it easier to breathe if the chest wall is immobilized with a sling and swathe (Figure 23.1). This method utilizes the arm as a splint for the unstable chest wall. The swathe should not be wrapped so tightly as to compress the chest and compromise the patient's ability to breathe.

Occasionally, the end of a fractured rib may puncture or lacerate the lung or the chest wall, causing a **hemothorax** or a **pneumothorax** (Figure 23.2). These two complications are discussed later in this chapter.

Flail Chest

When three or more ribs are broken, each in two places, the segment of the chest wall lying between

A   Laceration of chest wall

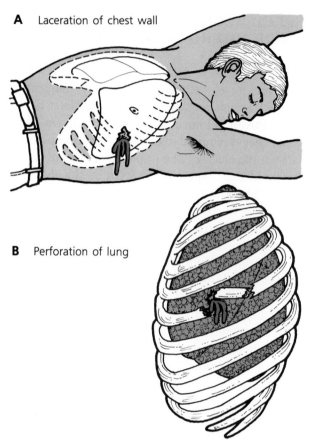

B   Perforation of lung

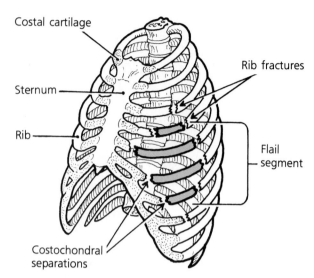

FIGURE 23.2   (a) A displaced rib fracture fragment may penetrate through the chest wall and create an open fracture. (b) More commonly, the fragment may penetrate (puncture) the lung and produce a hemothorax or a pneumothorax.

FIGURE 23.3   A flail chest results when several adjacent ribs are fractured in two or more places (fourth through seventh ribs on the left). With respiratory efforts, this segment will move paradoxically. Almost always this injury also results in severe contusion of the underlying lung.

the fractures becomes a free-floating segment. This segment will collapse rather than take part in the normal expansion of the chest wall each time the patient attempts to inhale. When the patient exhales, the segment will protrude slightly while the rest of the chest wall contracts. The motion of this floating segment is paradoxical because it is opposite to the normal movement of the rest of the chest wall. It is therefore called **paradoxical motion.** The portion of chest wall lying between the fractures is called the **flail segment** (Figure 23.3). Several terms are used to describe this injury. The proper one is **flail chest.** Other commonly used terms are **crushed chest** or **stove in chest.** Ordinarily, considerable pain is associated with the paradoxical motion of the flail segment.

Flail chest is a particularly serious injury. The lung immediately underneath the flail segment does not expand properly when the patient inhales, thus decreasing the efficiency of ventilation. Much more important, however, the amount of force that must be exerted on the chest wall to cause a series of ribs to fracture in several places and produce the flail segment almost always produces severe contusion of the lung tissue lying underneath the flail segment. Contusion of the lung causes immediate bleeding and swelling into the lung tissue and loss of respiratory function.

Flail chest can be diagnosed through close observation of the chest wall. The EMT will notice that the chest does not rise properly, despite the patient's most desperate efforts to inhale deeply. In some patients with this injury, severe hypoxia and cyanosis will rapidly result.

The emergency treatment of a flail chest requires vigorous respiratory support and the administration of supplemental oxygen. Pain associated with the paradoxical motion of the flail segment will limit the patient's voluntary breathing. Attempts should be made to stabilize the flail segment by applying firm support to it. The patient may breathe more comfortably if positioned with the flail segment against some external support such as the surface of the litter. Frequently, the flail segment will involve the central portion of the anterior chest wall with a frac-

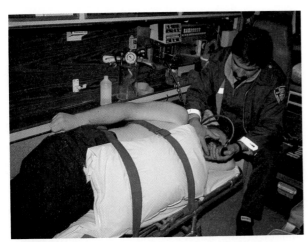

FIGURE 23.4 A flail anterior chest wall segment can be stabilized by having the patient hold a pillow firmly against the chest wall.

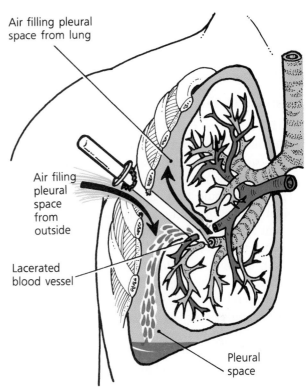

FIGURE 23.5 A penetrating injury caused by a knife. Damage to the lung, the heart, and/or the great vessels may occur with such penetrating injury.

ture of the sternum or fractures of ribs on both sides of the sternum. In this circumstance, the patient may breathe more readily when grasping a pillow and holding it up against the flail segment (Figure 23.4). Such support of the flail segment will lessen paradoxical motion and pain. The patient's vital signs must be monitored closely, and further respiratory support must be given as needed to maintain an adequate supply of oxygen. These patients should be transported with highest priority as promptly as possible to the hospital.

Penetrating Injury

Any sharp object, if driven with enough force, will produce a **penetrating chest injury.** Common examples of this type of injury are stab wounds and gunshot wounds (Figure 23.5). Occasionally the force will cause a rib fracture, and penetrating injury usually produces varying degrees of hemothorax and/or pneumothorax. Sucking chest wounds are also frequently created by these injuries. All of these complications of chest injury are described later in this chapter.

A penetrating object may injure any structure within the thoracic cavity. Gunshot wounds often have points of entrance and exit. There is significant danger of a laceration of the heart or the great vessels. In such instances bleeding may be massive, but rarely visible outside of the body because it remains contained within the chest cavity. The patient, in addition to having respiratory distress from the

injury, may be in shock from severe, rapid blood loss. Thus, a penetrating injury to the chest may be fatal, and vigorous treatment must be instituted promptly. The patient's airway must be maintained and ventilatory support and oxygen administered. The patient should be treated for hypovolemic shock by elevating the feet and applying a pneumatic antishock garment. Rapid transportation to the hospital may be necessary to save this patient's life.

Compression Injuries

Sometimes a patient sustains sudden, severe circumferential compression of the chest, which produces a rapid increase in intrathoracic pressure. Such injuries occur commonly when the chest is crushed by a heavy object such as a wall that collapses. Multiple fractures of the ribs can occur, and a flail chest may result. In addition, because of the increased intrathoracic pressure, the upper part of the body may become cyanotic and swollen, the neck veins may become distended, and the eyes may appear to be bulging. Severe intrathoracic injury is probable following this type of circumferential compression. Vigorous respiratory support and prompt transport to the hospital will be necessary.

Injuries of the Back of the Chest

Direct blows to the back of the chest produce contusions or rib fracture. Other common injuries of the back are muscular strains and lacerations. Any patient who complains of pain in the back following injury should be examined very closely for a spinal injury. In addition, it is imperative that the patient's airway and ventilatory status be monitored closely.

An uncommon injury to the back of the chest is a fracture of the scapula. The scapula is covered by very large muscles. Consequently, if a fracture of the scapula is suspected, the EMT must assume that the patient has sustained a particularly severe blow. This degree of force may cause injury to the underlying chest wall and lung. If a significant contusion, abrasion, or laceration of the shoulder region is observed, significant respiratory difficulty may result.

Direct blows to the lower rib cage in the region of the tenth through twelfth ribs can cause injury to the kidneys. This kind of injury is described in Chapter 25.

RESULTING COMPLICATIONS OF CHEST INJURIES

Many of the injuries just described have similar end results even though the cause of the injury may be different. The EMT should be aware that any of these injuries may result in the following complications. The treatment of each of these complications is also included in this section.

Pneumothorax

Pneumothorax means the presence of air within the chest cavity in the pleural space but outside the lung (Figure 23.6). In this condition the lung has been separated from the chest wall and is said to be "collapsed." The volume of the lung is diminished, and the amount of air that can be inhaled into it is reduced. As a result, hypoxia will occur and, as the degree of pneumothorax increases, respiratory distress becomes more severe. Pneumothorax can result

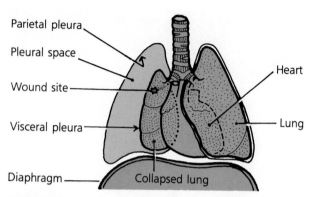

FIGURE 23.6 Pneumothorax occurs when air leaks into the pleural space from an opening in the chest wall or on the surface of the lung itself. The lung collapses as air fills the pleural space and the two pleural surfaces are no longer in contact.

from trauma as air enters the pleural space through an open wound in the chest wall. It can also be caused by air leaking from the lung into the pleural space following laceration of the lung by a fractured rib. In a pneumothorax, the normal mechanism by which the lung expands (the capillary adhesion of the pleural surface of the lung to the pleural surface of the chest wall) is lost, and the affected lung cannot expand with inhalation. For patients with an open wound of the chest, the amount of pneumothorax that develops can be minimized by rapidly sealing the open wound prior to transport.

In treating the patient suspected of having a pneumothorax, the EMT should clear and maintain the airway, administer oxygen, cover any open wound, and transport the patient to the hospital promptly.

Spontaneous Pneumothorax

In some people congenitally weak areas exist on the surface of the lungs. Occasionally, such a weak area will rupture (blow out) spontaneously, allowing air to leak into the pleural space. Usually this event, called **spontaneous pneumothorax,** is not related to any major injury but simply happens with normal breathing. The patient experiences sudden sharp chest pain and increasing difficulty in breathing. The affected lung collapses, losing its ability to expand normally. The amount of pneumothorax that develops will vary, and the patient with a spontaneous pneumothorax may be in mild, moderate, or severe respiratory distress.

The diagnosis of spontaneous pneumothorax should be suspected in a patient who develops the sudden onset of shortness of breath without a specific known cause. The treatment of this patient is the same as for the patient with a traumatic pneumothorax.

Tension Pneumothorax

A patient with a pneumothorax that results from trauma or from a spontaneous rupture of the lung may develop a **tension pneumothorax.** In this condition air continuously leaks out of the lung into the pleural space, expanding the space with every breath the patient takes. The air becomes trapped in the pleural space and cannot escape. Hence, with each breath the affected lung collapses more until it is completely reduced in size to a very small ball 2 or 3 inches in diameter. At this point, pressure in the affected chest cavity begins to rise, and the collapsed lung is pressed against the heart and the lung on the opposite side. The remaining uninjured lung in turn becomes compressed. As the pressure in the chest cavity rises further, it may exceed the normal pressure of blood in the veins returning to the heart (Figure 23.7). Blood can then no longer travel to the heart to be pumped out, and death can follow rapidly.

Tension pneumothorax cannot exist without an intact or well-sealed chest wall. However, it is not limited to closed chest injuries. A patient with an open wound of the chest and a severe lung laceration may develop a tension pneumothorax after the external chest wound has been effectively bandaged and sealed. In this situation, the lung continues to leak air into the now closed pleural space, and a tension pneumothorax may develop.

The signs of a tension pneumothorax are severe, rapidly progressive respiratory distress, a weak pulse, falling blood pressure, bulging of the tissues of the chest wall between the ribs and above the clavicle, distention of the veins in the neck, and cyanosis. The condition is rapidly progressive, and death may occur within a very few minutes.

Treatment of a tension pneumothorax is directed at relieving the increasing pressure within the pleural space. In closed chest injuries, decompression is accomplished by a physician or other appropriately trained medical personnel with advanced skills by placing a large bore needle into the pleural space to relieve the pressure.

If a tension pneumothorax develops following the bandaging of an open chest wound, simply releasing the dressing is often effective in relieving the tension pneumothorax. The air accumulated under pressure in the pleural space will rush from the wound once the dressing is released.

It must be emphasized that tension pneumothorax is one of the very few truly minute-by-minute emergencies. Prompt treatment of this patient will be lifesaving. Oxygen should be administered, and the patient should be transported rapidly to the hospital.

Hemothorax

Hemothorax means the presence of blood in the chest cavity within the pleural space (Figure 23.8). Hemothorax may occur in open or closed chest injuries. It is frequently accompanied by a pneumothorax. The bleeding may come from lacerated vessels in the chest wall, from lacerated major vessels within the chest cavity itself, or from a laceration of the lung. If the bleeding into the chest cavity is severe, the patient may develop hypovolemic shock.

In hemothorax, like pneumothorax, the chest cavity is filled with something other than the lungs. Normal lung expansion cannot occur, and the lung is compressed. Less air can be inhaled. In addition, there may be significantly less blood available in the

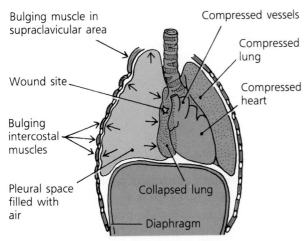

FIGURE 23.7 A tension pneumothorax develops when air becomes trapped in the pleural space and cannot escape to the outside. With each breath, more air accumulates in the pleural space. The trapped air compresses the injured lung and eventually the uninjured lung, the heart, and the great vessels.

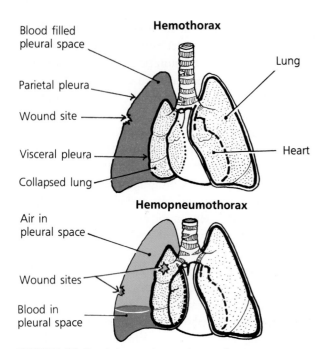

Hemothorax

Blood filled pleural space

Parietal pleura

Wound site

Visceral pleura

Collapsed lung

Lung

Heart

Hemopneumothorax

Air in pleural space

Wound sites

Blood in pleural space

FIGURE 23.8 A hemothorax is a collection of blood in the pleural space produced by lacerated blood vessels within the chest cavity.

circulation to carry this reduced amount of oxygen to the patient's vital organs.

The patient with a hemothorax will have signs and symptoms very similar to the patient with pneumothorax; in addition, the patient may be in hypovolemic shock as a result of the blood loss. The EMT should remember that the blood loss will not be obvious, as it accumulates out of sight within the chest cavity.

The patient with a hemothorax requires immediate ventilatory support, the administration of oxygen, and prompt transportation to the hospital.

Sucking Chest Wound

An open chest injury may produce a **sucking chest wound.** In this condition air from the environment is sucked through the wound when the patient inhales (Figure 23.9a). Ordinarily, the pressure inside the chest cavity is slightly less than atmospheric pressure. Inhalation further reduces this pressure. If there is an open wound in the chest wall, air will move through the wound just as it moves through the nose and mouth during normal respiration. The air that enters through the wound remains in the pleural space (a pneumothorax), and the lung does

not expand. When the patient exhales, air passes back through the wound. Such open chest wounds are called sucking chest wounds because each time the patient breathes there is a sucking sound at the wound, which is caused by the passage of air.

As an initial emergency step, it is imperative that sucking chest wounds be sealed with an airtight dressing (Figure 23.9b and c). The purpose of the airtight dressing is to seal the wound and prevent air from passing through it. Several sterile materials, including aluminum foil, vaseline gauze, or a folded universal dressing, may be used to seal the wound. A large enough cover must be used so that the dressing itself will not be sucked into the chest cavity. The dressing should be secured to the chest wall with tape to prevent any leakage of air around its edges.

Subcutaneous Emphysema

Laceration of the lung or disruption of any part of the tracheobronchial tree may allow air to escape into the soft tissues of the chest wall. The air will dissect into the tissues much as blood dissects into the tissues following a contusion. Small bubbles of air will be present in the subcutaneous tissue. This condition is called **subcutaneous emphysema.** Palpation over the area will result in a crackling sensation under the fingertips as the bubbles of air are pushed about. In very severe instances, subcutaneous emphysema can involve the entire chest, neck, and face. Fractured ribs, with laceration of the lung, are the most common cause of this condition. The presence of subcutaneous emphysema indicates significant loss of respiratory function. The patient should be given ventilatory support and oxygen and transported promptly to the hospital for evaluation and treatment.

Pulmonary Contusion

A **pulmonary contusion** is a bruise of the lung. It occurs in much the same way as bruises of any other tissue in the body. The lung is very fragile and very susceptible to contusion. When the blood vessels in the lung are injured, a considerable amount of blood oozes into the lung tissue. Edema fluid also accumulates in the lung tissue. In a contused area of the lung, the exchange of oxygen and carbon dioxide between the alveolus and the capillaries of the blood vessels cannot take place as it should.

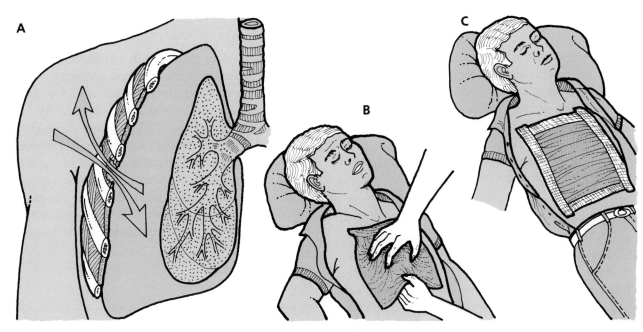

FIGURE 23.9 (a) With a sucking chest wound, air passes from the outside into the pleural space. (b) A sucking chest wound should be sealed with a large airtight dressing of aluminum foil or vaseline gauze. (c) The dressing should be secured to the chest wall with tape.

Pulmonary contusion is almost uniformly associated with blunt injuries to the chest as are seen in automobile accidents and severe falls. It occurs commonly after a direct blow to the chest and may cause severe respiratory distress. The size of the area of contusion is the most important factor in determining its effect on the patient's ability to breathe. Pulmonary contusion of a significant degree will result in hypoxia. The patient may be in significant respiratory distress with rapid respirations and even cyanosis. Emergency treatment includes adequate ventilatory support and the administration of oxygen.

Myocardial Contusion

Blunt injuries of the chest may produce **myocardial contusion,** or bruising of the heart muscle itself. This injury may not be detectable until fairly sophisticated laboratory and electrocardiographic studies have been done. Ordinarily, a severe myocardial contusion disturbs the electrical conduction system that controls the heart rate. In these circumstances, the heart is said to be irritable. The signs of such heart irritability are extra heartbeats which irregularly interrupt the normal pulse rhythm. The patient with a myocardial contusion will have an irregular pulse with occasional pauses and occasional beats coming very close together.

There is no specific treatment in the field for myocardial contusion. However, in any patient who has sustained a chest injury, the EMT must check the pulse carefully. Any abnormality noted in the pulse rate or rhythm should be reported promptly to medical control, along with the EMT's suspicion of a possible myocardial contusion. Any sign of a myocardial contusion requires prompt transportation of the patient to the hospital because persistent irregularity of the heartbeat may result in heart failure and death.

Pericardial Tamponade

In **pericardial tamponade,** blood or other fluid is present in the pericardial sac that surrounds the heart, exerting an unusual pressure on the heart itself. In patients with chest injuries, it almost always results from penetrating wounds of the heart that have opened one of its chambers so that with each heartbeat blood leaks out into the pericardial sac. The pericardial sac is a very tough, fibrous membrane that cannot expand. When blood leaks out of the heart, it is caught within this unyielding sac. As it accumulates within the pericardial cavity, it compresses the heart so that its chambers can no longer accommodate the blood normally returned to them through the veins. The signs of pericardial tamponade are:

1. Very soft and faint heart tones (hard to hear even with a stethoscope)
2. A weak pulse
3. Blood pressure readings in which the systolic and diastolic pressures come closer and closer together during successive readings
4. Congested and distended veins in the upper part of the body, particularly the veins of the neck

Pericardial tamponade is a rapidly progressive and life-threatening condition. The pressure of the blood accumulating within the pericardial sac must be relieved quickly or death will occur very rapidly. The patient should be given vigorous respiratory support and oxygen and transported rapidly to the hospital. The hospital should be notified of the possibility of the diagnosis of pericardial tamponade so that preparations can be made for its immediate treatment upon arrival.

Laceration of the Great Vessels

The chest contains several large blood vessels: the superior vena cava, the inferior vena cava, the main pulmonary artery, four main pulmonary veins, and the aorta with its major arteries distributing blood throughout the body. Injury of any of these vessels may be accompanied by massive, rapidly fatal hemorrhage. Any patient with a chest wound who is in hypovolemic shock may have an injury to one of these vessels. Frequently, the loss of blood is not obvious, as it remains within the chest cavity.

Emergency treatment of laceration of the great vessels includes pulmonary resuscitation with ventilatory support and the administration of oxygen. A pneumatic antishock garment should be applied. Here, particularly, rapid transport of the patient to the hospital may be life-saving. A few minutes have meant the difference between life and death for some of these patients.

YOU ARE THE EMT...

1. What is the difference between a hemothorax and a pneumothorax? What is the treatment for each?
2. One of the signs of chest injury is pleuritic pain. What is pleuritic pain? What are five other signs of chest injury?
3. Why is flail chest such a serious injury? What is the emergency treatment of flail chest?
4. How is tension pneumothorax treated in a closed chest injury? In an open chest injury?

The Abdomen and Genitalia

24

OVERVIEW

The abdomen is a large body cavity that extends from the diaphragm to the pelvis. It consists of several organs that make up the digestive system, the urinary system, and the genital system. All of these organs are susceptible to injury or illness. Some are better protected than others; some are more important than others. The EMT has to know where inside the abdominal cavity these organs are located. The EMT must also have a basic understanding of their various functions so that when illness or injury does occur, the seriousness of the situation can be assessed.

Chapter 24 begins with a description of the abdominal cavity — its boundaries and the organs that lie within it. Then the organs that make up the digestive system are more fully described. Next is an explanation of peristalsis, the wavelike contractions that propel food through the digestive tract. Then the organs of the urinary system are described. The last section of Chapter 24 is about the genital system — the male and female reproductive systems.

OBJECTIVES

The objectives of Chapter 24 are to

- identify the boundaries, the bony landmarks, and the location of organs in the abdominal cavity.
- know the function of the various organs of the digestive system and learn how food is converted into nutrients for use by the body's cells.
- understand how food is propelled through the digestive tract by wavelike muscular contractions called peristalsis.
- become familiar with the location and function of the organs of the urinary system.
- describe the organs of the genital system and understand their role in the reproductive process.

THE ABDOMINAL CAVITY

The superior boundary of the abdomen is the diaphragm. The inferior boundary is the level of an imaginary plane between the pubis and the sacrum. The anterior and posterior boundaries of the abdomen are the musculoskeletal body walls (Figure 24.1). The abdominal cavity is lined by the **peritoneum,** a glistening smooth layer of cells that covers the organs of the cavity and also lines the cavity wall.

The abdominal cavity contains the liver, gallbladder and bile ducts, spleen, stomach, and intestines (Figure 24.2). Immediately behind the peritoneum and between it and the major back muscles lie the kidneys with their drainage tubes (the ureters), the adrenal glands, the pancreas, and a portion of the duodenum of the small intestine. In this same area between the peritoneum and the back muscles (the **retroperitoneal space**) lie two major blood vessels, the aorta and the inferior vena cava. Many nerves and lymph glands lie near these large vessels (Figure 24.3).

The lowermost portion of the abdominal cavity, below the imaginary plane running from the pubis to the sacrum, is the **pelvic cavity.** In it lie the rectum, the urinary bladder, and in the female, the internal reproductive organs (Figure 24.4). Nearly all of the organs within the abdomen are suspended from the body wall by sheets of tissue called **mesentery.** The mesentery is a very delicate tissue formed from the peritoneum. It carries blood vessels and nerves to all of the organs. The organs hang fairly freely from their mesenteric attachments, which allows them to move about somewhat within the abdominal cavity. This mobility is necessary for the normal continuous muscular activity of the bowel (Figure 24.5). The peritoneum lining the abdominal cavity, like all other tissues, has a nerve supply. The peritoneum lining the walls of the abdomen can perceive the same sensations as the skin can; however, the peritoneum forming the mesentery and covering the organs of

A

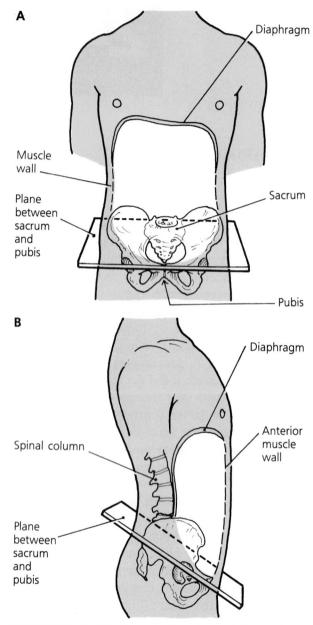

FIGURE 24.1 The boundaries of the abdominal cavity are the anterior and posterior abdominal walls, the diaphragm, and an imaginary plane between the pubis and the sacrum. (a) An anterior view; (b) a lateral view.

the abdomen cannot localize pain and is limited to the perception of tension or stretching. This varied innervation of the two parts of the peritoneum gives rise to the phenomenon of **referred pain,** which is discussed in Chapter 32.

In general, the organs of the abdominal and pelvic cavities and in the retroperitoneal space are either hollow or solid. **Hollow organs** are tubes

through which material passes. For example, the stomach and intestines conduct food through the body; the ureters and bladder conduct and store urine until it is expelled. The stomach, duodenum, small intestine, large intestine (colon), rectum, appendix,

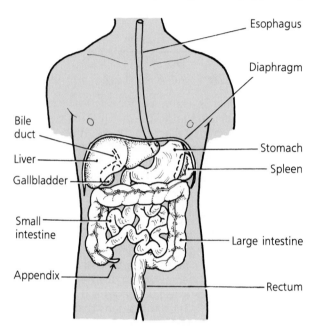

FIGURE 24.2 The major organs of the abdominal cavity.

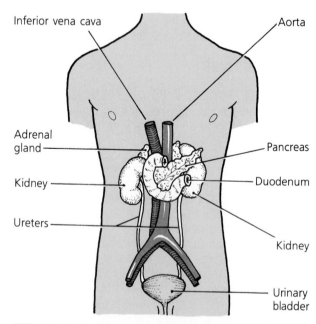

FIGURE 24.3 The major organs that lie in the retroperitoneal space between the peritoneum and the back muscles. The aorta and inferior vena cava also lie in this plane.

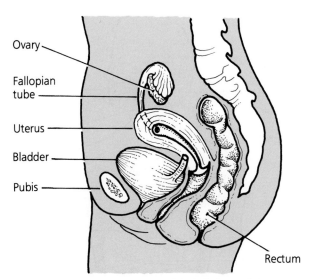

FIGURE 24.4 The major organs of the pelvic cavity, including the female reproductive organs.

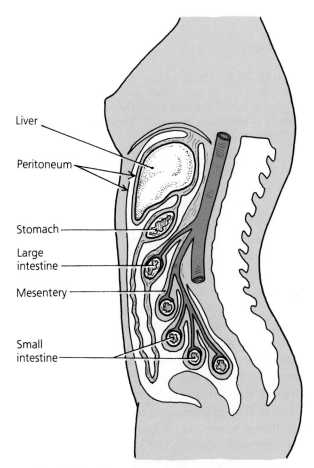

FIGURE 24.5 The abdominal organs are suspended from the body wall by tissue called mesentery. Within the mesentery are blood vessels that nourish the abdominal organs.

gallbladder, bile ducts, urinary bladder, ureters, and uterus are the hollow organs (Figure 24.6). **Solid organs** are solid masses of tissue where much of the chemical work of the body takes place. The liver, spleen, pancreas, kidneys, ovaries, and adrenal glands are the solid organs of this region (Figure 24.7).

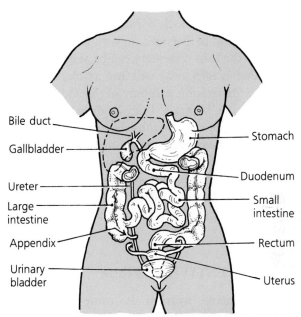

FIGURE 24.6 The hollow organs of the abdominal cavity, the retroperitoneal space, and the pelvic cavity.

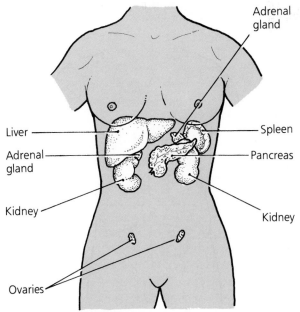

FIGURE 24.7 The solid organs of the abdominal cavity, the retroperitoneal space, and the pelvic cavity.

Injuries to the abdomen and pelvis can damage either hollow or solid organs. In general, hollow organs discharge their contents into the abdominal cavity when they are lacerated, while solid organs tend to bleed copiously. Spilled contents from the solid organs usually set up an intense inflammatory reaction, called **peritonitis,** which is very painful. Bleeding from solid organs may be rapidly fatal and frequently causes shock. Mesentery supporting hollow organs can be lacerated. In such instances bleeding from the torn mesentery can be severe, and the organ that is torn away will lose its blood supply.

The topographic anatomy of the abdomen was presented in Chapter 3. Bony landmarks in the abdomen include the **symphysis pubis,** the **costal arch,** the **iliac crests,** and the **anterior superior iliac spines.** The major soft tissue landmark is the **umbilicus,** which overlies the fourth lumbar vertebra. The abdomen is divided arbitrarily into quadrants by two perpendicular lines that intersect at the umbilicus (Figure 24.8).

THE DIGESTIVE SYSTEM

The **digestive system** is composed of the gastrointestinal tract (stomach and intestines), mouth, salivary glands, pharynx, esophagus, liver, gallbladder, pancreas, rectum, and anus (Figure 24.9). The function of this system is to process (digest) food so

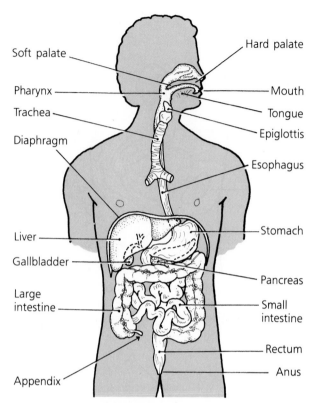

FIGURE 24.9 The digestive system lies within the head, thorax, abdomen, and pelvis. The many organs involved convert food through complex chemical processes into basic sugars, fatty acids, and amino acids.

that the individual cells of the body can be nourished. Digestion of food from the time it is taken into the mouth until essential compounds are extracted and delivered by the circulatory system to nourish all of the cells is a complicated chemical process. In succession, different secretions, primarily enzymes, are added to the food by the salivary glands, the stomach, the liver, the pancreas, and the small intestine to convert the food into basic sugars, fatty acids, and amino acids. These basic products of digestion are carried across the wall of the intestine and transported through veins to the liver. In the liver they are processed further and then transported to the heart through other veins. The heart then pumps the blood filled with these nutrients through the arteries to the capillaries where the nutrients pass through the capillary walls and the cell walls to feed all of the cells of the body. Digestion also produces many chemical compounds that are poisonous. They cannot be passed safely into the general body circulation until the liver has transformed them. All blood

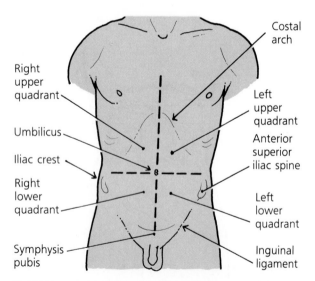

FIGURE 24.8 The bony landmarks and the major soft tissue landmark (the umbilicus) of the abdomen. The abdomen is divided into four quadrants.

leaving the intestine must pass first through the liver to ensure protection for the body against such compounds.

Mouth and Salivary Glands

The mouth consists of the lips, cheeks, gums, teeth, and tongue. A mucous membrane lines the mouth. The roof of the mouth is formed by the hard and soft palate. The **hard palate** is a bony plate lying anteriorly, while the **soft palate** is a fold of mucous membrane and muscle that extends posteriorly into the throat. It is designed to hold food that is being chewed within the mouth and to initiate swallowing.

Three paired **salivary glands** are located under the tongue, on each side of the lower jaw, and on each cheek. They produce nearly 1.5 liters of saliva daily. **Saliva** is approximately 98 percent water. The remaining 2 percent is mucus, salts, and organic compounds. **Mucus** serves as a binder for the chewed food being swallowed and as a lubricant within the mouth.

Ptyalin, a digestive enzyme in saliva, initiates the digestion of starches. Otherwise, in the mouth, food is converted into a soft mush mixed with mucus and saliva for easy swallowing.

Pharynx

The **pharynx,** or throat, is a tubular structure about 5 inches long that extends vertically from the back of the mouth to the esophagus and trachea. The **trachea** lies just in front of the esophagus. It is connected with the pharynx by the **larynx,** or voice box. The larynx is covered by a leaf-shaped valve called the **epiglottis.** An automatic movement of the pharynx permits the epiglottis to close over the larynx when swallowing is initiated so that liquids and solids are moved into the esophagus and away from the trachea.

Esophagus

The **esophagus** is a collapsible tube about 10 inches long. It extends from the end of the pharynx to the stomach and lies just anterior to the spinal column in the chest. Contractions of the muscle in the wall of the esophagus propel food through it to the stomach. Liquids will pass with very little assistance.

Stomach

The stomach is located in the left upper quadrant of the abdominal cavity, largely protected by the lower left ribs. Muscular contraction in the wall of the stomach and **gastric juice,** which contains much mucus, convert ingested food to a thoroughly mixed semisolid mass. The major function of the stomach is to receive food in large quantities intermittently, store it, and provide for its movement into the small bowel in regular small amounts. In 1 to 3 hours the semisolid food mass is propelled by muscular contractions into the duodenum, the first part of the small intestine. Poisoning or any reaction to trauma may paralyze gastric muscular action and cause the retention of food in the stomach for prolonged periods. One digestive enzyme, **pepsin,** is produced in the stomach. This agent initiates the digestion of proteins.

Pancreas

The **pancreas,** a flat, solid organ, lies below and behind the liver and stomach and behind the peritoneum on the spine and muscles of the back. It is firmly fixed in position, deep within the abdomen, and is not easily damaged. It contains two kinds of glands. One set of glands secretes nearly 2 liters of **pancreatic juice** daily. This juice contains many enzymes that aid in the digestion of fat, starch, and protein. Pancreatic juice flows directly into the duodenum through the pancreatic ducts.

The other kind of gland, called the **islets of Langerhans,** does not connect to any duct but secretes its products into the bloodstream across the capillaries. These islets produce a hormone, **insulin,** that regulates the amount of sugar in the blood.

Liver

The **liver** is a large solid organ that takes up most of the area immediately beneath the diaphragm in the right upper quadrant. It is the largest solid organ in the abdomen and consequently one of the most often injured. It has several functions. Poisonous substances produced by digestion are brought to it by the blood and are rendered harmless. Factors necessary for blood clotting and for the production of normal plasma are formed here. Between 0.5 and 1 liter of bile is made by the liver to assist in the normal digestion of fat. The liver is also the principal organ for the storage of sugar for immediate use by the body. It also produces many of the factors that aid in the proper regulation of immune responses.

Essentially, the liver is a large mass of blood vessels and cells that are packed tightly together. For this reason it is very fragile and relatively easily injured. Blood flow in the liver is very great since all of the blood that is pumped to the gastrointestinal tract passes through the liver before it returns to the heart. In addition, the liver receives a generous arterial blood supply of its own.

Biliary System

The liver is connected to the intestine by the **bile ducts.** The **gallbladder** is an outpouching of a bile duct that serves as a reservoir for bile produced in the liver. The gallbladder discharges bile into the duodenum through the common bile duct. The presence of food in the duodenum triggers the contraction of the gallbladder so that it can empty. It usually contains 2 to 3 ounces of bile. Stones can form in the gallbladder and can pass into the common bile duct and obstruct it. This obstruction will produce **jaundice.**

Small Intestine

The **small intestine,** the major abdominal hollow organ, is so named because of its diameter in comparison with the large intestine. It is made of three parts: the duodenum, the jejunum, and the ileum.

The **duodenum,** about 12 inches long, passes from the stomach to the jejunum. Most of this organ lies behind the peritoneum and closely curls around the pancreas. The duodenum is that part of the small intestine that receives food from the stomach. Here the food is mixed with secretions from the pancreas and liver for further digestion.

The **jejunum** and **ileum** together measure more than 20 feet on the average to make up the rest of the small bowel. The jejunum is the first half, and the ileum is the second half. The small intestine empties into the large intestine through the **ileocecal valve** between the ileum and **cecum,** the first part of the large bowel. This valve allows passage of bowel contents in only one direction — into the colon. The junction of the small and large bowel is normally in the right lower quadrant of the abdominal cavity.

The small intestine lies entirely free within the abdomen, hanging from its mesentery. Arteries from the aorta to the intestine and veins carrying blood to the liver lie in this mesentery. The cells lining the small intestine produce more enzymes and mucus to aid in digestion.

Bile, produced by the liver and stored in the gallbladder, is emptied as needed into the duodenum. It is greenish black in color but through changes during digestion gives feces their typical brown color. Its major function is the digestion of fat. Enzymes from the pancreas and the small intestine carry out the final processes of digestion. The products of digestion (proteins, fats, and carbohydrates), water, ingested vitamins, and minerals are then absorbed primarily across the wall of the lower end of the ileum into veins and then transported to the liver.

Large Intestine

The **large intestine,** another major hollow organ, consists of the cecum, the colon, and the rectum. About 5 feet long, it encircles the outer border of the abdomen around the small bowel. The major function of the **colon,** the portion of the large intestine that extends from the cecum to the rectum, is to absorb the remaining 5 to 10 percent of water from the intestine to form solid **stool,** which is stored in the rectum and passed out of the body through the anus.

Appendix

The **appendix** is a small tube that opens into the cecum (the first part of the large intestine) in the right lower quadrant of the abdomen. It is 3 or 4 inches long. It may easily become obstructed and as a result inflamed and infected. Appendicitis, which is the term for this inflammation, is one of the major causes of severe abdominal distress. The appendix has no major known function.

Rectum and Anus

The lowermost end of the colon is the **rectum.** It is a large hollow organ that is adapted to store quantities of feces until they are expelled. At its terminal end is the **anus,** a canal lined by normal skin and approximately 2 inches long. The rectum and anus are supplied with a complex series of circular muscles called **sphincters** that control the escape of liquids, gases, and solids from the digestive tract.

The Spleen

The **spleen,** a major solid organ, is smaller than the liver. It, too, is filled with large blood vessels and is even more fragile than the liver. It is found in the left upper quadrant of the abdomen, just beneath the diaphragm and immediately in front of the ninth to eleventh ribs. It is fixed in position by three strong ligaments. While it is well protected by the ribs, the supporting ligaments can easily be torn from the spleen in a blunt injury, and bleeding from the lacerated spleen may be very severe, controllable only by its removal. Injuries that produce fractures of the eighth through twelfth ribs on the left side are likely to cause lacerations of the spleen.

The spleen is not required for life, nor is it associated with the functions of the digestive tract. The major function of this organ lies in the normal production and destruction of blood cells. Its function, when removed, can be assumed by the liver and the bone marrow.

PERISTALSIS

There are two layers of involuntary (smooth) muscle in the walls of the entire gastrointestinal tract from the esophagus to the rectum. The outer layer of smooth muscle is oriented longitudinally, and the inner layer is circular (Figure 24.10). Contraction of these muscles is stimulated when they are stretched by food that is swallowed. This muscular contrac-tion is called **peristalsis.** Peristalsis starts at the esophagus and proceeds in a coordinated wavelike fashion to the anus, propelling food through the digestive tract (Figure 24.9). Once started, a wave passes entirely through the system. When peristaltic waves are especially strong or when they are inter-rupted by an obstruction so that the contents can-not be propelled along, the contraction causes a painful cramp that is called **colic.** Normal peristal-sis is responsible for the bowel sounds that can be heard if one listens to the abdomen with a stetho-scope. The sounds represent the passage of gas and fluid through the narrow, hollow digestive organs. The peristaltic contractions can be controlled by a set of voluntary sphincter muscles surrounding the anus. Thus, the healthy individual can control the time of the release of the products of digestion from the rectum.

THE URINARY SYSTEM

The **urinary system** controls the discharge of cer-tain waste materials filtered from the blood. In the urinary system the kidneys are solid organs and the ureters, bladder, and urethra are hollow organs (Fig-ure 24.11).

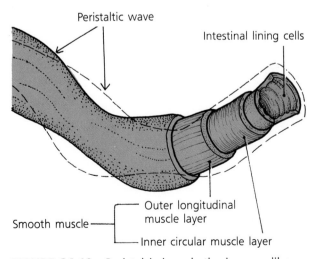

FIGURE 24.10 Peristalsis is a rhythmic, wavelike contraction of the smooth muscles in the wall of the intestine.

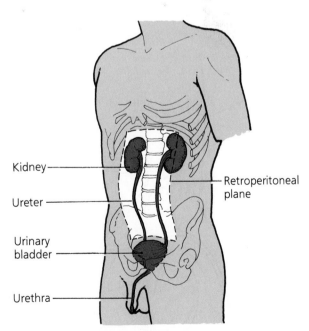

FIGURE 24.11 The urinary system lies in the retroperitoneal space behind the organs of the digestive system. The kidneys are solid organs, and the ureter, bladder, and urethra are hollow organs.

Kidneys

The body has two **kidneys.** They lie on the posterior muscular wall of the abdomen behind the peritoneum in the retroperitoneal space. These organs rid the blood of toxic waste products and control its balance of water and salt. If the kidneys are destroyed or no longer function adequately, a condition known as **uremia** occurs. Wastes accumulate within the bloodstream. The balance of salt and water is disturbed, and death will result.

Blood flow in the kidneys is high. Nearly 20 percent of the output of blood from the heart passes each minute through the kidneys. Large vessels attach the kidneys directly to the aorta and the inferior vena cava. Waste products and water are constantly filtered from the blood to form urine. The kidneys continuously concentrate this filtered urine by reabsorbing the water as it passes through a system of specialized tubes within them. The tubes finally unite to form the **renal pelvis,** a cone-shaped collecting area that connects the ureter and the kidney. Normally, each kidney drains its urine into one ureter through which the urine passes to the bladder.

Ureters

A **ureter** passes from the renal pelvis of each kidney along the surface of the posterior abdominal wall to drain into the urinary bladder. The ureters are small (diameter 0.5 centimeters), hollow, muscular tubes. Peristalsis occurs in these tubes to move the urine to the bladder.

Urinary Bladder and Urethra

The **urinary bladder** is situated immediately behind the pubic symphysis in the pelvic cavity. The two ureters enter posteriorly at its base on either side. The bladder empties to the outside of the body through the **urethra.** In the male the urethra passes from the anterior base of the bladder through the penis (Figure 24.12). In the female, the urethra opens at the front of the vagina (Figure 24.13).

The bladder is formed of smooth muscle with a specialized lining membrane. Urination is largely an automatic function that can, however, be controlled voluntarily. Just like around the anus, there are muscular sphincters over which we have voluntary control. When the bladder reaches a critical point of fullness, sensory cells in the bladder send messages to the brain notifying it that the bladder is ready to empty. The sensation is perceived as an urge or need to urinate (**void**). Under voluntary control, the sphincter muscles are relaxed, and the bladder involuntarily contracts and forces urine through the urethra to the outside of the body. The normal adult

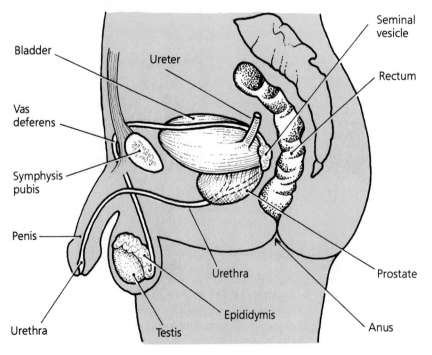

FIGURE 24.12 The male genitourinary system.

Bladder

Ureter

Vas deferens

Symphysis pubis

Penis

Urethra

Testis

Epididymis

Urethra

Seminal vesicle

Rectum

Prostate

Anus

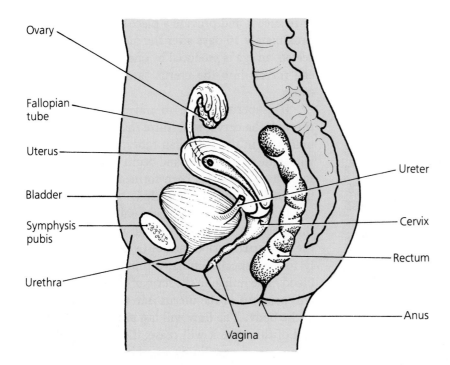

FIGURE 24.13 The female genitourinary system.

Ovary
Fallopian tube
Uterus
Bladder
Symphysis pubis
Urethra
Vagina
Ureter
Cervix
Rectum
Anus

forms 1.5 to 2 liters of concentrated urine every day. This waste is extracted and concentrated from the 1,500 liters of blood that circulate through the kidneys daily.

THE GENITAL SYSTEM

The **genital system** controls the reproductive processes from which life is created. The male genitalia, except for the prostate gland and seminal vesicles, lie outside the pelvic cavity (Figure 24.12). The female genitalia — uterus, ovaries, and Fallopian tubes — are contained entirely within the pelvis (Figure 24.13). The male and female reproductive organs have certain similarities and, of course, basic differences. They allow the production of sperm and egg cells and appropriate hormones, the act of sexual intercourse, and ultimately, reproduction.

Male Reproductive System and Organs

The male reproductive system includes the testicles, vasa deferentia, seminal vesicles, prostate gland, urethra, and penis (Figure 24.12). Each **testicle** contains specialized cells and ducts. Certain cells produce male hormones; others develop sperm. The hormones are absorbed directly into the bloodstream from the testicles. The **vasa deferentia** travel from the testicles up beneath the skin of the abdominal wall for a short distance. They then pass through an opening into the abdominal cavity and down into the prostate gland to connect with the urethra. The vasa deferentia carry the sperm from the testicles to the urethra. The **seminal vesicles** constitute small storage sacs for sperm and seminal fluid. The vesicles also empty into the urethra. **Semen,** also called **seminal fluid,** contains sperm cells carried up each vas from each testicle to be mixed with fluid from the seminal vesicles and prostate gland. The **prostate gland** is a small gland that surrounds the urethra where it emerges from the urinary bladder. Fluids from the prostate gland and from the seminal vesicles mix during **intercourse.** During intercourse, special mechanisms in the nervous system prevent the passage of urine into the urethra. Only seminal fluid, prostatic fluid, and sperm pass from the penis into the vagina during ejaculation.

The **penis** is a special type of tissue called **erectile tissue.** This specialized tissue is largely vascular and when filled with blood causes the penis to distend into a state of erection. As the vessels fill under pressure from the circulatory system, the penis becomes a rigid organ that can enter the vagina. Certain spinal injuries, and some diseases, cause a permanent and painful erection called **priapism.**

Female Reproductive System and Organs

The female reproductive organs include the ovaries, Fallopian tubes, uterus, and vagina (Figure 24.13).

The **ovaries,** like the testicles, produce sex hormones and specialized cells for reproduction. The female sex hormones are absorbed directly into the bloodstream. A specialized cell called an **ovum** is produced with regularity during the adult female's reproductive years. The ovaries release a mature egg, or ovum, approximately every 28 days. This egg travels through the Fallopian tubes to the uterus.

The **Fallopian tubes** connect with the uterus and carry the ovum to the cavity of the uterus. The **uterus** is a pear-shaped, hollow organ with muscular walls. The narrow opening from the uterus to the vagina is called the **cervix.**

The **vagina** is a muscular distensible tube that connects the uterus with the **vulva** (the external female genitalia). The vagina receives the male penis during intercourse, when semen and sperm are deposited in it. The sperm may pass into the uterus and fertilize an egg, causing **pregnancy.** Should the pregnancy come to completion at the end of nine months, the baby will pass through the vagina and be born.

The vagina also serves to channel the menstrual flow from the uterus out of the body.

Menstrual Cycle

The menstrual period is the end of the monthly female reproductive cycle. From the start of her first menstrual period at about age 12, until she passes through menopause at about age 50, a woman has monthly periods of **menstruation.** Each month the **endometrium** (lining of the uterus) is stimulated by the female sex hormones to form a special bed. This bed is prepared so that if a sperm and ovum unite to make a fertilized egg, the uterus will be ready to receive it and provide a place for it to grow. Approximately 15 days after the menstrual period has ceased, an egg is produced by one of the ovaries. This egg travels into the uterus through the Fallopian tubes.

If a sperm is able to travel from the vagina through the cervix to fertilize the egg, either in the uterus or in the Fallopian tubes, the fertilized egg will settle in the uterus and begin to grow in the lining where a bed has been formed since the end of the previous menstrual period.

If a fertilized egg does not embed in the wall of the uterus, a menstrual period will occur. During the menstrual period the uterus will shed its recently formed special lining, a thin layer of cells and blood. The lining, in the form of the menstrual flow, will pass out of the uterus into the vagina and out of the body. The flow will last about 5 days. At the end of this time it will cease; the uterus will begin to prepare a new lining as a bed to receive a new egg, and the cycle will be repeated.

YOU ARE THE EMT...

1. Most people think of the pancreas as the organ that supplies insulin. What does insulin do? What other product does the pancreas secrete and what is the role of this product?
2. What two major jobs does the liver perform?
3. Are the kidneys solid or hollow organs? Do they lie in the retroperitoneal space or the pelvic cavity? Are they part of the digestive system or the urinary system?
4. The spleen and the appendix are two abdominal organs that a person could live without. What is the function of each? What organs take over the functions of the appendix and the spleen if they are removed?

Injuries of the Abdomen and Genitalia

25

INJURIES OF THE ABDOMEN

Classification of Abdominal Injuries

Abdominal injuries may be closed or open, and they may involve hollow or solid organs. **Closed** or **blunt abdominal injuries** are those in which the abdomen is damaged by a severe blow, such as striking a steering wheel or being tackled in football, but in which the skin remains intact (Figure 25.1). **Open** or **penetrating abdominal injuries** are those in which a foreign body has entered the abdomen and opened the peritoneum-lined cavity to the outside. Stab wounds or gunshot wounds are examples of open injuries (Figure 25.2). Some penetrating injuries may be only a laceration of the abdominal wall itself. It may be hard to tell whether penetration extends through the peritoneum and into the abdominal

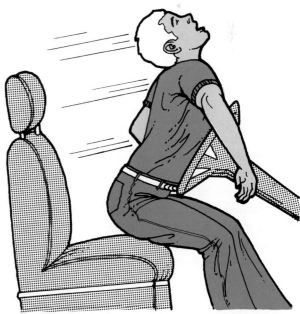

FIGURE 25.1 The steering wheel is a common mechanism of blunt abdominal injury. Even though it is a closed injury, it may result in a ruptured hollow organ, a lacerated spleen or liver, or a torn mesentery.

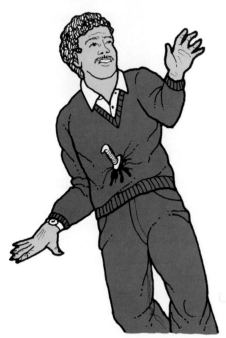

FIGURE 25.2 A common means of producing a penetrating abdominal injury is shown. The EMT, having no knowledge of the length of the penetrating instrument or the patient's position at the time of injury, must assume that penetration and visceral injury have been sustained.

cavity. When the injury is a gunshot or stab wound, the EMT must always assume that the bullet or knife has penetrated the peritoneum and entered the abdominal cavity. Emergency care should be carried out as if that were the case. In treating penetrating abdominal wounds, the only certain way to determine if organs have been injured is for the physician to explore the abdomen during an operation and look at each one. Emergency medical care for penetrating abdominal wounds is based on the assumption that penetration has occurred and that one or several organs have been injured.

The abdomen contains both hollow and solid organs, any of which may be injured. The hollow organs usually contain a stream of food that is in the process of being digested. Rupture or laceration of these organs will allow their contents to spill into the peritoneal cavity, where an intense inflammatory reaction (**peritonitis**) will be caused by the food (digested or undigested), the bowel contents, gastric juice, and the digestive enzymes that are present. This reaction produces prompt and severe abdominal tenderness, muscular rigidity, and intense pain.

There is also paralysis of bowel movement, and the abdomen becomes distended.

The solid organs have a rich blood supply; therefore, injuries of these organs usually cause severe hemorrhage. Laceration of the aorta or inferior vena cava in either closed or open abdominal injuries will also cause severe or fatal hemorrhage. Blood within the peritoneal cavity is not very irritating. Signs of these injuries may first be seen as changes in pulse and blood pressure, together with other signs that indicate shock — for example, an ashen, pale color and cold, clammy skin.

Evaluation of the Injured Abdomen

Abdominal injuries may be very simple to perceive or quite subtle. In general, the overriding complaint of a patient with abdominal injury is pain. For people who have sustained a blunt injury, bruises or tire marks may give clues as to the nature of the wounding agent (Figure 25.3). Patients with penetrating injuries will generally have abdominal wounds that are seen on visual inspection of the abdomen. Some external bleeding may be present, and a large wound may have bowel or fat protruding from it. In addition to the complaint of pain, patients are often nauseated and may have to vomit following any type of abdominal injury. Generally, patients who are developing peritonitis due to irritation of the peritoneal surfaces prefer to lie perfectly still because it hurts them to move.

The signs of abdominal injury are usually more definite than the patient's symptoms. Abdominal

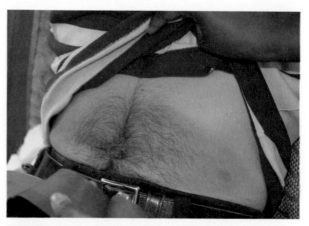

FIGURE 25.3 Bruises of the abdominal wall are strongly suggestive of significant blunt abdominal trauma.

tenderness, particularly localized abdominal tenderness, is a very important clinical sign. Difficulty in moving because of abdominal pain is another important clinical sign. Obvious wounds of both entry and exit are excellent clues for injuries; so are bruises. Altered vital signs such as low blood pressure, a rapid pulse, and rapid, shallow respirations are also important.

The method of evaluating an abdominal injury is the same for blunt and penetrating problems. The patient is permitted to lie supine as comfortably as possible, with the knees slightly flexed and supported. Clothes should be removed or loosened. First, the patient's vital signs are assessed. Many abdominal emergencies, aside from those that cause severe bleeding, can cause a rapid pulse and low blood pressure. It is absolutely essential that a record of vital signs be made as early as possible and that they be recorded periodically thereafter to help the physicians evaluate the progress and severity of the problem when the patient arrives in the emergency department.

A rapid assessment of the patient's condition can be made by simple inspection. The EMT should first note how the patient is lying. The patient with severe abdominal disease or injury prefers to lie still and usually lies with the knees drawn up. Rapid, shallow breaths prevent excessive movement of the abdominal contents. Motion of the body or the abdominal organs irritates the inflamed peritoneum and causes additional pain, which the patient instinctively tries to avoid.

Next, the abdomen should be inspected for skin wounds through which bullets, knives, or other missiles may have entered. The EMT should always check for corresponding exit holes in the patient's back or sides. Occasionally, if a very high velocity missile has been the wounding agent, the EMT will see a small, often harmless looking entrance wound with a huge, gaping exit wound on the back or side. Impaled objects such as knives should be left in place and stabilized with supportive bandaging. Bruises or tire marks, as mentioned earlier, are important clues of the cause and severity of any blunt injury. Steering wheels, seat belts, and arm rests can cause characteristic patterns of bruising of the abdomen or chest. The location of bruises or wounds provides a clue to the underlying organs that may be injured. With severe lacerations of the abdominal wall, in-

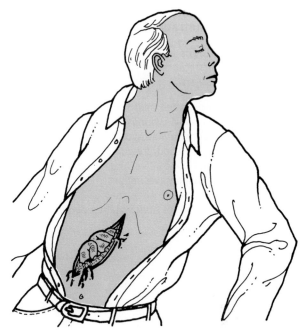

FIGURE 25.4 A large laceration of the abdominal wall will allow some abdominal contents to protrude through the defect.

ternal organs may be protruding through the wound. This condition is called **evisceration** (Figure 25.4).

The patient may tell the EMT how and where the abdomen hurts, may feel nauseated, or may vomit. A patient with abdominal injuries may have a stomach full of food or drink. If vomiting occurs, especially in a patient who is comatose or nearly so, it is imperative that the EMT keep the throat clear of vomitus so that it is not aspirated into the lungs. The EMT should turn the patient's head to one side and try to keep it lower than the chest. It is also important that the EMT note what has been vomited — undigested food, blood, mucus, or bile.

The purpose of the initial evaluation is to determine the type of injury — open (blunt) or closed (penetrating); its possible extent; and the presence of shock. Table 25.1 lists the signs and symptoms that occur in both blunt and penetrating abdominal injuries.

Treatment of Abdominal Injuries

Blunt Abdominal Wounds

Blunt abdominal wounds may cause severe bruises of the abdominal wall. Within the abdomen, the liver and spleen may be lacerated. The intestine

TABLE 25.1 Abdominal Injuries (Blunt or Penetrating) _

Signs and Symptoms
Signs
1. Bruises
2. Tire or seat belt marks
3. Entry and exit wounds (bullets)
4. Lacerations or stab wounds
5. Decreased blood pressure
6. Increased pulse
7. Rapid, shallow respirations
8. Ashen color
9. Local or diffuse abdominal tenderness
10. Distention
11. Shock
12. Vomiting
Symptoms
1. Pain (abdominal)
2. Pain (referred)
3. Nausea
4. Anxiety
5. Desire not to be moved

may be ruptured. Supporting mesenteries may be torn, with injury of the vessels within them. The kidneys may be ruptured or torn from their arteries and veins. The bladder may be ruptured, especially in a patient who has been drinking heavily and thus has a full and distended bladder. These patients may have severe intra-abdominal hemorrhage as well as peritoneal irritation and inflammation from the ruptured hollow organs.

The patient who has sustained a blunt abdominal injury should be placed supine in a comfortable position with the head turned to one side. The mouth and throat should be cleared of vomitus. The vital signs should be carefully monitored for any sign of shock: pallor, cold sweat, rapid thready pulse, or low blood pressure. All appropriate measures to combat shock should be instituted. Respiration may have to be assisted by clearing the airway and using oxygen when needed. The EMT must provide prompt transportation to the emergency department.

Injuries from Seat Belts and Shoulder Belts

Many thousands of injuries have been prevented and many lives have been saved by the use of seat belts. Patients who otherwise would have been thrown out of a smashed car literally owe their survival to the use of seat belts. However, the improper application of a belt occasionally causes a blunt injury of the abdominal organs.

Lap seat belts should be worn so that they lie below the iliac crests, snugly up against the anterior superior iliac spines of the pelvis. If the seat belt rides too high, sudden deceleration or an abrupt stop of the vehicle may cause an injury of the abdominal organs or of the great vessels as the belt squeezes them against the spine. Occasionally, fractures of the lumbar spine have been reported as a result of improper use of seat belts. It must be remembered, however, that the use of the belt in these cases usually converted what could have been a fatal injury into a manageable fracture.

In all current model automobiles, the lap and diagonal (shoulder) seat belts are combined into one so that they may not be used independently. In some older cars still in use, only lap belts or two separate belts are provided. Used alone, diagonal safety belts can cause injuries of the upper part of the trunk, such as a bruised chest, fractured ribs or sternum, a lacerated liver, or even decapitation. Far fewer head and neck injuries are seen, however, when this belt is used in conjunction with the lap belt and a head rest.

Penetrating Abdominal Injury

The penetrating abdominal wound presents a special problem. It is usually impossible to determine for certain without an operation if an instrument or a missile has penetrated the abdomen and if it has, what organs it has injured. The EMT must assume that major damage has occurred even if no obvious signs are present immediately. Signs of intra-abdominal injury often develop slowly. In penetrating wounds, hollow organs are usually lacerated, and their contents discharge into the abdominal cavity and produce peritonitis.

If major blood vessels are cut or if major solid organs are lacerated, hemorrhage may be rapid and severe. All of the steps taken for the care of a blunt abdominal wound should also be carried out for the penetrating ones. In addition, the EMT should note the area of the abdomen where penetration has occurred. The back and sides should be inspected for exit wounds. A dry, sterile dressing should be applied to all open wounds. If the penetrating instrument is still in place, it should be left in place and a stabilizing bandage should be applied to control external bleeding and prevent motion of the instrument.

Evisceration

Extensive lacerations of the abdominal wall may allow some abdominal organs to protrude through the wound. The EMT should not try to replace the organs within the abdomen. Instead, they should be covered with a moist, sterile dressing. Sterile gauze compresses should be moistened with sterile irrigating solution and secured with a sterile dressing. Covering the organs and keeping them moist and warm are of utmost importance. Never should extruding organs be covered with material that clings or loses its substance when wet, such as toilet paper, paper towels, or absorbent cotton. If there are no gauze compresses, the organs may be covered with sterile aluminum foil secured in place with a sterile bandage and tape. The aluminum foil will retain both moisture and heat (Figure 25.5). The EMT should give other necessary emergency medical care as already described and transport the patient promptly to the emergency department. Eviscerations are first priority emergencies.

INJURIES OF THE GENITOURINARY SYSTEM

Injuries of the Kidney

Injuries of the kidney are not common. They may result from blunt or penetrating trauma. The intensity of a blow required to damage a kidney is such that the injury is almost always associated with a fractured rib or other severely injured intra-abdominal organs. The kidneys lie in such a well-protected area of the body that a penetrating wound almost always involves other organs as well as the kidney.

A history or physical evidence of an abrasion, laceration, ecchymosis, or a penetrating wound in the region of the lower rib cage, the flank, or the upper abdomen should make the EMT suspect kidney damage. The patient found to have fractures on either side of the lower rib cage or of the lower thoracic or upper lumbar vertebrae may also be considered a likely candidate for a kidney injury (Figure 25.6).

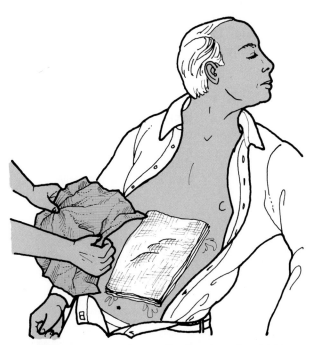

FIGURE 25.5 A moist sterile dressing should be applied to all exposed tissues following abdominal evisceration. Aluminum foil should be secured over the dressing to keep the tissues moist.

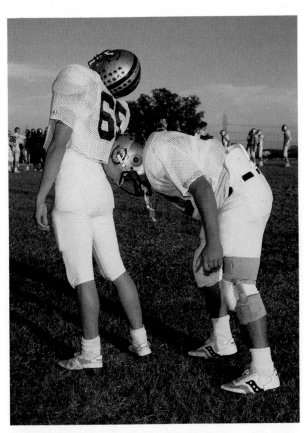

FIGURE 25.6 Blunt trauma to the lower rib cage or the flank can result in kidney injury.

Except for the signs of severe injury on the skin, such as bruises or lacerations, evidence of damage to the kidney will not be manifest on the external examination of the patient. Shock may be seen when the injury is associated with significant blood loss. Since the function of the kidney is the formation of urine, an injury will usually be associated with blood in the urine (**hematuria**). Thus, any urine passed by the patient while under observation by the EMT should be measured and saved for a detailed microscopic examination at the hospital.

When EMTs see a patient who, because of the nature of the injury or because blood has been passed in the urine, is suspected of having kidney damage, they should place the patient at total rest. Vital signs should be carefully monitored until arrival at the emergency department. Shock or other associated abdominal injuries may be present. The patient should be transported promptly to the hospital.

Injury of the Urinary Bladder

Injury of the urinary bladder, either blunt or penetrating, usually results in rupture. Urine is spilled into the surrounding tissues. Any urine that passes through the urethra is likely to be bloody. Blunt injuries of the lower abdomen or pelvis frequently cause an explosive rupture of the urinary bladder, particularly when it is full and distended. Fractures of the pelvis are commonly associated with rupture or perforation of the urinary bladder, which is torn by the sharp, bony fracture fragments (Figure 25.7). In the male, sudden deceleration can literally shear the bladder from the urethra. Penetrating wounds of the lower mid-abdomen or **perineum** (the pelvic floor and associated structures that occupy the pelvic outlet) can directly involve the bladder. A history of any of the above types of injury; evidence on physical examination of trauma to the lower abdomen, pelvis, or perineum; or blood at the urethral opening all point to a possible injury of the urinary bladder.

Any urine passed by a patient with suspected bladder injury should be saved for a detailed analysis in the emergency department. A small amount of blood in the urine will not cause it to turn red. Only microscopic examination will show the abnormal presence of red blood cells.

When the possibility of injury to the urinary bladder exists, the EMT should keep the patient at rest and monitor the vital signs. The presence of associated injuries or shock will dictate the urgency of transport to the emergency department.

Injuries of the External Male Genitalia

Injuries of the external male genitalia include all types of soft tissue wounds. Rarely are they life-threatening. They are uniformly extremely painful and generally a source of great concern to the patient.

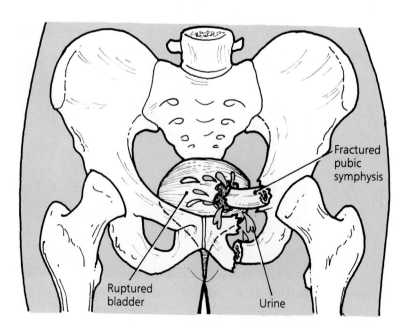

Fractured
pubic
symphysis

Ruptured
bladder

Urine

FIGURE 25.7 Fracture of the pelvis frequently results in laceration of the full bladder by the sharp fracture fragments. Urine then leaks into the pelvic cavity.

Avulsion (tearing away) of the skin of the penis, particularly in the uncircumcised male, can occur, especially in industrial accidents. When such an injury is encountered, the denuded penis should be wrapped in a soft, sterile dressing moistened with sterile saline solution before prompt transport of the patient to the emergency department. An effort should be made to salvage the avulsed skin and preserve it. One should not, however, delay treatment or transport for more than a couple of minutes to salvage a remnant of damaged tissue.

Amputation, partial or complete, of the penile shaft demands immediate attention to blood loss, which can be effectively managed with use of local pressure with a sterile dressing on the remaining stump. If a complete amputation has occurred, an effort must be made to locate the amputated part so that it can be used for surgical reconstruction. The recovered part should be wrapped in a sterile dressing, placed in a plastic bag, and transported in a cooled container. On very rare occasions, the EMT may see a patient who has amputated his own penis. This violent gesture is usually associated with severe mental disease. Treatment is as just noted, together with that appropriate for managing any disturbed patient.

The acute angulation of the erect penis with respect to the anterior abdominal wall can result in a "fracture" of the penis — a laceration of the supporting erectile tissues of this organ. The injury may occur during particularly active sexual intercourse. It is always associated with intense pain, bleeding into the tissues, and fear. Prompt transport to the emergency department is indicated since operative repair may be required.

Laceration of the skin about the head of the penis is an accident that usually occurs when the penis is in an erect state. These lacerations can be associated with profuse bleeding. Local pressure with a sterile dressing will usually be sufficient to stop the hemorrhage.

The foreskin sometimes gets caught in the zipper of trousers, a situation usually seen in children. If only one or two teeth of the zipper are involved, an attempt at unzipping should be made. If the child is agitated or a long segment of skin is trapped, the EMT should cut the zipper out of the trousers and make the patient more comfortable for prompt transport to the emergency department.

Urethral injuries in the male are uncommon. Lacerations of the urethra can result from straddle injuries, pelvic trauma, or penetrating wounds of the perineum. They can be associated with brisk bleeding. Direct pressure with a dry, sterile dressing will usually control the bleeding. Since the urethra is the channel for urine, the passing of any urine and the presence or absence of blood in it are facts of utmost importance. Any voided urine should be saved for a later examination at the hospital. Foreign bodies protruding from the urethra should be left for removal by emergency department personnel.

Avulsion of the scrotal skin with or without associated injury of the scrotal contents can occur. When possible, the EMT should recover and preserve the skin in a sterile dressing for possible use in reconstruction. The denuded scrotal contents or the perineal area should be dressed with a sterile, moist compress. Bleeding can be controlled with a local pressure dressing. The patient should be transported promptly to the emergency department.

Direct blows to the scrotum and its contents can result in rupture of a testicle or significant accumulation of blood about the testes. The EMT should apply an ice pack to the scrotal area while the patient is being transported.

A few general rules apply to the treatment of injuries involving the male external genitalia:

1. These injuries are extremely painful. Make the patient as comfortable as possible.
2. Use sterile, moist compresses to control bleeding and cover denuded areas.
3. Never move or manipulate impaled instruments or urethral foreign bodies.
4. If possible, always identify and bring detached parts with the patient.
5. Remember that these are rarely life-threatening injuries, and the presence and severity of other wounds dictate the priorities of care.

Injuries of the Female Genitalia

Internal Female Genitalia

The uterus, ovaries, and Fallopian tubes are subject to the same kinds of injuries as any other internal organ; however, they are rarely damaged because they are small and well protected by the pelvis. Unlike the bladder, they do not lie adjacent to the bony pelvis and are usually not injured when it is fractured.

External Female Genitalia

The external female genitalia include the vulva, the clitoris, and the major and minor labia (lips) at the entrance of the vagina. The female urethra enters the anterior vagina.

Injuries of the external female genitalia can include all types of soft tissue injuries. These genital parts have a rich nerve supply, and injuries are very painful. Lacerations, abrasions, and avulsions should be treated with moist compresses, local pressure to control bleeding, and a diaper-type dressing to hold dressings in place. Under no circumstances should dressings or packs be placed into the vagina.

Foreign bodies should be left alone after stabilization, and these patients should be transported promptly to the emergency department. Contusions and other blunt injuries all require careful in-hospital evaluation.

In general, although these injuries are painful, they are usually not life-threatening. Bleeding may be copious, but it can usually be controlled by local compression. Priorities of need for transport to the emergency department are dictated by associated injuries, amount of hemorrhage, and the presence of shock.

SEXUAL ASSAULT AND RAPE

Instances of sexual assault and rape are all too common. Often the EMT can do little beyond soothing and calming the patient and providing transportation to the emergency department. The genitalia should not be examined by the EMT unless obvious bleeding requires the application of a dressing. The patient should be advised not to wash, douche, urinate, or defecate until after a physician has had the opportunity to make an examination in the emergency department. All other injuries should be treated according to appropriate routine procedures and should dictate the urgency of transport to the emergency department. The EMT must obtain and record as clear a history of the incident as possible. Questioning and necessary treatment should be handled quietly, as speedily as possible, and away from onlookers. A calm, professional manner is appropriate, with no display of personal curiosity.

The EMT must be aware that the patient has the right to refuse assistance and to refuse to be taken to the emergency department. Such refusal sometimes occurs in cases of rape or sexual assault because the patient wishes to avoid publicity. Nor is it unusual for assistance to be refused after the EMT arrives at the scene, even though help may originally have been requested. This choice, too, is the patient's prerogative. Referral to a rape counseling center can often be helpful in these circumstances.

YOU ARE THE EMT...

1. What special problem does a penetrating abdominal wound present? How should you treat such a wound?
2. What two signs are suggestive of kidney injury?
3. What abdominal organ is commonly ruptured or perforated in conjunction with a fracture of the pelvis? How should you treat this injury?
4. What is peritonitis? What kinds of abdominal injuries would cause peritonitis? What characteristic symptoms does a patient with peritonitis exhibit?

SECTION 6

MEDICAL EMERGENCIES

26 Medical Emergencies

OVERVIEW

In the United States, the leading cause of death between the ages of 1 and 45 years is trauma. For this reason, much of the EMT's training focuses on the management of injuries and extrication. A large number of calls to any emergency medical service, however, have nothing to do with injury, accident, or violence. These calls are about medical emergencies — about people who have become suddenly and unexpectedly ill or who are experiencing symptoms brought about by the progress of a given disease.

EMTs are generally called upon to deal with medical emergencies at least as often as they have to respond to various instances of injury or accident. Frequently, knowing the exact cause of a given complaint is difficult. However, diagnosis of a specific condition is not the job of the EMT; rather, the EMT's responsibility lies in recognizing the existence of a significant medical complaint and instituting appropriate support and transportation procedures.

Chapter 26 describes some of the more common medical emergencies. The first half of the chapter focuses on the major causes of medical illness and disease. These range from medical causes to environmental causes to unknown or obscure causes. The symptoms and clinical signs of illness and disease are defined next. The last part of the chapter describes the chronology of medical illness and disease, which will help the EMT to decide whether a medical emergency is acute or whether it has resulted from a chronic disease or a periodic illness.

OBJECTIVES

The objectives of Chapter 26 are to

- understand the nature of a medical emergency and the usual causes of such events.
- relate each of these causes to its role in producing a medical emergency.
- distinguish between symptoms and clinical signs of medical illness and disease.
- identify acute, chronic, and periodic medical emergencies.

CAUSES OF MEDICAL ILLNESS AND DISEASE

Medical emergencies that arise from unexpected illness or symptoms brought about by the progress of a given disease usually result from one of the following causes:

1. Degeneration of normal, healthy tissues
2. Infection (bacterial, parasitic, or viral)
3. Neoplasm that both invades and destroys tissue
4. Endocrine (hormone) disturbances that alter tissue function
5. Obstruction of hollow organs
6. Congenital defects
7. The environment
8. Unknown or obscure causes

Degenerative Processes

As the population in the United States ages, we become increasingly aware of degenerative diseases that destroy tissue. No part of the body is immune to **degeneration** of normal, healthy tissues. Joints, for example, wear out in a process called **degenerative arthritis** and often require surgical replacement. As the joint gradually deteriorates, the patient develops pain and loss of function in the joint. Years of smoking, or simply inhaling city fumes, can destroy both lung and bronchial tissue, resulting in **chronic obstructive lung disease** and **emphysema.** Poor diet, smoking, high blood pressure, a relatively sedentary existence, and several other factors can result in one of the most common degenerative processes of all, **arteriosclerosis.** This is a disease that destroys small and large arteries in all tissues of the body and ultimately causes heart disease or stroke. Arteriosclerosis can also cause blood vessel damage in the legs and the internal organs, as well as in the head and heart. Symptoms of this degenerative blood vessel disease can show up in any organ of the body affected. The symptoms be-

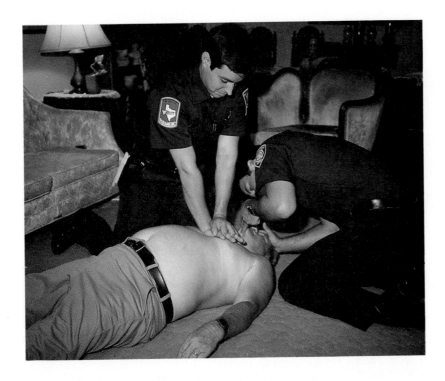

FIGURE 26.1 Many of the EMT's patients are victims of heart disease or stroke.

come more severe as the blood vessel degeneration progresses.

Heart disease is common today and ranges all the way from the person who suffers mild chest pain after exertion to the person who suddenly dies from a heart attack. Many patients have had operations to correct or control disease of the heart. The major cause of heart disease is degeneration and obstruction of the arteries that supply blood to the heart. The usual symptoms are chest pain, an irregular pulse, anxiety, and shortness of breath.

Degeneration of the blood vessels in the brain is referred to as **cerebrovascular disease.** If one of the arteries feeding the brain is blocked or if a damaged vessel within the brain ruptures, the supply of blood to parts of the brain may be suddenly interrupted, either partially or totally. The interruption of blood flow to an area of the brain is called a **stroke.** Strokes may cause a temporary loss of certain functions such as swallowing or speech, permanent paralysis of one-half of the body (**hemiplegia**), unconsciousness (**coma**), or even death. The usual cause of stroke is long-standing degeneration of blood vessels.

The EMT often has to take care of a person with heart disease or stroke (Figure 26.1). Treatment must be directed at the function most damaged. Often,

basic life support must be instituted to restore or maintain breathing and circulation.

Infectious Processes

Communicable (infectious) diseases are all around us. They range in severity from the common cold or viral "flu" to life-threatening infections such as meningitis or hepatitis. Much progress has been made in this century to control infectious diseases. Smallpox, for example, has been virtually eliminated in civilized countries, and tuberculosis is under strict control. New diseases take their place, however. **AIDS (acquired immune deficiency syndrome),** a life-threatening viral infection, was unheard of in 1975.

The human body provides an excellent environment for the growth of bacteria, viruses, fungi, and parasites. Rapid growth of infectious organisms saps the body's energy as they invade and destroy normal tissue (Figure 26.2). The body responds to infection in many different ways: Fever, chills, nausea, vomiting, diarrhea, coughing, shortness of breath, abdominal pain, local swelling and redness, and local tenderness are only a few of the many signs and symptoms that may accompany infection.

Most patients with infection require medical treatment. The EMT must be aware of the signs and

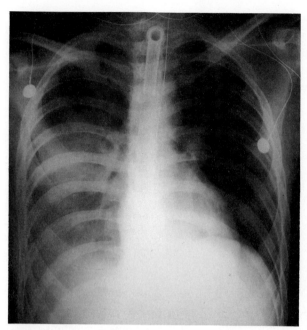

FIGURE 26.2 Chest x-ray of a patient with pneumonia, a bacterial infection of the lung. Note the destruction (whitened areas) of the right lung as compared to the clear left lung.

symptoms of infection to facilitate proper treatment. In addition, EMTs must be careful to protect themselves, their patients, and their vehicles from becoming contaminated while transporting an infected individual. A host of these diseases exist, and the chances are great that the EMT will encounter them often.

Neoplastic Processes

The word **neoplasm** means new growth. In the body new growth may be benign or malignant. Neoplasms always produce tumors or masses. **Benign** (nonmalignant) neoplasms tend to grow and expand locally, in the area of their origin. As they grow, they crowd and press onto adjacent organs. The symptoms of a benign neoplasm are those of a developing mass or of a disordered function of the organ being distorted. Usually they grow slowly, and rarely are they the cause of an emergency problem.

Malignant, or cancerous, neoplasms also develop as masses at their sites of origin; they, too, compress adjacent organs. Unlike benign neoplasms, however, they invade these adjacent organs and travel to distant parts of the body through veins and lym-

phatic vessels. There they take root, grow, and eventually invade other tissues. Malignant tumors destroy organs and tissues by invasion, replacement, and pressure.

From time to time, the EMT will treat a patient with **cancer.** The symptoms will depend on the location of the tumor and the extent of its growth. While any tissue may develop a malignant neoplasm, the common cancer sites are the lung, the colon, the breast, and the internal female genitalia. When cancer spreads, the most frequently involved organs are lymph nodes, liver, and lungs. Cancer is not a contagious disease, although it does appear with some predictability in certain families. There is also some indication that a few cancers may be caused by viruses. But cancer is not passed from one person to another like a common infection. In general, the EMT's responsibility toward a cancer patient is to provide support for the damaged functions such as breathing or circulation.

Complex Endocrine Processes

Some medical problems have a wide range of symptoms because they are the result of too much or too little hormone production by the **endocrine glands.** Each gland produces one or more **hormones.** Disease states are caused from over- or underproduction of each of these substances. In these diseases, specific bodily functions are increased, decreased, or absent. **Diabetes** is one such disease; because production of the hormone insulin is deficient, the body is unable to use sugar normally. The disease also damages the small blood vessels in the body. The tissue damage which results from the blood vessel disease is as much a part of diabetes as is the difficulty in regulating the amount of sugar in the blood.

Several other endocrine glands exist in the body beside those which produce insulin. Thyroxin from the **thyroid gland** controls the general **metabolism** of the body. The **parathyroid glands** control calcium levels in the blood, bone, and body fluids. The **adrenal glands** secrete hormones that control salt levels in the blood and some sexual function. The **ovaries** and **testes** control sexual development and reproduction.

Among the glandular diseases, the EMT will most frequently deal with diabetes, since it is a fairly common problem and often a cause of coma or insulin shock. The other complex endocrine problems are rarely the cause of acute emergencies.

Obstructive Processes

The body contains many different hollow organs and tubes that carry nutrients and waste products. When a blood vessel is obstructed, as with arteriosclerosis, the tissue it serves dies. Many things (stones, blood clots, tumors, or foreign bodies) can obstruct a hollow organ. Substances that flow through the organ slow or stop, causing the organ to bulge behind the point of obstruction (Figure 26.3). Cramping pain almost always occurs as a result of the bulging, or **distention,** because the muscle in the wall of the distended organ tries to overcome the obstruction by contracting. Infection often follows obstruction and persists for a long time.

When the bile duct or ureter is obstructed by stones, a prompt and specific colicky pain usually occurs and is often accompanied by fever and other signs of infection. (**Colic** is severe, intermittent pain in the abdomen caused by obstruction.) Sometimes the bronchi or the lungs become obstructed by mucus, a foreign body, or a tumor; if the obstructive process is not treated promptly, pneumonia may result. Obstruction in the gastrointestinal tract usually produces visible distention of the abdomen and colicky pain.

Often the EMT has to transport patients with pneumonia, bowel obstruction, kidney stones, or some other obstructive process. Treatment for these patients depends on the organ involved and the specific functions that have been lost.

Congenital Processes

Each year thousands of children are born with congenital defects. A **congenital defect** is a physical abnormality or deficiency that is present at birth. Some congenital defects are inherited; others develop as the fetus matures in the uterus. Congenital defects can involve any organ or system of the body. They range from the very common **inguinal hernia** to the rare absence of a given organ. Most defects are corrected immediately after birth and before the infant leaves the hospital. Some, however, are not. Among the symptoms they can produce are vomiting, yellow discoloration of the skin (**jaundice**), a "blue baby" (from certain heart defects), or difficulties with swallowing. Rarely do these defects cause extreme

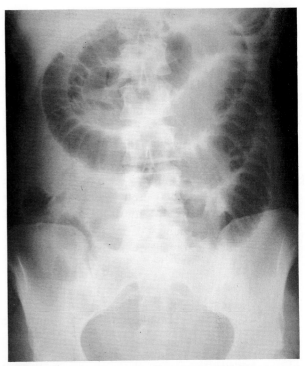

FIGURE 26.3 X-ray of patient with an acute bowel obstruction. Note the small intestine distended with gas.

emergencies for the EMT. However, such patients must be transported as quickly as possible for proper diagnosis and treatment.

Environmental Causes

Apart from the weather, water-related injuries, and electrical hazards, a great many medical emergencies have environmental causes. They are grouped in Chapter 27 as "Poisons, Stings, and Bites." The EMT in all likelihood will see several such problems. For example, many common household items when inhaled or ingested are poisonous. Stings and bites from snakes, bees, wasps, dogs, and other animals occur almost daily. And, the variety of allergies to pollens, food, injected toxins, and other agents is endless.

Symptoms and the extent of injury are directly related to the toxicity of the agent, the sensitivity of the patient to the substance, and the degree of exposure to the agent. Emergency treatment ranges from protecting patients from environmental hazards to providing cardiopulmonary resuscitation (CPR) to severely ill patients. Because of the frequency of medical emergencies due to environmental hazards, the EMT must become familiar with the symptoms and treatment of injuries and illnesses that result from poisons, stings, and bites.

Unknown or Obscure Causes

The cause of some medical emergencies is unknown or uncertain. Some diseases do not have clear-cut causes. **Epilepsy,** for example, is one such disease. Often it follows a specific brain injury, but it may be caused by a stroke, a brain tumor, or a high fever. More often there is no cause that can be specifically identified. Many different organs and body systems have diseases of unknown cause. Thus, not all medical emergencies can be categorized by specific causes.

SYMPTOMS AND CLINICAL SIGNS OF MEDICAL ILLNESS AND DISEASE

A **symptom** is a complaint voiced by the patient. It is subject to the patient's interpretation and is often a manifestation of the patient's fear. The same symptom can be interpreted very differently by different individuals. Examples of common symptoms include pain, fear, and difficulty with such functions as swallowing, breathing, or urinating.

A **clinical sign** is a physical finding that can be elicited or viewed by the physician or EMT. It is a sure, visible, often tangible, evidence of disease. Examples of common clinical signs are tenderness (local or diffuse), swelling, redness, or paralysis (inability to move).

TABLE 26.1 Medical Emergencies: Common Symptoms and Signs

Organ or System	Symptoms	Clinical Signs
General Body (Systemic)	Malaise (feeling unwell) Vertigo (lightheadedness) Nausea Chills	Fever Change in pulse rate Change in skin color Change in skin texture
Cardiovascular	Chest pain Shortness of breath	Pulse abnormality Hypotension Frothy or bloody sputum Cyanosis (bluish color of skin)
Cerebrovascular (Neurological)	Headache Dizziness Weakness	Alteration of consciousness Paralysis Loss of specific function Numbness Changes in pupil size
Gastrointestinal	Abdominal pain Nausea	Diarrhea Vomiting Blood in stool or vomitus Distention Abdominal tenderness Abdominal masses
Respiratory	Shortness of breath Chest pain	Change in respiratory rate Labored breathing Mucus production Frothy, bloody sputum Wheezing Rales
Genitourinary	Burning on urination Frequency	Blood in urine Changes in urinary flow abdominal masses

In general, symptoms and signs are associated with the system or organ involved. However, many medical emergencies are associated with **systemic** (generalized) symptoms and signs, such as fever, chills, and weakness. The signs and symptoms for which a specific patient will require treatment depend on which tissues are diseased and on the amount of function lost by the diseased tissues. A brief review of signs and symptoms is contained in Table 26.1.

CHRONOLOGY OF MEDICAL ILLNESS AND DISEASE

Many diseases progress slowly over several years and produce few, if any, symptoms during the early years. As the disease progresses, the symptoms become more frequent and more severe, usually forcing the person to seek medical treatment. For the EMT, this means that the patient will either have **acute symptoms** (sudden onset), **chronic symptoms** (slowly progressive), or **periodic symptoms** (recurring at intervals). A medical history of the disease process will aid the EMT in discovering the cause of the patient's symptoms. The history can be obtained from the patient, family, or friends at the scene.

Acute Medical Emergencies

Probably the best example of an acute medical emergency is the **acute myocardial infarction (AMI),** or heart attack. It occurs suddenly, often without any identifying history, and produces severe symptoms and signs that require prompt, aggressive treatment.

Chronic Disease

A chronic disease presents the EMT with a different situation. The patient with chronic obstructive lung disease or emphysema, for example, always has some difficulty in breathing. Although never free from the basic disease, the person usually is able to manage if no complicating factor is added to the problem. However, a minor infection, a cold, too much fluid, or a mild allergic response such as from hay fever may trigger an acute **decompensation** in breathing. A person with chronic disease almost always has a medical history on record, which is invaluable to the doctors handling the case. An alert EMT can often obtain this history.

Periodic Illness

Some problems are periodic — that is, they recur at intervals with no manifestation of the disease during the intervening period. The person with epilepsy, for example, is normal save for the occasional seizure. An individual with a specific, severe allergy is similarly normal unless exposed to the substance that produces the allergic reaction. In contrast to the patient who is chronically ill, the person with periodic illness is well most of the time with only temporary episodes of disease.

YOU ARE THE EMT...

1. You suspect the patient has cerebrovascular disease. Her symptoms are headache, dizziness, and weakness. Identify the possible clinical signs.
2. Your patient says he has diabetes. Is this disease related to neoplastic processes or endocrine processes? What part of the process dysfunctions?
3. You examine the patient and record her systemic signs and symptoms. What does that mean? Give some examples of systemic signs and symptoms.
4. Why is it important for you to identify a patient's symptoms as being either acute, chronic, or periodic?

27 Poisons, Stings, and Bites

OVERVIEW

Thousands of children and adults each year ingest, inhale, inject, or come into surface contact with poisonous substances. Most often these are accidental poisonings, although intentional poisonings and suicides also contribute to the statistics. The EMT has many responsibilities in dealing with poisoning cases. Chapter 27 examines these areas of responsibility, which range from identifying a toxic substance to treating various types of poisonings.

Chapter 27 also discusses stings and bites and their associated problems. While most stings and bites are more painful than injurious, some are potentially dangerous, even life-threatening. For example, some people are highly allergic to bees, wasps, and hornets. With dog bites, there is a worry about rabies. With snakes and spiders, the seriousness of the bite depends on whether the species is poisonous. Thus, much of Chapter 27 is devoted to identifying symptoms of serious reactions to bites and stings and distinguishing poisonous snakes and spiders from nonpoisonous varieties. The last part of the chapter discusses two often-neglected topics—human bites and marine animal injuries.

OBJECTIVES

The objectives of Chapter 27 are to

- become knowledgeable about the problem of accidental and intentional poisoning and the location of area poison control centers.
- recognize the symptoms of a poisoning and identify the toxic substance involved.
- learn the emergency treatment for ingested, surface, inhaled, and injected poisons.
- learn the emergency treatment for food poisoning and plant poisoning.
- identify the symptoms of stings from bees, wasps, hornets, and ants.
- become aware of the seriousness of an anaphylactic reaction to a bee, wasp, yellow jacket, or hornet sting.
- learn how to identify and treat scorpion stings and spider bites.
- distinguish poisonous snakes from nonpoisonous snakes and learn the emergency treatment for snake bites.
- understand the seriousness of rabies and its link to dog bites.
- learn the emergency treatment for human bites and marine animal injuries.

POISONS

A **poison** is defined as any substance which, when ingested, inhaled, or absorbed, or when applied to, injected into, or developed within the body, in relatively small amounts, by its chemical actions, may cause damage to structures or disturbances of function.[1] The key elements of this definition are the statements "in relatively small amounts," and "by its chemical action." Very small amounts of a poison can cause much damage or death. The injury within the body is chemical rather than physical as occurs with trauma. Poisons act by modifying the normal metabolism of cells or by actually destroying them. Poisoning can result from several routes of contact: ingestion, inhalation, injection, surface application, or absorption through the skin or mucous membranes.

Each year, thousands of children and adults come into some contact with poison. In 1977, accidental poisonings by solid or liquid materials caused 3,374 deaths. Two-thirds of these poisonings were from drugs. This is the most recent year for which full published statistics are available.[2] Intentional

1. *Dorland's Illustrated Medical Dictionary,* 24th Edition. W.B. Saunders Co., Philadelphia and London, 1965.
2. *Metropolitan Life Insurance Company: Statistical Bulletin,* 61(2), April-June 1980.

poisonings and suicides will increase this number. In 1977, it was noted that the death rate from poisoning in children under the age of 5 had dropped 60 percent and had markedly increased in the older groups. In 1982, poisoning from solid and liquid substances other than drugs caused 612 deaths: 474 males and 138 females.[3] In this year, 4 percent of those who died were under the age of 10; 12 percent, between 10 and 24 years; 36 percent, between 25 and 44 years; 37 percent, between 45 and 64 years; and 11 percent, above 65 years. These figures tend to confirm the shift in accidental poisoning away from the pediatric age group.

Roughly two-thirds of poisonings at all ages in 1977 were related to the use of drugs. No significant change has occurred in the distribution of poisonings since then.[4] Barbiturates constituted 9 percent of this number; opiates, 15 percent; and unspecified drugs, 51 percent. Previous figures have shown significant mortality related to barbiturate and opiate overdosing. These trends have changed, but only to reflect the availability of many more types of drugs than before. Some one-third of accidental poisoning deaths result from liquid and solid agents other than drugs. Age-related mortality from other agents closely parallels that for drug-related deaths.

Poison Control Centers

Several hundred poison control centers exist throughout the United States, many of them in the emergency departments of large hospitals. Many are independent. Telephone numbers of these poison control centers are readily available. The personnel who staff the poison control centers have access to information concerning virtually all of the commonly used drugs, chemicals, and substances that could possibly be poisonous. Information for each of these agents includes a specific **antidote,** or substance that will counteract the poison, if one is available and the appropriate emergency treatment for that particular poison. Most of the centers are staffed 24 hours a day; contact with them is mandatory whenever there is a poisoning problem. In general, they are able to provide information for specific agents under both trade and generic names. The EMT should know

3. National Center for Health Statistics, unpublished data.
4. National Clearing House for Poison Control Center: Poisoning Surveillance and Epidemiology Branch, unpublished statistics.

the location and telephone number of the nearest poison control center. Ordinarily, in an emergency situation, the EMT should notify dispatch concerning the nature of the specific case. The fact that a poisoning has occurred, the size, weight and age of the patient, and a description of the suspected agent should be included. Dispatch will contact the poison control center and relay specific instructions.

Occasionally, the poison control center will recommend that vomiting (**emesis**) be induced by the use of **syrup of ipecac.** The EMT should give this drug and proceed with arrangements to transport the patient. Generally, if one dose of ipecac does not produce results in 20 minutes, a repeat dose is given. The EMT should *not* delay transport to wait to give a second dose. Aggressive treatment of poisons, especially those that have been ingested, may be lifesaving. Such treatment is best provided at the emergency department.

Identifying Poisoning Victims and the Toxic Substance

The primary responsibility of the EMT is to recognize the likelihood that a poisoning has occurred. With even the slightest suspicion that someone has taken a poisonous substance, the EMT should contact dispatch with information for the poison control center and begin emergency treatment. Some of the more common symptoms and signs of various poisonings are nausea, vomiting, abdominal pain, diarrhea, dilation or constriction of the pupils, excessive salivation, sweating, difficulty in breathing, unconsciousness, or even convulsions. If respiration is inadequate, cyanosis will occur. Some chemical compounds will cause inflammation or burns of the skin or mucous membranes. Redness, blistering, or even severe burns may result. The presence of these injuries about the mouth is a strong clue suggesting an ingested caustic agent.

The EMT should next attempt to determine the nature of the poison. Objects at the scene such as overturned bottles, scattered pills, chemicals, or even an overturned or damaged plant may provide clues. The remains of any food or drink may also be important. Any suspicious material should be placed in a plastic bag and taken to the hospital. If the patient vomits, the material should be saved in a plastic bag and brought to the hospital for analysis. Bringing any suspicious materials, along with collected vomitus, may be the most important thing an EMT can do after resuscitating and instituting care for the patient.

Any containers for the materials that have been collected should also be brought. Specific ingredients are often listed on the labels. Also, the number of pills originally in a bottle is usually specified, together with the name of the drug and the concentration. Information concerning the content of the substances can be of great help to the doctors in the emergency department. Knowing how much material is left in any container may give the physician some idea of how much has been ingested. Brand names are known at most poison control centers, and specific chemical contents can be ascertained. Sometimes the manufacturer can be contacted for a specific description of the material in the container. By bringing the container with the patient, the EMT may be able to hasten the proper treatment and thus help save a life.

Ingested, Surface, Inhaled, and Injected Poisons

Most poisons do not have a specific antidote or remedy. Support for the patient may range all the way from reassuring an anxious parent to instituting cardiopulmonary resuscitation. In general, the most important treatment for poisons involves dilution and physical removal of the agent. This can be accomplished by surface flooding and washing for the skin, drinking water or milk and inducing vomiting for ingested poisons, or administering oxygen for inhaled noxious agents. Certain injected poisons may require a specific antidote. Injected poisons pose rather urgent problems since they are difficult to remove or dilute.

Ingested Poisons

Poisonous substances most likely to be ingested include drugs, drinks, household products, contaminated food, or plants. Children are often the victims of accidental household poisonings (Figure 27.1). With the exception of contaminated food, adults usually ingest poisonous agents as a method of committing suicide or as unsuspecting victims of murder. While drugs represent the majority of ingested poisonings, approximately one-third are caused by other liquid or solid agents, cleaners, soaps, acids, or alkalis. Plant poisonings are also prominent among children

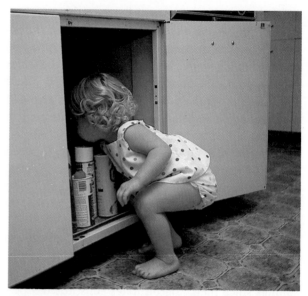

FIGURE 27.1 A curious child will try to taste or swallow almost any substance. A common victim of accidental ingestion of dangerous compounds is the unwatched toddler.

who like to explore and often bite the leaves of various bushes or shrubs. (Food poisoning, even though technically an ingested poison, and plant poisoning are covered in separate sections.)

The first step after determining that a poisoning with an ingested agent has occurred is to attempt to dilute the agent in the stomach. Water or a glass or two of milk may be given to drink if the poison is acting as a gastric irritant. The next step is to remove the poison physically by inducing vomiting in the patient. Vomiting may be stimulated if the patient is conscious and alert, and, especially, if the poison control center has so instructed. Vomiting is most easily induced by the oral administration of syrup of ipecac (one to two teaspoonsful for children under one year; three teaspoonsful for older children and adults), followed by a glass of water. The patient should be transported promptly after the dose of ipecac. Most patients will vomit after 15 to 20 minutes, frequently inside the ambulance. The vomitus should be saved. If vomiting has not occurred after 20 minutes, the dose should be repeated, but only once. Transport should not be delayed to administer a second dose. If vomiting fails after the second dose, the ipecac should be removed from the stomach by **gastric lavage** once the patient arrives in the emergency department. If the patient does vomit, the EMT should make sure that the airway remains clear. If the patient is lying down, the head should be turned to one side; if standing, the patient should be helped to lean over a basin or sink. Whenever a patient is vomiting, the EMT must be alert to prevent aspiration of vomitus.

The EMT should not induce vomiting under the following circumstances:

1. If the patient is unconscious, semiconscious, or having a convulsion.
2. If the poison is corrosive, such as a strong acid, lye, or drain cleaner, or has caused obvious burns on the lips or mouth.
3. If the poison contains any petroleum product such as kerosene, gasoline, lighter fluid, or clear furniture polish. These agents cause a serious **chemical pneumonia** if aspirated into the lungs.

Some substances are best managed by local adsorption onto **activated charcoal.** One tablespoon, well mixed and suspended in a glass of water, is the usual dose. This medication is given at the direction of the poison control center after the center has been provided with information as to the nature of the agent taken. Activated charcoal inhibits the action of ipecac; therefore, it should not be given after a dose of this medication. Many children are afraid to swallow this dirty, inky, messy substance. Often some coaxing is required to get them to do so. Never should the EMT force it into someone's mouth, however.

Most ingested poisonings are from drugs. Many of them are opiates, sedatives, or barbiturates. In these circumstances the EMT must expect central nervous system (CNS) depression and especially respiratory depression. These patients may require aggressive ventilatory support and even cardiopulmonary resuscitation, since absorption of some agents from the gastrointestinal tract is rapid. Prompt transportation to the emergency department is mandatory, since there is little the EMT can do beyond basic life support.

Surface Contact Poisons

Many corrosive substances cause damage of the skin, mucous membranes, or eyes by direct contact. Acids, alkalis, and some petroleum or benzene prod-

ucts are very destructive. Contact with these agents will cause inflammation, chemical burns, or specific rashes or lesions in affected areas.

The emergency treatment for contact poisoning is to remove the irritating or corrosive substance as rapidly as possible. Dry materials are dusted off thoroughly; then the affected area is washed with soap and water or flooded under a shower. When a large amount of material has been spilled on a patient, flooding may be the most rapidly effective treatment. All clothing that has been contaminated with poisons or irritating substances should be removed as rapidly as possible so the skin may be cleaned with running water. Chemical agents in the eyes must be treated by rapid and copious irrigation for several minutes. With eyes, at least 5 minutes of irrigation are needed for acid substances and 15 to 20 minutes for alkalis. This problem is discussed further in Chapter 39.

Time should not be spent attempting to neutralize substances on the skin. Rather they should be washed off immediately with water. This procedure is faster and more effective than attempting to neutralize a substance chemically.

The one exception to flooding the contact area with water is when the EMT knows the agent is one that chemically reacts violently with water. For example, phosphorus and elemental sodium are dry, solid chemicals that ignite when they contact water. The incidence of exposure to these elements is rare. As with other dry chemicals, they should be dusted off. The patient's clothing should be removed and dry dressings applied to any burn area. The patient should then be transported to the hospital for further care.

Inhaled Poisons

For inhaled poisons such as natural gas, carbon monoxide, chlorine, or other gases, the emergency treatment is to move the patient into fresh air. Patients exposed to prolonged inhalation may require supplementary oxygen and basic life support. Because it is easy to inhale noxious fumes in an emergency situation, EMTs must be careful to protect themselves as well as their patients.

Some inhaled poisons such as carbon monoxide are odorless and produce profound **hypoxia** without much damage to the lungs. Some such as chlorine are very irritating and induce **pulmonary edema** and airway obstruction. Oxygen is needed whenever hypoxia, pulmonary edema, or airway obstruction results from inhaled poisons. Supplemental suctioning and ventilatory support may also be necessary. These patients should be transported as quickly as possible because some inhaled agents cause progressive lung damage. Many times, these patients will require two or three days of intensive care until normal lung function can be reestablished.

Injected Poisons

Poisoning by injection is almost always the result of deliberate drug overdose — a problem that is discussed in Chapter 35. Other sources of injected poisons are the bites and stings of insects or animals. If the area around the site of an injection starts to swell, all rings, watches, or bracelets should be removed. A constricting band above and below the site of the injection should be applied. The band should be adjusted just tightly enough to occlude, or block, the flow of blood in the veins, creating a **venous tourniquet.** Arterial flow should not be cut off, however, and the patient's pulse should still be palpable distal to the constricting band. An ice pack may decrease local pain and swelling about the injection.

In general, injected poisons are impossible to dilute or remove. Usually they are absorbed quickly into the body or cause intense local tissue destruction. The EMT must be prepared, in the case of rapid absorption, to offer basic life support. With severe local tissue damage, complex operative procedures are needed. Thus, prompt transport to the emergency department is mandatory.

Food Poisoning

The term "ptomaine poisoning" was coined in 1870 and is used frequently in news accounts of episodes of food poisoning. Unfortunately, it is nonspecific and indicates little about the problem. Food poisoning is caused by the ingestion of **contaminated** food, or food that is carrying bacteria. There are two types: one type occurs when the bacteria themselves cause disease, and the other type occurs when the bacteria have produced **toxins** (poisons) that cause disease.

An example of the former is typhoid fever, which represents the ingestion of a bacterium — *Salmonella typhosa*. It produces characteristic gastrointestinal

problems that develop up to 72 hours after ingestion. Only ingested living bacteria can produce the disease. A variety of other organisms can also produce milder intestinal complaints. Usually, proper cooking will kill bacteria, and proper cleanliness in the kitchen will prevent the contamination of non-cooked foods. Some people are known as carriers of certain bacteria. In these instances, transmission of disease by these carriers has produced severe problems.

The ingestion of preformed bacterial toxins is probably the commonest cause of food poisoning. Far and away, the most frequent offender is food contaminated with staphylococcus; some strains can produce a potent toxin. This agent is responsible for the occasional episodes of food poisoning reported at church suppers or other large gatherings. It results from the early preparation of food which has been kept warm for many hours so that contaminating bacteria have a chance to grow and produce toxins. Usually, staphyloccal food poisoning results in the onset of violent gastrointestinal problems (nausea, vomiting, and diarrhea) within one to three hours after ingestion. In general, the episode is over in 6 to 8 hours.

The most severe form of toxin ingestion is **botulism.** Frequently fatal, this disease usually results from eating improperly canned food in which the spore of the bacterium has grown and developed its toxin. Symptoms develop as long as 24 hours after ingestion and may take weeks to subside if the patient survives.

In general, the EMT should not try to separate specific causes of acute gastrointestinal problems from one another. Transport to the emergency department is warranted for diagnosis. In obvious instances in which two or more individuals in one group have the same problem, it is wise to bring along the suspected food.

Plant Poisoning

Several thousand cases of poisoning from plants occur each year; some are severe. Many household plants are poisonous if they are accidentally ingested, especially by children who like to nibble strange-looking leaves. Some poisonous plants cause local irritation of the skin; others can affect the circulatory system, the gastrointestinal tract, or the central nervous system.

Circulatory Disturbances

Thirty to 50 minutes after ingesting a poisonous plant that affects circulation, the patient may show the classic signs of circulatory collapse: **tachycardia** (a rapid heart rate), falling blood pressure, sweating, weakness, and cold, moist, clammy skin. There are no effective antidotes for plant poisonings that cause circulatory collapse. The treatment is the same as for shock. The patient should be positioned lying down with the legs elevated, oxygen should be administered, and the patient should be transported promptly to the hospital. Vomiting should be induced with syrup of ipecac in the alert and conscious patient. The vomitus should be saved and brought to the hospital. The plant, or at least several loose leaves, should also be brought along for positive identification.

Gastrointestinal (GI) Disturbances

Small amounts of some plants can produce severe gastrointestinal disturbances. The usual symptoms of GI disturbance from plant ingestion are the same as those caused by any other toxic substance: vomiting, diarrhea, and cramps. Symptoms can occur within 20 to 30 minutes after ingestion. If the patient does vomit, the vomitus should be collected. Vomiting should be allowed as needed and the patient transported to the emergency department. Vomiting may be induced at the direction of the poison control center if the plant has been positively identified.

Some agents in plants are locally irritating to oral and throat mucosa. In these instances, it is unwise to increase the irritation. If gastrointestinal symptoms occur very soon after the ingestion, vomiting may help rid the patient of the substance; if symptoms are late, it is unlikely to do much good. Again, taking leaves or the whole plant to the emergency department may help identify the toxin.

Central Nervous System Disturbances

Poisonous plants sometimes affect the central nervous system. Signs of such problems include depression, hyperactivity, excitement, stupor, mental confusion, or coma. The treatment for this type of poisoning is basic life support. It may require complete ventilatory support during transportation. Vomiting should not be induced in patients who show any signs of stupor or coma. The patient should be brought promptly to the hospital, along with a sample of the plant or its leaves if possible.

Skin Irritants

Skin irritation certainly is the most common form of plant poisoning. Problems include itching, burning and local blister formation. One of the most common plants to produce such reactions is poison ivy (Figure 27.2). In general, skin irritation occurs after direct contact with the plant and from a spreading onto the skin of the plant's sap or juice. Contact with these plants rarely produces systemic symptoms such as tachycardia, hypotension, or respiratory distress. The emergency treatment of skin irritants is thorough cleansing with soap and water. This treatment is most effective if done within 30 to 60 minutes of exposure to the poison. Some patients occasionally need medical attention for prolonged symptoms.

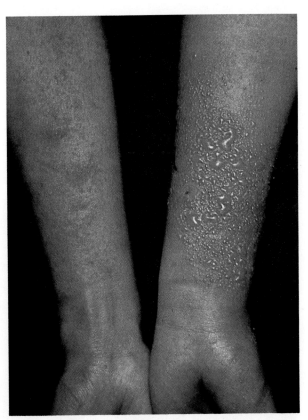

FIGURE 27.2 The sap or juice from poison ivy can cause itching, burning, and blister formation. Severe cases can become infected and require medical treatment.

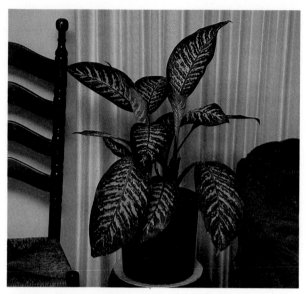

FIGURE 27.3 Dieffenbachia, also called "dumb-cane," is a common houseplant that can cause severe irritation and swelling of the mouth and throat if ingested.

A specific problem of skin or mucous membrane irritation occurs with dieffenbachia, a common houseplant (Figure 27.3). If a leaf of this plant is chewed, a severe irritation of the oral mucous membrane and the lining of the upper airway can occur. This irritation is enough to cause difficulty in swallowing, breathing, and speaking. Partial, and once in a while complete, airway obstruction can occur. For this

reason the plant has been given a conversational name: "dumb cane." The emergency medical treatment involves maintaining an open airway, giving oxygen, and transporting the patient as promptly as possible to the hospital for respiratory support.

STINGS

Many different kinds of insects can inflict pain from stings or bites. Some of these injuries are potentially dangerous. They are associated with stings or bites from bees, wasps, yellow jackets, hornets, certain ants, scorpions, and some spiders.

Bee, Wasp, Hornet, Yellow Jacket, and Ant Stings

There are over 100,000 species of hymenoptera, bees, wasps, hornets. Fatalities from the wide variety of stinging insects far outnumber those from snake bites; 65 percent are related to bee, wasp, and hornet stings. The stinging organ of most bees, wasps, or hornets is a small hollow spine that projects from the abdomen. **Venom** can be injected through this spine directly into the skin. The stinger of the honeybee is barbed so that it cannot be withdrawn. The bee must disembowel itself after stinging to fly away. Wasps or hornets, with unbarbed stingers, can sting repeatedly (Figure 27.4). Identification of the stinging insect is often impossible because it tends to fly away immediately after the injury.

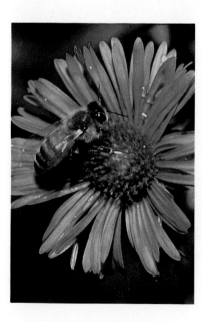

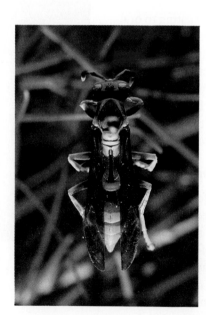

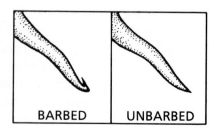

FIGURE 27.4 Most stinging insects inject venom through a small hollow spine that projects from the abdomen. The stinger of the honeybee (left) is barbed and so cannot be withdrawn. Wasps (right) have unbarbed stingers and can sting repeatedly.

Some species of ant, especially the fire ant, can bite repeatedly and often inject a particularly irritating toxin at the bite site. These bites usually occur on the feet and legs. It is not uncommon for the patient to sustain multiple bites within a very short period of time (Figure 27.5).

Symptoms associated with insect stings or bites usually occur at the site of injury. Local symptoms of stings and bites are sudden pain, swelling, heat, and redness about the affected area. Sometimes a whitish firm elevation of the skin (**wheal**) may occur, with itching (Figure 27.6). There is no specific treatment for these injuries; sometimes the application of ice may make them more comfortable. The swelling accompanying insect stings and bites may be considerable and sometimes frightens patients. However, the local manifestations of these stings are not serious.

The stinging organ of a honeybee with its attached muscle can continue to inject venom for up to 20 minutes after the bee has flown away because the stinger has remained in the wound. Anyone who is assisting a person who has been stung by a honeybee should gently attempt to remove the stinger and that portion of the abdomen of the bee by scraping it off the skin. Tweezers or forceps should not be used, as squeezing the stinger may only inject more venom into the patient.

Some insect bites are not noticed by the individual for some hours until a **cellulitis,** or spreading redness and swelling of the skin, has developed. These patients require transport to the emergency department with immobilization of the injured area. Warm, moist packs may produce some comfort. Typically, fire ant bites produce an acute inflammation and ulcerations that are slow to heal.

Anaphylactic Reaction to Stings

Approximately 5 percent of all people are allergic to the venom of the bee, hornet, yellow jacket, or wasp. This allergy accounts for approximately 200 deaths per year. Honeybee venom is commonly associated with allergy and very severe reactions. In an allergic person, the sting of such an insect will usually result in a hypersensitivity reaction called **anaphylaxis.** Generalized itching and burning, **urticaria** (hives) (Figure 27.7), swelling about the lips and tongue, bronchospasm and wheezing, chest tightness and cough, **dyspnea,** anxiety, abdominal

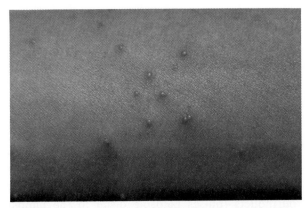
FIGURE 27.5   Fire ants, imported from Brazil, have become a serious problem in several southern states. They inject a particularly irritating toxin. They can bite repeatedly, and some patients sustain multiple bites within a short time.

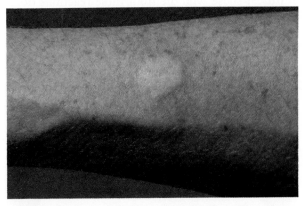
FIGURE 27.6   A wheal is a whitish firm elevation of the skin that occurs after an insect sting or bite.

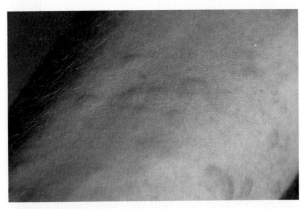
FIGURE 27.7   Hives that appear following a bee, hornet, or wasp sting are one of the warning signs of an impending anaphylactic reaction.

cramps, and occasionally respiratory failure can all occur. Such a reaction can even proceed, if untreated, to death from respiratory obstruction. The rapid development of skin wheals and hives and wheezing respiration should alert the EMT that a hypersensitivity reaction is taking place. Basic life support should be administered at once. This patient must be immediately transported to the hospital with first priority status. Oxygen should be given and preparations made to maintain an airway or give full cardiopulmonary resuscitation. If possible, venous tourniquets (pulses palpable distal to the bands) should be placed above and below the site of the sting to localize the spread of toxin. An attempt should be made to remove the stinger from the wound by gently scraping with the edge of a knife blade. An ice bag placed over the injury site may help to slow the rate of absorption of the toxin. More than two-thirds of those who die from these reactions do so within the first hour after the sting.

Patients who have a history of severe allergic reaction to stings may have at their disposal bee sting kits (Figure 27.8). Commercially manufactured, they are usually prescribed specifically for the hypersensitive person by a physician. The kits usually con-

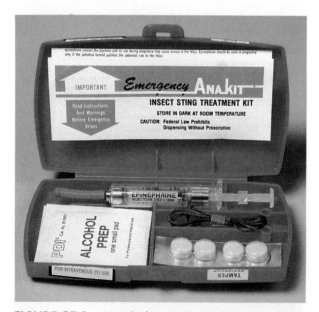

FIGURE 27.8 A typical prescription bee sting kit. The syringe is loaded with two, premeasured doses of epinephrine solution. Instructions for proper administration, including self-administration, are attached to the kit.

tain the medication epinephrine prepared in a syringe and ready for injection. **Epinephrine** is a rapidly acting agent which produces bronchodilation to reverse the effects of the allergen on the airway. It has a short period of action and produces acute relief. Most kits also contain some oral or intravenous **antihistamine.** These agents, of which a variety are available, are specific to counter the production of histamine, which is believed to be responsible for the attack. Usually, they are slower in onset of action and effective over a longer period than epinephrine. The patient who is able to do so should be assisted in administering these life-saving medications. Specific instructions for the use of epinephrine should be in the kit. In the absence of instructions, ½ ml of 1/1000 epinephrine solution should be injected **intramuscularly** (into a muscle) or **subcutaneously** (just below the skin). Frequently, more than one injection over a period of time will be required as an anaphylactic reaction develops and progresses. Injections may be needed at intervals of 5 to 15 minutes.

Having been injected with epinephrine, the patient will experience tachycardia and, on occasion, increased anxiety or nervousness. The emergency care outlined earlier for support for this patient should be completed and the patient transported promptly to the hospital.

Scorpion Stings

Scorpions and spiders are related, in that both are eight-legged insects from the same biological group (Arachnida). Scorpions are rare; they are found primarily in the Southwest and in deserts. Scorpions have a venom gland and a stinger at the end of their tail (Figure 27.9). Except for the sting of a specific scorpion in the desert of the Southwest, the Arizona scorpion, these injuries are ordinarily very painful but not dangerous. Only 4 percent of fatalities related to insect stings are associated with scorpions. Localized swelling, pain, and discoloration result from a scorpion sting. Arizona scorpion venom may produce a severe systemic reaction that brings about circulatory collapse, severe muscle contractions, excessive salivation, hypertension, convulsions, and cardiac failure. The emergency treatment for this sting is basic life support. **Antivenin,** a serum that contains antibodies that counteract the venom, is available but must be administered by a physician.

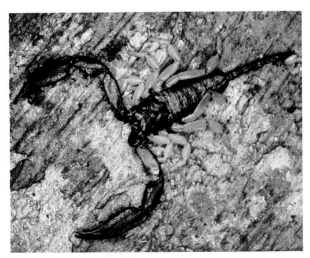

FIGURE 27.9 The sting of a scorpion is more painful than dangerous. A venom gland and stinger are located at the end of the scorpion's tail. Only the Arizona scorpion, which habitates the desert of the Southwest, is dangerous. Its venom can cause a severe systemic reaction.

An EMT who has a patient with a suspected sting from an Arizona scorpion should notify medical control as soon as possible. All of the elements of basic life support should be administered and the patient transported as rapidly as possible to the emergency department. Remember, however, that only the Arizona scorpion can cause this serious problem. This particular scorpion species does not reside anywhere else in the country.

BITES

Spider Bites

Thirty-one percent of fatalities associated with insect stings and bites are related to spiders. Spiders are numerous and widespread in the United States. Two species, the black widow spider and the brown recluse spider, are able to deliver serious, sometimes even life-threatening, bites. Most other spiders will bite, but these injuries do not produce serious complications.

Black Widow Spider

The black widow spider is approximately 1-inch long with its legs extended; it is not particularly large. It is glossy black and has a distinctive, bright red-orange marking in the shape of an hourglass on its belly (Figure 27.10). Black widow spiders are found in every state except Alaska. They prefer dry, dim places around buildings, in woodpiles, and among debris.

Commonly, a black widow spider bite is overlooked. The victim may not recall the bite itself, since the area may become numb after the bite. The venom is **neurotoxic** (poisonous to nerve tissue) and directly attacks spinal nerve centers. Thus, the major problem with these bites lies in their systemic manifestations. Severe cramps, with boardlike rigidity of the abdominal muscles, tightness in the chest, and difficulty in breathing occur over 24 hours. Abdominal symptoms are more commonly seen with bites in the lower half of the body. Chest symptoms tend to accompany bites on the upper extremities and the upper part of the body. Other complaints include dizziness, sweating, vomiting, nausea, and skin rashes. Generally, the signs and symptoms subside over 48 hours, but the muscle cramps and ensuing pain can be agonizing.

Although the complaints following the bites are severe, death is not common (63 recorded in ten years, from 1950 to 1960). A specific antivenin is available. Its use is reserved for very severe bites, the aged or very feeble, and children under the age of five. It will be administered, if necessary, by a physician.

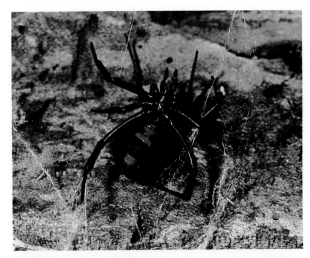

FIGURE 27.10 The bite of a black widow spider, distinguished by its glossy black color and bright red-orange hourglass markings on its abdomen, can cause severe, even life-threatening injuries.

In general, emergency treatment for a black widow spider bite is basic life support for the patient in respiratory distress who needs it. Much more commonly, the patient will require relief from pain. The individual often is unaware of having been bitten or where the bite is located. If the site can be identified, putting ice against it may slow the absorption of toxin. The EMT should transport the patient to the emergency department as soon as possible for treatment of the symptoms of pain and muscle rigidity. It is also important for the EMT, if possible, to identify the spider and bring it with the patient to the hospital.

Brown Recluse Spider

Dull brown in color, the brown recluse spider is somewhat smaller than the black widow (Figure 27.11). It has a dark violin-shaped mark on its back, which can be easily seen from above. Although found mostly in the southern and central United States, it is currently moving to other areas. The spider takes its name from the fact that it tends to live in dark areas, corners, old unused buildings, under rocks, and in woodpiles. It has moved indoors in cooler areas and inhabits closets, drawers, cellars, and old piles of clothing.

The bite from the brown recluse, in contrast to the black widow, produces local rather than systemic problems. The venom of the brown recluse spider causes severe local tissue damage, which will result

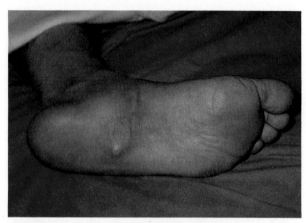

FIGURE 27.12 The venom from the bite of a brown recluse spider causes severe local tissue damage, which, if not treated promptly, can result in gangrene and a large, nonhealing ulcer.

in local gangrene and a large, nonhealing ulcer if not treated promptly (Figure 27.12). Typically, the bite is not painful initially but becomes so within hours. The area becomes red, swollen, and tender, and it develops a pale, mottled cyanotic center. A small blister may form. Over the next several days, a large scab of dead skin, fat, and debris will develop and deepen to produce a large ulcer.

Systemic symptoms and signs from brown recluse spider bites rarely occur. When they do, the emergency treatment is basic life support and transport to the emergency department. No specific antivenin exists for this toxin, and the only effective treatment to avoid the long-term painful ulceration is prompt surgical excision of the area. Thus, emergency treatment for a suspected brown recluse spider bite without systemic symptoms is also prompt transportation to the emergency department. Again, it is helpful if the spider can be identified and brought to the hospital along with the patient.

Snake Bites

Snake bite is a worldwide problem of some significance. More than 300,000 injuries from snake bites occur annually; 30,000 to 40,000 deaths result. The greatest number of the fatalities occur in Southeast Asia and in India (25,000 to 30,000), and in South America (3,000 to 4,000). Snake bites are fairly common in the United States: 40,000 to 50,000 are reported annually. Approximately 7,000 of them are caused by poisonous snakes. However, fatalities in

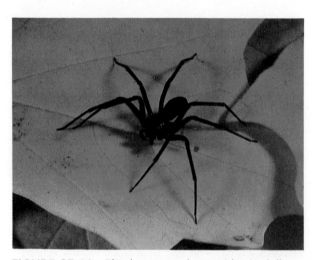

FIGURE 27.11 The brown recluse spider is dull brown in color and has a dark, violin-shaped mark on its back.

the United States from snake bites are extremely rare: about 15 a year for the entire country.

Of the approximately 150 different species of snakes in the United States, only four are poisonous: the rattlesnake, the copperhead, the cottonmouth (water) moccasin, and the coral snake. Only Alaska, Hawaii, and Maine do not have at least one species of venomous reptile. As a general rule, these creatures are retiring and timid. They usually do not bite unless provoked, angered, or accidentally injured (as when one steps on them). There are a few exceptions to these rules. Moccasins are often rather aggressive snakes, and certainly very little provocation is needed to annoy a rattlesnake. Coral snakes, on the other hand, are very shy and retiring and usually bite only when being handled.

Most snake bites occur between April and October when the animals are active. Most involve young males, and most occur within a very few states. Texas reports the largest number of bites. Other states with a major concentration of snake bites are Louisiana, Georgia, Oklahoma, North Carolina, Arkansas, West Virginia, and Mississippi. EMTs in these areas should be thoroughly familiar with the handling of snake bite problems.

When responding to a snake bite, it is extremely important for the EMT to identify whether **envenomation** (deposit of venom into the wound) has occurred. In one classification of all snake bites throughout the United States, 27 percent were found to have had no envenomation and an additional 37 percent were rated as minimal. Thus, only one-third of snake bites in general result in severe local or systemic problems. There are several reasons why envenomation does not occur. Most commonly, the snake recently has struck another animal and has exhausted its supply of venom.

Nonpoisonous snakes can also cause bites, which usually leave a horseshoe shape of tooth marks. With the exception of the coral snake, poisonous vipers in the United States all have hollow fangs in the roof of the mouth, which literally inject the poison from two sacs at the back of the head. The characteristic appearance of the poisonous snake bite, therefore, is two small puncture wounds, usually about a half-inch apart, with surrounding discoloration, swelling, and pain (Figure 27.13). Some poisonous snakes have teeth as well as fangs. The mere presence of tooth marks does not necessarily mean that a poisonous

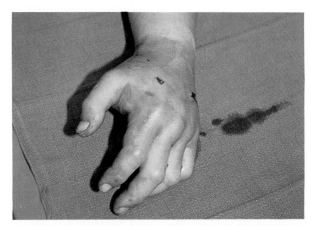

FIGURE 27.13 The presence of fang marks signal a poisonous snake bite. Swelling and discoloration of the hand indicate envenomation.

snake attack could not have occurred. Fang marks, on the other hand, are a clear indication of a bite by a poisonous snake. In this situation the EMT must look for signs of envenomation.

Pit Vipers

Rattlesnakes, copperheads, and cottonmouth (water) moccasins are all pit vipers (Figure 27.14). The head of the pit viper is triangular and flat; there is a small pit located just behind the nostril and in front of each eye. The pupil of the eye is vertical and slitlike. The pit is a heat-sensing organ that

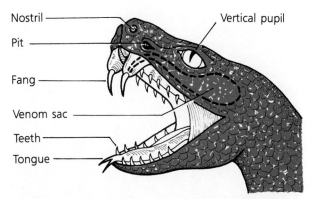

FIGURE 27.14 Rattlesnakes, copperheads, and cottonmouth (water) moccasins all have hollow fangs in the roof of the mouth, which inject poison from two sacs at the back of the head. These snakes are called pit vipers because they have small, heat-sensing organs (pits) located in front of their eyes that allow them to strike at warm targets, even in the dark.

allows the snake to strike accurately at any warm target, especially in the dark when it cannot see. Localization by the pits is much more accurate than that provided by the eye. The fangs of the pit viper normally lie flat against the roof of the mouth. When the snake is striking, the mouth opens wide and the fangs extend, so that if the mouth strikes an object, the fangs will penetrate. The fangs are hollow adapted teeth that act much like hypodermic needles. They are hinged to swing back and forth as the mouth opens. They are connected to a sac containing a reservoir of venom, which in turn is attached to a poison gland. The gland itself is an adapted salivary gland that produces powerful enzymes which digest and destroy tissue. A purpose of the venom is to kill the small animal the snake attacked and also to start the digestive process prior to the animal's being eaten by the snake.

Among the pit vipers, the commonest is the rattlesnake (Figure 27.15). Several different species of rattlesnake exist. Apart from the features of the pit vipers in general, rattlesnakes can usually be identified by the rattle on the tail. The rattle is actually numerous layers of shed skin which come to lie against a small nubbin on the end of the tail. Each year the skin is not completely shed; a small piece remains. As the snake sheds annually, the dried skin

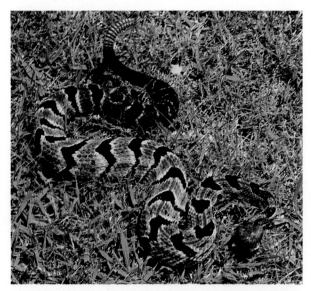

FIGURE 27.15 The rattlesnake is the commonest of the pit vipers. The "rattle" is actually layers of shed skin that lie against a small nubin on the end of the tail.

remnants that do not come off completely form the characteristic rattle. Generally, rattlesnakes have many patterns of color, often with a diamond pattern. They can develop to 6 feet or more in length.

Copperheads are smaller than rattlesnakes. They are usually 2 to 3 feet long and have a characteristic reddish coppery color with brown or red cross-bands (Figure 27.16). Shyer than rattlesnakes, they inhabit woodpiles and abandoned dwellings, often close to areas of habitation. They account for most of the venomous snake bites in the eastern United States. Fatalities are almost never seen with these injuries.

Cottonmouth moccasins grow to about 4 feet. Also called water moccasins, these snakes are olive or brown, with black cross-bands and a yellow under-surface (Figure 27.17). They are water snakes with a particularly aggressive pattern of behavior. Although fatalities from these snake bites are rare, tissue destruction from the venom may be severe.

The sign of envenomation by a pit viper is severe burning pain at the site of the injury, followed by swelling and discoloration. These signs are evident within 5 to 10 minutes after the bite has occurred and spread slowly over the next 8 to 36 hours. Bleeding under the skin (**ecchymosis**) causes bluish discoloration. An envenomated bite is painful and ecchymotic. Systemic signs, which may or may not occur, include weakness, sweating, fainting, and shock.

Occasionally, the patient bitten by a snake will faint. Usually this situation is corrected promptly when the patient is supine (lying flat). Consciousness returns, and the episode, triggered by fright, is temporary. A fainting spell should not be confused with shock, which ordinarily develops much later after the bite has occurred.

The venom of the pit viper causes localized destruction of all tissues: protein, fat, and entire cells. It can also interfere significantly with the body's clotting mechanism and cause bleeding at various distant sites. Tissue destruction locally starts from the moment of envenomation. If an hour has elapsed from the time the patient was bitten without local signs of envenomation (no swelling, no discoloration, no severe local pain), it is safe to assume that envenomation has not occurred.

The emergency treatment of snake bites from pit vipers is directed primarily at local containment of venom and then at the systemic effects. The EMT

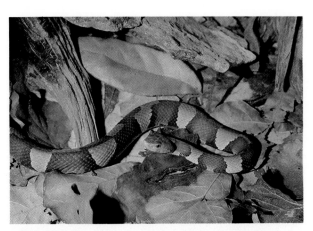

FIGURE 27.16 The copperhead is a reddish, copper-colored pit viper that accounts for most of the venomous snake bites in the eastern United States.

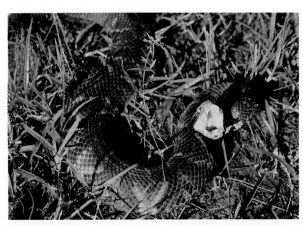

FIGURE 27.17 Cottonmouth (water) moccasins are pit vipers that live in the water. They are aggressive snakes whose bites cause serious tissue destruction.

should carry out the following steps when treating a bite from a pit viper.

1. Calm and reassure the patient. Place the patient supine and explain that staying quiet will decrease the spread of any venom through the system.
2. Locate the bite area; clean it gently with soap and water or a mild antiseptic.
3. Wrap soft rubber tubes about the extremity above and below the fang marks, and tighten them just enough to occlude the venous circulation (a venous tourniquet). The distal pulse in the extremity should not disappear. The purpose of this maneuver is to limit the spread of the venom through the veins of the extremity.
4. Immobilize the extremity with a splint.
5. Monitor the vital signs: blood pressure, pulse, and respiration.
6. If there are any signs of shock, place the patient in the shock position and give oxygen.
7. If the snake has been killed, as is often the case, bring it with you. Identification of the offending snake is extremely important in administering the correct antivenin.
8. Transport the patient promptly to the hospital. Notify the hospital that you are bringing in a snake bite patient; and, if possible, describe the snake.

9. Be alert for vomiting. Patients may often do so from anxiety rather than from the effects of the toxin itself.
10. Do not give anything by mouth, especially alcohol.
11. In the relatively rare instance of the bite occurring on the trunk rather than on the extremity, it will be impossible to use tourniquets and splinting. Keep the patient supine and as quiet as possible and transport as quickly as possible.

If the patient shows no sign of envenomation, basic life support should be provided as needed, a sterile dressing should be placed over the suspected bite area, venous constricting bands should be put above and below the bite, and the patient should be immobilized. The same procedure applies for the patient who shows early signs of envenomation but who can be delivered to the hospital in under 30 minutes.

The patient who shows early signs of envenomation but cannot be delivered to a hospital in under 30 minutes may require local removal of the venom by suction. This treatment should be carried out only on the specific instructions of a physician. After a bite, the venom remains locally in the tissue for about 30 minutes. Some of it can be mechanically removed by making a small, one-half-inch incision through the skin in the long axis of the extremity over the fang mark. The incision should be just deep enough to go through the skin so that subcutaneous fat is visible (one-quarter of an inch). To cut any deeper would risk injury of important tendons, nerves, or blood vessels. The suction cup from a snake-bite kit should be applied to suck out the poison mechanically.

This technique — incision and suction — should only be used on a bite of the extremity. It should never be used on the head or trunk. Nor should it be done without the direction of medical control. It is applicable only in the patient showing definite signs of envenomation less than 30 minutes after the bite. This process has come under much criticism because many snake bites deposit venom much deeper than the skin and subcutaneous fat. In these cases, signs of envenomation will be present, but the "cut and suck" technique offers little help because the venom has been deposited too deeply.

All suspected snake bite patients should be brought to the emergency department whether they show signs of immediate envenomation or not. Whether or not envenomation has occurred, these wounds are treated like all other deep puncture wounds to prevent infection. EMTs who work in an area where poisonous snakes are known to live should always keep a snake bite kit in the ambulance. They should also know the address of the nearest facility where antivenin is available. It may be a nearby zoo, the local or public state health department, or a local community hospital.

Coral Snake

The coral snake is a small, very colorful reptile with a series of bright red, yellow, and black bands that completely encircle its body (Figure 27.18). Many harmless snakes are colored in a fashion similar to the coral snake. The difference is that the red and yellow bands of the coral snake are next to another, completely encircling the body. There is a rhyme for remembering this fact: "Red on yellow will kill a fellow; red on black, venom will lack."

The coral snake lives primarily in Florida and in the desert Southwest. It is not found in the northern regions of the United States. In fact, it is only rarely found at all, since it is shy and will only bite when provoked or handled. The coral snake is not a pit viper; the head is not triangular, there are no pits, and there are no projecting fangs. A relative of the cobra, the coral snake has tiny fangs and injects

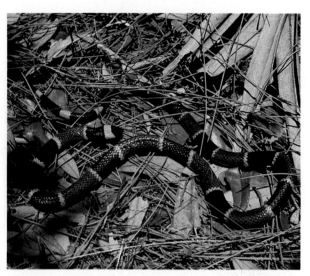

FIGURE 27.18   The coral snake is not a pit viper. It injects venom with its teeth, causing paralysis of the nervous system.

the venom with its teeth by a chewing motion, not an injection. Because of its small mouth and teeth and limited jaw expansion, the coral snake usually bites its victim on a small part of the body, especially a finger or toe. Following the bite of a coral snake, one or more punctures or scratchlike wounds can be found in the area.

The danger of this particular snake is that its venom is a powerful toxin that causes paralysis of the nervous system. Usually, there are minimal or no local manifestations of a coral snake bite. However, within a few hours bizarre behavior will occur, followed by progressive paralysis of eye movements and respiration as a result of the toxic effects on the nervous system.

Treatment, either emergency or long term, depends on positive identification of the snake. Antivenin is available, but most hospitals or doctors must order it from a central supply area, often in another city. Therefore, the need for it should be made known as soon as possible. The steps for emergency care of a coral snake bite are as follows:

1. Immediately quiet and reassure the patient.
2. Flush the area of the bite with one to two quarts of warm, soapy water to wash away any poison left on the surface of the skin.
3. Lightly apply soft rubber tubes around the extremity above and below the bite.

4. Splint the extremity to minimize movement and the spread of venom at the site.
5. Check the patient's vital signs and continue to monitor them.
6. Keep the patient warm and elevate the lower extremities to help prevent shock.
7. Give artificial ventilation with oxygen if needed.
8. Transport promptly to the emergency department, giving advance notice that the patient has been bitten by a coral snake.
9. Give nothing by mouth.

The incision and suction technique is not done in the case of a coral snake bite, as there is little local effect from this injury. The danger is to the central nervous system from an absorbed neurotoxin. Antivenin is the most effective means of control.

Dog Bites and Rabies

The exact incidence of dog bites is unknown. Most people who are bitten by dogs do not report the bite to a physician and do not require the services of an EMT. Dog bites, however, are potentially serious problems. The animal's mouth is heavily contaminated with virulent bacteria. If the bite occurs on the hand or the face, serious infection may result. All of the wounds are punctures which require **tetanus prophylaxis** (treatment to prevent tetanus, a potentially fatal infectious disease characterized by extreme body rigidity and muscle spasms). All dog bites should be considered as potentially infected wounds.

Often the patient is extremely upset and frightened. Most dog bites are not serious; therefore, calm reassurance on the part of the EMT is extremely important. Nevertheless, dog bites should be treated by a physician. Usually antibiotics are given. The wound may or may not need to be **sutured** (require stitches). Certainly, antitetanus measures must be considered for each patient.

The emergency treatment for dog bites of any severity is to place a dry, sterile dressing over the wound and transport the patient to the emergency department as promptly as possible. Occasionally, dog bites result in mangled, complex wounds that require much surgical expertise for repair.

A major concern with dog bites is the spread of rabies. **Rabies** is an acute viral infection of the central nervous system. Ordinarily, the virus is present in saliva of the infected carrier or host and is transmitted by biting or by licking an open wound. All warm-blooded animals can be affected. Once contracted and well established, rabies is almost always fatal. Prevention of the disease in a bitten person often requires long and complex treatment with antibiotics and vaccine. Although rabies is extremely rare today, particularly with widespread inoculation of pets, it still exists. There are still stray dogs that have not been inoculated and that could be carriers of the disease. Certain other animals — squirrels, bats, foxes, skunks, and raccoons — may also carry rabies. Each of these animals has been implicated in serious human bites.

Established rabies is still a very serious and fatal disease. Antibiotics do not prevent its development. Once the disease is well developed in an animal or patient, there is no effective treatment. A rabid animal (one with rabies) may act perfectly normal, may appear vicious, may salivate excessively, or may act in an abnormal way. One cannot tell for certain if an animal is rabid by its behavior. If the animal has been inoculated against rabies, it ordinarily will have a tag so stating on its collar. It is, therefore, very important to identify the fact if the animal can be located. Usually, in the case of dog bites, the dog is a pet and can be identified. If it does not have a rabies tag, it should be captured (not killed) by an animal control officer and turned over to the health department for observation. If the animal is then suspected of having rabies, it is killed and the brain studied. Results of this study (positive or negative) for rabies are needed to diagnose the presence of the disease in the bitten patient.

When the animal cannot be found or identified, then the patient usually must undergo a series of rabies inoculations. If started early enough, these inoculations will prevent rabies from developing. They are painful, possess some dangerous side effects, and are administered over a two-week period. In 1980, a new rabies vaccine was developed from material grown in human tissue. This new vaccine is much simpler to use and has fewer side effects. It is expensive and difficult to produce and may be in short supply. The EMT should know where the local rabies control center is located and also where the closest institution that has human rabies vaccine is located.

Human Bites

A somewhat neglected area of emergency medical treatment is the human bite. It is relatively uncommon but potentially one of the most severe injuries seen today. The human mouth contains an exceptionally wide range of bacteria, some of which live best without oxygen. The variety of germs contained in the human mouth is greater than the types found in the mouths of dogs or many other animals. For this reason, any human bite that has penetrated the skin must be regarded as a very serious injury. Similarly, any laceration caused by a human tooth may result in serious infection (Figure 27.19). If un-

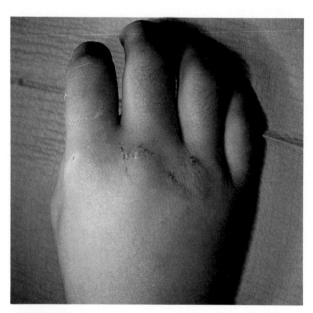

FIGURE 27.19 The human bite is a very serious injury because if left untreated, it will become the source of significant spreading infection.

treated, these wounds will almost certainly be followed by significant spreading infection. The emergency treatment for human bites is prompt immobilization of the area with a splint or bandage, application of a dry, sterile dressing, and transport to the emergency department for surgical cleansing of the wound and antibiotic therapy.

Injuries from Marine Animals

In recent years there has been a good deal of publicity concerning shark bites. They remain extremely rare. The emergency treatment of a large marine animal bite is the same as for any other major open wound. The patient should be removed from the water, hemorrhage controlled, dressings and splints applied, shock treated, and the patient transported to the emergency department promptly.

Many other injuries may result from marine animals, but none of them is as dramatic or as potentially life-threatening as the large marine animal bite. With the exception of the shark and barracuda, most marine creatures are not aggressive and will not deliberately attack. Injuries from these animals occur when they are accidentally stepped on or otherwise provoked.

The most frequent injuries from marine animals occur from swimming into the tentacles of a jellyfish, stepping on the back of a stingray, or falling on a sea urchin. EMTs should be familiar with marine life in their locality. Stings from the tentacles of a jellyfish, a Portuguese man-of-war, various anemones, corals, or hydras can be treated by removing the patient from the water and pouring alcohol on the affected area. The area is then sprinkled with meat tenderizer — a proteolytic enzyme — and finally with talcum powder. This treatment will inactivate the poison that has been deposited on the skin and usually is the only treatment necessary. Alcohol will fix or denature the toxins, and meat tenderizer will destroy them. On very rare occasions, a systemic allergic reaction may result from the sting of one of these animals. The patient should be treated for anaphylactic shock; basic life support must be given and the patient transported promptly to the hospital.

Punctures from the spines of urchins, stingrays, or certain spiny fish such as a catfish can best be treated by immobilizing the affected area and soaking it in hot water for 30 minutes. The water should be as hot as the patient can stand without risking a burn. Toxins from these animals are heat-sensitive, and dramatic relief from local pain often occurs just from the application of hot water. Also, allergic reactions may occur with injections from these animals. As with any other puncture wound, there is always the possibility that tetanus and other infections could develop. These patients should be taken to the emergency department for appropriate treatment for these problems.

Some sea animals may cause injuries by minor bites such as those from nonpoisonous water snakes.

These bites are treated as any other bites with sterile dressings and transport for evaluation and tetanus prophylaxis.

Many fish are poisonous if eaten. The emergency treatment of such poisoning is the same as for any other poisoning: basic life support, prevention of injury from convulsions, and prompt transport of the patient to the emergency department. Other rare conditions include shocks from electric eels or skin rashes from marine parasites. In general, these injuries are mild. Panic from contact with electric eels can be the most impressive part of this particular injury. Table 27.1 provides a quick reference for the management of common marine organism injuries.

TABLE 27.1   Guide to Diagnosis and Emergency Treatment of Marine Animal Injuries

Type of Injury	Marine Animal Involved	Emergency Treatment	Possible Complications

Trauma (bites and lacerations)	Major wounds by
	  Shark
	  Barracuda
	  Alligator gar
		Control bleeding
		Prevent shock
		Give basic life support
		Splint the injury
		Secure prompt medical care
			Shock
			Infections

	Minor wounds by
	  Moray eel
	  Turtle
	  Corals
		Cleanse wound
		Splint the injury	

Sting (by tentacles)	Jellyfish Portuguese man-of-war Anemones Corals Hydras	Inactivate the toxin with alcohol, meat tenderizer, and talcum powder[1]	Allergic reactions Respiratory arrest
Puncture (by spines)	Urchins Cone shells Stingrays Spiny fish (catfish, toad, or oyster fish)	Inactivate with hot water[2]	Allergic reactions Collapse Infections Tetanus Granuloma formation
Poisoning (by ingestion)[3]	Puffer fish Scromboids (tuna species) Ciguatera (large colored fish) Paralytic shellfish	Give basic life support; prevent self-injury from convulsions	Allergic reactions Asthmatic reactions Paresthesia, numbness Temperature reversal phenomena Respiratory arrest and circulatory collapse

Miscellaneous:
  Shocks
  Skin rashes
	Electric fish
	Marine parasites
		No treatment required; injuries usually self-limiting	Electric fish or electric eel may precipitate a panic reaction

[1]The intense burning pain resulting from the sting of the jellyfish is produced by nematocysts (stinging cells) on the tentacles. Even when the sea creature is washed up on shore, the stinging cells can remain potent for as long as several days. In treating the sting, 95-percent alcohol "fixes" the nematocysts on the skin and prevents further stinging, and the meat tenderizer neutralizes the protein toxin of the nematocyst. Powder dries the area and causes the cells to stick together so they can be more readily removed by scraping.

[2]A toxin is introduced with some of the puncture wounds from this group. In any case, the wounds are excruciatingly painful. It appears that the foreign material or poison introduced into the wound is heat-sensitive. Dramatic treatment results occur with soaking in quite hot water for thirty to sixty minutes. Be careful, however, not to scald the patient with water that is too hot, as the pain of the wound will mask the normal reaction to heat.

[3]Should ingestion of a poisonous fish be suspected, reference to Halstead's *Poisoning and Venomous Marine Animals of the World* or seeking immediate assistance from poison control centers is suggested.

YOU ARE THE EMT...

1. What circumstances would lead you to suspect that a poisoning has occurred? What should you do?
2. Describe when you would induce vomiting, how you would induce vomiting, and when you would *not* induce vomiting.
3. Your patient has been stung by a wasp and she tells you she is allergic to "bees." List the symptoms of an anaphylactic reaction and the emergency treatment you should be prepared to give.
4. A camper has been bitten by a water moccasin. Is this snake poisonous? If so, how do you determine if envenomation has occurred? Describe the steps needed to treat this patient.

Heart Disease

28

OVERVIEW

Heart attacks and other forms of heart disease strike over 4 million people a year in the United States. Currently, heart disease causes more than 700,000 deaths annually. Although death rates in recent years have tended to level off rather than increase, heart disease remains a leading cause of death. In fact, about one-third of the population will die as a result of heart disease. For EMTs, these statistics mean that on many occasions they will attend patients with some form of heart disease.

Chapter 28 begins with a basic definition of heart function and then explains how improper function results in heart disease. The chapter next describes angina (severe chest pain) and acute myocardial infarction (death of the heart muscle). The EMT must become familiar with the symptoms of these two major types of heart disease and with the emergency treatments each type calls for. Chapter 28 also deals with the symptoms and treatment of chronic congestive heart failure. The final section of the chapter discusses the emergency treatment of patients who have had prior heart surgery or who have a cardiac pacemaker.

OBJECTIVES

The objectives of Chapter 28 are to

- understand the function of the heart and how it meets demands for an increased output of blood.
- describe angina pectoris and learn how nitroglycerin is used to relieve the pain of angina.
- describe acute myocardial infarction (AMI) and its consequences.
- learn how to identify the signs and physical findings of AMI and how to approach the patient with suspected AMI.
- understand the causes and treatment of chronic congestive heart failure.
- learn how to treat AMI in the patient who has had a coronary artery bypass.
- learn how to treat the patient with pacemaker failure.

CARDIAC FUNCTION

In order to carry out its pumping function, the **myocardium** (heart muscle) must have a continuous supply of oxygen and nutrients. The coronary arteries carry oxygen and nutrients to the myocardium. When the heart must increase its work, as during periods of physical exertion and stress, the myocardium requires more oxygen and therefore more blood flow. In the normal heart, the increased need for blood is easily supplied by dilation of the coronary arteries, which increases blood flow. **Arteriosclerosis,** which is a thickening and destruction of the arterial walls caused by fatty deposits within them, interferes with the ability of the coronary arteries to dilate and to carry additional blood. Indeed, arteriosclerosis can cause complete **occlusion,** or blockage, of a coronary artery and thus cut off the supply of oxygen and nutrients to that part of the myocardium. **Acute myocardial infarction (AMI),** the death of the heart muscle, and **angina pectoris,** which is chest pain caused by an inadequate flow of blood to the heart muscle, are each conditions that occur from too little oxygen. Each represents a degree of coronary arteriosclerosis.

The **coronary arteries** originate at the first part of the **aorta,** just above the aortic valve. The right coronary artery supplies the right ventricle and, in most people, part of the left ventricle. The left coronary artery divides into the left anterior descending and the left circumflex arteries, and both supply the left ventricle (Figure 28.1).

Arteriosclerosis, the disease process that damages the coronary arteries, can attack other arteries of the body as well. The disease begins when a deposit of **cholesterol** is laid down just below the inner wall of an artery. Deposits may start accumulating as early as age 18. As a person ages, more of this fatty material is deposited, and the **lumen,** or the inside diameter of the artery, narrows. The deposits grow until they finally disrupt the inner wall of the artery. Blood clots can form easily on this damaged blood vessel lining.

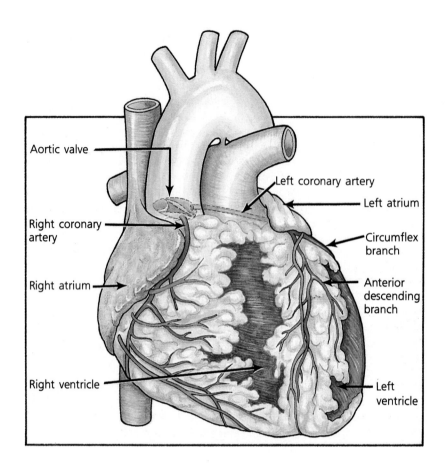

Aortic valve

Right coronary artery

Right atrium

Right ventricle

Left coronary artery

Left atrium

Circumflex branch

Anterior descending branch

Left ventricle

FIGURE 28.1 The coronary arteries carry the blood supply to the heart. The right coronary artery supplies the right ventricle, and the left coronary artery supplies the left ventricle.

Calcium deposited within the fatty material narrows the arteries still further (Figure 28.2) and significantly limits their ability to dilate. By age 40 or 50, damage of the coronary arteries may be so extensive as to limit their ability to increase blood flow at times of maximum need. Therefore, during physical activity or emotional stress, the oxygen supply to the heart can no longer meet the heart's requirement.

By no means is arteriosclerosis restricted to individuals over 40, even though in the United States, the peak incidence of heart disease occurs in the decades between 40 and 70. The EMT must be aware, however, that heart attack and angina can occur any time from the teens to the 90s. A 28-year-old person with chest pain is not "too young to have a heart attack."

Many risk factors have been identified as indicators of those who might suffer a heart attack. In general, they are divided into three groups:

1. Major factors that can be controlled
2. Major factors that cannot be controlled
3. Minor factors

The major controllable factors are high blood pressure, an elevated level of cholesterol in the blood, and smoking. The uncontrollable major factors are age, sex, heredity, and the presence of diseases such as diabetes. Minor factors include, among others, personality traits and obesity. The immediate cause of death is usually acute myocardial infarction (AMI) or death of the heart muscle. **Infarction** means the death of tissue because its blood supply has been cut off.

ANGINA PECTORIS

If the heart has too little oxygen for its needs for more than several seconds, severe chest pain will occur. The pain is characteristically crushing — it takes your breath away. Some people describe it as "squeezing" or "like somebody standing on my chest." This pain is called angina pectoris, or simply angina. Since the occurrence of angina pectoris indicates coronary artery disease, it is important to understand the pain and to recognize it.

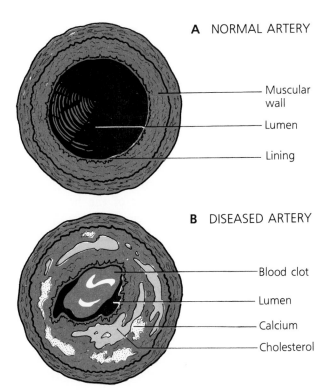

A NORMAL ARTERY

— Muscular wall

— Lumen

— Lining

B DISEASED ARTERY

— Blood clot

— Lumen

— Calcium

— Cholesterol

FIGURE 28.2 Cross-section of a coronary artery: (a) the lumen of a normal artery is unobstructed; (b) the lumen of a diseased artery is narrowed by cholesterol and calcium deposits and eventually obstructed by a blood clot.

Angina pectoris occurs when the need for oxygen by the heart exceeds the supply. It generally occurs at times when the heart is working hard — during periods of physical or emotional stress. The principal characteristic of angina pectoris is pain that comes on with exertion and is relieved by rest. The pain is usually felt under the **sternum,** or breast bone. It can radiate to the jaw, to the arms (especially the left arm), or to the **epigastrium** (the upper-middle region of the abdomen). The pain usually lasts from 3 to 8 minutes, and rarely longer than 10 minutes. It may be associated with shortness of breath, nausea, or sweating. It disappears promptly when the oxygen supply to the heart equals or exceeds the demand — that is, when stress lessens or ceases as the patient relaxes or when oxygen is given. Although angina pectoris is painful, it does not mean death of the myocardium. Nor does it lead to the death of the patient or to permanent heart damage. It is, however, an indicator that the person has some degree of destructive coronary artery disease.

Several variations of these specific symptoms may occur in patients with angina, and the EMT must be familiar with them. Occasionally, a patient will deny pain as such but will admit discomfort — the "squeezing" sensation or tightness in the chest mentioned earlier, or perhaps difficulty in breathing. Sometimes the patient complains of discomfort or pain not in the chest, but at a point of referral, such as the jaw, left arm, or epigastrium. Often such complaints are followed by the patient saying, "It's probably indigestion," or "My ulcer is kicking up." By no means is physical exertion the only cause of angina. Emotional stress, a large meal, or common anxiety may also trigger an attack. The EMT should keep this in mind if angina pectoris is suspected.

Angina is treated with a medication called **nitroglycerin.** It comes in the form of a small white pill, about one-half the size of an aspirin tablet (Figure 28.3). The pill is placed under the tongue and works

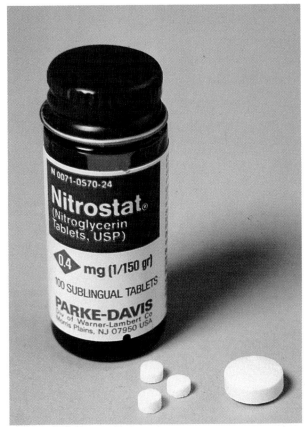

FIGURE 28.3 Nitroglycerin tablets are small white pills, about one-half the size of a standard aspirin tablet. They are placed under the tongue to relieve the pain of angina pectoris.

in seconds. Nitroglycerin relaxes vascular smooth muscle, dilates coronary arteries, and increases blood flow and the supply of oxygen to the heart muscle. It relieves the pain of angina pectoris. Nitroglycerin also relaxes and dilates blood vessels in the brain, sometimes causing a severe headache. In addition, it can be used to relax smooth muscle in the gastrointestinal tract.

ACUTE MYOCARDIAL INFARCTION (AMI)

If the narrowing of the coronary artery by arteriosclerosis is very severe, or if a blood clot forms inside the coronary artery, the oxygen supply in the area of the heart served by that artery can be so inadequate that the myocardium dies (Figure 28.2b). This condition, you will recall, is called acute myocardial infarction (AMI). AMI usually occurs in the left ventricle, the thick-walled chamber that produces the higher systemic blood pressure (Figure 28.4). The left ventricle requires more blood and much more oxygen than the lower-pressure right ventricle. The left ventricle therefore suffers the most from a lack of oxygen.

Consequences of AMI

Acute myocardial infarction has three major and serious consequences:

1. Sudden death from arrhythmia (unorganized, ineffective beating of the heart)
2. Congestive heart failure (CHF)
3. Cardiogenic shock

Sudden Death

Approximately 40 percent of all patients who suffer AMI die before they reach the hospital. These deaths occur because of sudden abnormalities in the heart rhythm called **arrhythmias,** which prevent any effective pumping action of the heart. The chance of an arrhythmia occurring after AMI is greatest within the first hour after the event; it diminishes to a very small risk after three to five days. Arrhythmias may produce completely disorganized quivering, called **fibrillation,** or no beat at all, called **asystole** (Figure 28.5). In either case, the heart is said to be in **cardiac arrest.** These situations require **cardiopulmonary resuscitation (CPR).**

A wide variety of arrhythmias are thought to be the result of AMI. Some of these include the following:

Tachycardia: Rapid but regular beating of the heart

Bradycardia: Unusually slow but regular beating of the heart

Atrial flutter: Beating of the atria up to rates of 300/minute not associated with equal beating of the ventricles

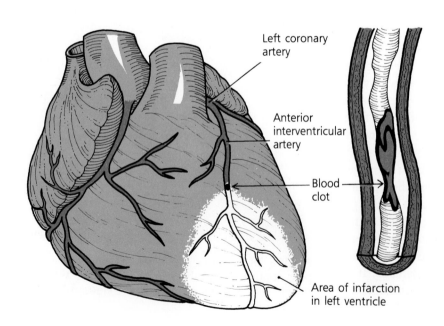

Left coronary artery

Anterior interventricular artery

Blood clot

Area of infarction in left ventricle

FIGURE 28.4 Acute myocardial infarction (AMI) usually occurs in the left ventricle after a blood clot obstructs the left coronary artery and prevents blood from reaching the left ventricle.

Atrial fibrillation: Disorganized, ineffective quivering of the atria

Ventricular extrasystoles: Additional beats of the ventricle interspersed with the regular rhythm

Ventricular fibrillation: Disorganized, ineffective quivering of the ventricles

Congestive Heart Failure (CHF)

Failure of the heart occurs when the heart muscle is so damaged by infarction (death of the tissue) that it can no longer pump enough blood for the needs of the body. **Congestive heart failure (CHF)** can occur any time after a myocardial infarction, but it usually happens between the first few hours and the first few days after a heart attack. These patients may develop **pulmonary edema,** which means their lungs fill up with fluid. Frothy pink **sputum** is a sign of pulmonary edema. People experiencing congestive heart failure may have difficulty breathing. They may also have generalized swelling in the body (**edema**), particularly in the legs and feet.

Cardiogenic Shock

Cardiogenic shock is an early complication of AMI that occurs within 24 hours of the event. It means that the heart has been so damaged that it is unable to sustain a normal systemic blood pressure. Consequently, tissue perfusion fails throughout the body and death may occur. Shock with AMI is an extremely grave sign. This condition is also discussed in Chapter 11.

Clinical Presentation of AMI

Acute myocardial infarction may have any of the following signs:

Sudden onset of weakness, nausea, and sweating without a clear cause
Chest pain (crushing or squeezing)
Sudden arrhythmia with fainting
Pulmonary edema
Sudden death

Unfortunately, the first sign of coronary heart disease may be sudden death; 40 percent of all patients with AMI never reach the hospital. Sudden death from AMI usually is the result of cardiac arrest from ventricular fibrillation. The chance to save such a patient exists only if someone begins cardiopulmonary resuscitation promptly (within four minutes of the event). Ventricular asystole, or the lack of any heartbeat, may also be a cause of sudden death. This is a hard problem to detect because many dangerous ventricular arrhythmias can rapidly evolve into asystole if no treatment is given. In general, fewer patients with ventricular asystole respond to resuscitation than those with ventricular fibrillation. Sudden death is greatest at the instant of myocardial infarction; therefore, this moment is the most dangerous time for the patient. However, rapid administration of basic life-support mechanisms has successfully resuscitated many a patient with cardiac arrest from AMI.

A

TM.07 ARRIII HR PR ⌐⌐ QRS ⌐⌐ ABN TIME 11:55

Ludlow 9600

B

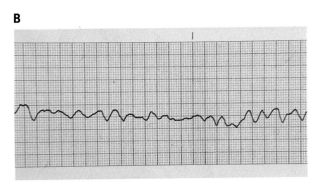

C

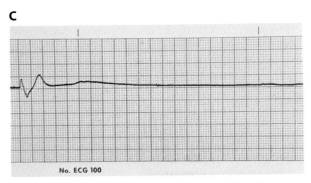

No. ECG 100

FIGURE 28.5 ECG (electrocardiogram) tracings show (a) normal heart rhythm, (b) arrhythmia from fibrillation, and (c) asystole (cardiac arrest).

The great majority of patients with AMI who do not die suddenly develop chest pain. Classically, this pain exhibits the following characteristics:

1. Is substernal in location
2. Is squeezing in character, or felt as a heaviness or pressure
3. Lasts longer than 30 minutes
4. Is not related to exertion, nor relieved by rest or nitroglycerin
5. Is perceived as radiating to the jaw, to the left arm, to both arms, or to the epigastrium

The pain of AMI differs from that of angina pectoris in two ways. First, the pain of AMI lasts longer than that of angina pectoris. Whereas anginal pain usually lasts no longer than from 3 to 10 minutes, the pain of AMI may last from 30 minutes to several hours. Second, the pain of AMI, unlike that of angina pectoris, may not be related to exertion or mental or emotional stress. Nor is it relieved by rest or nitroglycerin. The pain of AMI may come on at any time — perhaps waking the person from sleep or occurring when the individual is sitting quietly, reading.

About 90 percent of patients with AMI develop some sort of cardiac arrhythmia, usually extra beats in the damaged ventricle. These extra beats, called **ventricular premature contractions,** may group together and produce a series of disturbed, rapid, continuous beats, called **ventricular tachycardia.** If ventricular tachycardia persists, it can develop into ventricular fibrillation — the totally ineffective quivering of the cardiac muscle. Some patients with AMI do not feel pain but may notice the irregularity of their heartbeat. The episodes of ventricular arrhythmia may cause **syncope,** or fainting. Therefore, any patient who faints suddenly must be treated as suspect for AMI, especially if there was any chest pain or discomfort prior to or after the episode of syncope.

The sudden onset of left ventricular failure may cause pulmonary edema and **dyspnea,** which means shortness of breath. Pulmonary edema may be the first sign of AMI and should be treated as such. If the amount of damage caused by the infarction is great enough, the heart can no longer pump blood effectively. Since acute myocardial infarction occurs usually in the left ventricle, that ventricle will have a reduced pumping capability and cannot effective-

ly handle the blood coming from the lungs. The undamaged right ventricle, however, will continue to pump blood into the lungs. Therefore, pressure within the lung capillaries will rise, and fluid will pour out from the pulmonary blood vessels into the pulmonary alveoli. The lungs literally fill with fluid, and the patient feels a sensation akin to drowning. The patient cannot get enough oxygen from the air and experiences shortness of breath. Sometimes the fluid in the alveoli actually comes out of the mouth as a pink, frothy sputum (Figure 28.6). If the patient has no past history of dyspnea or heart failure, and if the pulmonary edema has come on suddenly, the EMT must provide emergency care for acute myocardial infarction. Such care includes positioning the patient with the head up. In addition, the EMT should administer supplemental oxygen and clear the airway.

When the left ventricular muscle is damaged by AMI, the amount of blood pumped per minute falls. Occasionally, a patient who has not complained of pain and who is not experiencing an arrhythmia might suddenly experience extreme weakness and feel unable to stand or walk. This extreme weakness is probably the result of falling cardiac output. Such an individual should be assumed to be having AMI and be so treated.

The Physical Findings of AMI

The physical findings of AMI are variable and will depend on the extent and severity of heart muscle damage. The following are the most frequent physical findings in acute myocardial infarction:

Pulse. Generally, the pulse rate increases as a normal response to stress, fear, or the actual injury of the myocardium. Since arrhythmias are the rule rather than the exception, an irregularity of the pulse may be noted. In some cases of acute infarction, bradycardia (an abnormal slowing of the pulse) develops rather than tachycardia (an abnormally rapid pulse).

Blood Pressure. Blood pressure falls as a result of diminished cardiac output and diminished capability of the left ventricle to pump.

Respiration. Respirations are normal unless pulmonary edema occurs. In this case, rapid shallow respirations are seen.

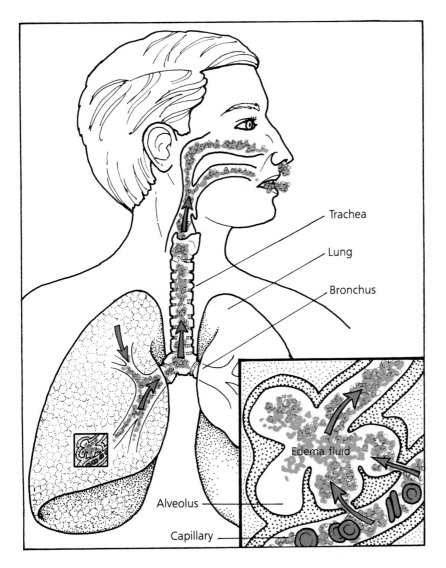

FIGURE 28.6 The lungs of a patient with pulmonary edema fill with fluid, and the person experiences shortness of breath. Some of the fluid may exit the mouth in the form of pink, frothy sputum.

Labels in figure: Trachea, Lung, Bronchus, Edema fluid, Alveolus, Capillary

General Appearance. The patient appears frightened. A cold sweat is frequently present. The patient may feel nauseated and may vomit. The skin is often ashen as a result of poor cardiac output and the loss of skin perfusion. Occasionally, **cyanosis** (a bluish tint to the skin) may be observed as a result of poor oxygenation of the circulating blood. In instances of acute congestive heart failure, the EMT may observe distended neck veins that do not collapse when the patient sits up.

Mental State. One of the unexplained aspects of acute myocardial infarction is that most patients have an almost overwhelming feeling of impending doom. They are convinced — almost resigned — that they are about to die.

Approach to the Patient with Suspected AMI

When treating a conscious patient in whom heart disease or acute myocardial infarction is suspected, the EMT should take the following steps:

1. *Reassure patient.* Act professionally. Be calm. Speak to the patient in a voice that is not too loud or too soft. Inform the patient that trained people are present to provide care and that he or she will soon be taken to the hospital. Remember, all patients are frightened. Some may act carefree, and some may be demanding; but all are frightened. The professional attitude of the EMT may be the single

most important factor in securing the patient's cooperation. Patient agitation and anxiety are directly related to the increased number and frequency of irregular or extra heartbeats. This arrhythmia may rapidly produce totally disorganized ventricular activity, fibrillation, and death. Apart from providing assurance and comfort, the calmness and poise of the EMT may help prevent a fatal worsening in the patient's condition.

2. *Take patient history.* Take a brief history from the patient. Friends or family members who are with the patient might have helpful information. As one EMT takes the history, the other should obtain and record vital signs — pulse, blood pressure, and respiratory rate. Note the exact time the vital signs are taken.

3. *Position patient.* If AMI is suspected, place the patient in a comfortable position, usually sitting, and well supported. Make sure the patient has no difficulty breathing and has no airway obstruction.

4. *Administer oxygen.* Administer oxygen by face mask. Explain to the patient that you are giving oxygen before positioning the face mask.

5. *Report to medical control.* Report to the hospital by radio. Give the patient's history, vital signs, medications being taken, and the treatment you are giving. Take care not to frighten the patient. Further treatment is undertaken only under the supervision of medical control.

6. *Transport patient to hospital.* The patient should be transported promptly to the nearest hospital. The hospital emergency department should be alerted as to the status of the patient and the estimated time of arrival. Give an oral report of the patient's condition to the emergency department staff upon arrival and leave a copy of the ambulance report form for the patient's hospital records.

CHRONIC CONGESTIVE HEART FAILURE

We already know that the pumping function of the left ventricle can be impaired by coronary artery disease. It can also be adversely affected by diseased heart valves or chronic hypertension. When the mus-cle can no longer contract well enough, the heart attempts in other ways to maintain adequate cardiac output. Two specific changes in heart function occur: (1) the heart rate increases, and (2) the left ventricle enlarges in an attempt to increase the amount of blood pumped each minute.

When these adaptations can no longer compensate for the decreased heart function, congestive heart failure eventually develops. It is called "congestive" heart failure (CHF) because the lungs become congested with fluid once the heart fails to pump the blood effectively. Blood tends to "back up" in the pulmonary veins, which increases the pressure in the capillaries of the lungs. When the pressure in the capillaries exceeds a certain level, fluid (mostly water) passes through the walls of the capillary vessels and into the alveoli. This condition, you will recall, is called pulmonary edema. It may occur suddenly, as in AMI, or slowly over months, as in chronic congestive heart failure.

When damage of the muscle of the right side of the heart has occurred, or when the right ventricle can no longer pump against the back pressure of a failed left ventricle, swelling takes place elsewhere in the body. Usually this fluid collects in both the feet and legs and is called **pedal edema.** It may occur suddenly over a few hours in acute problems or slowly over a long time. Beyond the sensation of uncomfortable swollen limbs, this swelling produces relatively few symptoms. Chronic pedal edema, however, even in the absence of pain or other symptoms, may indicate underlying heart disease.

Symptoms and Signs of CHF

Once fluid passes from the capillaries to the alveoli, the patient has a marked sensation of shortness of breath, or dyspnea. The fluid tends to make the lungs stiffer. Therefore, the patient breathes rapidly but with shallow respirations. The patient finds it harder to breathe lying down than standing or sitting. When the patient is lying down, the return of blood to the right ventricle and to the lungs increases and causes further pulmonary congestion.

The patient with chronic congestive heart failure generally has marked dyspnea, shows mild or pronounced agitation, and insists on sitting upright. Chest pain may or may not be present. The patient often has greatly distended neck veins that do not collapse even when the patient is sitting erect and

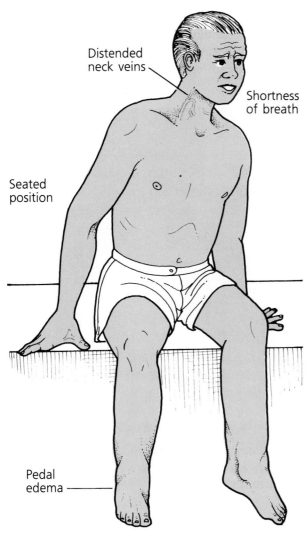

Distended
neck veins

Shortness
of breath

Seated
position

Pedal
edema

FIGURE 28.7 The patient with chronic congestive heart failure will be short of breath and prefer to sit to decrease the effort of breathing. Pedal edema and distended neck veins are commonly seen.

swollen limbs from pedal edema (Figure 28.7). Vital signs will reveal a normal or somewhat high blood pressure, a rapid heart rate, and rapid, shallow respirations. While listening to the patient's chest with a stethoscope, the EMT may hear the sound of air bubbling through the fluid in the alveoli and bronchi. This sound is called **rales,** a term that means rattles. The formal definition of rales is an abnormal sound indicating disease within the respiratory system. It is a sound much like sand falling on an empty tin can. The EMT might also hear **wheezing.** In severe congestive heart failure, these sounds can be heard from the apex to the base of

the lung. They are best heard by listening at the back of the patient's chest.

Treatment of CHF

The patient with chronic congestive heart failure is treated in the same way as the patient with AMI. The EMT takes vital signs, monitors heart action, and gives oxygen. The patient should be allowed to remain in an upright position with legs down. It is important to reassure and calm the patient. Many patients for whom this situation is chronic have specific medications for its treatment. The EMT should gather these and take them along. Prompt transportation to the emergency department is, of course, essential.

PATIENTS WITH PRIOR HEART OPERATIONS AND PACEMAKERS

In 1984, over 100,000 operations were performed to bypass damaged coronary arteries in the heart. In these **aorto-coronary bypass** operations, a vein from the leg or an artificial vessel is sewn directly from the aorta to a coronary artery beyond the point of the obstruction. The EMT is almost certain to have a patient with AMI or angina who has had such an operation. Usually these patients have a long scar on their chests over the sternum from the operation (Figure 28.8). The aorto-coronary bypass procedure produces remarkably good results in the treatment

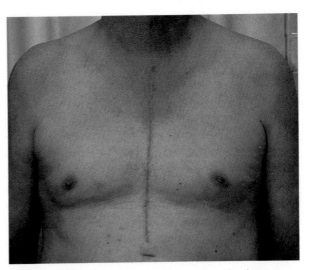

FIGURE 28.8 The scar on this patient's chest suggests an earlier aorto-coronary bypass operation.

of angina: 80 percent of patients achieve full relief, and 15 percent improve. No certain data exist regarding the rate of myocardial infarction after this operation. Some studies indicate that if an infarction does not occur at the time of the operation or during the time the patient is hospitalized, there is much less likelihood that AMI will occur within the next two or three years than in persons with similar histories who do not have a bypass. The debate over whether a bypass prolongs life significantly is not at all settled at this time.

In any event, AMI in a patient who has undergone a bypass procedure is treated exactly the same as in one who has not. All the previously mentioned procedures should be followed, and the patient should be transported promptly to the emergency department of the hospital. Even if CPR is required, it is carried out in the same way, regardless of the scar on the chest.

Many people with heart disease in the United States have cardiac **pacemakers.** These devices maintain a regular cardiac rhythm and rate by delivering an electrical impulse through wires that are in direct contact with the myocardium. The generating unit is generally placed under a heavy muscle or a fold of skin (Figure 28.9). Pacemakers are inserted when the electrical control system of the heart is so damaged that it cannot function properly.

Ordinarily, the EMT will not be concerned with pacemaker problems. The technology is such that an implanted unit will not require change or battery charge for some years. Wires are well protected and rarely broken. In past years, pacemakers sometimes malfunctioned when a patient got too close to an electrical radiation source such as a microwave oven. Those problems have been solved. Every patient wearing a pacemaker is fully aware of the precautions that must be observed for its optimal function.

If a pacemaker does not function properly, the patient may experience syncope, dizziness, or weakness. The pulse ordinarily will be slow (35 to 45) and irregular. In this situation, the heart is beating without the stimulus of the pacemaker and without the regulation of its own electrical system, which is damaged. The heart tends to assume a fixed slow rate that is not fast enough to allow the patient to

function normally. A patient with a malfunctioning pacemaker should be promptly transported to the emergency department because repair of the problem may require an operation.

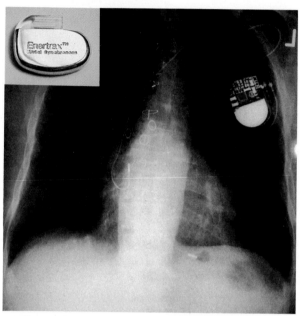

FIGURE 28.9 A pacemaker (inset) is a device implanted under the skin that delivers an electrical impulse to help regulate the heartbeat. The wire electrode can be seen on the x-ray from the pacemaker to the myocardium.

YOU ARE THE EMT...

1. On many occasions you will be called on to assist patients with AMI or angina. What role does arteriosclerosis play in these two serious heart problems?
2. You have a patient with chest pain. How can you decide if this person is suffering the pain of angina or the pain of acute myocardial infarction?
3. The patient is unconscious. You suspect AMI. What should you do? List the steps of emergency treatment.
4. You have a patient with congestive heart failure. What causes this condition and what are the signs and symptoms of CHF?

Stroke

29

OVERVIEW

Stroke is a medical problem that occurs when blood flow to the brain is interrupted long enough to damage the brain. The brain requires a continuous supply of oxygen and glucose, both of which are delivered via a continuous flow of blood to all parts of the brain. If that flow is interrupted for more than six minutes, irreversible damage can occur to that part of the brain which lost its blood supply. Since specific areas of the brain control specific functions of the body, the extent of the damage in the brain depends on the area destroyed. For example, a lack of blood flow in the motor control area on the right side of the brain will cause paralysis of the left side of the body.

Although brain damage following a stroke may be extensive, stroke patients usually do not die. Most gradually improve and after physical therapy experience partial or complete return of function.

Chapter 29 begins with a brief explanation of how blood circulates in the brain. The chapter then describes the three major causes of stroke: thrombosis, arterial rupture, or cerebral embolism. The symptoms and signs of stroke are discussed next. The final section focuses on the emergency treatment of stroke patients. Such treatment includes tender, loving care on the part of the EMT to alleviate the fear that can accompany a stroke and worsen its effects.

OBJECTIVES

The objectives of Chapter 29 are to

- understand how blood circulates in the brain.
- identify the three causes of stroke.
- recognize the symptoms and signs of stroke.
- learn the procedures for the emergency care of stroke patients.

CAUSES OF STROKE

Because the brain's need for a continuous blood supply is so critical, the **cerebral arteries** that feed the brain are large and originate close to the heart. Two **carotid arteries** anteriorly and two **vertebral arteries** posteriorly supply the brain. The two vertebral arteries unite at the base of the brain to form one large vessel called the **basilar artery.** The basilar artery has connections that link with the two carotid arteries at the base of the brain to form a circle of vessels around the brain stem. In this way a constant and rich blood supply is provided for the vital functions of the brain (Figure 29.1).

Stroke, the common term for **cerebrovascular accident (CVA),** is the set of symptoms and signs caused by any interruption of blood flow to the brain that lasts long enough to damage the brain. Although males and females are equally affected by cerebrovascular accidents, most strokes occur in elderly patients who have **arteriosclerosis,** mild chronic heart disease, or hypertension (abnormally high blood pressure). It is sometimes very difficult to sort out the specific cause of a stroke in these patients.

Interruption of cerebral blood flow may result from one of three events: (1) clotting of the cerebral arteries (**thrombosis**); (2) rupture of a cerebral artery (**arterial rupture**); or (3) obstruction of a cerebral artery by a clot that formed elsewhere in the body and traveled to the brain (**cerebral embolism**).

Thrombosis

Just as in coronary artery disease, progressive **occlusion,** or blockage, of a cerebral artery can result from arteriosclerosis. **Cholesterol** deposits in the vessel wall cause the **lumen** (the inside diameter of the artery) to narrow and promote the formation of a blood clot, or **thrombus,** which can completely cut off the flow of blood (Figure 29.2). Thrombosis is the most common cause of stroke.

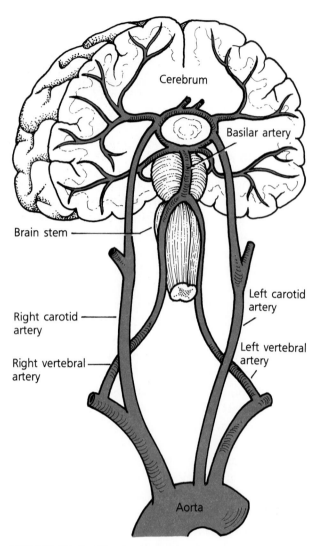

FIGURE 29.1 The brain receives a continuous supply of blood from the large carotid and vertebral arteries.

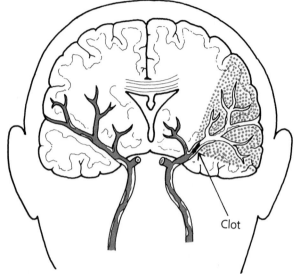

FIGURE 29.2 Arteriosclerosis can damage the wall of a cerebral artery, producing narrowing and clot formation. When the vessel is obstructed by a clot, blood flow to that portion of the brain stops and a stroke occurs.

that has been present since birth. Congenital arterial lesions are relatively common causes of stroke in young but otherwise healthy adults.

Occasionally, strokes are caused by hypertension. The bleeding is not caused by a weakened, damaged artery that ruptures easily; rather, excessive internal pressure forces a normal artery to give way.

Cerebral Embolism

A blood clot that forms elsewhere, usually within the heart, may travel to a cerebral artery and obstruct it. A blood clot that passes from its point of formation to another point in the body through the vascular system is called an **embolus.** Blood clots often form on damaged or diseased heart valves. Irregular cardiac rhythms, particularly **atrial fibrillation,** also allow clots to form within the heart. These clots can break loose and travel as emboli to the brain (Figure 29.4).

An embolus is not always clotted blood. Anything that enters the bloodstream as an object can travel from that point to another site through the blood vessels. Frequently, small particles from a degenerated arteriosclerotic blood vessel wall will break loose and travel as emboli to block a cerebral artery and cause a stroke.

Arterial Rupture

An artery that ruptures can cause bleeding, or **hemorrhage,** into the brain. The bleeding may cause a spasm in the leaking artery, which further diminishes blood flow within the vessel. Brain damage results directly from the hemorrhage into the tissue as well as from the impaired circulation. Generally, bleeding occurs at a weakened, dilated area of the wall of the blood vessel. The area of weakness, called an **aneurysm,** ordinarily occurs from arteriosclerotic damage of the arterial wall (Figure 29.3). An aneurysm may also be a **congenital lesion,** which is a weakened portion of the arterial wall

A

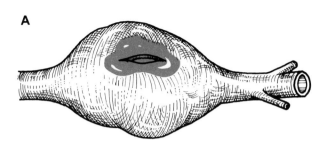

B

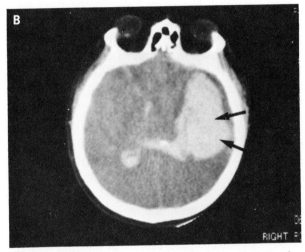

FIGURE 29.3 (a) A weakened, dilated portion of a blood vessel is called an aneurysm. The aneurysm can rupture, causing bleeding into the brain and cutting off the blood flow. (b) A CT scan of a ruptured aneurysm. The light area represents hemorrhage into the brain tissue (arrows).

Area of infarct

Clot

Clot origin on diseased aortic valve

FIGURE 29.4 An embolus, a blood clot usually formed on a diseased heart valve, can travel through the body's vascular system, lodge in a cerebral artery, and cause a stroke.

SYMPTOMS AND SIGNS OF STROKE

The three different events that can interrupt blood flow to the brain can cause three distinct clinical pictures. *Clotting* of cerebral arteries causes specific losses of body functions, generally without pain or seizures. The losses represent the area of the brain in which blood flow is interrupted. An *arterial rupture* is frequently accompanied by a sudden severe headache and rapid loss of consciousness; the pain is caused by a sudden increase in **intracranial pressure** from the brain swelling inside the rigid bony skull. A *cerebral embolism* may cause a sudden convulsion, paralysis, or loss of consciousness.

Regardless of the different presenting clinical symptoms of stroke, the final manifestation includes variable signs and symptoms, depending on the area

and the extent of the brain damaged. Strokes may produce the following effects:

1. Partial or complete paralysis of one or both extremities on one side of the body; rarely are both sides of the body paralyzed.
2. Diminished consciousness, varying from coma to confusion or dizziness.
3. Difficulty with speech or vision.
4. Convulsions (although many individuals with epilepsy experience convulsions from other causes without any damage of the brain).
5. Difficulty with swallowing or breathing.
6. Loss of facial expression or paralysis of facial motion.
7. Headache alone.

While a stroke patient usually experiences more than one of the above effects, even one of these signs and symptoms is sufficient evidence to suspect a cerebrovascular accident and to begin treatment.

EMERGENCY CARE OF A STROKE PATIENT

The EMT responding to a patient with a stroke should carefully observe vital signs, respiration, and blood pressure. Is respiration regular or irregular? Certain characteristic hesitancies in the breathing pattern occur in some patients with stroke. Others may have very rapid, but not labored, respiration. Is the frequency of breathing sufficient or will respiratory support be required? The EMT should always make certain that the airway is clear.

Paralysis of throat muscles occurs frequently following a stroke, and the patient may have difficulty maintaining an adequate airway. If the airway is difficult to maintain or if there is an irregular or slow respiratory rate, use supplemental oxygen, suction as needed, and prepare to establish an artificial airway. The airway should be assessed promptly, but not entered if it is clear and the patient is breathing well. This maneuver adds much to the discomfort of the patient who does not need it. The EMT should take the pulse both at the wrist and the neck. Observing early in the course of a stroke whether both carotid pulses (one on each side of the neck) are present can be helpful. The absence of a carotid pulse may indicate thrombosis of that vessel. When palpating the pulse, the EMT should note its rhythm. An irregularity of the pulse may indicate underlying heart disease and therefore suggest embolism as a cause of the stroke.

The blood pressure should also be taken. A very high blood pressure in combination with a slow pulse is often a sign of marked swelling of the brain. Because the brain is confined within the rigid bony skull, the swelling creates extreme pressure on the brain cells and destroys or permanently damages them. Such damage can occur in a matter of minutes. This patient requires immediate emergency care by a physician so that blood pressure and cerebral swelling can be controlled promptly.

A patient who is unable to speak and appears to be unconscious may still be able to hear and to comprehend what is taking place. Beyond avoiding unnecessary or inappropriate comments, the EMT must try to communicate with the patient by looking for signs indicating the patient understands the situation. Such indications may be very subtle indeed — a glance, a gaze, motion or pressure with the finger or hand, efforts to speak, or nodding of the head. The EMT who can establish effective communication with the patient often has an opportunity to calm the patient. The loss of the ability to communicate is a frightening experience which can add to a patient's problems. Allaying this fear can do much to help in treatment.

FIGURE 29.5 The semiconscious or unconscious stroke patient should be transported with the paralyzed side down and well protected with padding.

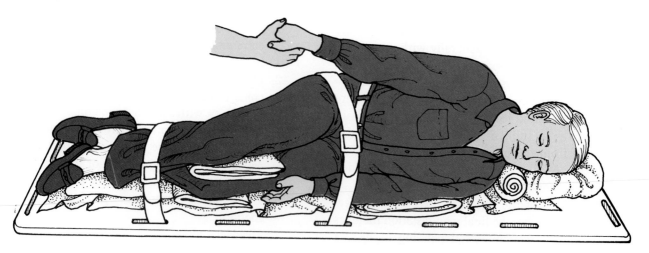

Stroke victims should not be given anything by mouth, because the muscles of the throat may be paralyzed. Even the conscious patient may be unable to swallow. Not infrequently, these patients will be choking on saliva or mucus, especially if they cannot swallow. The airway should be cleared by suction and oxygen given when necessary. Occasionally an oropharyngeal or nasal airway must be used if the tongue is **flaccid** (soft and limp) and obstructing. When inserting the airway, the EMT must be careful not to cause vomiting, which might cause greater airway obstruction. The patient should be transported to the emergency department gently and promptly.

The patient who is semiconscious or unconscious must be transported on one side, with the paralyzed side down (Figure 29.5). This position has the added benefit of freeing the conscious patient's useful extremities. Care must be taken, however, to adequately cushion and protect the paralyzed side from injury.

The way the EMT handles a patient with stroke as well as the patient's family is extremely important in the overall care. Anything that will increase the anxiety of the patient must be avoided. Energetic handling on the part of the EMT or the family may aggravate the effects of a stroke. The single most important aspect of the treatment for this patient is thoughtful, tender, loving care. In this time of crisis, both the patient and the family need calm reassurance. This point cannot be emphasized too much. A calm, professional attitude will reassure both the patient and the family and do much to prevent further damage.

YOU ARE THE EMT...

1. The patient is elderly, and his daughter tells you she thinks he has just suffered a stroke. What happens when a stroke is caused by a thrombosis? An arterial rupture? A cerebral hemorrhage?
2. You suspect stroke because the patient is paralyzed on one side. What are the other signs and symptoms of stroke?
3. Once you are sure you are dealing with a stroke patient, how do you proceed with emergency treatment? List the steps.
4. Why shouldn't you give a stroke patient anything to eat or drink?

30 Dyspnea

OVERVIEW

Dyspnea is the term for difficult or labored breathing, more commonly described as shortness of breath. It is a symptom the patient notes, and it may be accompanied by distinct signs of respiratory distress. Dyspnea may result from a variety of medical or traumatic causes. The traumatic causes of breathing difficulty are discussed in Chapter 23. Here, the discussion focuses on the nontraumatic, or medical, causes of dyspnea.

Chapter 30 begins with the physiology of the pulmonary system. The role of the lungs in exchanging oxygen and carbon dioxide is explained, along with the disorders that prevent or obstruct that exchange. Then the medical problems that produce dyspnea are described. These include infections of the upper or lower airway, acute pulmonary edema, chronic obstructive lung disease, asthma or allergic reactions, airway obstruction, pulmonary embolism, and hyperventilation. The last part of the chapter discusses the treatment of dyspnea in relation to whatever medical problems are involved.

OBJECTIVES

The objectives of Chapter 30 are to

- understand the physiology of the body's pulmonary system.
- identify the nontraumatic, or medical, causes of dyspnea.
- learn how to provide emergency medical care to patients with dyspnea.

PULMONARY PHYSIOLOGY

The major function of the lung is to provide oxygen to the blood and to take carbon dioxide from the blood to be expelled in the air that is breathed out. To carry out this exchange of oxygen and carbon dioxide properly, there must be no obstruction of the flow of air breathed in (**inspiration**) and air breathed out (**expiration**) to and from the pulmonary **alveoli** (air sacs). There must also be no interference with the passage of those gases between the alveoli and the **pulmonary capillaries.**

The alveoli are microscopic, thin-walled air sacs. They lie close against the pulmonary capillary vessels that connect the **pulmonary arterioles** and the **pulmonary venules.** The exchange of oxygen and carbon dioxide between air in the sacs and blood in the pulmonary capillaries is quick and easy (Figure 30.1).

In most disorders of the lung, one of the following situations exists:

1. The pulmonary vessels are physically separated from the air sacs by fluid or infection.
2. The air sac is damaged and cannot transport gases properly across its own wall.
3. The major air passages are obstructed by **spasm** or **mucus.**

All these conditions prevent the proper exchange of oxygen and carbon dioxide. In addition, abnormalities of the pulmonary blood vessels themselves may interfere with blood flow and thus with the proper transfer of oxygen and carbon dioxide.

Any type of lung disease that causes too little oxygen to enter the blood is harmful to the body. An excessive level of carbon dioxide also has an adverse effect. The major, principal stimulus that causes an individual to breathe is the level of carbon dioxide in the arterial blood. If the level of carbon dioxide in the blood drops too low, the person

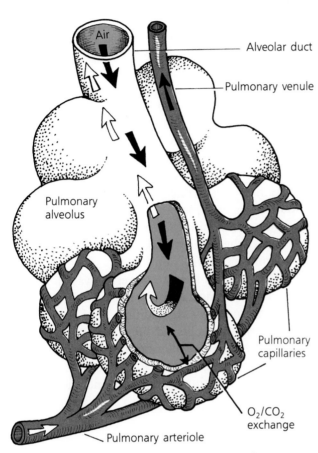

FIGURE 30.1 An enlarged view of a single alveolus (air sac) showing where the exchange of oxygen and carbon dioxide between air in the sac and blood in the pulmonary capillaries takes place.

Air

Alveolar duct

Pulmonary venule

Pulmonary alveolus

Pulmonary capillaries

O_2/CO_2 exchange

Pulmonary arteriole

automatically breathes at a slower rate and less deeply. This response, which causes less carbon dioxide to be expired, allows carbon dioxide to rise in the blood to a normal level. On the other hand, should the level of carbon dioxide rise above normal in the arterial blood, the person breathes at a more rapid rate and more deeply, "blowing off" the gas and thereby lowering its amount in the arterial blood. The arterial level of carbon dioxide is controlled, breath by breath, and is regulated so automatically that very little variation occurs in the normal, healthy person. Normal values are 40 to 46 millimeters of mercury (mm Hg).

The level of carbon dioxide in the arterial blood can rise for a number of reasons. The "blowing off" process itself may be impaired by various types of lung disease. Also, the normal body production of carbon dioxide may increase, either acutely in some diseases, or chronically over a long time. If the arterial carbon dioxide level slowly rises to a high level and remains there, the **respiratory center** (the area in the brain stem that senses the level of carbon dioxide and controls respiration) may become **narcotized** (depressed, with lower than normal activity, as though affected by a narcotic drug). **Carbon dioxide narcosis** may be so severe and the respiratory center become so depressed that the patient has no stimulus to breathe at all from the increased arterial carbon dioxide concentration. Respiration will then cease unless a secondary drive to stimulate it exists. Fortunately, there is a second stimulus. A low level of oxygen in the blood will also compel one to breathe, although the stimulus of falling oxygen is not as strong as the "drive" of rising carbon dioxide.

A fairly definite physiologic danger exists in this situation. Much time is required to treat carbon dioxide narcosis and to get the respiratory center used to gradually higher levels of the gas. On the other hand, a few breaths of air that are heavily enriched with oxygen will raise arterial levels of this gas to normal or higher. In that situation, both carbon dioxide and oxygen drives to stimulate breathing are lost. Thus, one can appreciate the apparently contradictory advice of not giving too much oxygen to the chronically ill patient with pulmonary problems.

If the carbon dioxide level rises rapidly, the patient generally is in acute respiratory failure and desperately ill. These situations usually occur in the hospital, but they can sometimes be seen with acute injuries or respiratory paralysis. Carbon dioxide narcosis, on the other hand, requires a long time to develop and occurs with severe, longstanding pulmonary disease.

CAUSES OF DYSPNEA

Medical problems in which **dyspnea,** or evidence of breathing difficulty, is present include the following:

1. Infections of the upper or lower airway
2. Acute pulmonary edema
3. Chronic obstructive lung disease
4. Asthma or allergic reactions
5. Obstruction of the airway
6. Pulmonary embolism
7. Hyperventilation

Infection of the Upper or Lower Airway

Infectious diseases causing dyspnea may affect all parts of the airway. They range from those causing mild discomfort to those showing signs of acute obstruction that require a full range of respiratory support. In general, in all of these situations, the problem is obstruction, either to the flow of air in the major passages (colds, diphtheria, epiglottitis, and croup), or to the exchange of gases between the alveoli and the capillaries (pneumonia). The common cold is usually associated with swollen **nasal mucosa** and the production of fluid from the **sinuses** and the nose. Dyspnea is not severe, and the common complaint is "stuffiness" or difficulty in breathing. Despite years of research, no sure treatment exists for colds; conversely, they rarely if ever pose severe emergency problems.

Diphtheria, although well controlled in the past decade, is still highly contagious and severe when it occurs. A product of the disease is the formation of a membrane lining the pharynx which is composed of debris, inflammatory cells, and mucus. This diphtheritic membrane can rapidly and severely obstruct the passage of air into the larynx. **Acute epiglottitis,** a bacterial infection of the epiglottis, can produce severe (two to three times normal) swelling of this flap over the larynx, especially in children (Figure 30.2). Acute and complete airway obstruction can occur from this swelling. Acute epiglottitis is further discussed in Chapter 37.

Croup is an inflammation and swelling of the lining of the larynx, where the airway is normally at its narrowest. The common sign of croup is **stridor** — a high-pitched, rough sound heard on inspiration. It signifies further narrowing of the air passage of the larynx and occasionally may progress to significant obstruction.

Pneumonia is acute bacteria invasion and infection of the lung itself. The infection damages and destroys lung tissue. In addition, fluid accumulates in the surrounding normal lung tissue separating the alveoli from their capillaries. As a result, the lung's ability to exchange oxygen and carbon dioxide is impaired. The breathing pattern does not indicate major obstruction but may show a significant increase

FIGURE 30.2 Dyspnea from infection of the upper airway. The epiglottis in (a) is normal; air clearly outlines the pharynx, upper airway, and epiglottis (arrow). The epiglottis in (b) is massively swollen and almost fully obstructs the upper airway.

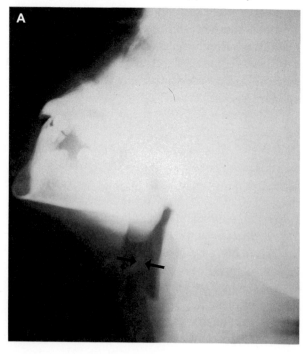
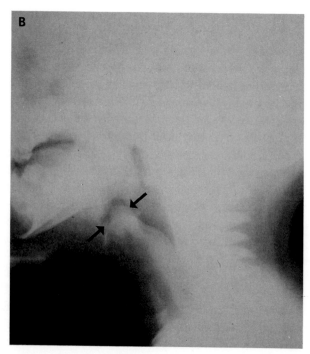

in rate (**tachypnea**) to compensate for the reduced amount of normal lung tissue.

Acute Pulmonary Edema

Acute pulmonary edema usually occurs following an **acute myocardial infarction,** when the heart muscle has been so damaged that it cannot circulate blood properly. In this case, the left side of the heart cannot remove blood from the lung as fast as the right side delivers it. Fluid then builds up within the alveoli and between them and the pulmonary capillaries in the lung tissue itself. This accumulation of fluid is called **pulmonary edema.** It physically separates alveoli from pulmonary capillary vessels and thus interferes with the exchange of carbon dioxide and oxygen (Figure 30.3). The patient usually experiences dyspnea with rapid, shallow respirations. There is not enough room left in the lung after fluid has been added to allow slow deep breaths. In very severe instances, a frothy pink **sputum** is apparent at the nose and mouth.

In some instances, the EMT will see patients who have pulmonary edema without heart disease. Acute smoke inhalation, the inhalation of irritating toxic chemical fumes, or sudden compression injuries can all produce it. In these cases pulmonary edema occurs from direct lung or bronchial damage or irritation. The result, however, is the same: fluid collects in alveoli and lung tissue.

Chronic Obstructive Lung Disease

Chronic obstructive lung disease is a common problem in the United States. It is a slow process, which over several years results in disruption of the normal airways, the alveoli, and the pulmonary blood vessels. The process itself may be a result of direct lung damage from repeated infections, from the inhalation of toxic agents such as industrial gases, or from cigarette smoking. Most commonly, the combination of damage from cigarette smoking and frequent lung infection is the cause. Although much has been said about cigarettes as being a direct cause of lung cancer, their role in the development of chronic obstructive lung disease is far more significant. Tobacco smoke is itself a bronchial irritant. All these substances create chronic irritation of the trachea and bronchi (**chronic bronchitis**). Excess mucus is constantly produced and obstructs small airways and air sacs. Pneumonia easily occurs when

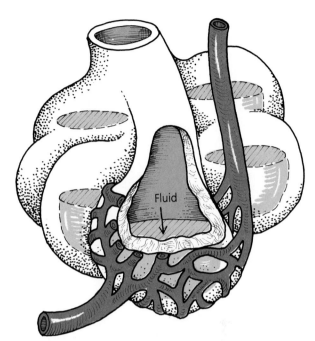

FIGURE 30.3   Dyspnea from acute pulmonary edema. Fluid fills the alveoli and separates the capillaries from the alveolar wall.

these passages are persistently obstructed. Ultimately, repeated episodes of pneumonia cause scarring in the lung itself and dilation of the obstructed alveoli, a condition called **emphysema** (Figure 30.4). Gradually, the patient's arterial oxygen level falls, and the carbon dioxide level rises.

If an acute infection of the lung is added to an already chronic lung condition, the arterial oxygen level may fall rapidly. In many patients, the arterial carbon dioxide level is high enough to produce narcosis of the respiratory center. Patients with chronic obstructive lung disease cannot handle pulmonary infections well because the existing airway damage makes them unable to cough up the mucus or sputum produced by the infection. The chronic airway obstruction makes it difficult to breathe deeply enough to clear the lung. These patients require respiratory support and careful administration of oxygen.

Patients with chronic obstructive lung disease usually are older, often **cyanotic,** and have a history of recurring lung problems. They may complain of chest tightness and constant fatigue. Quite often they are long-term smokers. Cigarette habits for patients are measured in **pack years.** One package of cigarettes per day per year is a one-pack year. It is not

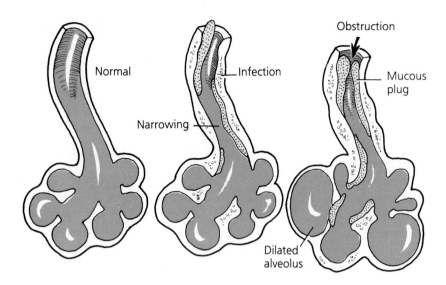

FIGURE 30.4 Dyspnea from chronic obstructive lung disease. Chronic irritation of the smaller airways results in partial or complete obstruction from infection and mucous plugs. The alveoli enlarge and become scarred, and their ability to exchange oxygen and carbon dioxide is impaired.

uncommon to find a 60-year-old patient with a 100-pack-year-history of cigarette use. There is a direct relationship between numbers of pack years and incidence of chronic obstructive lung disease.

Asthma or Allergic Reactions

Asthma is an acute spasm of the smaller air passages (**bronchioles**) associated with excessive mucus production (Figure 30.5). It produces a characteristic wheezing as the patient attempts to exhale through the partially obstructed air passages. These same bronchioles open easily during inspiration. In some instances, the actual work of exhaling is very tiring and the patient may become cyanotic.

Asthma, which can occur at any age, usually results from inhalation, ingestion, or injection of some agent to which the patient has become sensitized (**allergic**). The reaction in the airways is an intense exaggeration of the normal protective mechanisms set off by the **allergens** (agents to which the patient is sensitive). Between attacks, patients have normal lung function. An allergic response to a bee sting or to any other substance may produce an acute asthmatic attack. In its severest form, this allergic reaction can produce **anaphylactic shock,** which may cause respiratory distress severe enough to result in coma and possibly death. (Anaphylactic shock is also discussed in Chapters 11 and 27.)

A much milder and much more common allergy problem is "**hay fever.**" In some areas of the country where pollen is present in the air throughout the year, it is almost a universal illness. Generally, it pro-duces no major emergency problems but a host of difficulties such as upper respiratory tract infection — stuffy, runny nose, and sneezing.

Obstruction of the Airway

Obstruction of the airway may occur in semi-conscious and unconscious individuals as a result of the position of the head, obstruction by the tongue, or **aspiration** of vomitus. Opening the airway with the head-tilt/chin-lift may solve the problem. The maneuver may be done only after a head or neck injury has been ruled out. If simple opening of the airway does not correct the breathing problem, a search for upper airway obstruction must be made. Foreign body, upper airway obstruction must be considered as a first diagnosis in any dyspneic patient who has been eating just before the onset of the problem or in young children, especially crawling babies, who might have swallowed and choked on a small object.

Strictly speaking, acute upper airway obstruction is a much more traumatic cause of dyspnea than other causes, since it is rarely associated with disease. The techniques for handling the acutely obstructed airway, both in adults and children, are reviewed in Chapter 6. The important consideration for the EMT is to suspect the cause and move expeditiously to treat it.

Pulmonary Embolism

An **embolus** is anything in the circulatory system that passes from its point of origin to lodge at a distant site, remaining within the system. In gen-

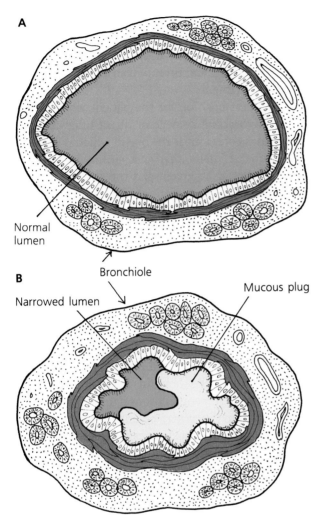

A

Normal
lumen

Bronchiole

B

Narrowed lumen

Mucous plug

FIGURE 30.5 Dyspnea from asthma. In (a) the bronchiole is normal. In (b) the bronchiole is in spasm with a mucous plug; the excessive mucus partially obstructs the bronchioles in the lungs of an asthma patient.

eral, circulation beyond the point of obstruction is cut off or markedly decreased. Emboli can be blood clots in the arteries or the veins. They can also be foreign bodies which enter the circulation, such as a bullet or a bubble of air. An embolus that causes an obstruction is called an **embolism.** Needless to say, embolisms are very serious and can cause sudden death.

Pulmonary embolism is the passage of a clot formed in the venous side of the circulation through that system, through the right side of the heart, and into the pulmonary artery where it becomes lodged. Pulmonary emboli almost always arise as a result of

slow blood flow, damage of the lining of vessels, or a tendency for blood to clot unusually fast. Usually they are seen in patients confined to bed when blood flow decreases and veins are often collapsed. Almost always, they arise in the veins of the legs or pelvis which are long and straight, thus affording the opportunity for a large, long clot to develop. The dislodging of the clot, so that it passes to the pulmonary artery, gives rise to the symptoms of the problem and is called pulmonary embolism. The large, long clot can significantly interrupt pulmonary artery blood flow.

The degree of patient awareness of this problem is directly related to the amount of lung tissue damaged. Complete, sudden obstruction of the right heart output results in sudden death. Damage of the lung, with inflammation of the pleural surface, frequently causes **pleuritic chest pain** (sharp, stabbing pain) with each breath. Significant obstruction of the pulmonary artery or its main branches means that, even though a lung is actively involved in inhalation and exhalation of air, no exchange of oxygen or carbon dioxide takes place in the areas of blocked blood flow because there is no effective circulation. In this circumstance, the level of arterial carbon dioxide usually rises, and oxygen may drop sufficiently to cause cyanosis.

Pulmonary emboli are fairly common and difficult to diagnose. In the United States, approximately 650,000 (estimated) instances occur yearly; 10 percent will be immediately fatal and 90 percent will not. Most often, pulmonary emboli are never noticed by the patient. Symptoms and signs when they do occur include acute pleuritic chest pain, **hemoptysis** (coughing up blood), cyanosis, and tachypnea. Almost anything that imposes undue inactivity or low blood flow on a lower extremity will predispose to a pulmonary embolus — bed rest, dehydration, a cast, traction, or a direct injury. Usually, however, pulmonary emboli arise with hospitalization. Only very rarely do they occur in active, healthy individuals.

Hyperventilation

Dyspnea occurring in a patient without lung abnormalities is called hyperventilation. **Hyperventilation** is described as overbreathing to the extent that the level of arterial carbon dioxide falls way below normal. When excessive breathing "blows off" too much carbon dioxide, the blood pH (a measure of blood acidity) rises above normal and becomes **alkaline. Alkalosis** develops and is the cause of many of the symptoms associated with hyperventilation. This response is common in psychological stress — almost as common a reaction as a headache or an upset stomach. Some of the symptoms can be self-induced by breathing as deeply and as rapidly as possible for three to five minutes; most people undergoing this exercise would not be aware that they had been hyperventilating. In general, the symptoms are numbness, tingling of the hands and feet, and, despite the rapid breathing, a sense of shortness of breath. Respiratory rates generally rise above 40 or 50 per minute. Recent studies indicate that this type of "panic attack" can be associated with significant differences in blood flow in specific areas of the right and left sides of the brain. A specific organic defect may exist to explain this reaction.

TREATMENT OF DYSPNEA

Infection of the Upper or Lower Airway

Dyspnea associated with acute infectious processes is quite common and rarely very serious. The acute congestion and stuffiness of a common cold rarely require emergency care. In fact, people with colds usually treat themselves with over-the-counter medications.

When acute infections obstruct the upper airway, even the very skilled anesthesiologist finds it extremely difficult to visualize the larynx, let alone intubate it. Nasal and oropharyngeal airways are designed to support a flaccid tongue — not to bypass a grossly swollen epiglottis or diphtheritic membrane. Supplemental oxygen that is warm and thoroughly saturated with moisture should be administered, and gentle suction should be used to keep the airway clear of mucus.

The dyspnea of pneumonia is not caused by upper airway obstruction but by the loss of lung volume and a need for more rapid air exchange. It will not be helped by the use of artificial airways but will improve with the administration of oxygen.

Acute Pulmonary Edema

Dyspnea caused by acute pulmonary edema usually is associated with a heart attack. The treatment is outlined in Chapter 28. When the problem is not associated with cardiac disease but with direct lung damage, the patient will require supplemental oxygen, clearing of the usually copious secretions from the airway, and prompt transport to the emergency department.

The best position for the patient who has sustained myocardial damage or direct lung irritation and who is conscious is the one in which it is easiest to breathe. Usually that is a sitting-up position. Oxygen should be given, and the airway carefully suctioned of heavy secretions. Rarely will artificial airways be needed since no upper airway obstructive problem exists. The unconscious patient with acute pulmonary edema may require full ventilatory support, an airway, oxygen, and suctioning.

Chronic Obstructive Lung Disease

People with chronic obstructive lung disease (emphysema or chronic bronchitis) are generally older. Their chests often have a barrellike appearance because air has been gradually and continuously trapped within the lung in increasing amounts. Generally, these people lose weight slowly and are therefore thin. They may be only semiconscious or unconscious from hypoxia or carbon dioxide narcosis, may appear in respiratory distress, and may be cyanotic. The patient with chronic obstructive lung disease may be using accessory muscles to breathe, including those in the neck and shoulders. The lips will be pursed in an attempt to puff air out (Figure 30.6).

The history of the person with lung disease will usually reveal a sudden increase in shortness of breath with a long history of dyspnea; rarely, however, is there any history of chest pain. The patient probably has had a recent "chest cold" and may remember having a recent fever as well as the inability to cough up mucus. The patient who can produce sputum will cough up thick, green or yellow sputum. The patient will usually be a smoker.

The blood pressure of patients with chronic obstructive lung disease will be normal. The pulse, however, will be rapid and occasionally irregular. Particular attention must be paid to the respiratory rate. It may be rapid, or it may be very slow, as in carbon dioxide narcosis. When listening to the chest, the EMT will hear **rales** (crackling breath sounds), **wheezes** (whistling sounds), and **rhonchi** (rough, gravely sounds). Sounds of breathing are frequently

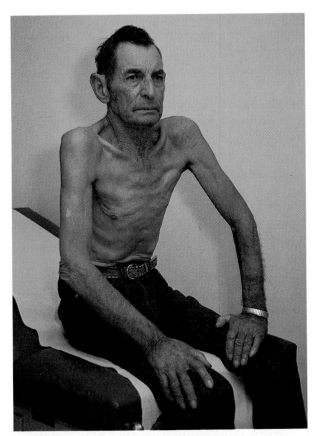

FIGURE 30.6 The typical appearance of a patient with chronic obstructive lung disease. Notice the barrel-shaped chest, pursed lips, and the use of the accessory muscles of respiration.

hard to hear and often are detected only high up on the posterior chest.

The patient's initial vital signs should be noted and recorded with particular attention to the respiratory rate. The EMT should speak with assurance and assume a concerned, professional approach. Oxygen usually should be given, although great care must be taken to monitor the respiratory rate after oxygen treatment has been started. The EMT must reevaluate the respiratory rate and the patient's response to oxygen repeatedly — at least every five minutes — until the patient reaches the emergency department. This monitoring is important, for the supplemental oxygen can cause the level to rise rapidly, which, in turn, can abolish the secondary respiratory oxygen drive while the carbon dioxide level still remains high. It takes a long time to correct a high arterial carbon dioxide level and narcosis of the respiratory

center. The oxygen content, however, may rise at once when enriched air is given. If the patient is depending only on a low oxygen level to sustain breathing, the rapid rise might abolish this stimulus and cause respiratory arrest.

For this reason, the best system to use when providing supplemental oxygen to a patient with chronic obstructive lung disease is a **venturi mask** (Figure 30.7). With this system, 100 percent oxygen is delivered to a mask, usually at a low (2 to 5 liters per minute) flow. Inside the mask, the tube caliber widens, and ports, open to room air, exist. The widened tube caliber causes a low pressure within the mask. Room air is sucked through the ports to dilute the 100 percent oxygen. Depending on the initial oxygen flow and the size of the ports, a given concentration of inspired oxygen can be administered (24 percent, 28 percent, 35 percent, and up to 50 percent).

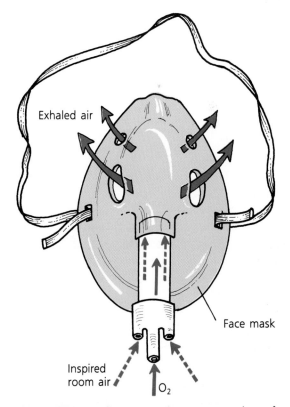

FIGURE 30.7 A diagrammatic representation of the functions of the venturi mask. Room air is inhaled, along with 100 percent oxygen. The room air dilutes the pure oxygen to a specific concentration, minimizing the risk of exposure to high oxygen concentrations.

The advantage of the venturi mask is the production of a high volume, high flow of inspired air at a controlled, fairly low concentration of inspired oxygen. It is impossible to determine beforehand what concentration of inspired oxygen may raise arterial levels enough to interfere with the breathing drive. Therefore, when a mask system is used, the EMT must watch the patient's response very carefully, give assistance when the respiratory rate declines, urge the patient to breathe deeply, and transport the patient as promptly as possible to the emergency department. Patients with chronic obstructive lung disease are more comfortable in the sitting position during transport (Figure 30.8).

Asthma or Allergic Reactions

The asthma patient may be young or old. Respiratory distress is obvious; the wheezing on expiration can be heard without the stethoscope. While the individual can breathe in without much difficulty, expiration is greatly impeded because of bronchospasm and mucus production. The obstruction causes the person literally to labor to push each breath out. The effort to breathe out is tiring and frightening. The history of the asthmatic is one of episodic attacks of shortness of breath, with the patient usually completely normal between them. Since the public generally tends to call all lung trouble "asthma," it is important for the EMT to confirm whether the patient has recurrent attacks of this nature but can breathe normally at other times. The patient or family should always be asked to describe what "asthma" means.

Chest pain is rarely present in asthma patients. The pulse rate will be normal or elevated. The blood pressure may be slightly elevated as a consequence of tension and anxiety experienced by the patient or from a medication that the patient may have taken in an attempt to alleviate the attack. The respiratory rate will be increased. Vital signs should be assessed and a history obtained. Reactions of this type that occur following a bee or wasp sting may progress rapidly to full anaphylactic shock. Thus, finding out what brought on the attack is very important. Oxygen should be given, and the person should be allowed to sit up, as breathing will be much easier in this position. As in other emergencies, reassurance from the EMT will relieve the tension and anxiety that make these attacks worse.

Many persons with asthma or known sensitivities

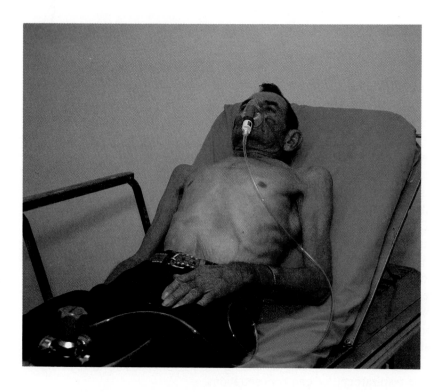

FIGURE 30.8 The patient with chronic obstructive lung disease and dyspnea should be transported in the sitting position. A venturi mask can provide supplemental oxygen at a controlled concentration, but the respiratory rate must be rechecked every five minutes.

to bees or certain food products have medications to take when an attack occurs. These medications should be obtained and administered with the help of the EMT. Many individuals also wear or carry medical identification tags that may help provide a clue in the most extreme cases. The person with full-blown anaphylactic shock may rapidly become unconscious and require assisted respiration as well as supplemental oxygen. All such patients require prompt transport to the emergency department. Kits are now available for the subcutaneous or intramuscular injection of ½ ml of 1:1,000 **epinephrine.** The use of this agent may rapidly reverse or reduce an anaphylactic reaction. Many patients who know their sensitivities keep such kits readily available. The EMT should know how to help the patient with a kit to administer the agent promptly, as it may be life-saving. Epinephrine is a very potent agent that has a number of significant side effects, so the user must be certain of the diagnosis and clear as to the history of the episode.

In the absence of coma, the EMT must be prepared to handle the production of large amounts of mucus with appropriate suctioning, and administer oxygen. If the patient is in a coma, airway maintenance may be needed. Occasionally, full CPR is required for an episode of anaphylaxis.

Obstruction of the Airway

In crawling children, or in patients known to have been eating just before dyspnea developed, the EMT must assume that the acute breathing difficulty arose from an inhaled or aspirated foreign body. The first thing to do is clear the upper airway. Supplemental oxygen and prompt transport to the emergency department are indicated, especially if the EMT is unsuccessful in clearing the air passage. Airway management from this cause is discussed in Chapters 6 and 37.

Pulmonary Embolism

Usually, pulmonary embolus is not a problem for the EMT since it is most likely to occur in hospitalized patients. The common signs and symptoms are acute pleuritic chest pain on respiration, which may limit breathing, varying degrees of hypoxia and carbon dioxide retention, and tachypnea. Occasionally, the patient experiences hemoptysis.

The airway usually does not need to be cleared since no obstruction exists. Supplemental oxygen is mandatory since a considerable amount of lung tissue may be nonfunctional. The patient should be placed in a position of comfort, usually sitting, and given breathing assistance. Hemoptysis, if present, is usually not copious but must be cleared. The EMT should also expect an unusually rapid heartbeat, which may also be irregular. Acute reflex responses to pulmonary emboli may produce cardiac arrest that will require full life support. When this diagnosis is suspected, prompt transport to the emergency department is indicated, along with respiratory support as outlined.

Hyperventilation

The hyperventilating patient is generally hysterical, terrified of dying, and has the feeling that it is impossible to get enough air into the chest, despite the fact that a larger quantity than usual is being exchanged. Dizziness is common. Often the person experiences the sensation of numbness or tingling in the hands and feet, which may also be described as "being cold." Sticking, stabbing chest pains that increase with respiration may occur. Vital signs reveal rapid breathing and a high pulse rate (**tachycardia**), with normal blood pressure. Cyanosis is not seen, which may be the key that hyperventilation is the cause of the dyspnea.

Other illnesses may cause a reaction that looks like simple overbreathing. The principal means within the body for maintaining a stable, normal level of acid within the blood (the pH) is to vary the respiratory rate. If blood pH falls (**acidosis**) and becomes too acidic from **diabetic ketoacidosis** (severe, out-of-control diabetes), shock, or from ingesting acid, the body attempts to return the pH to normal by blowing off carbon dioxide with overbreathing. Pulmonary embolus can also cause hyperventilation.

It is thus important when responding to a suspected case of hyperventilation that the EMT assess the patient's status and obtain a history. The presence or absence of chest pain, cardiac problems, the coughing of blood, and diabetes may easily be noted. In the absence of any other cause for hyperventilation, the best treatment begins with reassurance from the EMT. In most of the foregoing diseases or conditions, carbon dioxide in the blood rises and the pH

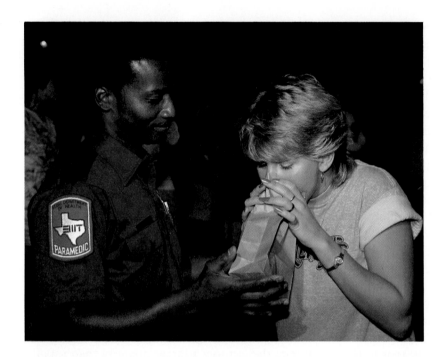

FIGURE 30.9 Simple hyperventilation can be treated effectively by rebreathing exhaled air from a paper bag.

falls (acidosis). In hyperventilation, carbon dioxide is exhaled rapidly and the pH rises (alkalosis). A maneuver designed to build up the level of carbon dioxide in the blood is to have the patient breathe into a paper bag (Figure 30.9). This technique forces the patient to rebreathe the expired air and thus raise the level of arterial carbon dioxide. There is no need to be concerned about a lack of oxygen, because expired air is not exclusively carbon dioxide (only 5 percent); it contains at least 16 percent oxygen. The hyperventilating patient should be transported to the emergency department, especially if the incident has never occurred before. It is easy for an experienced observer, as well as an EMT, to make an incorrect diagnosis. All of these patients should be carefully examined to allow the most accurate treatment possible.

YOU ARE THE EMT. . .

1. Which of the causes of dyspnea can be quickly ruled out and why? Which of the causes must you focus on and why?
2. Why should you be careful about not giving an elderly patient with chronic obstructive lung disease too much oxygen?
3. You have been called to treat a patient who reportedly is hyperventilating. Upon arrival, you notice that someone is already holding a paper bag and telling the patient to breathe into it. Should you continue this treatment? Why or why not?
4. The patient is having an asthma attack. What does that mean? What will you do if the attack progresses to anaphylactic shock?

Diabetes

THE ROLE OF GLUCOSE AND INSULIN

All cells require **glucose,** or sugar, to function properly, and some cells will not function at all without it. In the absence of glucose, or with very low levels, brain cells rapidly sustain permanent damage. In fact, sugar is as important to the brain as oxygen.

Glucose is carried to the cells through the bloodstream. However, glucose cannot enter the cells without the action of insulin. **Insulin** is a hormone produced by the specialized cells in the pancreas called **beta cells of the islets of Langerhans.** Insulin's specific function is to allow glucose to enter the cells of the body. Thus, insulin is absolutely necessary for the body cells to function normally.

Diabetes mellitus, often called sugar diabetes, is a disease in which the body is unable to utilize glucose normally as an energy source because of a deficiency or total lack of insulin. When there is not enough insulin, glucose in the blood cannot be used by tissues of the body because it cannot enter the cells. Glucose is then retained in the blood and will gradually rise to an extremely high level. At a sufficiently high level, usually three times the normal level (300 mg/deciliter) or more, glucose is excreted by the kidney. Glucose excretion by the kidney causes an excessive loss of both sugar and water in the urine, since more water must be excreted to allow the sugar to pass. The loss of sugar and water in large amounts, in turn, causes the classic symptoms of uncontrolled diabetes: **polyuria** (frequent and copious urination) and **polydipsia** (frequent drinking of liquid to satisfy continuous thirst).

Since without insulin glucose cannot be used as an energy source by cells, other sources must be found. Fat is usually the one. **Acetone** and other metabolic products, called **ketones** and **fatty acids,** are formed when fat is used for routine energy needs instead of glucose. (When glucose is used, the end products are carbon dioxide and water.) Acetone and ketones can be detected in the urine and the blood. Together with fatty acids they can produce the dangerous level of **acidosis** seen in uncontrolled diabetes. Severe, uncontrolled diabetes results in **diabetic ketoacidosis,** the signs of which are vomiting, stomach pain, and deep and rapid breathing. If the person is not given fluids and insulin, ketoacidosis will progress to **diabetic coma** (unconsciousness) and eventually death.

Diabetes mellitus is treatable. When there is an insufficient amount or a total lack of insulin production by the pancreas, insulin can be replaced by daily injections of insulin that has been extracted from animals or, more recently, by injections of synthetic insulin. Diabetics who have to take one or more injections of insulin every day are said to be **insulin-dependent diabetics.** Children who have to take insulin every day are called **juvenile diabetics.**

All children with diabetes are insulin-dependent. However, not all adults are. Some adults have a milder form of the disease. Insulin is usually still produced, but at a lower, insufficient level. Many of these people can control their diabetes by diet alone, limiting the sugar intake to the insulin their bodies still produce. Others do well with pills that stimulate the pancreatic cells to produce more insulin. This milder form of diabetes is called **adult onset diabetes.**

Ordinarily, most diabetic patients check their urine daily for the presence of sugar and acetone. The balance of insulin and food should be such that no sugar or only a trace and no acetone at all are detectable in the urine. Many patients now use **self-blood-glucose monitoring** to measure the level of sugar in the blood. A drop of blood from the fingertip or ear lobe is placed on a thin strip of chemically treated paper. The color the paper turns is compared with the color chart that comes with the strips. The patient gets a measurement of the amount of glucose currently present in the blood. The readings are in milligrams per deciliter of blood; the normal blood glucose level is 100 to 150 mg/deciliter. Devices for pricking the fingertip with a fine needle are now available, as well as meters for reading the strips (Figure 31.1).

DIABETIC COMA AND INSULIN SHOCK

The patient with diabetes may develop an acute emergency situation because of one of two conditions: diabetic coma or insulin shock. The problem for the EMT is that the symptoms of both conditions are quite similar. Therefore, the EMT has to know how to tell the difference between the two and what to do when unsure of which condition exists.

Diabetic Coma

The waste products from the body's use of fat for normal energy requirements markedly increase the acidity of blood. If the loss of fluid from frequent urination and the increase in acidity are severe

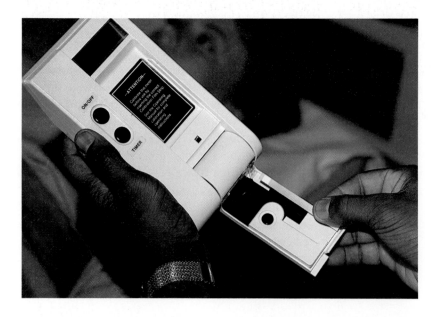

FIGURE 31.1 Self-blood-glucose monitoring. A drop of blood from the fingertip is obtained using a small, hand-held device. The chemically treated strip with the blood on it is inserted into the meter, which measures the amount of glucose currently present in the blood.

enough, diabetic coma will occur. Although the sugar level in the blood is very high (the condition called **hyperglycemia**), too much sugar does not directly cause the coma. Ketoacidosis, the presence of acid waste products in the blood, and the loss of fluid cause the coma.

Diabetic coma occurs in the patient who is not under medical treatment, who takes insufficient insulin, who markedly overeats, or who, although well controlled, undergoes some sort of stress, such as an infection or illness. Usually, ketoacidosis develops over a long period of time — hours or days. The patient may ultimately be found comatose with the following physical signs:

1. Air hunger, manifested by rapid and deep sighing respirations (**Kussmaul respiration**)
2. **Dehydration,** or excessive loss of body water, manifested by a dry, warm skin and sunken eyes
3. A sweet or fruity (acetone) odor on the breath caused by the acid in the blood
4. A rapid, weak ("thready") pulse
5. A normal or slightly low blood pressure
6. Varying degrees of unresponsiveness

Insulin Shock

Insulin shock occurs in the patient who has taken too much insulin, who has taken a regular dose of insulin but has not eaten enough food, or who has exercised excessively and used up all the available glucose. Sugar is then rapidly driven out of the blood and into the cells for energy. Not enough sugar remains in the blood to provide a continuous supply to the brain. Since the brain requires as constant a supply of glucose as it does oxygen, unconsciousness and permanent brain damage can quickly occur if the blood sugar remains low. Insulin shock develops much more quickly than diabetic coma — in some instances, in a matter of minutes.

Insufficient sugar in the blood, the condition called **hypoglycemia,** is associated with the following signs and symptoms:

1. Normal or rapid respiration
2. Pale, moist skin (clammy)
3. **Diaphoresis** (sweating)
4. Dizziness, headache
5. Full, rapid pulse
6. Normal blood pressure

7. Fainting, seizure, or coma
8. Aggressive or unusual behavior
9. Hunger

Diabetes and the Alcoholic

Occasionally, a patient who is diabetic is mistakenly identified as an alcoholic and confined without treatment in a "drunk tank" for over 24 hours. Usually the patient dies. Certainly, diabetes and alcoholism can coexist in any patient. The EMT, however, must be alert to the fact that the signs and symptoms of acute alcoholic intoxication are quite similar to those of diabetic coma and insulin shock. Sometimes in situations such as this, a "medic alert" bracelet or card may help save the patient's life. Often, only a blood sugar test in the emergency department will allow final determination of the problem.

DIAGNOSIS AND TREATMENT OF DIABETIC EMERGENCIES

It may be difficult for an inexperienced person, even one who knows the patient has diabetes, to tell the difference between diabetic coma and insulin shock. In either case, the patient who has not yet reached coma may feel sick or be semiconscious. Such a patient can frequently inform the EMT about the exact cause of his or her illness.

In taking care of an ill diabetic, the EMT must ask the patient or the family these two questions:

1. Have you eaten today?
2. Have you taken your insulin today?

If the patient has eaten but has not taken insulin, the problem is probably diabetic coma. If the patient has taken insulin but has not eaten, the problem is probably insulin shock. The diabetic patient will often know what the trouble is. Listen carefully.

If the patient is unconscious, the EMT must decide on the basis of the signs and symptoms just discussed whether the problem is diabetic coma or insulin shock. The primary visible difference will be the patient's breathing — deep, sighing respiration in diabetic coma and normal or rapid respiration in insulin shock. The diabetic patient who is unconscious and having convulsions is more likely to be in insulin shock. All noticeable differences are compared in Table 31.1.

TABLE 31.1   Findings in Diabetic Emergencies

	Diabetic Coma	Insulin Shock
History		
Food intake	Excessive	Insufficient
Insulin dosage	Insufficient	Excessive
Onset	Gradual	Rapid, within minutes
Skin	Warm and dry	Pale and moist
Infection	Common	Uncommon
Gastrointestinal Tract		
Thirst	Intense	Absent
Hunger	Absent	Intense
Vomiting	Common	Uncommon
Respiratory System		
Breathing	Air hunger	Normal, or rapid
Odor of breath	Sweet, fruity	Normal
Cardiovascular System		
Blood pressure	Low	Normal
Pulse	Rapid, weak	Normal, or rapid and full
Nervous System		
Headache	Absent	Present
Consciousness	Restless merging to coma	Irritability, seizure, or coma
Urine		
Sugar	Present	Absent
Acetone	Present	Absent
Treatment Response	Gradual within 6 to 12 hours following medication and fluid	Immediate after glucose

When testing a patient with suspected signs of diabetes, the EMT should first check to see if the patient has an emergency medical identification symbol, which may be found as a wallet card, necklace, or bracelet. It will advise if the patient has a known problem and can probably save the EMT from having to grope for a diagnosis. The patient in diabetic coma (blood sugar too high) needs insulin, complex intravenous fluids, and probably other medications. The EMT should transfer the patient to the hospital promptly for further medical care.

The patient in insulin shock (blood sugar too low) needs sugar. For the still-conscious patient, sugar cubes, granulated sugar, maple syrup, honey, candy, fruit juice (sweetened with granulated sugar if available), or soft drinks will reverse the reaction within one to two minutes (Figure 31.2). The EMT should not be afraid to give too much sugar. In fact, the problem probably won't reverse itself if only a sip of juice or pinch of sugar is given. An entire candy bar or glass of juice is better. However, do not give sugar-free drinks sweetened with saccharin or nutrasweet®. Even if the person responds after receiving sugar, the EMT should transport the patient to the hospital as soon as possible. Whether hospitalization is required is a decision for the physician to make.

If there is any doubt about whether a diabetic is in insulin shock or a diabetic coma, *give sugar,* even though the final diagnosis may be diabetic coma. The reason for giving sugar is that untreated insulin shock will result in unconsciousness and can quickly cause brain damage or death. As a matter of priority, the patient in insulin shock is in a far more critical condition and far more likely to develop brain damage than the patient in a diabetic coma. Thus, giving sugar to a still-conscious patient in insulin shock could save a life or prevent brain damage. If the EMT gives sugar to a patient in a diabetic coma, there is very little risk of seriously worsening the patient's condition. Permanent damage or death will occur, if at all, only after a long period. Diabetic coma requires hours of insulin and fluid therapy, which should be done only under a physician's care.

The patient in insulin shock (or suspected insulin shock) who is unconscious or becomes unconscious during treatment cannot swallow. Therefore, no attempts should be made to give the patient juice or sugar, as it may be aspirated into the lungs. Intravenous glucose will be given at the emergency department. The basic EMT is not responsible for starting an intravenous solution; rather, the EMT's responsibility is to provide prompt transport of the patient so that care may be given in this very urgent situation.

In the past it has been recommended that "instant glucose," a prepared jelly, or glucose tablets be placed under the tongue or in the mouth of the unconscious patient. The substances may be used when no other treatment is at hand and transporta-

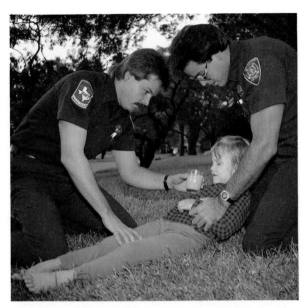

FIGURE 31.2 Juvenile diabetics frequently experience insulin shock because their activity level varies more than that of adults. This person needs sugar — lots of it, quickly — to offset the effects of too much insulin in the body. Pure sugar, candy, or fruit juice will reverse the reaction in one or two minutes.

tion will be prolonged. In general, however, this practice is probably not wise. Recent studies indicate that very little sugar administered in this way is absorbed.

The risk of choking or aspirating liquid into the lungs probably outweighs the benefits. The only way of giving sugar to these patients is intravenously. Prompt transport to the emergency department is the appropriate step.

YOU ARE THE EMT...

1. You know that glucose is as important to the brain as oxygen. Explain why the combination of too much insulin and too little food deprives the brain of glucose.
2. Juvenile diabetics are much more likely to go into insulin shock than adults, even though mother and dad carefully control their diet and injections. What is hard to control is the activity level of children. Why does this factor contribute to insulin shock?
3. The patient is semiconscious, and you believe he is suffering from hyperglycemia. Describe the signs and symptoms that led you to conclude he is hyperglycemic. How will you treat this patient?
4. You have been called to a college frat party. One of the girls seems to have had too much to drink and is talking incoherently. Her friends are worried because they know she is a diabetic. What should you do?

32 The Acute Abdomen

DEFINITION OF ACUTE ABDOMEN

Acute abdomen is a medical term that indicates the presence of some abdominal process that causes the sudden irritation of the **peritoneum,** the thin membrane that lines the entire abdominal cavity. Called **peritonitis,** this condition causes severe pain. The signs are abdominal tenderness and **distention** (swelling). All penetrating abdominal wounds and all blunt injuries severe enough to damage abdominal organs result in an acute abdomen. Certain diseases can also cause an acute abdomen.

The term **abdominal catastrophe** is used less frequently to denote the most severe form of an acute abdomen. Neither term — acute abdomen or abdominal catastrophe — is exact. Nor does either term refer to any specific disease or organ. Both mean the presence of a severe intra-abdominal problem that causes peritonitis. Both mean that a combination of certain signs and symptoms exists in a patient, regardless of the cause. Since many diseases in many different organs result in the same signs and complaints of pain and tenderness in the abdomen, it is possible to consider them all under the term "acute abdomen." Frequently, even a skilled surgeon has a hard time determining exactly what is causing an acute abdomen. The EMT need not know the exact cause and should not waste time attempting to make a diagnosis. Rather, the EMT's responsibility lies in being able to recognize the existence of this condition.

THE SIGNS AND SYMPTOMS OF THE ACUTE ABDOMEN

The following are common signs and symptoms of an acute abdomen arising from irritation or inflammation of the peritoneum:

1. Abdominal pain, local or diffuse
2. Abdominal tenderness, local or diffuse

3. Anorexia, nausea, vomiting
4. Patient lying rigid because it hurts to move
5. Rapid, shallow breaths because it hurts to breathe
6. Rapid pulse
7. Low blood pressure
8. A tense, often distended, abdomen
9. Referred (distant) pain
10. Fever
11. Constipation

The patient with peritonitis complains of abdominal pain even when lying quietly. There is extreme tenderness when the abdomen is palpated or when the patient moves. The degree of pain and tenderness usually is related to the severity of the peritoneal inflammation within.

The peritoneum is separated anatomically into two parts. The **parietal peritoneum** lines the walls of the abdominal cavity, and the **visceral peritoneum** covers the surface of all the abdominal organs. The nerve supply to these two parts of the peritoneum is different. The parietal peritoneum is innervated by the same nerves that innervate the skin in the abdominal region. Sensations perceived by the parietal peritoneum are similar to those felt by the skin: pain, touch, pressure, heat, and cold. Thus, the sensory nerves of the parietal peritoneum can identify and localize a point of irritation well.

In contrast, the visceral peritoneum is supplied by the **autonomic nervous system.** These nerves are far less able to localize any sensation. Sensations that are felt arise from activation of stretch receptors caused by distention or forceful contraction of the abdominal organs. This type of sensation is usually interpreted as **colic,** a severe, intermittent cramping pain.

The autonomic innervation of the visceral peritoneum gives rise to the phenomenon of **referred pain.** This means that an irritated peritoneal surface of a distended or inflamed organ may cause pain at a distant point on the body surface. This phenomenon occurs because one part of the spinal cord supplies nerves to two different body parts: sensory nerves to the skin and autonomic nerves to the abdominal organs. For example, **acute cholecystitis** (inflammation of the gallbladder) may cause pain in the right shoulder. The autonomic nerves to the gall-bladder originate at the same level of the spinal cord as the sensory nerves that supply the skin of the shoulder (Figure 32.1).

Peritonitis always causes **ileus** or paralysis of the muscular contractions that normally propel matter through the intestines. Often, retained gas and feces cause abdominal distention. In the presence of such paralysis, nothing that is eaten will be passed out of the stomach or through the bowel. Vomiting (**emesis**) is the only way in which the stomach can empty itself. Peritonitis almost always is associated with nausea and vomiting. These are nonspecific complaints, seen with almost every situation of gastrointestinal disease or peritonitis. Nausea is nearly universal and usually precedes emesis. Similarly, **anorexia** (loss of hunger or appetite) is a nonspecific symptom. It, too, is almost universal in gastrointestinal and abdominal disease but not specific for any one disease. Its absence usually indicates that the problems are not as serious as they might be. Diarrhea is rarely seen in patients with an acute abdomen because of the bowel paralysis. Varying degrees of constipation are much more frequent.

Peritonitis is always associated with the loss of body fluid into the abdominal cavity. The loss results

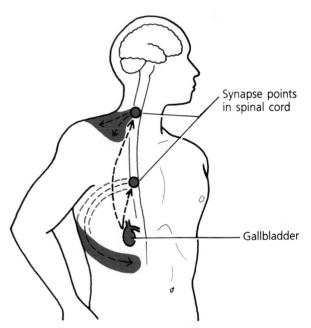

FIGURE 32.1 Acute cholecystitis causes referred pain in the shoulder as well as abdominal pain.

in a decrease in the volume of the circulating blood and may eventually cause **hypovolemic shock.** Depending on the stage of the development of peritonitis, the patient may have normal vital signs or may have a very rapid pulse (tachycardia) and low blood pressure (hypotension). If peritonitis is associated with hemorrhage, the signs of shock are much more severe.

Depending on the cause of the acute abdomen, fever may be present. Patients with **diverticulitis** (an inflammation of small pockets in the colon) or cholecystitis may have substantial temperature elevations. On the other hand, patients with acute **appendicitis** may not have fever until the appendix has ruptured and an abscess starts to form.

The acute abdomen is accompanied by varying degrees of abdominal pain and tenderness. Pain may be sharply localized or diffuse. Localized pain gives a clue to the cause. Tenderness may be minimal, or it may be so great that the patient will not allow the abdomen to be touched. In some instances, the muscles of the abdominal wall are absolutely rigid. This boardlike spasm of the abdominal muscles is seen with major problems such as a perforated **peptic ulcer** or **pancreatitis** (inflammation of the pancreas). Usually, there are varying decrees of **guarding** by the abdominal muscles in the irritated areas. In some diseases, patients can obtain comfort only by lying in one position. The position of the patient may provide an important clue. The patient with appendicitis, for example, may draw up the right knee. The patient with pancreatitis may lie curled up on one side. Each position tends to relax muscles adjacent to the inflamed organ and to lessen the pain.

Peritonitis may also cause painful breathing, since it hurts to move the inflamed peritoneal surfaces. Pulse and blood pressure may undergo radical change or none at all. Pulse and blood pressure readings usually reflect the severity of the process and its duration. Distention can easily be gauged by looking at the patient's abdomen, for it begins within a few hours after muscular contractions of the bowels have ceased.

The abdomen can be examined quickly using the following steps:

1. Determine whether the patient is restless or quiet, whether motion causes pain, or whether any characteristic position, distention, or abnormality is present.

2. Feel the abdomen gently to see whether it is tense (guarded) or soft.
3. Determine whether the patient can relax the abdominal wall on command.
4. Determine whether the abdomen is tender when touched. Such an examination will yield much information, but it should not be prolonged. The physician will do a much more detailed examination in the hospital. Abdominal palpation should be done very gently. Occasionally, an organ within the abdomen will be enlarged and very fragile, and rough palpation could cause further damage.

CAUSES OF ABDOMINAL DISEASE

The abdominal cavity contains the solid and hollow organs that make up the **gastrointestinal** and **genitourinary** systems. These organs, you will recall, are completely covered by the peritoneum; the parietal peritoneum lines the inside of the abdominal cavity, and the visceral peritoneum covers the surface of the organs. The entire cavity normally contains a very small amount of peritoneal fluid bathing the organs. Any condition that allows pus, blood, feces, urine, gastric juice, intestinal contents, bile, pancreatic juice, amniotic fluid, or other material to lie within or adjacent to this cavity can give rise to the signs of an acute abdomen (Figure 32.2).

Among the common diseases that produce these signs are acute appendicitis, perforated peptic ulcer, cholecystitis, and diverticulitis. The list of diseases that can produce an acute abdomen includes nearly every abdominal problem. The more common emergency problems and the location of the direct and referred pain produced are listed in Table 32.1.

Because the peritoneum is richly supplied with nerves that are sensitive to the presence of irritation, disease or inflammation of organs that lie behind or beneath the abdominal cavity can also cause the signs of peritonitis. These signs and symptoms are similar to those produced by actual inflammation within the abdominal cavity itself. Pancreatitis, for example, can produce a severe reaction that is hard to distinguish from a perforated ulcer. Kidney stones that cause ureteral colic are frequently associated with paralysis of bowel action, or ileus. One of the very common causes of an acute abdomen in the female is **pelvic inflammatory disease,** an infection in the

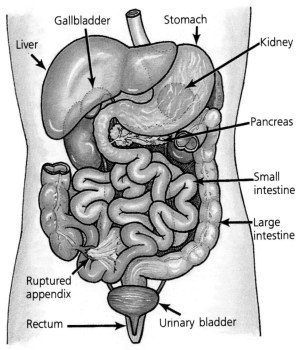

Liver, Gallbladder, Stomach, Kidney, Pancreas, Small intestine, Large intestine, Ruptured appendix, Rectum, Urinary bladder

FIGURE 32.2 Pus from a ruptured appendix has entered the abdominal cavity and caused peritonitis.

Fallopian tubes and the surrounding tissue of the pelvis. It is one of the major diseases that must be distinguished from appendicitis in female patients. Infections of the urinary tract may also cause peritoneal irritation.

The **aorta** lies immediately behind the peritoneum on the spinal column. In older people the wall of the aorta sometimes develops weak areas that swell and form an **aneurysm.** The development of an aneurysm is rarely associated with symptoms because it occurs slowly, but if the aneurysm ruptures, massive hemorrhage may occur. Some of the signs of acute peritoneal irritation may then arise, along with severe back pain, because the peritoneum is rapidly stripped away from the body wall by the hemorrhage. In such instances, peritoneal signs are usually associated with profound shock because of the associated bleeding.

EMERGENCY CARE OF THE PATIENT WITH AN ACUTE ABDOMEN

The signs and symptoms of an acute abdomen justify a working diagnosis of some serious abdominal surgical emergency. There should be no delay in trans-

porting the patient to the emergency department. The following steps should be carried out as quickly as possible prior to transport:

1. Do not attempt to make a specific diagnosis.
2. Clear and maintain the airway.
3. Anticipate vomiting.
4. Give oxygen.
5. Anticipate the development of hypovolemic shock.
6. Do not give anything by mouth.
7. Do not administer any sedative or analgesic agent.
8. Record all pertinent information: onset, type, severity, and duration of symptoms.
9. Position the patient comfortably for transport.

Vomiting is not uncommon in these patients, as the emergency frequently develops just after the patient has eaten a large meal or had much to drink. The patient's throat and airway must be cleared of vomited material and kept clear. Pain makes breathing physically difficult. Thus, supplemental oxygen should be used to compensate for small respiratory volumes.

TABLE 32.1 Common Diseases That Cause Acute Abdomen and Localization of Pain

Disease	Localization of Pain
Appendicitis	Around navel (referred); right lower quadrant (direct)
Cholecystitis	Right shoulder (referred); right upper quadrant (direct)
Duodenal ulcer	Upper mid-abdomen or upper back
Diverticulitis	Left lower quadrant
Aortic aneurysm (ruptured)	Low back and right lower quadrant
Cystitis (bladder inflammation)	Lower mid-abdomen (retropubic)
Kidney infection	Costovertebral angle
Kidney stone	Either right or left flanks, radiating to genitalia
Pelvic inflammation (female)	Both lower quadrants
Pancreatitis	Upper abdomen (both quadrants); back

Under no circumstances should a patient with acute abdominal signs be given anything to eat or drink. Food or fluid will only aggravate many of the symptoms. In the presence of peritoneal irritation and intestinal paralysis, food does not pass out of the stomach. If an emergency operation is required, the presence of food in the stomach will make the operation much more dangerous.

No matter how much pain the patient is experiencing, the EMT should not give any medication to relieve pain or sedate the patient. The examining physician must know exactly where and how severe the pain is. Medication frequently masks these findings and may delay an ultimate diagnosis until it is too late to correct the problem.

In cases of acute abdomen, the EMT should not attempt to diagnose the patient's disease. Rather, the EMT should listen to the description of the location of pain and tenderness and the severity of symptoms. The presence of abdominal tenderness, distention, or guarding should be noted. The patient's description of how the process started should be recorded, along with the vital signs, so that the physician may know what these were when the patient was first seen. Shock is common in these cases and must be recognized early. Its presence makes prompt transport to the hospital even more imperative. The patient should be made as comfortable as possible; body heat should be conserved using blankets. Finally, the patient should be gently and promptly transported to the emergency department.

YOU ARE THE EMT...

1. You believe the patient's severe abdominal pain is from acute cholecystitis. The patient also has referred shoulder pain. What abdominal organ is affected? Explain why the patient is experiencing referred shoulder pain.
2. You were complimented for recognizing acute appendicitis and getting the patient to the hospital before his appendix ruptured. Why is a ruptured appendix considered such a serious medical emergency?
3. Acute abdomen, you know, can occur if body fluids that do not belong in the abdomen enter it and cause inflammation. Identify eight bodily substances that could by their presence cause an acute abdomen.
4. Your patient has all the signs and symptoms of an acute abdomen. Describe the emergency treatment you will administer.

Common Medical Complaints

33

OVERVIEW

The EMT will attend many patients who have not been injured in an accident or become severely ill from an acute abdomen, diabetes, stroke, or a heart attack. These patients will have any one of a number of less severe complaints that are serious enough to interfere with their normal daily activities.

Emergency complaints involving the gastrointestinal (GI) tract include difficulty in swallowing, vomiting, vomiting blood, diarrhea, passage of blood in the stool, jaundice, colic, heartburn, constipation, and the eating disorders bulimia and anorexia nervosa. Emergency complaints involving the genitourinary (GU) tract include pain or burning during urination, passage of blood in the urine, frequency of urination, lack of bladder control, urinary retention, urethral discharge, vaginal bleeding, kidney stones, and pregnancy outside the uterus.

Chapter 33 discusses all of these GI and GU problems, as well as two additional ones: vertigo and hiccough. While generally not life-threatening, many of these problems are perceived as being serious by the patient. Elderly patients are especially upset by many of the symptoms of these problems. The chapter therefore concludes with a discussion of the special concerns of geriatric patients.

OBJECTIVES

The objectives of Chapter 33 are to

- identify and describe common gastrointestinal complaints not associated with injury or an acute abdomen.
- identify and describe common genitourinary complaints not associated with injuries.
- define vertigo and hiccough and describe their causes.
- understand the special concerns of geriatric patients.

THE GASTROINTESTINAL TRACT

Dysphagia

Dysphagia is the sensation of sticking or discomfort when swallowing. It is caused by obstructing lesions in the esophagus, which can range all the way from swallowed foreign bodies to tumors. The condition may be severe and acute, as with a foreign body, or slowly progressive, as with cancer. In general, the patient complains of a sensation of food sticking under the sternum or at the back of the throat.

Dysphagia is a complaint ignored by many people until the problem becomes very serious. For example, at first only chunks of meat may have given problems. Most individuals can treat such swallowing difficulties with a drink of water at meals. They then tend to forget about the problem until the next meal, since dysphagia usually does not cause pain. Eventually, however, only liquids or very soft foods can be tolerated. When the person finally gets to a physician, the problem is often severe and has interfered with the patient's nutrition.

The EMT should recognize that dysphagia has either come about because of a long-standing disease which has recently become intolerable or it has come on quickly and is thus an acute, severe problem. In either instance, professional help must be obtained promptly. While not usually an emergency condition in itself, dysphagia is a complaint that is often associated with very serious illness which has been neglected or ignored. It becomes an emergency once the patient can no longer swallow at all. Then there is a danger that food or saliva will be aspirated into the lungs. Prompt transportation to the emergency department is called for.

Vomiting and the Aspiration of Vomitus

One of the commonest GI complaints is vomiting, or **emesis.** It is the stomach's response to a stimulus — irritation, infection, or obstruction. It is to be distinguished from **regurgitation,** which is a "burp" of air and fluid that comes back up as the result of the stomach's being too full.

Vomiting has many causes. One cause is any situation that produces **peritonitis** or an **acute abdomen** that can stop **peristaltic contraction** in the GI tract — that is, when the muscles that propel the contents of the intestines stop working. Vomiting then becomes the only way the stomach can empty. Or, any disease that causes inflammation of the lining of the GI tract, especially the stomach, will cause vomiting. **Gastroenteritis,** a viral or bacterial infection of the stomach or the intestine, is another common cause. The ingestion of irritating agents can also cause vomiting, especially among those who have heavily indulged in an alcoholic beverage. Alcohol is a stimulator of gastric juice production as well as an irritant of the lining of the stomach. Food poisoning often causes vomiting as the stomach attempts to rid itself of the noxious agent. Contaminated food and alcohol are not the only irritants. The excessive use of certain drugs such as aspirin may also cause inflammation of the stomach lining and vomiting. Finally, mechanical obstruction to the passage of material through the GI tract will also cause vomiting. Mechanical obstruction can be produced by tumors or by swallowed foreign bodies.

Vomiting is very common among children. Often, a baby's contented "burp" after a full bottle will produce a "swallowful" of regurgitated milk and much air. Some infants will experience severe, unremitting and forceful vomiting from a condition called **pyloric stenosis,** an obstruction of the outlet of the stomach. Most of the time, vomiting in children is from a bacterial or viral gastroenteritis.

Vomiting is always serious, since the EMT has no real knowledge of its cause. It may be much more complex than gastroenteritis or too much whiskey. In adults, vomiting that continues for several days may result in a dangerous loss of water and nutrients. Serious metabolic problems can then occur, particularly **dehydration.** In infants and small children, vomiting may produce these changes within 24 hours. In such situations, the patient may actually be in shock because of the significant fluid and salt loss. (Shock is dealt with in Chapter 11.)

The alert patient who is vomiting because of illness is rarely, if ever, in danger of aspirating the vomitus. All the protective reflexes of the airway are active. However, a very small drop of irritating saliva or gastric juice will usually cause severe **laryngospasm** and violent coughing. The patient must be assisted to vomit as is necessary and placed in a position of comfort. The EMT must be alert for more vomiting during transport. An emesis basin or other receptacle and clean towels should be available to the patient.

The sleepy, unconscious, or drunken patient may aspirate vomited material into the airway. Normal reflex protection in these patients is often depressed or absent. Once aspirated, material is rarely coughed out by the patient because the cough reflex is also depressed. Acidic gastric juice will destroy lung tissue rapidly. Alveoli and small bronchi can literally be digested away. The damaged lung tissue is easily infected, and **pulmonary abscess** usually follows.

In treating a vomiting patient who is not fully alert, the EMT must pay special attention to the airway. Aspiration of vomitus can occur in a matter of seconds, and the EMT must be prepared to clear and maintain the airway. The patient should be placed on one side, with the head lower than the feet. Nothing must be allowed to accumulate in the pharynx. Large-bore suction catheters should be at hand to clear vomitus as it occurs. The airway should be maintained manually using the jaw thrust or chin-lift technique (Figure 33.1).

Many times, the EMT will arrive after vomitus has been aspirated into the lungs. Sometimes this event produces few symptoms and signs. More often, however, the patient will be breathing rapidly and have a large volume of tracheal secretions. The patient may be cyanotic. In this instance, prompt transport to the emergency department is absolutely essential. En route, the patient should be given supplemental oxygen. Full ventilatory support, including assisted breathing, may be required. Surgical removal of the aspirated vomitus within 30 to 60 minutes may save the patient's life or prevent abscess formation in the lungs.

The vomiting patient who is in shock (dehydrated, lethargic, low blood pressure, and rapid, thready pulse) as a result of emesis alone is seriously ill and demands prompt hospital care. This patient has lost as much fluid, electrolytes, and plasma as the patient with a severe burn or with extensive hemorrhage. After all the needed measures for airway protection and initial support have been completed, the patient should be given oxygen and

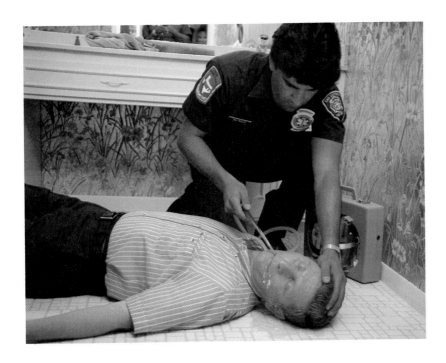

FIGURE 33.1 The airway must be kept clear, particularly in the semiconscious patient. Here, the EMT is using a large-bore suction catheter to keep the airway patent.

transported as promptly as possible to the emergency department.

In each of the above instances, the EMT should note the nature of the vomited material (what it contains), its frequency, its volume, and the character of the vomiting process (forceful, projectile, or regurgitant).

Hematemesis

The vomiting of blood, called **hematemesis,** is a particularly disturbing event for the patient. In general, it is associated with diseases in the esophagus or stomach. The three most common disorders causing hematemesis are stomach ulcers, ruptured esophageal varices, or gastritis.

Stomach ulcers have a variety of causes. Most patients will have a history of upper abdominal pain and may be taking antacid medication to relieve these symptoms. Many have had a previous history of vomiting blood. **Esophageal varices** are dilated veins in the wall of the esophagus, which develop in patients with liver disease. Scarring in the liver impairs its normal blood flow, and the blood is shunted to the veins in the esophagus. The veins become quite enlarged, and their very thin walls rupture easily. Bleeding from esophageal varices is sudden, heavy, bright red, painless, and frequently fatal.

Gastritis, which is inflammation or irritation of the stomach lining, is produced by emotional stress and by chemical irritants such as alcohol, aspirin, and other drugs. The patient will usually have vague, moderate upper-abdominal pain and tenderness with gastritis.

Hematemesis can occur as **"coffee-grounds" vomitus** in relatively small quantities or as large quantities of very bright red blood. Coffee-grounds vomitus is so called because the material produced looks like coffee grounds suspended in the clear mucus and liquid of normal gastric juice. It indicates a slow rate of bleeding into the stomach. Small quantities of blood are digested and turn dark brown from the hydrochloric acid that is present in the stomach. Large quantities of bright red blood, on the other hand, mean that very brisk bleeding is taking place.

With either form of hematemesis — bright red bleeding or coffee-ground vomitus — the patient should be transported promptly to the emergency department. The amount of blood vomited should be estimated and recorded. If possible, a sample of the vomitus should be collected and taken with the patient to the hospital. In addition, vital signs should be monitored closely, the airway should be protected and maintained, and provisions should be made for further vomiting while en route to the hospital.

Diarrhea

Just as there are a number of causes of vomiting, so are there a number of causes of **diarrhea,** which is a term describing an abnormally large number of bowel movements of abnormally liquid character. Anxiety, gastroenteritis, the common viral "flu," severe infections with bacteria such as typhoid fever, or parasitic infestation as with amoebae can all cause diarrhea. A number of inflammatory diseases in the bowel for which causes are unknown, such as **ulcerative colitis,** can also cause diarrhea. In the elderly person, one of the most common causes is a partial obstruction of the bowel by a **fecal impaction.** In this apparently contradictory situation, the fecal impaction allows only watery material to pass, which produces the complaint of diarrhea.

Very rarely is diarrhea the cause of an acute emergency problem. If it has been present for several days and if the patient has been unable to take sufficient food or fluid to balance the amount lost, then dehydration and lethargy may be present. This patient, just like the neglected vomiter, may have unstable vital signs and may be developing **hypovolemic shock.**

The EMT must recognize that uncontrolled diarrhea or vomiting, if it has lasted over a period of several days or more, may result in serious metabolic changes. The patient with diarrhea serious enough to necessitate an emergency call should be transported to the emergency department for an assessment of the cause of the problem.

Melena and Hematochezia

The term **melena** is derived from a Greek word meaning black. It describes a dark, black **stool** that is very tarry or sticky in consistency. It has a characteristic, particularly foul odor. The black color is due to the presence of blood that has been digested within the GI tract. In general, melena is caused by slow, continuous bleeding in the upper part of the GI tract from ulcers, polyps, or tumors. Some medications (bismuth and iron-containing compounds) may give the same dark color to the stool but not the tarry consistency or foul smell. Melena is not an emergency situation unless it has persisted and been ignored for a long time. Under those circumstances the patient could exhibit signs of hypovolemic shock. Melena is, however, a cause for grave concern because the bleeding source must be identified as expeditiously as possible.

The passage of bright red blood in the stool is called **hematochezia.** Hemotochezia has a number of causes that range from the very serious problem of colon or rectal cancer to the common problem of **hemorrhoids.** The EMT should keep in mind that sometimes patients mistake vaginal bleeding for rectal bleeding. Bright red blood in the stool is not ordinarily an emergency medical problem, although it may be very alarming to the patient. Except in a very few instances, the bleeding is customarily not massive. It is, however, a distinctly abnormal situation that requires prompt medical evaluation to diagnose the cause.

The EMT who has responded to a complaint of melena or hematochezia must monitor the patient's vital signs and then transfer the patient to the emergency department for appropriate examination and diagnosis of the cause. An accurate description of the characteristics and the volume of bloody stool passed will be helpful to the evaluating physician.

Jaundice

Occasionally, the EMT will be called to see a patient who is jaundiced. **Jaundice** is a term derived from a French word meaning yellow. It is not a disease; rather, it describes a yellow color of the skin. Many problems may cause jaundice, almost all of them related to some malfunction of the liver or the biliary tract. The liver produces **bile,** a yellow compound that plays an essential role in the digestion of fat in the GI tract. Bile is excreted from the liver into the duodenum through the **biliary tract.** A considerable portion of the excreted bile is reabsorbed in the intestines and returned to the liver. The rest of the bile is excreted. It is responsible for the normal brown color of feces.

Any disease that interferes with the normal function of the liver so that bile cannot be made or excreted will cause jaundice. Common causes of abnormal liver function are infection (**hepatitis**) and poisoning of liver cells from alcohol and other toxic substances. Chronic alcohol abuse causes permanent liver damage, which is called **cirrhosis.** In addition, any situation in which the outflow of bile from the liver to the GI tract is blocked will cause jaundice. For example, a stone (**gallstone**) that forms in the gallbladder can block the biliary tract; cancers of the

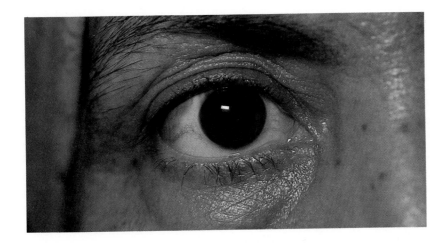

FIGURE 33.2 Careful inspection of the sclera, or normally white portion, of the eye in good lighting will reveal even mild degrees of jaundice.

bile duct, pancreas, or duodenum can also block the biliary tract.

Although severe jaundice is evident by simply looking at the patient, the early and mild stages are only detected by using good lighting to look at areas of the body that are normally white. The best place to look for jaundice is in the sclera of the eye, particularly in darkly pigmented individuals (Figure 33.2). When examining any patient, the EMT should check the sclera for a yellow color (**scleral icterus**).

Jaundice always indicates a potentially serious medical condition. Therefore, all patients with jaundice must receive a thorough medical evaluation by a physician. Because the jaundice may be caused by hepatitis, the EMT must be particularly careful when handling the patient (see Chapter 34).

Colic

Colic is a characteristic, intra-abdominal pain that is caused by obstruction of one of the hollow organs. The pain is intermittent; it rises sharply to an excruciating peak and then relents fairly suddenly as the muscle in the wall of the organ relaxes. Colic occurs in individuals with obstruction of the GI tract by tumors, polyps, foreign bodies, or adhesions. Obstruction in the small bowel is generally noted as colic felt around the **umbilicus** (the area around the belly button). In the right or left colon, obstruction produces a pain that is felt in the same flank. Individuals who have a urinary stone obstructing a ureter, called a **kidney stone,** experience a characteristic radiation of pain from the flank and into the genitalia. The pain from a kidney stone is excruciating.

Colic is a very common complaint among children, where it represents very active peristalsis in the GI tract. It is also a relatively frequent complaint in the adult in association with flu syndrome and vigorous diarrhea. Again, in this situation, it is associated with extreme hyperperistaltic activity of the GI tract. Frequently, the patient will describe colic as a cramp or a "gas pain."

The EMT should be familiar with the term *colic* and be able to recognize the pain when it is described. It is a very distressing complaint for the patient, and its cause must be assessed by a physician.

Heartburn (Esophageal Reflux)

The esophagus is lined with tissue that is similar to the skin. Because it does not produce mucus, it has no capacity to protect itself from the potent corrosive action of the digestive enzymes in gastric juice. Occasionally, gastric juice will reflux into the lower esophagus and attack its lining. The damage to the lining will range from mild irritation to deep ulcers and even perforation of the esophagus in extreme cases. **Esophageal reflux** causes a typical burning pain referred to as **heartburn,** under the sternum. Usually, the pain occurs after heavy meals, much drinking, or at night when a person is lying in bed. It occurs most frequently in the obese, short patient and is aggravated by straining, squatting, or lifting. Anything that increases the intra-abdominal pressure (such as pregnancy) will aggravate it.

Esophageal reflux is a common problem but not an emergency. However, the symptom of substernal chest pain can be caused by other, more serious, disorders. The EMT must be alert to the patient complaining of "indigestion" or "heartburn" whose symptoms may be due to an acute myocardial infarction.

Bulimia and Anorexia Nervosa

Bulimia is defined as an abnormal increase in the sensation of hunger. Bulimia results in significant overeating followed by self-induced vomiting. In this way, the bulimic individual maintains a relatively normal weight. Often this situation comes to light only when the family realizes the grocery bills have increased enormously. **Anorexia nervosa,** as contrasted with bulimia, is defined as lack or loss of appetite. Characteristically, the patient takes less and less food and may become seriously emaciated and malnourished.

Bulimia may occur at any age, but it is rare in older individuals. Anorexia nervosa is much more common in younger females. Neither is a strict emergency situation, although the EMT may be called if anorexia has caused severe problems in nutrition. Each situation is a manifestation of rather severe underlying psychological disorders. Each requires skilled treatment for a prolonged period of time. The EMT should recognize the need for this type of care in these patients. Emergency transport ordinarily will be needed only by the neglected, severely dehydrated, and starved anorexic patient, or by the bulimic individual who is experiencing a specific problem related to vomiting.

A warning for EMTs is that significant instances of drug abuse with **syrup of ipecac,** a drug traditionally used to induce vomiting in patients who have swallowed a poisonous substance, are now being reported in bulimic patients. Drug abuse of this type is rarely suspected. Ambulance supplies of this medication should therefore be carefully supervised.

Constipation

Constipation in the older individual is a frequent and generally progressive phenomenon. As patients become less and less physically active, bowel activity similarly tends to decrease. Much more important is that the older person's diet tends to become softer and include less fresh fruits, vegetables, and bulk. The person perhaps loses teeth, has some difficulty in swallowing, and automatically tends to turn to softer and mushier foods. Not surprisingly, many individuals in this age group subsist on soup, tea, and toast. This type of diet produces a very small, hard stool, which takes considerable effort to pass. Many individuals, especially those bedridden or in nursing homes, cease to make the effort.

After some time, the colon (large bowel) becomes greatly distended with accumulated feces. Ironically, constipated patients may develop watery diarrhea, which is caused by the substantial fecal impaction. In this situation, the only material that can pass down the GI tract and around the impaction is liquid; the liquid literally flows around the obstruction. Fecal impaction is one of the most common problems of the older patient. It is often a cause of partial bowel obstruction.

Unfortunately, in the older patient the rather common complaint of chronic constipation frequently masks a very serious cause of progressive constipation and obstruction — cancer of the colon. A common presenting complaint of colon cancer is difficulty passing stools, up to and including complete obstruction. For this reason alone, the elderly patient who complains of increasing and severe constipation should be taken to the emergency department for diagnosis.

THE GENITOURINARY TRACT

Dysuria

Dysuria is the sensation of pain, burning, or itching that occurs during urination. It generally indicates an inflammatory process or infection within the lower urinary tract, which includes the external urethral opening, the urethra, and the bladder. Dysuria is a relatively common symptom in females because of the higher frequency of urinary tract infections in females than in males. Although dysuria is symptomatic of a problem that should be evaluated and treated, it is not a significant emergency situation.

Hematuria

The passage of blood in the urine is called **hematuria.** Occasionally there is enough of it to be visible to the naked eye. More frequently, however, it is identified only by microscopic examination of a urine specimen. Hematuria has a number of causes: tumors of the urinary tract, stones causing abrasions and bleeding from the kidney or the ureters, and trauma are some of the more common causes. If called for this problem, the EMT should transport the patient to the emergency department for an appropriate diagnostic workup. Except following injury, hematuria is not an emergency situation. However, if it is easily evident to the unaided eye, it may point to a very serious problem within the urinary tract. Expeditious diagnosis is demanded, especially if the patient has no pain. Hematuria associated with pain, burning, or itching usually means infection. Hematuria caused by trauma is discussed in Chapter 25.

Any urine passed by the patient with significant urinary complaints should be brought to the emergency department for careful analysis. Frequently, it can provide the necessary clue for diagnosis.

Frequency

The term **frequency** describes an abnormally high number of **voiding** (urinating) episodes during any 24-hour period. Frequency associated with dysuria usually indicates a bladder infection. Infection causes the passage of very small quantities of urine at very frequent intervals. Generally, the urine associated with a bladder infection smells unusually bad.

In the aging male a situation commonly develops in which the **prostate gland,** which surrounds the upper portion of the urethra, enlarges. As this gland enlarges, it encroaches on the urethral passage and partially obstructs it. A sign of this obstruction is urinary frequency, which persists not only during the day but throughout the night as well. The passage of urine at night is called **nocturia.** Congestive heart failure is another problem which can often cause frequency and nocturia in the older patient.

Urinary frequency is not necessarily an emergency situation, but its presence should be recognized by the EMT. Its significance is the indication of an underlying disorder.

Incontinence

The uncontrolled passage of urine or feces resulting in soiling of one's clothing is called **incontinence.** It may occur in several emergency conditions. For example, the patient undergoing an epileptic seizure frequently experiences incontinence during the seizure. In this situation it does not indicate significant urinary or bowel disease. The patient with a spinal cord injury resulting in paraplegia has lost control of the muscular sphincters which control both urinary and fecal discharge.

Episodic incontinence is frequently associated with unconsciousness or semiconsciousness, as in an alcoholic binge. The elderly patient may be incontinent as a result of generalized senile degeneration of the brain cells that provide control. Incontinence that is sudden, unexpected, and not associated with any obvious cause may signal the presence of a significant disorder in the lower urinary tract or rectum. Such incontinence is a reason to transport the patient to the hospital for diagnosis.

Urethral Discharge

Any material that passes out of the male urethra other than urine or semen is called a **urethral discharge.** It is an abnormal condition that requires medical attention. Urethral discharge is the most common indication in the male of venereal disease — an extremely common problem in the United States today. The penile urethral discharge may be thin and watery or it may be grossly **purulent** (containing pus).

If the EMT is called for the patient whose only complaint is a urethral discharge, the situation is not an emergency. But treatment for the cause of the discharge should be sought immediately, because these diseases can become chronic and can have devastating effects for the individual years later.

Renal Colic

A fairly common clinical problem is the formation of kidney stones. Once formed, the stones cannot be dissolved by the body. As long as the stones are in the kidney they do not cause pain. At the most, they may produce hematuria, which may not be apparent unless the urine is examined microscropically for red blood cells.

A stone that passes from the kidney into the **ureter** can obstruct this very small caliber tube. Urine is formed continuously in the kidney. Approximately one liter of it is passed out of each kidney through the ureters into the bladder every day. Since there is no reservoir for urine above the bladder and since the capacity of the ureters and the collecting system of the kidney is very small, this liter of urine must pass quickly through the ureter into the bladder without impediment. When a ureter becomes obstructed by a stone, a characteristic severe pain

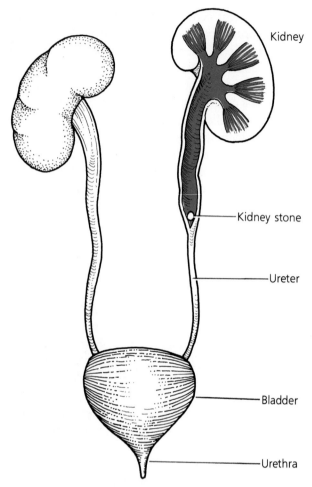

Kidney

Kidney stone

Ureter

Bladder

Urethra

FIGURE 33.3 A kidney stone produces excruciating pain called renal colic when it passes from the kidney where it is formed and into the ureter. The stone obstructs the ureter and causes distention.

(**renal colic**) occurs as the muscular ureter tries to overcome the obstruction by very vigorous peristalsis close to the stone (Figure 33.3). The colic is perceived as an excruciatingly sharp pain in the flank on the right or left side of the back. As the stone progresses down the ureter, the pain may radiate to the groin and the external genitalia. Once the stone enters the bladder, the renal colic ceases. Renal colic, as mentioned earlier, is one of the severest forms of pain known. Relief requires very vigorous treatment.

The patient suffering from renal colic can describe the type of pain, its location, and its radiation. This patient is generally restless and forever seeking a position of some comfort — getting up or lying down. The situation is not a life-threatening

one for the patient. It is, however, an urgent situation in which the patient demands and requires relief from pain. The EMT called to see a patient suffering from renal colic should transport the patient promptly to the emergency department. Ordinarily, no significant measures for support of other body systems are necessary. Any urine passed should be collected, saved, and presented for analysis at the hospital.

Acute Urinary Retention

Occasionally, and almost always in the older male patient, the EMT will encounter **acute urinary retention.** Ordinarily, this situation occurs as an event in a long history of urinary difficulty characterized by gradual loss of force of the stream, increased urinary frequency, and nocturia. Usually it results from a slowly progressive enlargement of the prostate gland so that the urethral outlet of the bladder is obstructed. This enlargement can be benign (**prostatic hypertrophy**) or the result of cancer.

The pain of acute bladder distention is intense, and the urge to void is overwhelming. As more urine is produced by the kidneys, the bladder may enlarge to lie as high as the umbilicus. This situation develops over a matter of a very few hours and requires prompt transport to the emergency department. Relief will be obtained only by inserting a tube directly into the bladder, called **catheterization,** by skilled medical personnel. Ordinarily, the catheter will be left in until the obstruction can be corrected.

Vaginal Spotting, Bleeding, and Discharge

A normal menstrual cycle produces a monthly, regular, bloody, menstrual, **vaginal discharge** in all healthy, nonpregnant women after puberty and before menopause. The characteristics of the bleeding vary from patient to patient and are usually well known to the individual (length of flow, amount of material discharged, presence or absence of cramps, onset and termination). Any other vaginal discharge is abnormal.

Far and away the most common causes of abnormal vaginal discharge are fungal or bacterial infections. The complaint of a vaginal discharge is not an emergency condition, and emergency transport to the hospital is not necessary. But medical care and advice should be recommended and sought.

Any bleeding from the vagina, other than menstrual, is abnormal. The most common and least serious cause relates to abnormalities of the menstrual cycle. However, this type of bleeding may be the only sign of malignant disease within the female reproductive system. Bleeding after sexual contact may be a sign of a tumor of the vagina or cervix.

In general, vaginal bleeding is not a medical emergency because the volume of blood lost is usually quite small. The bleeding, however, indicates the possibility of a serious problem requiring prompt diagnosis. Unfortunately, as with many other problems, the patient tends to ignore bleeding if there is no pain. For these reasons, the EMT should encourage the patient to seek medical evaluation and even offer transport to the emergency department for diagnosis. The EMT should not examine the female genitalia or vagina, or pack or put anything into the vagina.

Ectopic Pregnancy

Ectopic pregnancy is the development of a fetus in an abnormal location, usually in the Fallopian tube. It occurs on rare occasions when an ovum, after being discharged from the ovary, becomes fertilized early in its passage to the uterus through the Fallopian tube. The ovum sometimes comes to rest within the tube rather than in the cavity of the uterus. The Fallopian tube is a relatively thin-walled structure with little muscular content. It does not have the capacity to expand to encompass the developing fetus. If the fertilized ovum lodges there, the Fallopian tube can support the growth of the fetus and its placenta for approximately six weeks. Then the tube, stretched beyond its capacity to expand, ruptures.

Rupture of the Fallopian tube causes severe bleeding into the abdominal cavity. The patient will have lower abdominal pain and tenderness and may develop hypovolemic shock very rapidly. The young female who can give a history of appropriate sexual exposure, with one or two missed menstrual periods, who is in shock, and who has a tender lower abdomen is highly suggestive of an ectopic pregnancy. The emergency medical treatment for this patient is based on anticipating and treating shock. All the measures needed for the correction of hypovolemic shock must be instituted. Prompt transportation to the hospital is mandatory since the bleeding usually continues and may become life-threatening. This patient will require an emergency operation to control the problem.

VERTIGO AND HICCOUGH

Vertigo

The problem of **vertigo,** or dizziness, is relatively common, especially among the aging population. It usually is caused by arteriosclerosis of the cerebral blood vessels, which produces impaired circulation to the brain. Injuries of the inner ear can also cause vertigo. In these cases, the vertigo is usually accompanied by **tinnitus** (ringing in the ear). Certain medications are available to counteract vertigo even when the exact cause is unknown.

In general, vertigo is not an acute emergency problem. It can be so severe, however, that the patient is literally confined to bed, unable to walk or sit safely. When vertigo is this severe, the cause should be identified and the patient transported to the emergency department. It is not uncommon for these patients to be nauseated, so the EMT should be alert for vomiting. Ordinarily, no care other than keeping the patient lying flat and comfortable is needed. Vertigo in which there is an actual sensation of rotating in space should be distinguished from lightheadedness or giddiness, which is a much more common complaint.

Hiccough

Hiccough, a common complaint that arises from a variety of causes, is a sudden inspiration of air that is rapidly checked by closure of the epiglottis of the larynx. In the healthy individual it results from acute distention of the stomach, from anxiety, or, occasionally, from a central neurological problem. Irritation of the diaphragm, particularly the presence of an abscess in a postoperative patient, will cause persistent hiccough. Very rarely is hiccough an emergency medical problem. It becomes so only if it has lasted for several hours or days and interferes with eating and sleeping. A number of treatments exist ranging from rebreathing inspired air to the use of intravenous sedative medication. In general, if the symptoms are severe and persistent enough to warrant calling an emergency medical service, transportation to the emergency department is indicated.

SPECIAL CONCERNS FOR GERIATRIC PATIENTS

Most of the problems discussed in this chapter occur in adults. A few of them are much more complicated in the older, or **geriatric,** patient. The EMT should keep in mind that sudden changes or rapid moves from familiar surroundings may easily disorient or terrorize geriatric patients. They may respond with a combative, hostile, or surly attitude. Not infrequently, they stubbornly refuse to accept the most obviously needed methods of treatment. In these situations, the cooperation of friends and family, along with patience and a calm approach on the part of the EMT, is absolutely necessary. Generally, the wishes of the patient and the patient's family must be respected unless the emergency is obviously life-threatening.

YOU ARE THE EMT...

1. The patient is in shock as a result of long hours of vomiting. Why is this condition as serious as that resulting from a severe burn or uncontrolled internal bleeding?
2. You have been called to a medical emergency in which a female patient is vomiting blood. Identify and describe the three possible causes of hematemesis.
3. You have probably heard a lot about anorexia—it seems to be a popular ailment of movie actresses, models, and teenage girls. What is anorexia and how does it differ from bulimia? Why do you think it occurs more often among the females just described?
4. What are kidney stones, and why do they cause such terrific pain?

Communicable Diseases

34

OVERVIEW

Communicable diseases go back to the origins of man. In epidemic proportions they have killed more people than wars or natural disasters. Smallpox, typhoid, and influenza have been catastrophic enough to change the course of history. Medical research, vaccines, and improvements in sanitation have eradicated many communicable diseases, but germs still exist and are transmitted to humans by other humans or by insects and animals. And old diseases have been replaced by new ones. AIDS, for example, is the communicable disease perhaps most feared today.

EMTs, doctors, nurses, and other medical personnel are sometimes exposed to communicable diseases. It is very important that they become knowledgeable in lessening the risk of exposure and taking preventive actions after exposure. Chapter 34 thus begins by presenting the terms and definitions that EMTs are expected to know when dealing with communicable diseases. The chapter next explains how communicable diseases are transmitted and how to prevent their transmission to the EMT. Part of prevention is identifying infectious disease patients — often a difficult task. The chapter next describes five communicable diseases that are apt to cause problems for EMTs and other care providers: hepatitis, herpetic whitlow, meningitis, tuberculosis, and AIDS. The last section of Chapter 34 reviews risk and prevention procedures that should be followed by EMTs.

OBJECTIVES

The objectives of Chapter 34 are to

- understand communicable diseases and the infectious process.
- understand the role of the EMT in treating a patient with a communicable disease.
- become familiar with the characteristics and basic epidemiology of common communicable diseases.

TERMS AND DEFINITIONS

The following terms are routinely used to describe **communicable (infectious** or **contagious) diseases,** or diseases that can be transmitted from one person to another. The EMT must be thoroughly familiar with these terms.

Infection: The invasion of a host or host tissue by organisms such as bacteria, viruses, or parasites.

Contamination: The presence of infective organisms on or in objects such as dressings, water, food, or the patient's body surface.

Communicable (infectious or contagious): Capable of transmitting disease.

Reservoir: A place where infectious organisms live and multiply, such as stagnant water or a sewer.

Source of infection: The origin of the infection or infectious agent; it may be a person, object, or any substance carrying bacteria, viruses, or parasites (occasionally a reservoir is a source of infection).

Period of communicability: The time during which an infectious agent may be transmitted to a host from another carrier.

Incubation period: The time between exposure of the host to the infectious agent and the appearance of symptoms of that infection.

Carrier: An animal or person who may transmit an infectious disease but does not display any symptoms of it.

Transmission: The manner by which an infectious agent is spread: contact, airborne, by vehicles, or by vectors.

Host: The organism or individual attacked by the infecting agent (the host is infected).

ROUTES OF TRANSMISSION

The term *communicable (infectious) disease* refers to an illness that can be transmitted from one person to another. The method of transfer is called the **mode of transmission;** it can take place in one of four ways (Figure 34.1).

1. **Contact transmission.** There are two methods of contact: direct and indirect. Direct physical contact takes place between an individual and the infected person. Indirect physical contact takes place between an individual and inanimate objects that may have infectious organisms on them — for example, vehicle surfaces, dressings, equipment, or linens.

2. **Airborne transmission.** The infective organism is introduced into the air by a patient who is coughing or sneezing. Droplets of mucus that carry bacteria or other organisms can then be inhaled by another individual.

3. **Vehicle transmission.** The infective organism is introduced directly into the body through the ingestion of contaminated food, or water, or by the infusion of contaminated drugs, fluid, or blood.

4. **Vector transmission.** The infective organism is transmitted to an individual by animals; for example, mosquitoes transmit malarial parasites, and ticks transmit rocky mountain spotted fever. Vector-borne diseases rarely present a great risk to prehospital care providers.

Vehicle and vector transmission present little additional risk for an EMT. The greatest opportunity for acquiring an infectious or communicable disease is through direct or indirect contact. When rendering care, care providers often do not take the time to wash hands thoroughly following contact with a patient or contaminated materials. When this simple procedure is omitted, the opportunity for infection increases, especially if the care provider engages in hand-to-nose or hand-to-mouth activity.

Airborne transmission can present a risk of infection; but it is less likely than with direct or indirect contact. The method of organism transfer and the duration of exposure to the patient play major roles. In general, there must be contact with a coughing or sneezing patient, direct contact with sputum produced, or prolonged exposure to the patient. In most areas, transport times and conditions do not fulfill these requirements. For instance, if an EMT transports a patient and later finds out that the patient had tuberculosis, the risk to the EMT is minimal.

Whether or not an infection develops depends on three factors:

1. The dose of the organism present
2. The degree to which the organism survives when exposed to light and air, or its **virulence**
3. The individual's resistance to infection

These factors can best be related by a formula:

$$\text{infection} = \frac{\text{dose} \times \text{virulence}}{\text{resistance of the host}}$$

Each part of this formula should be considered when evaluating exposure in a particular situation. In most instances, simply having transported a patient with a communicable disease will not put one at risk. The *actual* risk, in any situation, arises when there is direct contact with the infective organism for a given disease. In general, actual risk is much less than *perceived* risk in any infectious situation. Knowledge of how each disease is spread and how to block the spread is an EMT's major protective measure.

PREVENTION

All persons involved in the care of patients are at risk for acquiring an infectious or communicable disease. The risk can be minimized, however, by using basic protective measures. EMTs are responsible for protecting themselves, other personnel, and other patients.

Prevention begins with maintenance of the EMT's personal health. Regular yearly health examinations should be required for all personnel. A history of all childhood infectious diseases (for example, measles, mumps, whooping cough, or chicken pox) experienced by the EMT should be recorded and kept on file. If the EMT has not had one of these diseases, appropriate immunizations should be offered. Immunizations should be kept up

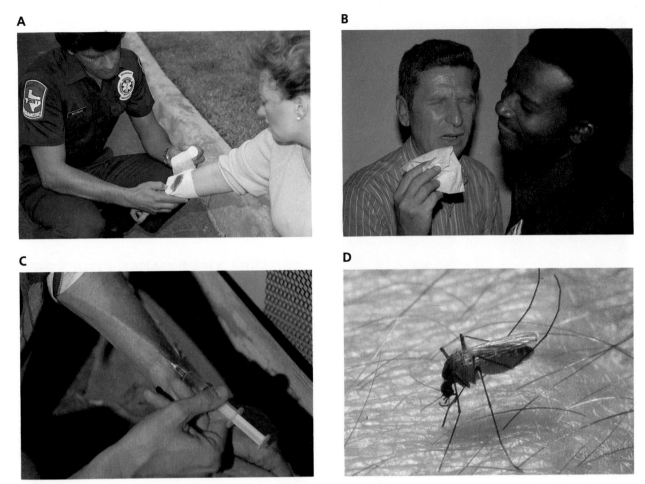

FIGURE 34.1 There are four major methods of transmission of infectious diseases: (a) contact — touching materials contaminated by infectious organisms; (b) airborne — inhaling droplets containing infectious organisms; (c) vehicle — using contaminated needles or other instruments; and (d) vector — being bitten by an animal or insect that is carrying disease.

to date and recorded in the EMT's health file. Recommended immunizations include:

Rubella (German measles) vaccine
Tetanus-diphtheria boosters
Mumps vaccine
Influenza vaccine (yearly)
Hepatitis B vaccine

All EMTs should be skin tested for tuberculosis (PPD) prior to employment to identify those who have been exposed to the disease in the past.

Knowing beforehand that a patient to be transported has a communicable disease is a definite advantage. This is when an EMT's health record will

be valuable. An EMT who has already had the disease or been vaccinated against it is, of course, not at risk. Otherwise, appropriate protective measures must be taken. Not all patients with a communicable disease will be identified initially, however. Therefore, preventive measures must be practiced whenever possible.

Many times patients can be carriers of diseases and not exhibit symptoms. For example, an EMT may treat a patient who is bleeding and not realize that the patient has hepatitis. If the EMT had an open cut anywhere, the virus could enter and cause infection. Hand washing is the single most important measure for self-protection. It should be carried

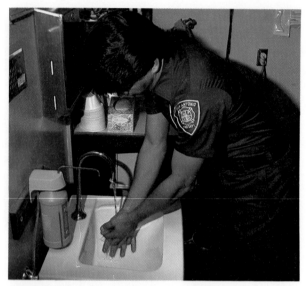

FIGURE 34.2 The single most important measure for self-protection against contagious disease is thorough hand washing.

out before and as soon after contact as possible. Some hand-washing agents, such as those that have an alcohol base, do not require running water. They are a good first line of defense until a proper hand-wash procedure can be done (Figure 34.2).

IDENTIFICATION OF INFECTIOUS DISEASE PATIENTS

Identifying a patient as having a possible communicable disease is often difficult. Ordinarily, EMTs do not have an established diagnosis and must respond based on presenting symptoms. Table 34.1 details general protective measures that are appropriate when communicable disease could be a threat.

In any instance in which exposure is documented or suspected, there should be an established protocol for the care provider. The protocol should list the steps to be followed to ensure proper follow-up for the EMT. Care should begin with the completion of an incident report to document the specific events. Specific information regarding the patient will be available from the hospital. The infection control practitioner at each hospital is a valuable resource person who can review the events of the exposure, evaluate the EMT's contact with the patient, and provide initial information regarding the need for ad-

ditional follow-up. Follow-up and documentation of work-related illnesses or exposure are each very important.

EMTs should not take field exposures lightly. An example of a field exposure that is often ignored by the care provider or the hospital is a needle stick injury. A puncture wound from a needle stick should never be ignored. The needle may itself be contaminated, and the risk of contracting hepatitis is high. Every hospital has a needle stick protocol. EMTs should be familiar with the procedures followed in their area and make sure they are followed whenever a needle stick injury occurs.

DISEASES THAT CAUSE CONCERN

Several infections or communicable diseases raise concern among prehospital care providers. They include, among others, hepatitis, herpetic whitlow, meningitis, tuberculosis (TB), and AIDS (acquired immune deficiency syndrome). In most cases, the risk to the prehospital care provider is minimal.

Hepatitis

Hepatitis can be caused by chemicals, alcohol, or drugs, as well as by viruses. The first three forms of the disease are not communicable and are relatively

TABLE 34.1   Protective Measures Against Possible Signs and Symptoms of Communicable Disease

Signs and Symptoms	Protective Measures
Presence of fever and rash	Mask
Diarrhea	Hand washing; use disposable gloves when in contact with stool; wash hands after gloves are removed
Draining wounds (pus or blood oozing)	Hand washing; use disposable gloves when touching drainage; wash hands after gloves are removed; apply dressing to wound
Jaundice (yellow tinge to the skin or sclera of eyes)	Hand washing; use disposable gloves when touching blood or secretions; wash hands after gloves are removed

common. Several viral types of hepatitis also exist and are communicable. The major ones are:

1. Type A (viral or infectious)
2. Type B (serum)
3. Type Non-A, Non-B (transfusion)

Hepatitis A is a disease usually seen in children. Most children who have it do not show any symptoms. They do pass it to their parents (during close contact, especially diaper changes). Hepatitis A does not have serious complications, and the patient usually recovers without difficulty. Hepatitis A can also be acquired by the ingestion of the virus through contaminated shellfish or water.

Hepatitis B, also known as **serum hepatitis,** is caused by a virus that is spread through blood-to-blood contact (transfusion, needle stick), mucous membrane (saliva or sputum contact), or sexual contact. The virus is hardy; it can survive for long periods of time in the environment. It has been found alive on surfaces for six weeks and longer.

The patient with hepatitis B can be very hard to identify because many individuals who have the disease do not demonstrate the primary symptoms or signs. The primary symptoms and signs are nausea, vomiting, fatigue, abdominal pain, and jaundice. Many individuals will have only "flu" symptoms, which are often overlooked. The incubation period for hepatitis B is very long — from 42 to 200 days after exposure.

Serum hepatitis is a disease that has been shown to have long-term serious effects for many of the individuals who acquire it. Many patients become carriers or develop chronic hepatitis. There has been a relationship established between the incidence of hepatitis B and liver cancer. Thus, one can appreciate the efforts to eradicate this disease through vaccination in high-risk groups. There is no specific treatment for hepatitis B nor is there a cure for the disease once it has been acquired.

Because prehospital care personnel have a high degree of contact with blood from patients, vaccination for them is recommended. To protect against exposure to hepatitis B, the EMT should carry out the following steps:

1. Practice good hand-washing technique.
2. Wear disposable gloves whenever possible when in contact with blood or oral secretions.

3. Clean blood-contaminated areas in the vehicle with a bleach solution.
4. Use proper technique for needle disposal. Do not recap needles and do not cut them; dispose of them in a puncture-resistant container.

Non-A, Non-B hepatitis presents itself in a similar manner as the other types. Infection with this strain of virus is usually related to a transfusion or contaminated needle stick. This strain is called Non-A, Non-B because there are no laboratory tests available to identify the causative virus.

Herpetic Whitlow

Another recognized occupational health risk is **herpetic whitlow.** Herpetic whitlow is a **herpes virus** infection of the finger. It is acquired when a care provider has breaks in the skin of the hands and has direct contact with the oral secretions of a patient actively infected with herpes virus. Like other herpes viral infections, there is no cure for this disease. It will recur from time to time. The incubation period is 2 to 12 days following exposure, but it may vary with each individual. The symptoms are redness, swelling, pain, and nerve impairment of the finger or hand. Treatment is supportive, to relieve the pain. Since there is no cure, prevention is especially important. Measures for protection include good hand washing, especially if there are breaks in the skin, and the wearing of disposable gloves when in contact with a patient's oral secretions.

Meningitis

Meningitis, an inflammation of the meningeal coverings of the brain, may be caused by either a virus or a bacterium. The patient who has **viral meningitis** does not present a significant risk to the EMT. The viral form of the disease is usually transmitted via food or water. **Bacterial meningitis** does carry a risk for transmission, especially if there is direct contact with nasopharyngeal secretions from suctioning the patient, from giving mouth-to-mouth ventilation, or from the patient's coughing into the EMT's face. Even under these circumstances, only a few forms of meningitis from very specific bacteria are transmitted — and these only rarely. In each of these instances, there would be a recommendation for follow-up care. The EMT should also follow the local guidelines for exposure to communicable diseases.

Tuberculosis

Tuberculosis (TB) is another of the diseases that create concern for those involved in the care of the patient. However, TB is not a highly communicable disease. The organism that causes tuberculosis is known to reside in the lungs. If the patient is not coughing and creating droplets, the disease is not communicable. There must be direct contact with a coughing patient, or the patient's sputum, to be considered at risk. Simply transporting a patient does not constitute a high risk. Care providers who work in an area where the incidence of tuberculosis is high should undergo skin testing and follow-up.

Acquired Immune Deficiency Syndrome

Acquired immune deficiency syndrome (AIDS) is caused by the human immunodeficiency virus (HIV), which was discovered in 1983. HIV attacks and destroys certain white blood cells of the immune system, the T4 lymphocytes. The loss of these cells makes the HIV-infected individual prone to further infection by organisms which do not commonly cause disease in humans (opportunistic infections). The virus does not survive outside of the body in sufficient numbers to cause infection and is easily killed by drying and most commonly used disinfectants.

Epidemiologic studies since 1981 have shown that HIV is transmitted by direct contact with HIV-infected blood, semen, or vaginal secretions; it can also be transmitted across the placenta to offspring of HIV-infected mothers. In addition, it is likely that cerebrospinal, pericardial, joint, and amniotic fluids are capable of transmitting HIV infection. There is no scientific documentation that HIV infection is caused by contact with tears, sweat, saliva, sputum, urine, feces, vomitus, or nasal secretions, *unless* those fluids contain grossly visible blood. AIDS is *not* transmitted by handshaking, kissing, toilet seats, telephones, hot tubs, swimming pools, or mosquitoes. It is possible, but unlikely, that a human bite could transmit HIV infection. However, the Centers for Disease Control (CDC) advises EMTs who come in contact with body fluids in situations where distinguishing fluid types is difficult to "treat all body fluids as potentially hazardous."

AIDS is clinically described in stages, depending on how the immune system is affected by the disease. Once HIV infection has occurred, the body begins to produce antibodies to the virus. These antibodies can be detected by the ELISA blood test 6 to 12 weeks after infection. In some cases, the ELISA test is incorrectly positive for HIV infection: a false-positive. Therefore, a positive ELISA test should be confirmed by another test, the Western Blot Test. Another test, an antigen test, is designed to directly detect the virus and is pending FDA approval. Combined with the ELISA and Western Blot tests, this antigen test should yield more conclusive information.

The CDC has divided HIV infection into four clinical classes:

Group 1 **Acute Infection:** Individuals experience a flu-like illness and the ELISA and Western Blot tests subsequently become positive ("sero-positive");

Group 2 **Asymptomatic Infection:** Individuals are "sero-positive" and have changes in T4 cell counts;

Group 3 **Persistent Generalized Lymphadenopathy:** Patients have swollen lymph glands at two or more sites which persist for more than three months; and

Group 4 **Other Illnesses:** Patients experience one or more of the following: mental disorientation (dementia), muscle wasting and weakness (myelopathy), peripheral nerve numbness and weakness (neuropathy), fever, and/or diarrhea for more than one month, and/or more than 10 percent weight loss.

Over 95 percent of all AIDS cases are found among intravenous (IV) drug users who share needles, homosexual and bisexual men, and sexual partners of HIV-infected persons. Other high-risk groups are hemophiliacs, those who have received transfusions of HIV-contaminated blood, and those born to HIV-infected mothers. According to the CDC's statistics on health care workers exposed to AIDS, the maximum chance of contracting HIV infection from a known AIDS patient by occupational exposure (needle stick) to blood is 0.5 percent. As of May 1989, only one paramedic has become HIV infected as a result of occupational exposure; that case is listed in the "undetermined" risk category by the CDC. EMTs who observe the CDC's recommended "Universal Blood and Body Fluid Precautions" for infection control are at minimal risk. However, a completely risk-free environment is impossible.

Universal Precautions is a new concept in health care and infection control. It stresses that all patients should be assumed to be infectious for HIV and other blood-borne disease-causing organisms (pathogens). The precautions include:

1. Wear gloves when handling all patients. When cleaning contaminated equipment, general-purpose utility gloves (e.g., rubber household gloves) are recommended. Heavy leather or "bunker gloves" are recommended for use where broken glass and sharp edges are likely to be encountered, such as when extricating persons from automobile accidents.
2. Wear protective eyewear and mask when body fluid splatter is anticipated.
3. Do not recap, cut, or bend used needles; place them directly into a puncture-resistant container designed for "sharps."
4. Follow cleaning and infection control protocols closely.
5. Wear gowns when uniforms may become extensively soiled with body fluids.
6. Change contaminated clothes and wash exposed skin thoroughly.
7. Use face shields, pocket masks, or other airway adjuncts.
8. Wash hands following glove removal as a means of self-protection. Change gloves between patients.

If contact with a patient's high-risk body fluids occurs on an unprotected area of the body, inform the responsible medical authority and follow appropriate local protocols. These protocols should include: (1) submitting an incident report; (2) notifying the appropriate medical advisor; (3) obtaining counseling for the pre-HIV test and informed consent for baseline testing; (4) retesting at 6 weeks, 12 weeks, and 6 months; and (5) obtaining post-test counseling.

The most problematic aspect of this disease is that there are no outward markers. A patient with AIDS looks no different than any other patient suffering from a chronic debilitating illness. The EMT cannot discriminate against any patient, because to delay or refuse care is not only unethical but is gross negligence, abandonment, and malpractice. With Universal Precautions, there should be little fear of increased risk in caring for HIV-infected patients.

ACTUAL RISK AND PREVENTION PROCEDURES

Consideration of the hepatitis virus and HIV clearly leads one to the conclusion that exposure to blood puts the EMT at risk. The importance of handwashing and careful handling of blood-related problems cannot be overemphasized. Blood-contaminated equipment and work areas should be cleaned as a first step in infection control. Blood-covered areas should be cleaned with a fresh solution of one part bleach to 100 parts water (1:100). Gloves should always be worn during cleaning.

TABLE 34.2 Common Childhood Diseases

Disease	Signs and Symptoms	Mode of Transmission
Bacterial Meningitis	fever, severe headache, stiff neck, sore throat	direct contact with oral, nasal secretions
Chickenpox (Varicella)	fever, rash, cutaneous vesicles	airborne, direct contact with vesicle drainage
German Measles (Rubella)	fever, rash	airborne, direct contact with oral secretions
Hepatitis A	fever, loss of appetite, jaundice, fatigue	direct contact with urine, stool, or oral ingestion of virus
Measles (Rubeola)	fever, rash, bronchitis	airborne, direct contact with secretions
Mumps	fever, swelling of salivary glands (parotid)	airborne, direct contact with saliva
Whooping Cough (Pertussis)	violent cough at night, whooping sound when cough subsides	airborne, direct contact with oral secretions
Scarlet Fever	fever, headache, nausea, vomiting	airborne, direct contact with oral secretions

TABLE 34.3 Common Adult Diseases

Disease	Signs and Symptoms	Mode of Transmission
AIDS	fever, night sweats, weight loss, cough	sexual contact, blood, needles
Gonorrhea	discharge from urethra or vagina, lower abdominal pain, fever	sexual contact
Hepatitis B	fever, fatigue, loss of appetite, nausea, headache, jaundice	blood, oral secretions, sexual contact
Hepatitis Non A–Non B	fever, headache, fatigue, jaundice	blood
Malaria	cyclic fever, chills, fever	blood-mosquito vector
Mononucleosis	fever, sore throat, fatigue	mouth-to-mouth kiss
Pneumonia	fever, cough	airborne
Syphilis	genital and cutaneous lesions, nerve degeneration (late)	sexual contact, blood
Tuberculosis	fever, night sweats, weight loss, cough	airborne

Routine rescue vehicle cleaning is an essential part of the prevention and control of infectious/communicable disease. Cleaning will remove surface organisms and should be accomplished after each run and on a daily basis. "High contact areas" are those which were in direct contact with the patient's blood/body fluids or those which the EMT touched after contact with the patient. These areas must be cleaned after each run.

Cleaning solutions recommended by the CDC are either an Environmental Protection Agency (EPA)-approved germicide which is effective against the tuberculosis (TB) bacterium or a 1:100 solution of household bleach. Avoid the use of aerosol spray products. A solution in a bucket or a pistol-grip spray bottle is recommended. Alcohol is not a recommended cleaning solution.

Contaminated disposables (paper sheets, needles, dressings, and other infectious waste) should be handled in strict accordance with local health department procedures. Hospital infection control personnel or the local medical director should be consulted, and written protocols should be followed. EMTs should be aware of the local infection control regulations and procedures.

Handwashing is extremely important. It should be completed as soon as practical. While it is recommended that a waterless antiseptic hand cleanser should be kept on responding units to use when handwashing facilities are not available, handwashing with soap and water should be accomplished as soon as practical after every patient contact.

Knowledge of disease processes and the consistent following of infection control protocols remain the best defenses for the EMT against communicable disease. Tables 34.2 and 34.3 summarize this information for common childhood and adult diseases.

YOU ARE THE EMT...

1. Malaria is a vector-borne disease that is transmitted to humans by mosquitoes. Identify three other modes of transmission of communicable diseases. Give an example of a disease spread by each mode.
2. You have just suffered a needle stick injury in the field. What should you do?
3. You just found out that one of the patients you transported yesterday has serum hepatitis. You're not worried, though, because you have followed all the steps to protect against exposure. What are they?
4. AIDS is not only a serious disease; it is also a controversial social issue that is at the forefront of media attention. What are the *facts* concerning the mode of transmission of this disease? How can you protect yourself against infection from an AIDS patient?

Substance Abuse

35

OVERVIEW

The term "substance abuse" has been introduced in recent years because the medical and non-medical preparations that are used and abused today far exceed those of past years, which were pretty much limited to alcohol and narcotic drugs. The abuse of readily or illegally obtained materials involves millions of persons and billions of dollars. The indirect cost of substance abuse to society cannot be calculated. The EMT will treat many patients whose problems can be traced to some type of substance abuse. Among them will be the usual "skid row" drunks, arthritics whose problems arise from the overuse of aspirin, bulimics who suffer from self-induced vomiting, and narcotic or hypnotic drug addicts.

Chapter 35 begins by defining the terms the EMT must be familiar with in order to understand the range of problems of substance abuse. The chapter then describes the two major forms of substance abuse: alcohol abuse and drug abuse. The symptoms of alcoholism, the effects on the body of too much alcohol, and the treatment of alcohol abuse patients are all discussed. Drug abuse is a broader subject that begins with a description of the various types of drugs that are abused and progresses to the problems of drug abuse and the emergency treatment of the drug abuser. The chapter concludes with a brief discussion of other forms of substance abuse — specifically, aspirin, laxatives, vitamins, and food abuse.

OBJECTIVES

The objectives of Chapter 35 are to

- define the terms *substance abuse, drug, addiction, dependency,* and *tolerance.*
- review the general effects of alcohol on a patient under the influence of alcohol.
- learn the emergency treatment for injuries and illnesses that occur as a result of alcohol abuse.
- review the general problems related to drug abuse, including the nature of the drug itself, the route of administration, the use of more than one drug at a time, and the tolerance and sensitivity that can develop in a drug user.
- know the specific acute treatment for the problems associated with several types of drug use and with drug withdrawal.
- become familiar with other forms of substance abuse.

THE MEANING AND IMPLICATIONS OF SUBSTANCE ABUSE

When we mention substance abuse, we commonly think of specific narcotic addiction. While narcotic addiction is a major social and public health problem in the United States today, it is by no means the only form of drug abuse. Alcohol, laxatives, emetics, and routine medications such as aspirin and vitamins are significantly abused (Figure 35.1).

A common thread uniting all the agents used is that they are self-administered, without medical control or consideration for proper or sterile preparation. The agents are self-prescribed for their supposed effects by the user. Generally, no medical indication for the use of the agent exists. In time, continued compulsive use produces addiction. An unfortunate result of the widespread use of drugs is that many crimes are committed by individuals who need money to purchase them. Many agents in widespread use are freely available and inexpensive. Others can only be obtained legally with a prescription. Still others cannot be obtained legally at all. Fulfilling the demand for the latter group has produced a flourishing black market drug trade that nets traffickers billions and billions of dollars. Into this trade have come substances with little or no medical use, such

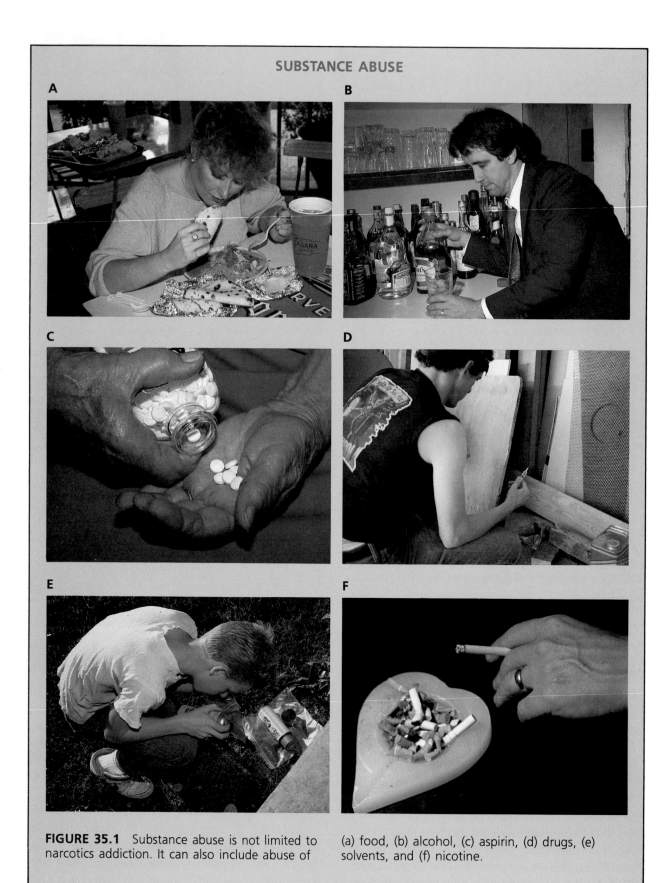

SUBSTANCE ABUSE

FIGURE 35.1 Substance abuse is not limited to narcotics addiction. It can also include abuse of (a) food, (b) alcohol, (c) aspirin, (d) drugs, (e) solvents, and (f) nicotine.

as marijuana, as well as legitimate pharmacologic agents like Seconal® or morphine.

The indiscriminate use of drugs has produced varying degrees of dependency and addiction among users. Addicts cannot live without their drug support and are willing to exhaust any means to obtain it. In general, the treatment of addiction and substance abuse is long, frequently unsuccessful, and one that requires patience, persistence, and dedication.

Most drugs that are knowingly misused are taken for their effects on the mind: they can be described as stimulatory, depressant, or hallucinatory. In the United States the use of such agents proliferated widely in the late 1960s and 1970s; 40 percent of military personnel serving in Vietnam are said to have experienced significant drug use in that country.

Several patterns of initial drug contact exist. Sometimes the drugs are given legitimately for a bonafide medical reason such as the treatment of pain. Sometimes the drugs are used for recreational purposes or in response to group or peer pressure. The general pattern is for drug use to be tapered or stopped by an individual. Use itself is not equated with addiction. In fact, the greater percentage of initial users do not become addicts.

Overall, substance abuse presents many different patterns and a wide spectrum of effects. One common theme, however, is that it is detrimental to individuals and society. Direct costs related to alcohol abuse alone have been estimated at $60 billion annually. Indirect costs in other lives affected, opportunities lost, toxic effects on newborn children, and the like are incalculable.

In order to fully comprehend the various effects of substances that are commonly abused, the EMT should be familiar with the following terms:

Substance abuse: The knowing misuse or overuse of any material that can be ingested, injected, or otherwise taken to produce an effect greater than or different from that experienced with the normal use of the agent. Agents that are abused include alcohol, food, legitimate drugs, illegal drugs, proprietary medications, vitamins, laxatives, and items like solvents, gasoline, and aerosol propellants.

Drug: Any substance that is given with the intention of preventing or curing disease or otherwise enhancing the physical or mental welfare of humans or animals. Any drug can produce undesirable side effects or adverse reactions apart from its desired effect, and any drug can be used to excess to enhance its effect.

Addiction: A state characterized by an overwhelming desire or need (compulsion) to continue the use of a drug and to obtain it by any means whatsoever. There is a tendency to increase the dosage gradually and continually, a psychological and, usually, a physical dependence on its effects, and a detrimental effect on the individual and society. The addict has a compulsive need for the agent used.

Dependency: The combined psychological and physical state of an individual in which the usual or increasing doses of a drug are required to prevent the onset of withdrawal symptoms. If no withdrawal symptoms occur when the use of the drug stops, addiction does not exist. An individual may be dependent on a given agent yet not addicted. For example, an individual may be dependent on antacids to control pain from a gastric or duodenal ulcer. If the ulcer heals, the antacid is no longer needed and can be withdrawn without difficulty. There is no compulsion to continue or increase its use after the problem is solved.

Tolerance: An individual's increasing resistance to the usual effects of a drug, resulting from its continued administration, as in the case of a drug addict. Tolerance is characterized by necessary increases of the doses of the drug taken as well as the frequency of its administration to obtain the same effect.

ALCOHOL ABUSE

The most commonly abused drug in the United States is alcohol. It affects 10,000,000 people annually and causes 200,000 deaths. It is the third greatest national health problem after heart disease and cancer. Alcoholism is not, by any means, limited exclusively to destitute drunks. Executives, housewives, business people, and laborers can all become victims of this disease. It is a powerful central nervous system (CNS) depressant. More than 50 percent of all traffic fatalities or injuries involve alcohol; 67 percent of murders and 33 percent of suicides involve the use of alcohol. It is a significant factor in the development of mental retardation in children of alcoholic mothers. All in all, it is a devastating agent in society.

Effects of Alcohol

Alcohol, like all other drugs, produces tolerance. Patients who are addicted to it require more and more alcohol to produce the same mental effect. In general, it dulls the sense of awareness, slows reflexes, and increases reaction time. Patients under the influence of alcohol may exhibit the same signs as patients with physical injuries or illnesses, such as head injuries, toxic reactions, or uncontrolled diabetes. When attending a patient who may be suffering from the acute effects of alcohol, the EMT should always bear in mind that the patient could have a physical illness as well. A patient should be brought to the emergency department even if there is the slightest question that illness or injury is involved in addition to the direct, observable effect of alcohol. Sometimes a physician has difficulty sorting out the effect on a patient of injury or illness from that of alcohol. Often the family or acquaintances will be able to provide some information about the patient's drinking habits up to the time of the emergency situation.

The drunken patient may engage in aggressive and inappropriate behavior, fall easily, or be combative. Self-injury is common and often not perceived by the inebriated patient. The EMT may have to search for injuries and fractures. Occasionally, a patient will have consumed so much alcohol that signs of serious central nervous system depression appear. In such cases complete respiratory support may be necessary. Death can result from this degree of excessive consumption of alcohol.

Alcohol in large amounts is a gastric irritant. Patients who have consumed too much alcohol may vomit, usually forcefully. Sometimes these patients will vomit blood, a condition called **hematemesis.** Hematemesis can occur when the lower part of the esophagus is lacerated by repeated forceful vomiting or from direct irritation of the stomach wall (**gastritis**). It can also occur from the rupture of dilated veins in the lower esophagus (**esophageal varices**) that have become enlarged because of alcoholic liver disease (**cirrhosis**).

Long-term, chronic abuse of alcohol produces muscular incoordination, memory loss, apathy, and other evidences of chronic brain deterioration. A very specific syndrome occurs when a patient who is used to a constant supply of alcohol withdraws from it. This condition may occur if a patient can no longer buy alcohol, is ill, or for some other reason is cut off from the source. The alcoholic withdrawal syndrome may manifest itself as **alcoholic hallucinations** or as **delerium tremens (DTs).**

Alcoholic hallucinations are the awareness or perception of fantastic figures, often walking on the wall and sometimes giving the appearance of attacking the patient. Hallucinations may be frightening but are usually only temporary. They usually precede delirium tremens, a much more severe complication. Delirium tremens may occur from one to seven days after withdrawal. They are characterized by restlessness, fever, sweating, confusion, disorientation, agitation, delusions, hallucinations, and convulsions. A history of chronic alcohol ingestion, with a period of one or more days of withdrawal, can usually be obtained from the patient's family or acquaintances. Patients with DTs are extremely ill; the mortality rate from this problem is very high.

Treatment of Alcohol Abuse

Given the widespread use of alcohol, one cannot conclude that an acute episode of alcohol intoxication is reason for emergency medical care. Those patients whom the EMT is called to treat will usually be acutely intoxicated and have another major problem such as CNS depression, respiratory difficulty, vomiting, aspiration, hematemesis, or an injury. These patients must be taken to the emergency department with care given to the major associated medical problem. Occasionally, complete ventilatory support is needed. The EMT must always be alert for vomiting and its consequences with these patients. Injuries or bleeding are treated as noted elsewhere in this text.

Individuals suffering from hallucinations or DTs are acutely ill patients. Hallucinations and restlessness may precede the development of convulsions. Should convulsions occur, they should be treated like any other seizure. The patient should not be restrained, although adequate protection must be provided to prevent self-injury. Oxygen should be given and the patient watched for vomiting. These patients may also be hypovolemic from sweating, fluid loss, insufficient fluid intake, or vomiting. Should signs of hypovolemic shock develop, the patient should be promptly transported. The EMT should elevate the feet slightly, clear the airway, and turn the head to one side to minimize the chance of aspiration. These patients are usually irrational and will respond inappropriately to suggestions or conversation; however, they are frequently frightened. Each one should be approached in a calm and relaxed manner with assurance and the necessary emotional support.

The chronic alcoholic patient rarely needs emergency support unless mental deterioration leads to an injury or to unusual exposure such as falling asleep in an unprotected, exposed area, doorway, or park bench. This type of patient may frequently require emergency care for hematemesis as a result of esophageal variceal rupture. In these circumstances, treatment and transport are dictated by the associated illness or injury.

DRUG ABUSE

Types of Drugs

Aside from alcohol, drugs that are abused for their subjective effects on a person's mental state include:

> Opium compounds
> Central nervous system (CNS) depressants
> CNS stimulants
> Nicotine
> Marijuana
> Hallucinogens
> Inhalants

Opium Compounds

The **opium analgesics** (pain medications) are all natural or synthetic derivatives of opium from poppy seeds. They include heroin, morphine, Demerol®, Dilaudid®, and Methadone®. The very mild agent codeine is also in this group. In general, these drugs are all pain relievers and have a wide range of legitimate medical applications. Individual use may have started with an appropriate medical prescription or as a recreational venture.

Of these agents, the use of heroin is absolutely illegal in the United States. The remainder can be obtained by medical prescription, with the exception of codeine. In most, but not all of the United States, codeine is an **exempt narcotic.** This means that a given amount in a given period of time may be sold over the counter without prescription. As such, codeine is the basic drug in many nonprescription cough preparations. Some states have abolished the exempt status of codeine because of drug abuse problems.

The EMT is expected to know which narcotic agents may be purchased locally without prescription. Intravenous administration of these drugs is associated with a characteristic "high" or "kick." These agents are all CNS depressants and cause respiratory depression. Tolerance develops rapidly with their use so that massive doses are being taken by some users. In general, emergency medical problems will be related to respiratory depression and general CNS malfunction.

CNS Depressants

The **barbiturates** and other sedative drugs, called CNS depressants, generally have effects remarkably similar to that of alcohol. They depress the nervous system. They do not relieve pain. Nor do they produce a specific "high." Frequently, they are used with alcohol or with the opium analgesics to augment the effects of a weaker product.

In street jargon, barbiturates are known as "Goof Balls" (Figure 35.2). The short-acting agents pento-

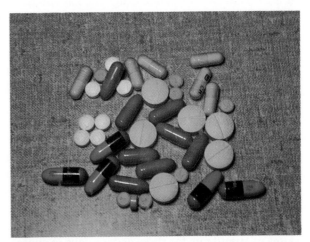

FIGURE 35.2 "Goof Balls" (barbiturates), "Yellow Jackets" (pentobarbital), "Red Devils" (secobarbital), and other CNS depressants alter the state of consciousness so that the individual appears drowsy or peaceful.

barbital ("Yellow Jackets") and secobarbital ("Red Devils") are preferred over the long-acting, more stable phenobarbital. A host of other nonbarbiturate agents are included in the average drug menu: meprobamate, glutethimide, methylprylon, methaqualone, and various other tranquilizers. Older sedative agents, such as chloral hydrate and paraldehyde, have been replaced by more effective and palatable compounds.

These agents all depress CNS activity and alter the state of consciousness so that the individual may appear drowsy or peaceful. In general, the agents are taken by mouth or by injection. The EMT who is involved with these patients will usually find problems of significant nervous system depression, insufficient respiration, and coma.

CNS Stimulants

The effects of CNS stimulants on the individual depend on the route of administration, the drug, its dose, and the circumstances. **Amphetamines** are commonly taken orally by truck drivers, students, and others to produce a general mood elevation, improve task performance, suppress appetite, or prevent sleepiness. They may just as well produce irritability, anxiety, and lack of effective concentration. A host of these agents exist. Amphetamine, methamphetamine, and benzedrine ("speed," "uppers," or "Bennies") are the characteristic drugs. Caffeine, found in coffee and cola drinks, is a mild stimulant, as are certain antiasthmatic drugs such as adrenalin and aminophylline. Nasal decongestants, such as ephedrine and isoproterenol, are also mild stimulants. These drugs will cause tachycardia (increased heart beat), increased blood pressure, rapid breathing, an excited state, agitation, headaches, sleeplessness, and a sense of euphoria or well-being. Disorganized behavior may also accompany the use of these agents.

When attending a patient who has taken large doses of stimulants over a rather brief period, the EMT will usually find an agitated individual who is exhibiting irrational or paranoid behavior. Occasionally, chest pain is experienced with large doses of stimulants. The individual who has taken large doses of stimulants for three or four days in succession ("a run") and is forced to stop because of the effects, may fall into a deep sleep to awake hungry, lethargic, and depressed. Sudden withdrawal may also produce coma.

Cocaine is classed with the CNS stimulants. In the street it is known as "coke." It is a more powerful stimulant than amphetamines, with effects remarkably similar. It induces an extreme state of euphoria. Legitimately, it is a potent local anesthetic used in eye and nose operations. Taken as a stimulant, it is often inhaled. Chronic inhalant use results in destruction of the nasal septum with perforation. The EMT will usually deal with acute effects similar to those of CNS stimulants and often more severe.

Nicotine

Cigarette smoking is so widespread and such a common phenomenon in the United States today that no one takes it other than as a routine activity. In fact, it does fit all the criteria for drug dependence and should be so regarded. There is general agreement that **nicotine** is the agent that contributes to the continuing use of cigarettes by many. Nicotine is a mild CNS stimulant, although it is not as powerful a self-reinforcer as the opium compounds or the CNS depressants.

Compulsive smokers report a range of withdrawal effects from no particular problems to irritability, hostility, and depression. The role of the EMT in dealing with this problem is in handling the effects of long-term smoking on the tracheobronchial system. Smoking is by far the most effective means of inducing chronic obstructive pulmonary disease, since cigarette smoke is a bronchial irritant. Side effects of smoking are linked to lung, airway, and bladder cancer and the aggravation of peripheral vascular disease. Although none of these effects is directly related to nicotine, nicotine is the major effective agent that keeps people smoking — even those who wish they could stop.

Marijuana

A variety of names are associated with the active agent from the flowering hemp plant called *Cannabis sativa*. In the United States, the extract from the plant top is called **marijuana** or "pot" (Figure 35.3). In Africa, the Far East, and India, it is called hashish. Other names, bhang and charas, refer to less powerful extracts from the stems and leaves. Inhaling marijuana as smoke from a cigarette produces euphoria, relaxation, and drowsiness. The drug does impair the capacity to do complex work and also short-term memory. In some people euphoria can

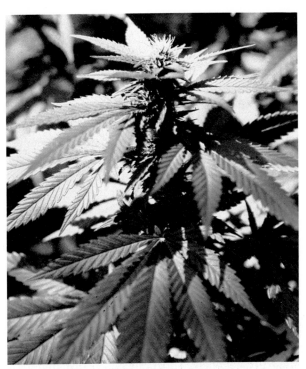

FIGURE 35.3 Marijuana is known as "pot" in the United States and "hashish" in other parts of the world. Extracts obtained from the plant tops are inhaled as cigarette smoke and produce euphoria, relaxation, and drowsiness. Despite its popularity, marijuana is known to produce acute anxiety, impaired memory, and hallucinations.

give way to depression and confusion. An altered perception of time is common, and anxiety approaching panic can occur. With very high doses, hallucinations akin to toxic psychoses are seen. Marijuana use is common: Estimates are that in the United States one-quarter of the population uses this drug, and 20,000,000 people continue to use it daily.

No known beneficial medical effect is associated with marijuana use, although recently, extracts of the active agent in marijuana have been found to control nausea in patients undergoing long-term cancer chemotherapy treatment. These results are experimental as yet. In view of the widespread popularity of marijuana, the EMT will undoubtedly encounter problems associated with its use — probably acute anxiety and the hallucinatory effect the drug can produce. Both conditions should be treated in the same way that problems arising from the use of hallucinogens are treated.

Hallucinogens

Hallucinogens cause an alteration of the patient's sense of self-awareness or self-perception. They frequently result in dangerous psychiatric symptoms and behavior, attempts at suicide, or panic reactions. Patients often describe feelings of seeing something that is not there or hearing someone speaking who is not present. Their perceptions regarding themselves and their capabilities are altered. For example, they may think they can fly or safely leap out of a window. Fatal accidents, which appear as suicides, may be the result of such perceptions. Among the common hallucinogens are lysergic acid diethylamide (LSD), peyote, ololiuqui (morning glory seeds), psilocybin (mushrooms), and mescaline. The agents are usually taken orally and induce in some instances visual, musical, or colored hallucinations. The role of the EMT in the care of these patients ordinarily will be in managing the "bad trip" or acute panic reactions.

Inhalants

An additional problem, outside the realm of specific drug use, is associated with the inhalation of agents to produce an intoxicating effect. Inhalants include solvents, such as acetone or toluene that are found in glues, gasoline, and various halogenated hydrocarbons that are used as propellants in aerosol sprays. None of these agents is a pharmacologic item. They all produce CNS effects remarkably similar to the effect of alcohol. They are all CNS depressants.

A variety of improvised containers have been devised as inhaling devices by individual users; some are as simple as breathing vapors within plastic bags (Figure 35.4). Most of the time, the EMT may be handling a "sniffer" who appears to be drunk. If, however, the patient has become unconscious while sniffing, the apparatus that was used may have caused significant or complete airway obstruction. In this case, the EMT may have a patient with profound hypoxia and its associated problems, including cardiopulmonary arrest.

Long-term effects of the use of inhalants include destruction of liver cells, as seen in various forms of hepatitis that is caused by exposure to toxic organic compounds, and destruction of cells in the central nervous system. At this time, it is unclear whether central nervous system cellular destruction is due to the inhaled agent itself or to hypoxia.

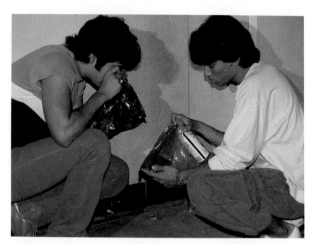

FIGURE 35.4 Inhalants such as paint spray are "sniffed" using improvised, closed containers. The simplest device is a plastic bag. Inhalants are CNS depressants that can destroy liver cells as well as cells in the central nervous system.

General Problems with Drug Abuse

Problems arising from drug abuse relate to the specific nature of the drug taken, its effects on the patient, the route of administration, and the combined effect of other agents used at the same time. Certainly, individual tolerance and sensitivity to a given agent have a bearing on the severity of the problem.

Nature and Effect of the Drug Itself

Almost every patient who abuses drugs does so because they alter the state of consciousness. Many of these agents cause CNS depression. The EMT is likely to see all stages of depression, from mild drowsiness to coma. Other potential problems include the likelihood of vomiting and subsequent aspiration, respiratory depression or arrest, and self-injury. Sometimes patients fall asleep in odd positions, with an arm or leg curled under or hanging over a chair or couch. Compression of the blood vessels reduces circulation in the extremity for hours. This decreased blood flow can result in permanent injury. Sometimes severely depressed patients fall and sustain mild or severe injuries of which they are unaware. These injuries may be neglected for long periods of time.

Stimulants induce restlessness in the user and sometimes severe anxiety. When this state is un-

manageable, it becomes similar to an acute psychosis with paranoia. The EMT may very well encounter a patient with an acute fright reaction who exhibits paranoid or totally wrong thinking. Or, acute depression might be evident in the patient who has suddenly stopped using stimulants. Convulsions may occur with extreme use of stimulants.

Hallucinogens induce very specific perceptual alterations that are related to sound, sight, or the other senses. The user, of course, anticipates that the altered sensory state will be pleasurable. Frequently, this is not so; instead, the induced hallucination or perception is terrifying. Again, the EMT is almost certain to encounter someone who is having a "bad trip."

Route of Administration

Many agents are taken by mouth. Ordinarily, the oral route of administration poses no particular problem for the patient. Other agents are injected by needle, intravenously, subcutaneously (just under the skin), or into muscles. Illegally obtained drugs often are not prepared with regard to sterility or to proper composition for injection. They are frequently "cut" or diluted by agents such as sugar which are not sterile. Addicts are endless experimenters who are willing to take any drug by any route to experience a new "high." Thus, many agents not designed for injection are being given by needle. Frequently, a group of addicts will share the same needle. Usually, one individual will use a single needle for several injections.

The results of such practices can be devastating. Infection can be introduced into a vein, subcutaneous tissue, or muscle at each injection. Tissue can be destroyed by the direct action of the injected material upon it. **Phlebitis** (an infection of the vein) or both superficial and deep subcutaneous abscesses commonly occur. Even more lethal to the patient are the severe systemic infections, hepatitis, brain abscess, or **endocarditis** (infection of the valves of the lining membrane of the heart) that can develop. An additional risk is **AIDS (acquired immune deficiency syndrome),** a life-threatening disease that can be transmitted through blood contact. When many individuals use one needle with no sterile precautions, they are at a high risk for contracting any of these diseases if one among them has or is carrying the disease.

Other Agent Use

Using more than one agent at one time is a common practice with some addicts. Generally, these drugs will have a complementary effect, such as alcohol and tranquilizers. Occasionally, stimulants and depressants are mixed or hallucinogens are used with each. The results in many instances are unpredictable. The EMT who finds such a situation should gather as much evidence and information about the agents used as possible. Often, it is difficult for the doctors at the emergency department to assess the major problem.

Tolerance and Sensitivity

Tolerance to some agents rapidly develops in users. Additionally, cross-tolerance to other agents may occur. The result of tolerance is that the abuser uses extremely large doses to achieve the desired effect. During a period when the drug is not used, tolerance is often lost as rapidly as it developed (usually within weeks). Thus a user returning to an accustomed habit after a period of abstinence or withdrawal may dangerously overdose on what was previously a routine amount of drug. The EMT may certainly see instances of this effect and note greatly exaggerated (for the patient) results of a single routine dose.

Any individual may have or may develop *sensitivity* to any drug or to any of the materials mixed with it. In the most acute form, an allergic or sensitivity reaction to an agent results in anaphylaxis. Anaphylaxis is characterized by the rapid development of skin itching and burning, **urticaria** (hives), chest tightness, cough, and respiratory wheezing. It can occur following the administration of a substance by any route (orally, intravenously, subcutaneously, or otherwise). The major response in anaphylaxis is bronchospasm and a copious outpouring of mucus into the airway. Respiration is difficult and may become impossible. Anaphylaxis is a relatively rare occurrence in the addicted population; however, it is a constant risk with the use of any substance.

Treatment of the Drug Abuser

Assessment

A few general rules apply for the EMT faced with a situation of drug abuse. Information is absolutely necessary for the doctor at the emergency department. Bottles, needles, and whatever appliances or drug paraphernalia are about the patient should be collected and brought with the patient to the hospital. Unprescribed drug use is illegal in the United States. Each state has regulations about turning the equipment over to police. In some states, the sale of equipment for the preparation of cocaine and other agents is legal, although the use of the drug is not. The EMT must be thoroughly knowledgeable about state and federal drug laws.

When drug use is suspected, the EMT should look for signs that will identify the substance. The presence of spoons, lamps, or pipes may give a clue that an agent is indeed being used (Fig. 35.5). Examination of the patient may reveal further clues. The chronic user of the opium analgesics, for example, usually has small constricted pupils that do not constrict any further with light. Barbiturate users have dilated pupils, again relatively insensitive to light. The presence of intravenous puncture sites or multiple, small, continuous abscesses on the arms or legs is also a sign of a chronic drug abuser (Figure 35.6).

Depressants

The moderately depressed patient should be stimulated by talking, gentle pinching, or light shaking. The EMT cannot know whether the patient is on the way to further depression or is awakening.

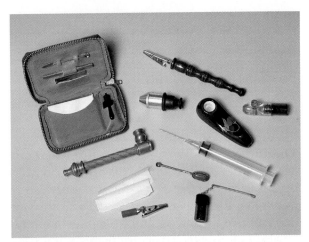

FIGURE 35.5 Drug paraphernalia may provide a clue to identifying the substance when the EMT suspects drug use. Any bottles, needles, and appliances should be brought to the hospital with the patient.

A

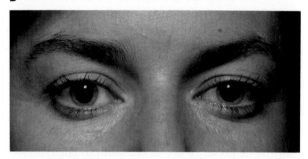

B

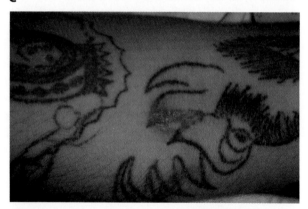

C

FIGURE 35.6 Signs of a chronic drug abuser: (a) small constricted pupils (an opium user); (b) large dilated pupils (a barbiturate user); (c) intravenous needle marks or small cutaneous abscesses on the arms or legs.

The danger in further depression is that it may produce respiratory arrest. Thus, the patient should be kept awake during transport to the emergency department. The EMT should be ready to assist respiration and be alert for vomiting. The use of oxygen is beneficial. Even if certain that the agent was taken orally, the EMT should never induce vomiting in a semiconscious or drowsy patient. The patient should be transported promptly and any information made available to the appropriate personnel at the emergency center. The patient with respiratory depression needs ventilatory support and must be transported as quickly as possible while receiving it.

Stimulants

The anxious, excited, or paranoid patient on stimulants should be handled in a calm, professional manner. Often a quiet attitude and gentle approach will help "talk him down." Gaining the patient's confidence with a pleasant manner often works. Restraints should not be used unless the patient is likely to get hurt or injure others. Restraints are usually difficult to apply and may require more than two EMTs to do so. At the very least, they will increase a patient's anxiety and fear. The patient on stimulants should never be left alone during transport or even placed alone in the ambulance where difficult behavior cannot be controlled.

The patient on stimulants who is convulsing must be protected from injury. Oxygen should be given and the airway kept clear with gentle suction. This patient will require complex, intravenous drug treatment at the hospital and must be taken there as quickly as possible. Occasionally, the patient taking stimulants will undergo severe reactive depression if withdrawn suddenly from any drug. Usually, the withdrawal symptoms include listlessness, apathy, and hunger.

Hallucinogens

The patient who is experiencing a bad trip from an hallucinogenic agent is treated just like the one on stimulants. Individuals rarely take a dose sufficient to induce coma or significant depression. These patients require a calm, mature manner and much emotional support. Unless absolutely needed, restraint should not be used. These patients must never be left unattended. Hallucinations or odd perceptions can occur suddenly, and patients have been known to leap from cars or windows under the influence of various agents. They must be carefully watched until arrival at the hospital.

Inhalants

The patient in severe distress from inhalants is usually hypoxic. Hypoxia is caused by the device, often of makeshift construction, that is used to inhale the active vapors. Frequently, substances are inhaled from within a closed plastic bag. With hypoxia, the EMT must be prepared to render all possible support: oxygen, artificial ventilation, and even cardiopulmonary resuscitation. In the absence of severe hypoxia, the patient should be treated as one with an overdose of a CNS depressant. Vomiting should be watched for and treated. Oxygen may be needed. The patient should be transported to the emergency department along with the agent inhaled, if at all possible. It might be an aerosol can, a bottle of glue, or a tin of gasoline.

Injuries

A rapid assessment of the physical status of the drug user is absolutely essential. Injuries not sought are often overlooked. Fractures must be splinted. The swollen cyanotic limb that has been compressed must be splinted and positioned as naturally and comfortably as possible. Head injuries must be recognized promptly since their effects frequently mimic drug use. Prompt transportation is indicated for the drug user who has sustained any injury.

Infections

In addition to the effects of the drugs, the drug user may develop major systemic or local infectious problems. The local problems are almost always abscesses or **cellulitis.** Cellulitis is characterized by redness, swelling, warmth, and tenderness. It usually occurs in an extremity at the site of drug injection. An infected limb should be splinted and the patient transported promptly since hospitalization and intravenous antibiotic treatment will probably be required. Abscesses, especially if they have ruptured spontaneously and are draining, should be dressed with sterile bandages and treated with all the precautions for open draining wounds (see Chapter 34).

The individual with a major systemic infection usually shows signs of that problem. Seizures, coma, or other neurological manifestations, and fever occur with a brain abscess, and acute cardiac failure and fever occur with endocarditis. These patients require prompt transport to the hospital. Handling the jaundiced patient with suspected hepatitis or AIDS is covered in Chapter 34.

Multiple Drug Use

The EMT should be alert to the fact that a drug user may have used as many as three or four different agents. The use of drugs in conjunction with alcohol also occurs frequently. In situations in which the drugs complement one another, the effects on the patient are generally much greater than when each drug is used alone. Sometimes drugs with opposite effects are taken. In general, unless a given agent is a specific antagonist of one drug, opposing effects do not cancel each other. They usually result in panic reactions from acute stimulation that has been imposed on an altered mental state.

Anaphylaxis

A drug user undergoing an acute anaphylactic reaction is a priority-one emergency patient who requires major respiratory and ventilatory support. The most expeditious transport to the emergency department is indicated.

Drug Withdrawal

Patients who are addicted to drugs — that is, who are psychologically and physically dependent on a constant supply of a drug — may experience a severe reaction when the drug is withdrawn. These reactions are characterized by anxiety, nausea and vomiting, convulsions, delirium, profuse sweating, tachycardia, hallucinations, and severe abdominal cramps. Ordinarily, the EMT is not required to treat acute withdrawal. However, if a patient has suddenly become unable to procure a regular supply, acute withdrawal may occur. Usually the patient can tell the EMT what the problem is.

Individuals experiencing acute withdrawl are as urgently ill as those suffering from a drug overdose. They should be transported promptly to the emergency department where controlled withdrawal is almost always done, with constant medical and psychological support. Except for nicotine, planned withdrawal is rarely attempted on an ambulatory or out-patient basis.

OTHER FORMS OF SUBSTANCE ABUSE

Virtually anything that can be taken as an agent, eaten or drunk, has been used to excess. There are compulsive water drinkers, over-the-counter "pill poppers," and abusers of a variety of agents and foods. The EMT will undoubtedly meet people who exhibit this type of behavior. In every instance, the characteristic is the obsessional, compulsive need of the patient to do whatever it is that is being done, even if it is to the patient's obvious detriment. Some specific problems are described below.

Aspirin

One of the most widely used, and useful, medications available today is aspirin (acetylsalicylic acid). Found in a variety of compounds, it is an effective pain reliever. Because of its availability, many people take aspirin for a wide variety of reasons. Despite its usefulness, aspirin can produce two specific toxic effects on the body. It can irritate the lining of the stomach and the small intestine, which can cause inflammation and ulcers that bleed. It can also interfere with platelet function and impair the blood-clotting mechanism. The EMT may be called to see a patient with hematemesis (vomiting blood) caused by too much aspirin. The emergency treatment would be the same as for upper gastrointestinal bleeding.

Laxatives

A variety of laxatives and stool softeners, both potent and mild, are available without prescription. Some individuals use them to the extent that significant diarrhea occurs and is sustained. In these instances, the EMT must focus on the result of the laxative use. For example, a patient may be in profound dehydration as a result of the diarrhea. Emergency transportation then is called for, with treatment directed at metabolic shock.

Vitamins

Nearly every pharmacy and supermarket has a huge stock of every available vitamin. Well-described disease states are associated with excessive use of as well as lack of vitamins. Sometimes the clinical picture of vitamin abuse is indeed bizarre. Ordinarily, vitamin abuse is not a concern of the EMT; however, it is a widespread problem in the United States.

Food Abuse

In the United States, morbid obesity as a result of food abuse is a major area of malnutrition that involves millions of individuals. These patients routinely consume in excess of 5,000 calories per day. Many seek and require surgical control of their obesity. Emergency problems for this group of people occur when their weights reach a level that in-

terferes with normal breathing or other activities. The compulsion to eat may not be controllable by the individual and has been likened to alcohol addiction.

Some individuals with a compulsion to eat control their weight with vomiting, a disorder called **bulimia.** For them, a second addiction to syrup of ipecac or other **emetic** (medication to induce vomiting) in addition to that for food is becoming recognized. Other individuals, concerned with figure and weight, cannot bear the sight of food and literally starve themselves, a condition called **anorexia nervosa.** They often become addicted to a variety of appetite suppressants.

One of the responsibilities of the EMT is to recognize the widespread nature of substance abuse in the United States and the great variety of presentations it can have. It is likely that in a few months of routine work the EMT will encounter more than one of the situations discussed. Each has a specific treatment pattern and each must be met logically for support to be effective. In general, the problems of substance abuse represent for the patient much more severe, deep psychological needs. The EMT who is aware of the spectrum of disability associated with substance abuse can more easily cope with its manifestations.

YOU ARE THE EMT...

1. You have been called to treat a patient who "passed out" at a beer bash. His friends were going to let him "sleep it off," but they don't think he looks right. What are some of the problems you should be looking for?
2. The patient has overdosed on "Goof Balls." Are these a central nervous system depressant or stimulant? What kinds of problems is this patient likely to experience?
3. Your patient is on a "bad trip." He thinks he is Superman. What type of drugs is he probably taking? How should you treat him?
4. Your patient is a 15-year-old girl who is screaming that her family is trying to kill her. Her parents tell you she has never been on drugs, but the younger sister pulls out some pills she says she found in her sister's room. What will you say to the parents? What kind of drugs does her behavior indicate she might be using? How will you treat this patient?

Unconsciousness and Epilepsy

36

INITIAL EMERGENCY CARE OF UNCONSCIOUSNESS

All unconscious patients require similar emergency medical treatment, regardless of the specific cause of the unconsciousness. In general, the EMT should follow these six steps:

1. Secure and maintain an airway.
2. Resuscitate and institute CPR when necessary.
3. Observe the incident; record history when it is available; note any items that might serve as evidence regarding the cause of the unconscious state.
4. Attempt to define the specific cause of unconsciousness in the patient.
5. Observe and record vital signs and the level of consciousness.
6. Transport the patient promptly to the emergency department.

For every unconscious patient, the first and foremost treatment is to assure an open airway and to provide respiratory support when necessary (Figure 36.1). A supine (lying flat), unconscious patient is in danger of aspirating vomitus or other oral contents, or of suffocating from an obstructed airway. The airway should be opened and the unconscious patient placed on one side with the head lower than the feet. Steps must be taken to keep the airway open. The patient must be transported in this position with continued monitoring of respiration and vital signs. When a neck injury is suspected following an accident, the first step in emergency care is to stabilize the spine (Chapter 6 and Chapter 20). Then attention is directed to the airway.

When the unconscious patient has sustained a full cardiopulmonary arrest and when it is known that this state has lasted fewer than 10 minutes at normal body temperature, **cardiopulmonary resuscitation (CPR)** must be started (Figure 36.2).

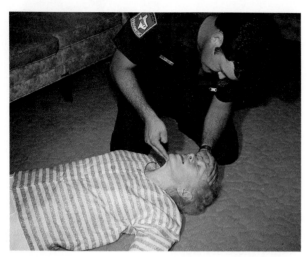

FIGURE 36.1 Securing an airway is the first and most important emergency treatment for an unconscious patient.

Many patients with **acute myocardial infarction** have been saved by the timely application of CPR immediately after the attack. Resuscitation should not be offered to patients when it is known that an arrest has lasted for appreciably longer periods of time.

Once cardiopulmonary function has been restored and stabilized, a medical history should be obtained (Figure 36.3). The EMT is in an excellent position to retrieve and accumulate information concerning the cause of a patient's problem. The EMT should question the patient, relatives, and bystanders about previous episodes of unconsciousness, epilepsy, any medical illness, details of drug use, the possibility of a drug overdose, or any type of poisoning. The EMT should also look for medical identification symbols that may suggest the cause of the unconscious state. Environmental causes of unconsciousness, such as electrical shock or exposure to excess heat or cold, should be noted. Evidence of head injury should be sought. The EMT should also look about and gather any plants, bottles, evidence of drugs, or any other materials that might be linked to the patient's unconsciousness and take them along with the patient to the emergency department. Such materials might help emergency department personnel to complete the patient's medical history.

Vital signs should be recorded, and any injuries noted and described. The time of the onset of unconsciousness should also be noted — whether it was sudden or slow — along with any subsequent changes. The level of consciousness should be assessed and recorded using the AVPU scale described in Chapter 19. A determination should be made of whether the pupils of the eyes are constricted or widely dilated. The pupillary response to light should be evaluated and recorded. Finally, the patient should be transported promptly to the emergency department.

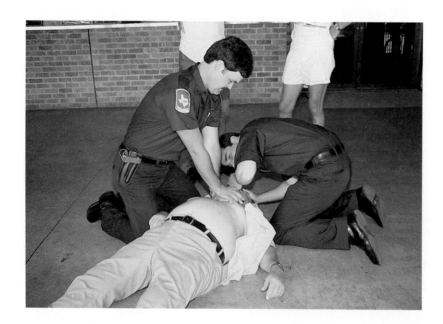

FIGURE 36.2 CPR should be started on an unconscious patient who has sustained a full cardiopulmonary arrest for less than 10 minutes at normal body temperatures.

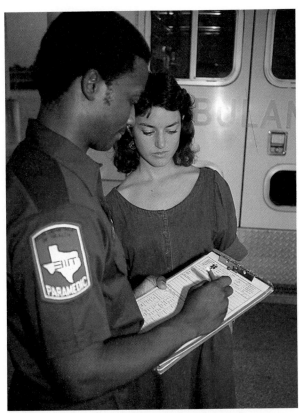

FIGURE 36.3 Any information concerning the patient's medical history that the EMT can provide will help emergency department personnel.

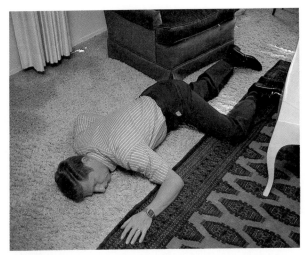

FIGURE 36.4 Unconsciousness can be caused by injuries, epilepsy, injected or ingested agents, environmental causes, diseases, and emotions.

CAUSES AND TREATMENT OF UNCONSCIOUSNESS

The first consideration after resuscitation for the EMT who is dealing with an unconscious patient is to determine the cause of the unconsciousness. In general, unconscious patients take highest priority in **triage.** Once the cause has been determined, medical treatment designed to reverse the unconscious state can be started. Unconsciousness can be caused by diseases, injuries, emotions, environmental causes, injected or ingested poisonous agents, and epilepsy (Figure 36.4). Table 36.1 lists some of the most common problems causing unconsciousness, their pathophysiology, the emergency medical treatment, and the chapter of reference in this book for each one.

Diseases

The common diseases that may produce unconsciousness are **diabetes mellitus** and **arterio-**

sclerosis. In diabetes, unconsciousness may quickly occur if too much insulin is taken without enough food so that the blood sugar level drops. In this situation (**insulin shock**), not enough glucose is available for routine brain function. A headache, followed by unconsciousness, develops rather quickly. This situation is a pressing emergency if permanent brain injury is to be avoided. In the opposite state — that is, when the blood sugar is too high because of insufficient insulin — unconsciousness results after a long period of time during which the patient develops a condition known as **diabetic ketoacidosis** (also called **diabetic coma**). Unconsciousness in this situation occurs because of excessive fluid and sugar loss from the kidneys, which produces dehydration and a gradual accumulation in the blood of metabolic waste products. Insulin shock and diabetic coma are more fully discussed in Chapter 31. The EMT should be thoroughly familiar with emergency medical care for each of them.

Arteriosclerotic blood vessel disease can attack every artery in the body. When the disease damages and subsequently blocks the arterial vessels that supply the myocardium (the heart muscle), a heart attack may follow. Loss of consciousness may be sudden because of the sudden disordered beating of the damaged heart. In this situation, CPR may be life-saving. Heart attack and its many presentations are more fully discussed in Chapter 28.

TABLE 36.1 Causes of Unconsciousness and Emergency Medical Management

Problem	Cause	Pathophysiology	Management	Chapter Reference
General loss of consciousness	Injury or disease	Shock, head injury, other injuries/diabetes, arteriosclerosis	Need for CPR; triage, priority one	36
Diseases: Diabetic coma	Hyperglycemia and acidosis	Inadequate use of sugar, acidosis	Transport; complex treatment for acidosis	31
Insulin shock	Hypoglycemia	Excess insulin	Sugar; transport	31
Myocardial infarct	Damaged myocardium	Insufficient cardiac output	Oxygen, CPR, transport	28
Stroke	Damaged brain	Loss of arterial supply to brain or hemorrhage within brain	Support, gentle transport	29
Injury: Hemorrhagic shock	Bleeding	Hypovolemia	Control external bleeding, recognize internal bleeding, CPR, transport	11
Respiratory insufficiency	Insufficient inspired O_2	Paralysis, chest wall damage, airway obstruction	Clear airway, supplemental O_2, CPR, transport	6
Cerebral contusion, concussion, or hematoma	Blunt head injury	Bleeding into or around brain, concussive effect of blow	Airway, supplemental O_2, CPR, careful monitoring, transport	19
Emotions: Psychogenic shock	Emotional reaction	Sudden drop in cerebral blood flow caused by vasodilation	Place supine, make comfortable, observe for injuries	36
Neurological problems: Epilepsy	Brain injury, scar, genetic predisposition, disease	Excitable focus of motor activity in brain	Support, protect patient, transport in status epilepticus	36

Similarly, when arteriosclerotic vascular disease damages the arteries that supply blood to the brain, **thrombosis** or rupture of the vessel may cause a **stroke.** Although a stroke rarely causes sudden death, it may result in partial or complete loss of consciousness. Considerations in handling the partially conscious patient with a stroke are unique to this condition and are presented in Chapter 29.

Injuries

Many injuries result in loss of consciousness. All injuries that cause excessive blood loss may bring about **hypovolemic shock.** This means that there is not enough blood left in the vascular system to supply the brain and heart. Loss of consciousness from hypovolemic shock occurs late, only after much of the circulating blood volume has been lost. This patient is critically ill and will require the most rapid possible transport to a source of medical care.

Unconsciousness that results from insufficient oxygen intake, for whatever reason, presents a very serious situation for the patient. Injuries of the chest wall, for example, cause severe pain, which restricts breathing and limits the oxygen supply to the lung.

TABLE 36.1 (continued)

Problem	Cause	Pathophysiology	Management	Chapter Reference
Injected or ingested agents:				
Alcohol	Excess intake	Cerebral depression	Support, CPR, transport	35
Drugs	Excess intake	Cerebral depression	Support, CPR, transport (bring drug)	35
Plant poisons	Contact, ingestion	Direct cerebral or other toxic effect, local irritant effect	Support, recognition, CPR, identify plant, local wound care, transport	27
Animal poisons	Contact, ingestion, injection	Direct cerebral or other toxic effect, local irritant effects	Recognition, support, CPR, identify agent, local wound care, transport	27
Environment:				
Heatstroke	Excessive heat, inability to sweat	Brain damage from heat	Immediate cooling, support, CPR, transport	41
Anaphylaxis	Acute contact with agent to which patient is sensitive	Allergic reaction, bronchospasm, excess bronchial secretions	Intramuscular epinephrine, support, CPR, transport	27
Electric shock	Contact with electrical current	Cardiac abnormalities (fibrillation, standstill)	CPR, transport, do not treat until current controlled	39
Systemic hypothermia	Prolonged exposure to cold	Diminished cerebral function, cardiac arrhythmias	CPR, rapid transport, warming on the way	41
Drowning	$O_2\downarrow$, $CO_2\uparrow$, breath holding, H_2O inhalation	Cerebral damage	CPR, rapid transport	42
Air embolism	Intravascular air	Obstruction to arterial blood flow by air bubbles	CPR, transport, recompression	42
Decompression sickness	Intravascular nitrogen	Obstruction to arterial blood flow by nitrogen bubbles	CPR, recompression	42

As described in Chapter 23, **hemothorax** or **pneumothorax** from a perforated chest wall or lung reduces the actual volume and capacity of the lung to accept and transport oxygen. Cervical spinal cord injuries result in a paralysis of some or all of the muscles of respiration. With all of these injuries, the primary responsibility of the EMT is to provide an airway when needed and supplemental oxygen as soon as possible.

Injury of the head that produces **cerebral concussion, contusion,** or **hematoma** is probably the most common overall cause of loss of consciousness.

The most important consideration in dealing with the person who has sustained a head injury is to observe the level of consciousness at the time the patient is first seen and at intervals thereafter. Often, changes in the level of consciousness occur very rapidly in these patients. For this reason a person with a head injury should be transported to the emergency department as rapidly as possible. Frequently, an immediate operation to correct the situation is necessary. During transport the airway should be restored and maintained, the cervical spine should be protected, and oxygen should be given.

Emotions

The common faint is an emotional reaction that results in a temporary but sudden general dilation of blood vessels without increase in cardiac output. Momentarily, an adequate blood supply for the brain is lost and its function impaired. In general, consciousness is restored promptly once the patient becomes supine. The EMT must be alert for injuries that might have occurred if the patient fell during a fainting episode.

Environmental Causes

Environmental causes for loss of consciousness include excessive heat, cold, electricity, water, the exposure to gases under extreme pressure, and anaphylaxis (an allergic reaction in its most extreme form). Generally, unconsciousness due to extremes of heat (**heat stroke**) or cold (**systemic hypothermia**) are easily diagnosed by virtue of the circumstances and the patient's body temperature. General support of the patient is mandatory, plus appropriate cooling or warming. Specific details of these problems are contained in Chapter 41.

With patients who have sustained **electric shock,** the EMT must think first of self-protection. The patient, if still charged, is a good electrical conductor and may transmit the full volume of current to the EMT. Control of the electric current must be achieved before any treatment can be given. The patient may have sustained a cardiopulmonary arrest as a result of the shock and require CPR as an initial step. A detailed review of handling the patient injured by electricity is contained in Chapter 39.

In general, drowning patients require basic life support measures and transport to the nearest emergency department. A detailed statement of the treatment for water-related problems is presented in Chapter 42.

Patients who are suspected of having either **air embolism** or **decompression sickness** usually require treatment in a recompression chamber. They may need support up to and including CPR. Prompt transportation to the emergency department, where the recompression treatment can be arranged, is mandatory. Details concerning these problems are presented in Chapter 42.

The very special situation of anaphylaxis, which results from acute contact either by injection, inges-tion, or inhalation of some agent, is a manifestation of an allergic reaction in its most extreme form. Anaphylactic shock can produce death from respiratory failure in a matter of minutes. The usual problem is severe spasm of the bronchi, compounded by a flood of mucus into the bronchi. Each of these responses makes breathing difficult and markedly reduces the amount of inhaled oxygen. A great number of patients who are sensitized to specific agents know it and carry kits for the injection of intramuscular or subcutaneous **epinephrine** as an antidote. Anaphylaxis is discussed in detail in Chapters 11 and 27.

Injected or Ingested Agents

All manner of agents, including alcohol, drugs, and plant and animal poisons, may be injected or ingested. Some are very toxic in very minute amounts. Some, such as alcohol, are used as routine daily items by a large portion of the population and may be used to great excess by a few. In general, each of these agents has a direct toxic effect on the brain. Usually, emergency medical care for injection or ingestion of toxic agents includes support up to and including CPR and prompt transport to the emergency department. If it is possible to do so quickly, and without jeopardizing the care of the patient, the EMT should try to identify the agent causing the unconsciousness and either bring it or report its existence to the emergency department personnel.

The medical treatment for all toxic overdoses — alcohol, drugs, or other agents — is support of the patient's basic life functions until the drug has been cleared and metabolized by the body. In some cases, treatment may include the use of a specific antagonist to the toxic substance. Occasionally, syrup of ipecac will be used to induce vomiting of an ingested toxin. In most overdose situations, respiratory function is depressed, and vomiting should not be induced if there is a risk of vomitus being aspirated. The airway must be cleared carefully and artificial ventilation given as needed.

If there is a fall in blood pressure in an overdose situation, the patient's legs should be elevated 10 to 12 inches. The response of the pupils to light should be noted. Widely dilated pupils are characteristic of overdose with drugs such as barbiturates; constricted pupils, on the other hand, occur with the use of narcotics such as heroin, morphine, and Demerol®. Detailed discussions of the handling of substance abusers are contained in Chapter 35.

EPILEPSY

Epilepsy is a common condition that is characterized by recurrent episodes of seizures. One out of every 200 people will have epilepsy. Its frequency is increasing as more individuals survive episodes of head injury, meningitis, or brain abscess. It is usually easily controlled by medication. When uncontrolled, epilepsy is manifested by seizures. In general, most people take the term **seizure** to mean generalized, uncoordinated muscular activity associated with loss of consciousness. However, seizures can take a variety of forms from severe convulsions to simply "blacking out" for a few seconds. Seizures may occur as a result of a recent or old brain injury, a brain tumor, a cerebral embolus that is causing an acute block of blood flow within the brain, infection, fever, or simply a genetic predisposition. They are usually caused by an abnormal focus of electrical activity in the brain that produces severe motor activity and changes in the level of consciousness. Most seizures involve altered states of consciousness that last for variable periods of time. Most seizures are followed by a **postictal state** of sleepiness or unconsciousness for a varying length of time. Patients with epilepsy who have recurrent seizures can frequently be identified by medical identification tags or by close questioning of family members.

Not all seizures are due to epilepsy; many other serious illnesses can cause them. It is especially important to determine the cause in the patient who has had no history of previous seizure activity. Identification of the cause may require an extensive medical work-up in the hospital.

Classification of Seizures

Seizures are generally classified according to the degree and location of abnormal electrical activity in the brain. Seizure episodes are classified in two categories: generalized seizures and partial seizures. In a **generalized seizure** (**convulsive** or **tonic-clonic seizure**), most of the brain is involved. There are usually three phases of a generalized seizure: the aura, the convulsion, and the postictal state.

The **aura** is a sensation that something is about to happen; it precedes the convulsion in many pa-

tients with epilepsy. It can take many forms (a sound, a twitch, a feeling of dizziness or anxiety, or a characteristic smell), but for an epileptic patient it is always the same and serves as a warning that a seizure is about to begin. The aura lasts only a few seconds and is followed by the **convulsion.** During the convulsion, the jaw muscles contract, which may lead to biting the tongue or lips. Loss of bowel or bladder control is common, and involuntary urination or defecation often takes place. Sustained, **tonic** (rigid) **muscular contractions,** which can cause odd posturing of the body, may last several minutes. **Clonic** (repetitive) **muscular activity,** or spasms, may be superimposed on the rigid muscular contractions. After one to several minutes, the convulsive phase is followed by the postictal state that was mentioned earlier. The postictal phase is a period of exhaustion and recovery following the convulsion. During this phase, which may last for 10 to 30 minutes, the patient's level of consciousness is depressed, the airway may become obstructed by mucus, vomitus, or the relaxed pharyngeal muscles, and respirations may be slowed.

Partial seizures involve less extensive areas of the brain. The seizure activity may be limited to one or more extremities or one side of the body, called a **simple partial seizure.** Consciousness may be clouded, or the patient may display automatic behavior such as chewing, fumbling with clothes, walking aimlessly, muttering, or unresponsiveness, called **complex partial seizures.**

Management of Seizures

The important first step in the management of a generalized seizure is to keep the patient from inflicting self-injury during the attack. When an epileptic patient says that a seizure is about to occur (the aura), immediate action should be taken. The patient should be helped to lie down on the ground away from danger to minimize chances of injury during the seizure. The patient's head, arms, and legs should be protected, but not rigidly restrained. Clothes should be loosened. Nothing should be forced into the patient's mouth, especially if the teeth are clenched or if the patient is convulsing. Padded "bite sticks" made by taping tongue depressors together have been popular to prevent biting of the lips, cheeks, or tongue. Sometimes, however, these have been bitten in two by the patient, or sometimes they have lodged in the pharynx and obstructed the airway. If an object is used to prevent biting, it should be placed between the molars, not the front teeth. Fingers should never be put in the patient's mouth.

Contraction of the chest muscles may cause the patient to appear to have an airway obstruction and to become cyanotic. Normal respiration almost always follows the seizure activity. Lack of respiration during the attack rarely presents a problem unless several convulsions follow one another in quick succession. The airway can best be kept open by putting the patient on one side, head down, so that gravity will aid in keeping the tongue out of the pharynx and any vomited material will not be easily aspirated.

Following the phase of excessive muscular activity, the patient will be lethargic, perhaps disoriented, and only partially conscious (the postictal phase). At this point the airway should be assessed; any mucus or vomitus should be cleared and the airway adequately maintained until the patient is fully awake. Once vital signs are assessed and recorded, a secondary survey of the patient should be performed. The EMT should look for any injuries that may have occurred during the seizure.

The patient who has a history of epilepsy and who has frequently recurring seizures usually achieves complete recovery of function soon after the seizure, and transportation to the hospital is not necessary. Following the seizure, this patient requires a period of rest to allow full recovery. Patients without a history of previous seizures, however, must have a thorough medical evaluation in the hospital. If the EMT's evaluation during the postictal state reveals any abnormality (airway difficulty or injury as a result of the seizure), even the patient with a history of seizures should be transported to the hospital for continued evaluation and treatment. Since most seizure patients take some type of medication, all drugs being taken by the patient should be brought to the hospital.

A few patients with epilepsy experience **status epilepticus,** in which one seizure closely follows another, with no return of full consciousness between them. Potentially, this situation is serious since the patient does not have time to breathe well and recover from the stress of the initial seizure. The same problem can occur if a single seizure lasts longer than

ten minutes. The EMT who is faced with a prolonged convulsive spell (greater than 10 minutes) or repeated seizures closely following one another (status epilepticus) must give supplemental oxygen and transport the patient promptly to the hospital. Under these circumstances, the seizure may not be controlled without an intravenous infusion of medication given over a prolonged period of time.

In the management of partial seizures, the same general rules apply as for convulsive seizures. A problem may arise in diagnosing a complex partial seizure, as it may be mistaken for intoxication, drug abuse, or another medical condition causing abnormal behavior. A cardinal rule concerning the handling of a patient with aberrant behavior is that the patient should not be physically restrained unless it is essential for safety. A patient may react violently to restraint. During a complex partial seizure, which may last 15 minutes or longer, the patient is in a confused state but is usually amenable to suggestions and comments given in a friendly manner. It is usually possible to control the person for the duration of the seizure. The EMT must stay with the patient, provide reassurance, and observe the patient carefully until the abnormal behavior ceases. A thorough medical evaluation in the hospital will be needed to evaluate and diagnose the cause of this type of seizure.

YOU ARE THE EMT...

1. You have responded to a construction accident. A worker has fallen off a ladder and is unconscious. What are the first three steps you should take in administering emergency care?
2. As you know, stroke can cause unconsciousness because the supply of blood to the brain is interrupted. Explain how the following problems can cause unconsciousness: insulin shock, air embolism, hemorrhagic shock.
3. With epilepsy, how can you tell whether the patient is having a tonic-clonic seizure or a partial seizure? How would you manage each type?
4. The patient has just suffered an epileptic seizure and is in a postictal state. What does that mean? What should you do during this time?

Pediatric Emergencies

37

THE PEDIATRIC PATIENT

An entire segment of professional medical practice, called **pediatrics,** is devoted to the care of the young. Many problems in children are unique, and similarly, many common problems of adults simply do not exist in this population. Thus, medicine has come to consider pediatrics as a separate discipline.

Handling a sick or injured child can be extremely difficult. It is almost always a trying emotional experience to confront a seriously ill or injured child, and not everyone is comfortable doing so. The EMT must approach a child with a calm, professional manner; hard as it is, personal feelings must be kept in check. Although helping ill or injured children may not be easy, it has rewards that few other activities can match.

Traditionally, pediatrics has encompassed children up to age fifteen. Very recently, however, interest has been expressed in extending the upper age limit to the time of entrance into college. This is the time that many children sever family ties. Further, it seems reasonable to provide an individual with continuous care from infancy to adulthood. Within this long time span, some specific divisions exist. The neonatal period covers the first 30 days after birth.

In this group, the commonest causes of death are problems related to the birth (prematurity, for example) or congenital defects. Until the age of one year, a child is regarded as an infant; among these pediatric patients, congenital defects are the major cause of death. From age one to age eight, the individual is considered a young child; and from eight to fifteen, an older child. Among these latter groups, the commonest cause of death is trauma from motor vehicle accidents, falls, household accidents, and poisonings.

Pediatric diseases are by no means limited to the common infectious problems such as measles, mumps, or chicken pox. Cancer, while uncommon, is a real and very serious problem. Some viral and bacterial infections can also be severe. And injury, accidental or not, is another common and serious childhood problem.

BASIC LIFE SUPPORT

Like adults, children cannot tolerate cerebral hypoxia (lack of oxygen) for more than a few minutes before permanent brain damage occurs. Therefore, the rules of basic life support are no different for children than for adults. The techniques of basic life support must be adapted because of the child's size and metabolic requirements. Chapters 6 and 8 should be reviewed to refresh the EMT's understanding of the principles of basic life support.

Cardiopulmonary arrest in an adult is usually caused by heart attack. In contrast, primary heart disease is rare in children unless there is a major congenital defect. Such defects are usually identified at birth. In the majority of instances, infants and children first sustain a respiratory arrest. Then they may undergo cardiac arrest as a result of the lack of oxygen produced by the respiratory problem. It is therefore very important for the EMT to secure and maintain an airway and to adequately ventilate the child with respiratory problems. Specific causes of cardiopulmonary arrest in children include suffocation caused by the aspiration of a foreign body, near drowning, infections of the airway such as **croup** (acute bacterial or viral laryngitis) or **acute epiglottitis** (bacterial infection and swelling of the epiglottis), injuries about the head and neck, accidental poisonings, and **sudden infant death syndrome (SIDS).**

The basic difference in the management of a child with cardiopulmonary arrest as compared with an adult is the size of the patient. This factor dictates the specific techniques of resuscitation. For children above eight years of age, techniques used in an adult will be effective. In patients under the age of eight (infants and younger children), modified techniques of resuscitation must be used. These divisions are not rigid; for example, a small nine- or ten-year-old should be managed as a child. The specific techniques for cardiopulmonary resuscitation (CPR) in infants, children, and adults are described in Chapters 6 and 8. They will not be repeated in detail here.

AIRWAY OBSTRUCTION

Airway obstructions can usually be relieved by placing the child supine, tilting the head, and lifting the chin in the usual fashion (the head-tilt/chin-lift maneuver). In infants and some small children, forced cervical hyperextension may actually obstruct the airway because of the suppleness of the neck. These children may breathe better if the neck is held straight rather than hyperextended (Figure 37.1). If the child has vomited, the EMT should clear the pharynx with a finger or suction and turn the head to one side.

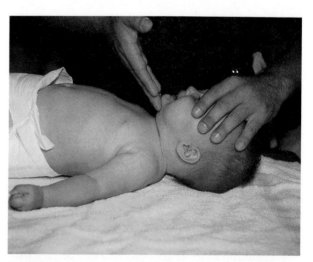

FIGURE 37.1 Airway obstruction may be relieved in a young child or infant by keeping the neck straight rather than hyperextended. Hyperextension, the technique for adults and older children, could possibly contribute to airway obstruction because of the suppleness of the infant and young child's neck.

The airway must be clear before assisted ventilation can be given. Because infants and small children are primarily nose breathers rather than mouth breathers, the EMT must pay particular attention to keeping the nasal passages open.

Obstruction of the airway by a foreign body is an especially common problem in young children, particularly among those who are crawling and exploring their environment. Sometimes the foreign body is aspirated into the lung and must be removed under anesthesia at the hospital. If a foreign body is only partially obstructing the airway, the child usually will still be able to breathe in and out, although with some difficulty. If the foreign body is clearly visible in the mouth and can be easily removed, the EMT should do so. However, if it is lodged in the upper airway, cannot be easily seen, or cannot be easily dislodged with a finger, it should not be removed if the child can still breathe air past the obstruction. Improper manipulation of a foreign body can turn a partial obstruction into a complete one.

Children with partial airway obstruction should be transported promptly to the hospital. Oxygen should be given by gently placing the oxygen mask over the child's mouth and nose. Children are often afraid of anything placed over their mouths or faces.

The EMT should explain what the mask is and how it will help the youngster to breathe. It should not be held close to the face to achieve an airtight seal. Rather, it should be held a bit away, with a high flow of oxygen, so that the inspired air is substantially enriched (Figure 37.2).

The EMT must only attempt to dislodge a foreign body when there is complete airway obstruction or when there is partial obstruction with poor air exchange that does not improve with the use of 100 percent oxygen (when cyanosis persists). In the past, recommendations for removing foreign bodies from the airway included giving four rapid back blows as an initial step. At the 1985 Conference on Emergency Cardiac Care, sponsored by the American Heart Association, much new information was presented. The participants agreed that in children, as in adults, a foreign body could only be dislodged by applying energy to it. The evidence showed that an **abdominal-thrust maneuver** reliably imparts the most energy, in the right direction, to dislodge the body. Back blows provide a short spurt of energy, which might dislodge the body or might drive it farther down the airway. Thus the conference adopted the abdominal-thrust maneuver, modified for size, as the best method of dislodging a foreign body in the airway of a child.

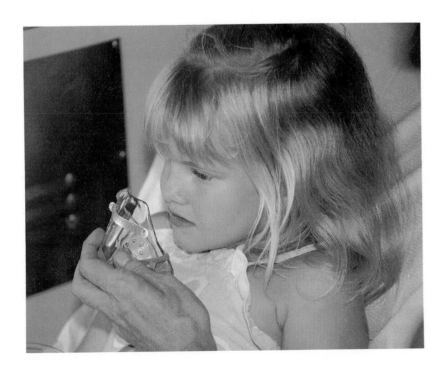

FIGURE 37.2 An oxygen mask should be held slightly away from a child's face instead of over the mouth or face. A high flow of oxygen will enrich the air the youngster breathes.

The EMT who has to remove a foreign body because of complete airway obstruction or persisting cyanosis should follow these steps:

1. First attempt to pull the foreign body out of the airway with your fingers.

2. If direct manual extraction does not work, use the abdominal-thrust maneuver. Place the child supine and deliver four abdominal thrusts as described in Chapter 6. In the child under one year, some concern exists that the abdominal thrust might injure the liver. For this group of patients, the **chest-thrust maneuver** can be used. Sometimes, given the size of the EMT's hands and the size of the patient, abdominal thrust combined with chest compression will provide the best results in the very young patient.

3. If the foreign body is obstructing the airway of an infant, place the baby supine on your thigh, with the head lower than the chest. This maneuver can be accomplished by supporting the head, neck, and back with one hand and the chest with your other hand. When the infant is placed on your thigh, you are now in a position to deliver four chest thrusts with the hand about the infant's thorax (Figure 37.3).

4. Once the obstructing foreign body has been dislodged using one of the above methods, open the airway again using the tongue-jaw-lift maneuver and remove the dislodged foreign body with your fingers.

5. Maintain the open airway and assist ventilation as necessary. If the infant or child begins to breathe spontaneously, give oxygen and transport the patient promptly to the hospital, even if the foreign body appears to have been completely removed.

6. If these maneuvers fail to dislodge the foreign body or to open an adequate airway, repeat a full series once and arrange to transport the child or infant as quickly as possible to the hospital.

Croup and Epiglottitis

Two illnesses may cause airway obstruction in children because of swelling of the tissues of the airway itself. They are croup, a viral illness that causes

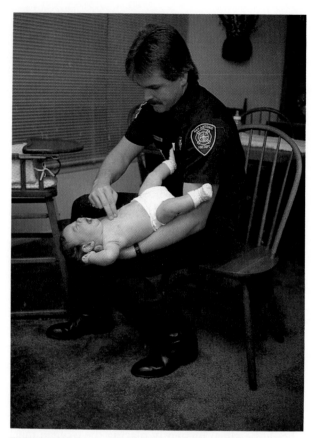

FIGURE 37.3 In the infant with complete airway obstruction, the foreign body can be expelled most effectively by applying four chest thrusts with the infant held in the position shown.

extensive edema of the lining of the larynx, and acute epiglottitis, a bacterial infection that produces severe swelling of the epiglottis (Figure 37.4). Children with these illnesses have fever, show progressive respiratory difficulty, and generally have a barking, brassy cough and hoarseness. There is a progressive and excessive muscular effort with breathing.

The EMT should never put a tongue blade, a finger, or an artificial airway into the mouth of such a child. Often this type of intervention will cause spasm of the larynx and complete a partial airway obstruction. Airways (oral or nasal) are designed to support a flaccid tongue — not to bypass a swollen epiglottis, and they do not help in croup, since the obstruction in this condition is beyond the reach of the device. Back blows and chest thrusts — the techniques for dislodging a foreign object — obviously will be of no benefit in these children and should

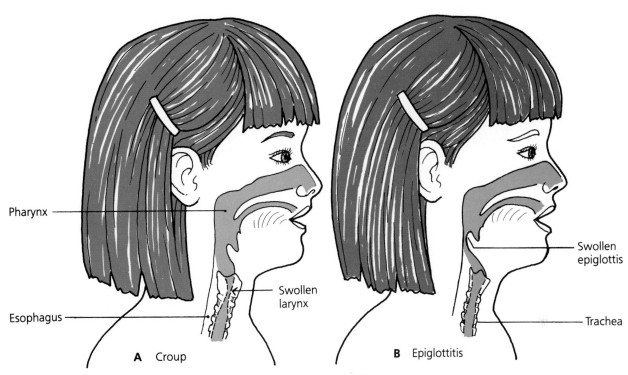

Pharynx

Esophagus

Swollen larynx

A Croup

Swollen epiglottis

Trachea

B Epiglottitis

FIGURE 37.4 (a) Airway obstruction caused by croup, a viral illness that causes extensive swelling of the lining of the larynx; (b) epiglottitis, a bacterial infection that produces severe swelling of the epiglottis.

be avoided. Instead, the infant or child should be placed in a position in which breathing is most comfortable, usually sitting up. Warm, moist oxygen should be administered. Any secretions should be gently removed with suction. The child should be transported as promptly as possible to the hospital for treatment.

Airway Maintenance

An unconscious infant or child should have an appropriately sized **oropharyngeal airway** inserted between the tongue and the palate. The proper length of the oropharyngeal airway for these patients is roughly equal to the distance from the corner of the patient's mouth to the earlobe (Figure 37.5). A semiconscious child may accept an airway or may expel it. The child who expels it can probably breathe adequately without it. This child has retained adequate reflex responses to protect the airway. Complicated equipment should not be used on little children. Mouth-to-mouth, or mouth-to-nose-and-mouth, resuscitation is usually very effective and easier than using a bag and mask.

TRAUMA

The automobile is the major killer of American children today. Many more children are injured as pedestrians, on bicycles, on motorcycles, or as passengers in cars. Occasionally, a serious injury results from athletics or recreational activity. The basic principles that apply to the management of trauma in adults also apply to trauma in children: establish an airway, control bleeding, and splint musculoskeletal injuries.

Shock

Shock in an injured child almost always results from blood loss. A child, with a smaller blood volume, can tolerate far less actual blood loss than an adult. The total circulating blood volume in an infant is only 300 to 500 ml. A late but important indicator of the presence of shock is a low systolic blood pressure. If the systolic blood pressure is below 50 in a child under five years of age, under 60 in a child of between five and twelve, or under 70 in a teenager or young adult, the patient is in shock.

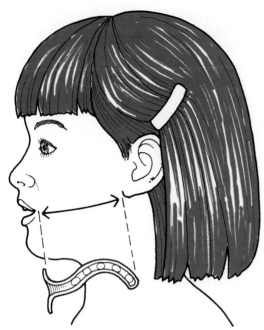

FIGURE 37.5 Technique of approximating the proper size of oropharyngeal airway to insert in a child. The length of airway should be equal to the distance from the corner of the mouth to the earlobe.

Remember, many other physiologic changes precede the actual fall in blood pressure. These changes are mechanisms that help sustain blood pressure in the early postinjury state. When the blood pressure finally becomes low, the condition is serious. To measure the blood pressure properly, three different sizes of pediatric blood pressure cuffs should be available at all times. A cuff that will cover about two-thirds of the length of the child's arm between shoulder and elbow should be used.

Treatment for the child in shock consists of controlling the airway, dressing any obvious wound to stop bleeding, splinting fractures, elevating the feet, and handling the patient gently. The child who has been in an accident should not be given anything by mouth. In the event that the child needs an emergency operation, the stomach should be completely empty. Often these children will ask for water, particularly if they are in shock. The EMT must say "no" in a kindly way.

Head, Neck, and Spinal Injuries

Injuries of the head, neck, and spine usually are caused by vehicular accidents, falls, or diving mis-

haps. The EMT should assume that any unconscious child who has been involved in an accident has a neck injury. The child should be treated and transported in the same manner as any other patient with a suspected spinal fracture:

1. Do not bend the neck or back.
2. Secure an adequate airway and immobilize the head, neck, and trunk on a spineboard before moving the child.
3. Offer assisted ventilation as the need arises and be alert to control vomiting.
4. Avoid the urge to pick up and cradle an injured child unless there is an overriding need to move quickly, such as a fire or other threatening environmental problem. Rarely is it necessary to move an injured person, adult or child, before adequate splinting and control of external bleeding are achieved.
5. Transfer children with head injuries with the head slightly elevated and supported on the spineboard. All the basic rules for managing the patient with a head injury (Chapter 19) apply equally in children.
6. Monitor the patient's level of consciousness. This is one of the most important duties after resuscitation and control of injuries. From the time you first see the patient until you deliver the patient to the emergency department, make periodic notations regarding the patient's level of consciousness. Use the AVPU scale and record your observations every 5 minutes. Report and record any change in the level of consciousness. A patient with a head injury may pass from an alert state to a comatose state in 15 or 20 minutes and require an urgent, lifesaving operative procedure. Assessing the level of consciousness and its change is the single most important measure the EMT can take in the management of head injury patients, pediatric or adult.

Extremity Injuries

In general, extremity injuries are not life-threatening. Open soft tissue wounds should be treated with a dry, sterile compression dressing. Open fractures tend to bleed considerably in children as well as in adults. Prompt control of bleeding is especially important in children. Bleeding can almost always be controlled by local compression; using a tourniquet for extremity bleeding is almost never necessary. In those rare circumstances when a tourniquet must be used to supplement control of bleeding, the same rules apply as for an adult (see Chapter 10). If a blood pressure cuff is used as a tourniquet on a child, inflation of the cuff to 100 mm Hg will usually secure complete control of the bleeding.

Splinting of a child's extremities should be carried out in the same manner as for an adult. Of course, the small extremity of a child requires appropriate size splints. A supply of pediatric splints must be maintained in the ambulance (see Chapter 15). Prior to placing a splint or aligning an injured extremity, the distal neurovascular function (pulse, capillary refill, sensation, and motor function) should be assessed. The neurovascular status should continue to be monitored after splinting until the patient reaches the hospital.

Injuries of the Trunk

Penetrating abdominal or chest injuries are uncommon in children. When they occur, however, the principles of management are identical with those for adults. Blunt injuries from falls or vehicular accidents are far more common. Blunt abdominal trauma may result in a serious internal injury such as rupture of the liver, spleen, or kidney. The child with this kind of injury may complain of abdominal pain and develop signs of shock, even without obvious external blood loss. These injuries are often difficult to diagnose. A child who has sustained a blunt abdominal injury and is complaining of abdominal pain should be transported promptly to the emergency department to be examined by a physician. The vital signs must be carefully monitored. Shock must be anticipated and treated promptly. The EMT should also be alert for vomiting.

Blunt injuries of the chest may cause serious cardiac or pulmonary injury. All children who have sustained a chest injury require immediate transport to the emergency department. Prehospital care is identical to that for adults.

SPECIFIC PEDIATRIC EMERGENCIES

A few emergency situations occur in children that do not exist or are seen only rarely in adults. They include high fevers with convulsions, certain conditions that cause abdominal pain, poisoning by various household substances, specific contagious diseases, and sudden infant death syndrome (SIDS). Any of these conditions may be quite serious, and all will be frightening to the parents.

Fever

A child responds to many illnesses by very rapidly developing a high fever. Temperatures of 103 degrees F (39.4 degrees C) and higher are common in children. In general, the EMT should not attempt to measure rectal temperature in small children or infants. The rectum is small and can be damaged easily by the thermometer. In these patients, high fever is usually obvious. The child is flushed, crying, and feels warm to the touch. In older children, oral or rectal temperatures should be taken using the appropriate type of thermometer.

Fever is not a disease itself, but rather the sign of an underlying problem, usually infectious. Most fevers in children are not serious and do not cause permanent brain injury, even though they might be frightening. About 5 percent of children with fever will develop **febrile convulsions.** These seizures are of short duration, usually are not dangerous, and require no special treatment beyond airway maintenance. The underlying cause of the fever must be determined by a physician so that proper treatment of the principal disease can be instituted.

The most dangerous fevers in children are those caused by **heat stroke.** In the treatment of heat stroke, the same principles apply for the care of children as for adults (see Chapter 41). The temperature of the body must be reduced as quickly as possible. A child who has been in the sun, in an extremely warm, poorly ventilated room, or in a closed, parked car, and who has hot, dry skin may be suffering from heat stroke. These children should be undressed, cooled in a tub of cold water, and transported promptly to the emergency department. Covering the child with cool, wet sheets and using fans will also help lower temperature quickly. Children with heat stroke must be carefully monitored. The surface area of a child is large with respect to the child's volume, and temperature may change rapidly. Sponging is not necessary for children with fever other than fever caused by heat stroke; it is not very effective. Treatment is best directed at the cause of the fever.

Occasionally, a child who has **epilepsy,** an underlying seizure disorder, may have a fever and develop a prolonged epileptic attack. The child with epilepsy whose attack is triggered by fever needs a prompt diagnosis of febrile disease. In contrast to the usual febrile seizures, which are extremely brief (one to two minutes), a true epileptic seizure of this nature will last longer. The EMT who is treating a child having a seizure who is cyanotic must attempt to restore the airway, although doing so may be extremely difficult. The EMT should never place fingers in the mouth, as the convulsing child may bite. Nor should the EMT try to pry the jaws open. It will usually do more harm than good. Gentle extension of the neck will open the airway partially. Ventilation through the nose in the patient with clenched teeth should be facilitated by keeping the nasal passages clear. Oxygen should always be administered by face mask. Following the seizure, the child will be in a postictal state — that is, somewhat depressed, with slow respirations, and perhaps difficult to rouse. The EMT should maintain the airway, continue to administer oxygen, and transport this child promptly to the hospital. The general treatment for patients with epilepsy is outlined in Chapter 36.

Another cause of febrile convulsions in childhood is **meningitis,** a viral or bacterial infection of the covering membranes of the brain and spinal cord. This is an extremely serious disease but not usually a very contagious one. These children will be hot and obviously sick. A sore throat or upper respiratory problem may have preceded the current illness. Headache and a stiff neck are common complaints. Children with these symptoms should be brought to the emergency department as quickly as possible.

Abdominal Pain

The most serious cause of abdominal pain in childhood is **appendicitis.** While it can occur at any age, appendicitis is usually seen between the ages of ten and twenty-five. The older child may give a history of progressive abdominal pain. It starts over the umbilicus and is crampy in nature. It moves to the right lower quadrant of the abdomen in a matter of hours and becomes steady and severe. Usually the child is nauseated and has no appetite. Occasionally, vomiting occurs. The child tends to be irritable or fussy, and fever is common.

The major difficulty in identifying appendicitis in pediatric patients occurs with the younger child or infant who can give no clear history. In this situation, the clinical picture is almost identical with viral or bacterial **gastroenteritis** ("flu"). Diagnosis is difficult for the doctors and may be delayed. A good rule for the EMT to follow is to transport every child with a sore or tender abdomen to the emergency department if only for appropriate diagnosis. Never should the EMT attempt to make a distinction between appendicitis and gastroenteritis.

Dehydration (loss of body fluids) is a common problem in infants and children. It is frequently seen in association with situations that cause abdominal pain. Diarrhea or vomiting can each bring about dehydration in small patients much more quickly than in adults. Sometimes gastroenteritis produces diarrhea that persists for days before medical aid is sought. Dehydration may be a cause of shock in infants and children. The dehydrated child is lethargic with dry skin and mucous membranes. Because of the potential for shock, the dehydrated child must be transported to the emergency department promptly.

Poisoning

Little children are curious and like to sample the contents of brightly colored bottles or cans thinking that they contain something good to eat or drink. Sometimes a considerable amount of substance is swallowed before the child or parent realizes that a dangerous substance has been ingested. Many common household items are poisonous. The EMT who responds to a poisoning should take these steps:

1. If caustic (irritating) material has been spilled on the child, wash it off with water. If it has spilled on the child's clothes, remove them. If any of the material is in the child's eyes, flush the eyes thoroughly with water for several minutes.
2. If the child has swallowed tablets from a medicine bottle, gather any spilled tablets and replace them in the bottle so that the number can be counted. The emergency department physician will then have an idea of how many tablets the child may actually have taken.
3. If the child has swallowed any substance, identify it, attempt to estimate the amount

taken, and gather the remainder. Bring any bottle or any other container of the substance with you to the emergency department.

4. As soon as you are certain that a poisoning has occurred, notify dispatch and medical control. Identify the patient, the child's age and size, the agent, and the suspected amount taken. The dispatch center will contact the local poison control center and relay specific treatment instructions to you. Your job is to care for and transport the patient safely and promptly and to gather critical information about the ingested substance for the emergency department personnel.

5. If the poison control center recommends that vomiting should be induced, give one tablespoon of syrup of ipecac in a glass of water and transport the child promptly to the hospital. If the child does not vomit in 20 minutes, the dose may be repeated once. If the level of consciousness deteriorates, do not give any more ipecac. Do not delay transport to await the onset of vomiting.

6. Do not attempt to induce vomiting in a child who has swallowed strong acid or strong alkali (such as lye or Drano®), or any petroleum product.

7. Do not attempt to induce vomiting in a child who is unconscious or partially conscious. The danger of vomitus being aspirated into the lungs is too great. If the poisoned child does vomit, suction the material out of the mouth and pharynx and collect it for analysis at the hospital.

8. Transport the patient to the emergency department promptly. Be prepared to give all needed support up to and including full CPR. Many ingested items, especially medications, promptly produce respiratory depression. In all children who have ingested poisonous substances, close monitoring of respiration is critical and support of impaired breathing is essential. Anticipate vomiting in these patients also. Many substances that are ingested are very irritating to the stomach and induce vomiting by themselves.

A statement of the proper emergency treatment for various poisonous agents is contained in Chapter 27.

Contagious Disease

Occasionally a child who is suffering from one of the common infectious childhood diseases must be transported by the EMT for some other medical reason. A contagious disease is usually easy to spot. Measles (rubeola), German measles (rubella), and chicken pox produce specific types of rash; mumps causes swelling and tenderness of the parotid glands directly in front of the ears.

The EMT should notify the hospital that a child is arriving who appears to have a contagious disease. Masks can serve a useful purpose if the child has fever and a rash. As a general rule, however, children with these diseases are not particularly infectious for the EMT, who probably has had the disease or has been immunized against it. Careful hand washing, cleaning of exposed surfaces and equipment in the vehicle, and appropriate use of masks will usually protect the EMT. Specific information regarding a variety of contagious diseases is contained in Chapter 34.

Sudden Infant Death Syndrome (SIDS)

Approximately 10,000 infants per year die in the United States from sudden infant death syndrome (SIDS). The exact cause is unknown, but it is suspected to be a viral infection. It usually occurs during sleep in an otherwise healthy infant and thus has been called **crib death.** In such a situation, the EMT is going to encounter anguished, severely disturbed parents. Some time and effort must be spent on comforting the parents. At the same time, however, every effort must be made to revive the baby, even if the infant's death preceded the EMT's arrival by some prolonged period of time. Basic life support measures should be instituted before and during transportation to the hospital, even if the baby seems to be dead. Resuscitation efforts should be continued until the baby is pronounced dead by a physician. The emergency department should be notified in advance of the nature of the problem.

SPECIAL PEDIATRIC PROBLEMS

Child Abuse

The exact incidence of **child abuse** is unknown. What is known, however, is that child abuse is a far greater problem than was once suspected. The deliberate, intentional injury of a child physically and emotionally is, unfortunately, not rare in our society today. Child abuse is progressive — that is, the child may be continually abused with increasing severity, until death ultimately results. Child abuse can occur in any family and is found at all socioeconomic levels.

An abused child is often brought to the hospital for medical attention, or the EMT is called because of a supposed accidental injury. Child abuse should be suspected if the history given by the person who called does not appear to fit the child's injury. Characteristically, the abused or battered child will have many injuries, all at different stages of healing. The child may appear withdrawn, fearful, or hostile, and may or may not be undernourished. Occasionally, the child's parent or caretaker will reveal a history of several "accidents" in the past. the abuser may be a parent, relative, or baby sitter. Sometimes, particularly if the child is living with a single parent, the abuser is an acquaintance of that single parent.

The EMT who suspects child abuse should not attempt to make a diagnosis. Instead, what history is given should be carefully recorded and the child transported promptly to the hospital, even if the injuries appear relatively trivial. Most states have laws requiring health care personnel to report cases of suspected child abuse to various social service or police agencies. Ordinarily, this responsibility lies with the physician. Thus, the EMT who has special information or who suspects child abuse should report it to the physician at the hospital. Often a child who is a suspected victim of abuse will be admitted to the hospital for protection, even though the injuries alone are not severe enough to warrant hospitalization.

An EMT, however, cannot bring the child to the hospital without the parent's consent. Sometimes the parents can be persuaded if the EMT tells them that the child may need special x-rays or tests. The EMT should not accuse anyone of child abuse, even if it appears obvious. Maintaining a professional approach is not easy for an EMT, as an obvious case of child abuse arouses strong emotions and challenges one's ability to think and act clearly.

The ultimate determination of child abuse is made in the courts, often after a long and complicated legal process. The responsibility of all health-care professionals is to identify suspicious instances of child abuse early so that necessary steps can be taken. EMTs should be knowledgeable about the specific laws in their states regarding the reporting of child abuse.

Sexual Abuse of Children

Sexual abuse is another problem that can occur in children as well as adults. It may occur in infants, young children, adolescents, and to both boys and girls. Most victims of rape are over ten years of age, although, unfortunately, younger children are sometimes victims as well. The EMT should not examine the young child's genitalia unless there is obvious bleeding or other injury that must be treated. An examination that allows the EMT to place the proper dressing for the injury is sufficient. Sometimes a child will have been beaten and will also have bruises or even fractures. These injuries should be treated appropriately.

When sexual abuse is suspected, the child should not wash, urinate, or defecate before any examination is carried out by the physician at the emergency department. If the molested child is a girl, a male EMT should enlist the aid of a female EMT or police officer to assist him. A professional composure should be retained throughout. A concerned, caring approach to these children is extremely important. They should be shielded from onlookers and curious passersby. As much history as is possible should be obtained from the child and any witnesses. The child may be hysterical or unwilling to give any story at all, especially if the abuser is a sibling, relative, or family friend. The EMT is in the best position to retrieve the most accurate first-hand information concerning the incident, so any information should be recorded carefully and completely. All information should be written in clear and accurate detail on the ambulance report form. All child victims of sexual assault should be transported to the emergency department. Sexual molestation of children is a crime, and the EMT should cooperate with law enforcement officials in their investigations.

TRANSPORTATION OF CHILDREN

Infants and small children are very susceptible to temperature changes. Their body surface area is very large in relation to their total body volume. Thus, they lose body heat more rapidly than adults and

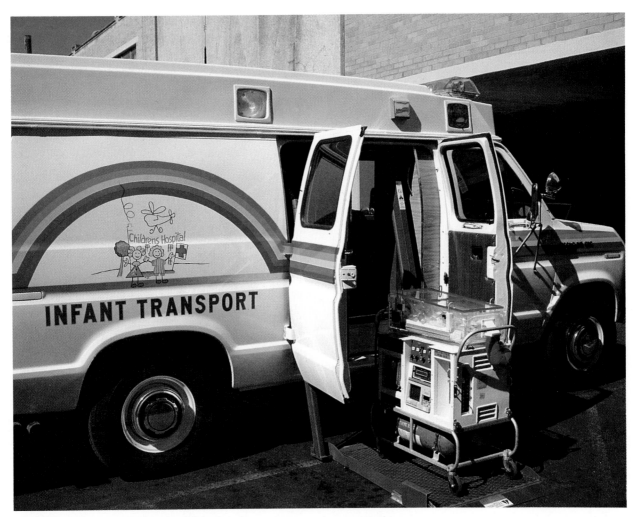

FIGURE 37.6 A specialized vehicle for the emergency transportation of premature, ill, or high-risk infants.

must always be transported well wrapped in blankets. Very young and sick children are also extremely susceptible to infection. The EMT should thus avoid breathing or coughing directly on a small, sick child. The child should be as isolated as possible from bacterial contamination, particularly from the EMT's own nose, mouth, and hands.

An infant carrier should provide access to the child so that the airway may be kept clear and artificial ventilation maintained if necessary. If oxygen is given, it should be warm. Carriers and their accessories are described in Chapter 38.

Newborns should be transported in special incubators that will allow oxygen enrichment and control of humidity and temperature. If such an in-

cubator is not available, the newborn should be wrapped in blankets except for the face, and carried in a warm ambulance. Many large medical centers maintain specially equipped vehicles for the transportation of infants and small children. The EMT should know the location and availability of these vehicles (Figure 37.6).

An older child may comprehend, to some degree, that an emergency event is taking place but not the exact nature or severity of the problem. Children are easily frightened, and, as such, often behave in a belligerent or hysterical fashion. Whenever possible, the child should have a familiar person or familiar object close by. Parents, relatives, or close friends are invaluable in dealing with frightened children.

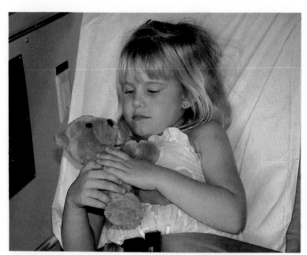

FIGURE 37.7   The young child will be less frightened if allowed to take a favorite stuffed animal or blanket during transport to the hospital.

Treasured objects such as dolls, teddy bears, or a blanket may be necessary in helping to secure the cooperation of these young patients. The child should be allowed to take such objects to the hospital (Figure 37.7). The EMT should help prevent the child's getting separated from the parents. The child's siblings should be assigned to the care of a responsible neighbor or relative who can keep them informed and safe, yet away from interfering with the care of the patient.

YOU ARE THE EMT...

1. Your patient is a young child with croup who is gasping for breath. Should you insert an artificial airway, give oxygen, or both? Why?
2. What are the common causes of shock in a child? How do you treat a child in shock?
3. You have been called to treat a child with a very high temperature. The mother is perplexed because the youngster did not seem to be sick. You notice the child has a sunburn and you suspect heatstroke. What are the other symptoms of heatstroke? What emergency care will you give this patient?
4. Your patient is a two-year-old child who has fallen out of his crib. After a thorough examination, you are confident that he has no broken bones or head injuries, but you have noticed lots of "old" bruises. You begin to suspect child abuse, but there is no real evidence. What will you do?

CHILDBIRTH

38 Childbirth

OVERVIEW

Childbirth, especially the not-making-the-hospital-in-time version, has for years been the subject of TV drama. The woman is in great pain, there is always a storm or an accident, and someone comes to the rescue and orders everyone to boil water. The baby is adorable, the mother is exhausted, and the baby's stand-in doctor — the father or the star of the show — is elated.

In real life, this situation occurs infrequently. Most babies in the United States are born in hospitals. Rarely is the EMT called to see a pregnant woman when the birth process is well along and there is not time to get her to a hospital. Once in a while, however, it does happen, and the EMT must be prepared to move quickly and efficiently. A sterile emergency delivery pack replaces the boiling water, but a number of potential problems replace the drama. The cord could be wrapped around the baby's neck. The baby could have difficulty breathing. The mother might have excessive bleeding. Fortunately, most emergency births are trouble free, but even so, the EMT must be very knowledgeable about the whole process of childbirth.

Chapter 38 begins with a description of the developing fetus and an explanation of what can go wrong during pregnancy. The chapter next describes the onset of labor and how an EMT decides whether an emergency delivery is needed. Then the three stages of labor are presented in detail. The last part of the chapter discusses abnormal deliveries and complications, including failure of the amniotic membrane to rupture, breech deliveries, prolapsed umbilical cord, excessive bleeding, abortion or miscarriage, twins, delivery without sterile supplies, and premature infants.

OBJECTIVES

The objectives of Chapter 38 are to

- understand the basic anatomy of the developing fetus.
- recognize the complications of pregnancy.
- identify the onset of labor.
- know how to assess the need for an emergency delivery of a baby.
- describe the three stages of labor and the role of the EMT in assisting the mother during the childbirth process.
- know the procedures for handling both abnormal deliveries and complications of childbirth.

THE DEVELOPING FETUS

The developing baby, or **fetus,** grows inside the mother's womb (**uterus**) for nine months. During this time, the mother's abdomen grows larger as the uterus enlarges with the growing fetus. As the fetus grows, it requires more and more nourishment. The **placenta,** also called the **afterbirth,** develops on the wall of the uterus and is connected to the fetus by the **umbilical cord.** The close attachment of the placenta to the wall of the uterus allows oxygen and other nutrients to cross from the mother's circulation into the placenta and then along the umbilical cord to support the fetus as it grows. The fetus develops inside a fluid-filled sac called the **amniotic sac** (Figure 38.1).

COMPLICATIONS OF PREGNANCY

As the time for delivery approaches, certain complications can occur. Convulsions that result from severe hypertension (**eclampsia**) are treated by laying the mother on her side, maintaining an airway, and providing supplemental oxygen. If vomiting occurs, the airway should be suctioned. The pregnant patient with convulsions should be transported promptly to the hospital.

Most pregnant women are healthy, but some may have medical diseases along with being pregnant. Heart or lung disease, if present, may be safely treated with oxygen without harm to the fetus. Hemorrhage from the birth canal (**vagina**) that occurs before labor begins may be very serious. In early pregnancy, bleeding may be a sign of an **abortion (miscarriage)**. In the later stages of pregnancy, hemorrhage may indicate problems with the placenta, among them placenta abruptio and placenta previa. In **placenta abruptio,** the placenta separates prematurely from the wall of the uterus. In **placenta previa,** the placenta develops over and covers the mouth of the uterus (**cervix**). In both instances, sudden, often painless, bleeding will result.

Any bleeding from the vagina in a pregnant woman is a serious sign and should be treated in the hospital promptly. If the patient shows signs of shock,

she should lie on her side during transportation. A pregnant woman is usually more comfortable lying on her side than on her back. A sterile pad or sanitary napkin should be placed over the vagina and replaced as often as necessary. The pads should be saved so that the hospital personnel can estimate how much blood has been lost. Nothing should be put into the vagina. Any tissue that may be passed from the vagina should also be saved.

Sometimes a pregnant woman is involved in an automobile accident. Such a situation can be very serious, as severe hemorrhage may occur from injuries to the pregnant uterus. A pregnant woman who has been in an accident should be evaluated and transported to the hospital promptly.

THE ONSET OF LABOR

The onset of **labor** is the beginning of the delivery process. It begins with the characteristic labor pains, which are contractions of the uterus. The total time of labor varies greatly, but it is usually longer in a woman who is having her first baby (**primagravida**) and becomes progressively shorter with each successive baby. (A pregnant woman who has previously given birth is called a **multigravida.**) Other signs indicating the beginning of labor are the appearance of the bloody show and rupture of the amniotic sac (breaking of the bag of waters). These events may occur before the onset of labor pains. The **bloody show** is a small plug of blood-stained mucus that forms in the cervix and is expelled when labor begins. Rupture of the amniotic sac allows the amniotic fluid to gush out of the uterus through the vagina. At term, there is normally about one liter of amniotic fluid.

Labor pains become stronger and more regular as the baby begins to move down the birth canal. The mother will feel increasing pressure in her lower abdomen and may feel she has to move her bowels. This sensation is normal and means that the baby's head is pressing on the rectum. As delivery nears, the cervix of the uterus opens, called **dilation of the cervix,** so that the baby's head can pass through into the vagina.

There are three stages of labor. The first stage begins with the onset of labor pains and ends when the cervix is fully dilated. The second stage begins when the cervix is fully dilated and ends when the baby is born. The third stage begins with the birth

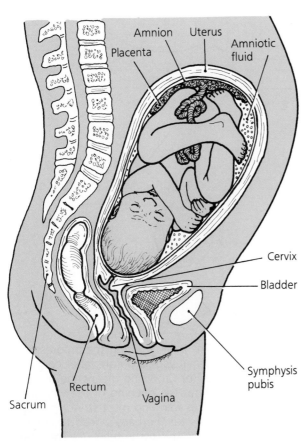

FIGURE 38.1 Anatomic structures of the pregnant woman.

of the baby and ends with the delivery of the placenta. During the first stage there is usually time to transport the mother to the hospital. If the mother is in the second stage, the EMT should consider delivering her at home. If the third stage is occurring and the baby has been born, the placenta will usually deliver within 30 minutes, and the mother usually should not be transported during that time.

ASSESSING THE NEED FOR AN EMERGENCY DELIVERY

Once the EMT has determined that the woman is indeed in labor, the next major decision is whether to have her deliver at home or transport her to the hospital. The EMT should consider delivering the mother under the following circumstances:

1. When delivery can be expected within a few minutes.
2. When the hospital cannot be reached because of a natural disaster or traffic accident.
3. When there is no transportation available.

The EMT can make a determination of whether the delivery is going to occur within a few minutes by asking the mother certain questions and looking for crowning. The patient should first be asked if she is a multigravida. A multigravida can often tell the EMT if she is about to deliver. If she says yes, the EMT should believe her and make immediate preparations for delivery. The patient should also be asked if she feels as if she has to move her bowels. This means that the baby's head is pressing on the rectum and that delivery is about to occur. The EMT should also inspect the vagina to see if the baby's head is visible, the phase of labor called **crowning.** To do this, the EMT has to spread the mother's legs apart gently, reassuring her that this is being done in order to help decide if she should be delivered immediately or transported to the hospital. Crowning means that delivery is about to occur (Figure 38.2).

Once labor has begun, there is no way it can be slowed down or stopped. The mother's legs should never be held together. To do so would only complicate the delivery. Nor should the mother be allowed to go to the bathroom. Instead, she must be assured that the sensation of needing to move her bowels is normal and that it means she is about to deliver.

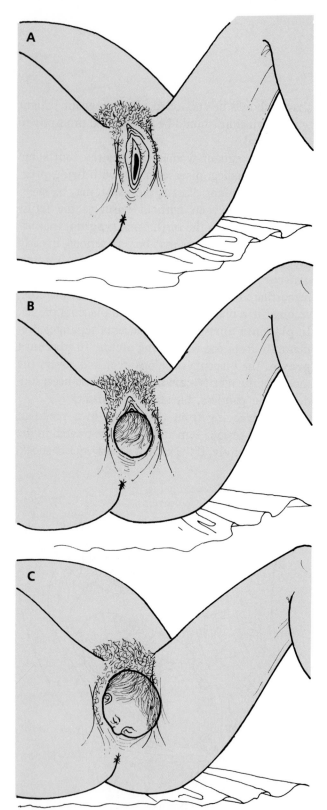

FIGURE 38.2 The vagina during the progress of labor. (a) The normal vagina before labor commences is closed. (b) Crowning means the head of the baby is visible at the opening of the vagina. The vaginal tissue is thin and must stretch enough during contractions for the baby's head to come through. Sometimes this tissue tears. (c) The head is delivered, usually with the baby's face pointing to the right or left posterior.

THE FIRST STAGE OF LABOR

Once the EMT has decided to deliver the baby at home, steps must be taken quickly but calmly. Delivery will usually require the assistance of two people. If only one EMT is available, he or she must seek assistance from a nurse, police officer, or even a family member or neighbor who may have had experience in childbirth. The EMT should never leave the patient once the decision has been made to deliver her at home. Someone else should seek outside help if it is needed. Remember, the mother, *not* the EMT, delivers the baby. The EMT helps, guides, and supports the baby as it is born.

The emergency vehicle should always be equipped with a sterile **emergency delivery pack** containing the following items:

    1 pair surgical scissors
    3 hemostats or special cord clamps
    umbilical tape
    small rubber bulb syringe
    5 towels
    1 dozen 4×4 gauze sponges
    3 or 4 pairs of rubber gloves
    1 baby blanket
    sanitary napkins

The mother should be placed on a spine board that is padded with blankets, folded sheets, or towels.

If delivery is occurring in an automobile, the mother should lie on the seat, with one foot on the floor and the other on the seat, with the knee and hip bent (Figure 38.3).

If the emergency delivery is occurring at home, the mother should be moved to a sturdy table if at all possible. The EMT will find it easier to work there than if the mother is in bed. Both her hips and knees should be flexed, and her head should be supported with one or two pillows. Her legs should be spread apart. Placing newspapers or sheets on the floor around the delivery area will help soak up the amniotic fluid that will be released when the amniotic sac ruptures (Figure 38.4).

The EMT's assistant should sit at the mother's head to comfort and soothe her and to reassure her during the delivery. She may want to grip someone's hand. She may have to vomit. In that case, the EMT's helper should turn her head to the side so that her mouth and airway can be cleared. The EMT should be positioned at the mother's right side if he or she is right-handed, or her left side if left-handed. About 2 feet of the table should extend beyond the mother's buttocks. This will be a convenient surface on which to place the newborn baby.

The EMT should place the emergency delivery pack on a chair or table close to the patient so that it can be reached easily. The delivery pack should be opened carefully so that its contents remain sterile;

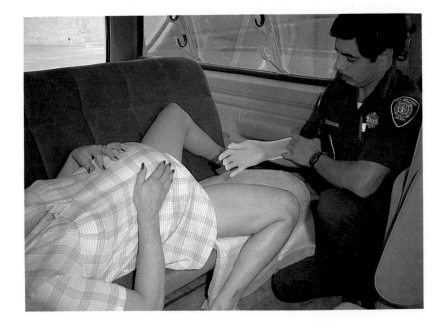

FIGURE 38.3 The setup for an emergency delivery in an automobile.

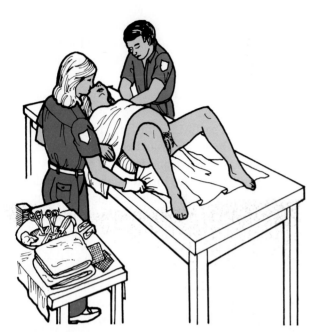

FIGURE 38.4 The setup for an emergency delivery in the home. The setup shown is for a right-handed EMT. Note the projection of the surface beyond the mother's vagina so that the baby may be placed there after delivery.

after a thorough hand washing, the EMT should put on the sterile gloves. One sterile folded towel should be placed under the patient's buttocks using a sterile, gloved hand. Another sterile towel should be placed between her legs, just below the vagina. The third towel should be spread across her abdomen.

The EMT should stand so that the vagina is in view at all times. The mother's contractions should be timed from the beginning of one to the beginning of the next. In between contractions, the mother should be encouraged to rest. She should be reminded not to strain with the contractions and to breathe deeply through her mouth.

THE SECOND STAGE OF LABOR

Delivery

The EMT should watch the head as it comes out of the vagina. Once it is obvious that the head is coming out farther with each contraction, the EMT should place his or her right hand (or left hand if left-handed) over the emerging head and exert very gentle pressure. This will allow the head to come out smoothly and prevent the head and baby from

suddenly popping out of the vagina during a strong contraction, possibly causing injury.

The head is usually tilted to one side or the other rather than straight up and down. A baby's head has two soft areas — one near the front (**brow**) and one near the back (**occiput**). They are called the **fontanelles.** The brain is covered only by skin and membranes at these places. The EMT must be careful not to push his fingers into the fontanelles. The head should be gently held in the EMT's palm. Gentle pressure should be maintained during contractions and decreased between contractions. It may take two, three, or more contractions for the delivery of the head to occur from the time it presents (Figure 38.5).

The head has to be supported as it is born. As soon as the head is delivered, the EMT can use the index finger of the other hand to feel if the umbilical cord is wrapped around the neck. A cord that is wound tightly around the neck could cause the baby to strangle and must therefore be released from the neck immediately. Usually, it can be slipped over the baby's shoulder. If not, and if it feels tightly wound around the neck, it must be cut. The cord must be clamped with two clamps placed about 2 inches apart. The cord is cut between the clamps. Then the EMT can unwrap it from around the neck. The cord is fragile and easily torn. It must be handled very carefully. The clamps should not come off until the ends of the cord have been tied. Usually, the cord is *not* around the baby's neck and does not have to be cut until after the birth (Figure 38.6).

The EMT should support the baby's head with one hand as the mother continues to deliver the baby. As soon as the chin, and, therefore, the whole head, is born, the baby's face will turn sideways. At this point, once the whole face is visible, the mouth and nose should be suctioned. A bulb syringe is squeezed and gently inserted into the baby's mouth about 1½ inches; any accumulated mucus, blood, water, or amniotic fluid is sucked out and squirted onto the towel across the mother's abdomen. The suctioning must be repeated two or three times in the mouth and two or three times in each nostril. The newborn baby is a nose breather, so particular attention must be paid to clearing the nose (Figure 38.7).

By the time suctioning is finished, the upper shoulder will be visible in the vagina. The baby's head is the largest part of the body. Once it is born, the rest of the baby usually delivers easily. The head

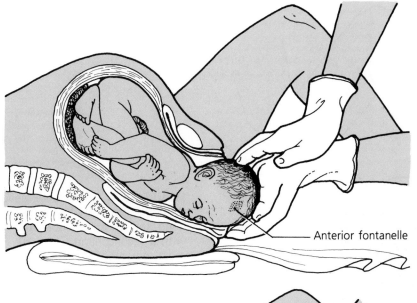

FIGURE 38.5 A side view as the baby's head leaves the vagina. The face is pointed posteriorly and to one side. The EMT supports and exerts gentle pressure to prevent rapid expulsion of the baby.

Anterior fontanelle

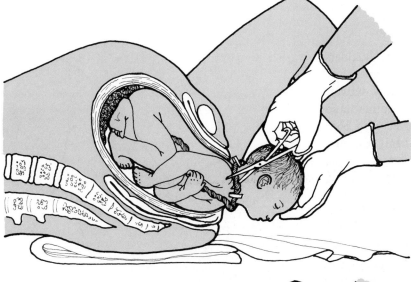

FIGURE 38.6 If the umbilical cord is wrapped tightly around the baby's neck, it must be freed, clamped, and cut.

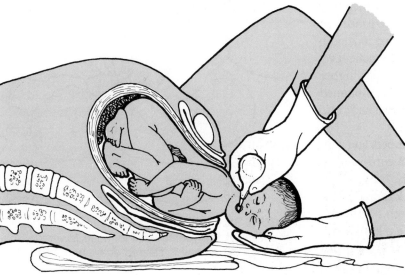

FIGURE 38.7 Once delivery of the head is complete, the mouth and nostrils of the child can be suctioned for the first time.

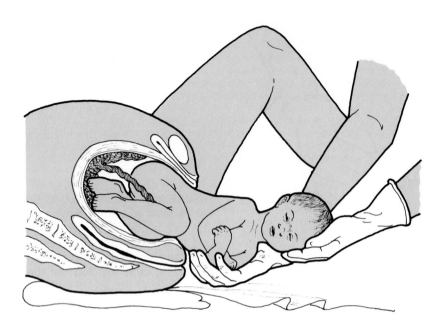

FIGURE 38.8 The infant's head should be supported with one hand and the trunk supported with a second hand. The EMT must remember that the baby is quite slippery and must be held firmly but gently.

and upper body should be supported as the shoulders deliver. Then the abdomen and hips will appear and be delivered. Once the abdomen and hips deliver, the EMT should support them with his other hand so that now the baby is being supported with both hands. The baby should be handled firmly but carefully. It will be slippery. Particular care should be taken not to squeeze the neck or chest while holding the baby (Figure 38.8).

As soon as the entire baby is born, it should be placed immediately on a towel, on its back, on the space on the table or bed that was set aside for this purpose. The baby's head should be kept slightly lower than the rest of its body, and turned slightly to one side. The EMT should use a sterile gauze pad to wipe the baby's mouth and again suction its mouth and nose. The baby should be kept at the same level as the mother's vagina. If the baby is held higher than the mother's vagina, blood will be siphoned from the baby through the umbilical cord back into the placenta (Figure 38.9).

Next, the umbilical cord is clamped and cut. Once the baby is born, the umbilical cord is of no further use to either the mother or the baby. Using the two clamps in the emergency kit, the EMT clamps the cord about halfway between the mother and the baby. The clamps should be placed about 2 to 3 inches apart. Once they are firmly in place, the cord between them should be cut using the sterile

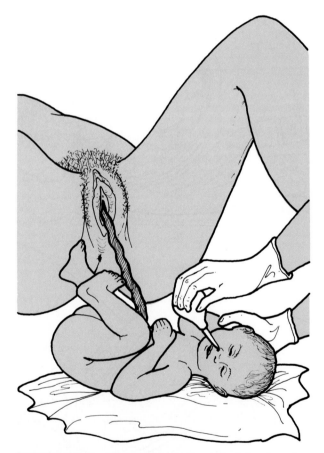

FIGURE 38.9 After delivery, the infant is placed at the level of the vagina with its head lowered slightly. The airway is cleared again with the bulb syringe.

scissors. There is no rush to cut the cord once it is clamped. The procedure should be done with care for the cord is fragile and easily torn. If it is handled too roughly, it could be torn from the baby's abdomen, which would result in a fatal hemorrhage. Once the cord is cut between the two clamps, the end coming from the baby should be tied. If the cord was cut earlier to get it out from around the baby's neck while the head was being delivered, now is the time to tie it. The emergency childbirth kit contains special umbilical tape for tying the cord. Ordinary string or twine should not be used as it will cut through the soft, fragile tissues of the cord. A loop of the tape should be placed around the cord about 1 inch nearer to the baby than the clamp. The tape should be tightened slowly so that it doesn't cut the cord and then tied firmly with a square knot. The ends of the tape should be cut, but the clamp should not be removed. Nor should the clamp on the end of the cord coming out of the mother's vagina be removed. This part of the cord is attached to the placenta and will be delivered when the placenta delivers (Figure 38.10).

The baby should be wrapped in a blanket or towel so that only the face is exposed. The baby can be cradled in the EMT's arm while its mouth and nose are being suctioned rather than leaving it on the flat surface. Newborn babies are very sensitive to cold, so if possible the blanket should be kept warm (to about 90 degrees Fahrenheit) before it is used. By now the baby should be pink and breathing on its own.

Evaluating the Newborn

A rough guide to the status of the newborn baby can be obtained using the **Apgar score.** This system assigns a number value to each of five areas of activity of the baby: cardiac rate (pulse), respirations, muscle tone, reflex irritability, and color. The numbers are then added up. A perfectly healthy baby will have a total score of ten. Most babies have a score of seven or eight at one minute after birth. The Apgar score should be calculated at one and five minutes after birth. By five minutes, most babies have a score of eight to ten (Figure 38.11).

Cardiac Rate

The newborn's pulse rate should be over 100 beats per minute. If a stethoscope is unavailable, the

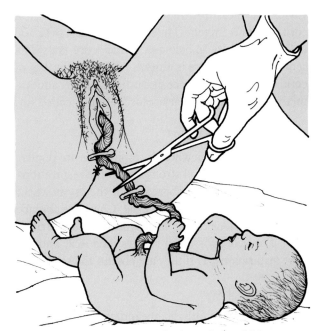

FIGURE 38.10 The umbilical cord should be clamped with two sterile clamps, 3 inches apart, placed halfway between the baby and the mother's vagina. The cord is cut between the clamps. As an extra safeguard against bleeding, it is tied again closer to the naval with umbilical tape.

APGAR SCALE	1 min.	5 min.
Cardiac Rate (>100 = 2, <100 = 1, 0 = 0)	2	2
Respiratory Rate (Rapid = 2, Slow = 1, Absent = 0)	2	2
Muscle Tone (Good = 2, Fair = 1, Absent = 0)	1	2
Reflex Irritability (Strong = 2, Weak = 1, Absent = 0)	2	2
Color (All pink = 2, Some pink = 1, No pink = 0)	1	2
TOTAL	8	10

FIGURE 38.11 The Apgar score is calculated for each birth at 1 and 5 minutes. In this example, at 1 minute the infant had only fair muscle tone and some cyanosis of the feet. By 5 minutes, muscle tone and color had improved, giving an Apgar score of 10 — a sign of normal function.

EMT can measure the pulsations in the umbilical cord using his fingers. The score for a pulse over 100 is 2. If the pulse is below 100, the score is 1. The score is 0 if the pulse is absent. Absence of pulse, of course, indicates absence of cardiac activity, and immediate cardiopulmonary resuscitation is called for.

Respiratory Effort

Normally, the newborn's respirations are regular and rapid, with a good strong cry. If the respirations are slow, shallow, or labored, or if the cry is weak, respiratory insufficiency may exist. Complete absence of respirations or crying is obviously a very serious sign. The score for rapid respirations is 2, and for slow respirations, 1. If they are absent, the score is 0.

Muscle Tone

The degree of muscle tone indicates the oxygenation of the baby's tissues. Normally, the hips and knees are flexed, and the baby will resist, to some degree, attempts to straighten them out. If this is the case, the score is 2. If the baby has some muscle tone but only weakly resists attempts to straighten out the knees or hips, the score is 1. If the baby is completely limp, with no muscle tone, the score is 0.

Reflex Irritability

This part of the Apgar scale measures the baby's response to a stimulus. It calls for snapping a finger against the sole of the baby's foot. If the baby cries and tries to move the foot away, the score is 2. A weak cry is scored 1, and no cry or reaction is scored 0.

Color

Most babies are blue at birth but become pink very rapidly. The feet and lips should "pink up" within a few minutes of birth. If the entire baby is pink, the score is 2. If the body is pink but the feet and lips remain blue, the score is 1. The score is 0 if the entire baby is blue or pale. Skin color cannot be used as a guide in black babies. Instead, the lips and tongue are used. They may be blue at birth but should "pink up" within a few minutes.

On occasion, the EMT may be called to assist in a delivery and find that the delivery has already taken place and that the baby is in trouble. The first thing the EMT should do is to quickly calculate the Apgar score to establish a baseline evaluation of the baby's vital functions. One way to help remember the five components is to use the name Apgar as follows:

A   appearance (color)
P   pulse
G   grimace (reflex irritability)
A   activity (muscle tone)
R   respirations

THE THIRD STAGE OF LABOR

The third stage of labor begins after the baby is delivered. The EMT gives the baby, wrapped in a warm blanket, to his or her assistant. Now the EMT must assist the mother with delivery of the placenta. The placenta should never be removed by pulling on the end of the umbilical cord. The placenta, like the baby, delivers itself; the EMT only assists. The placenta usually delivers itself within a few minutes of the baby's birth, but it may take as long as 30 minutes. Delivery of the placenta may be speeded up by gently massaging the mother's abdomen with a firm, circular motion. The abdominal skin will be wrinkled and very soft. The EMT should be able to feel a firm, grapefruit-sized mass in the lower abdomen. This is the uterus, with the placenta inside. As the uterus is massaged, it will contract and become firmer. If the baby is breathing well and is in good condition, it can be put to the mother's breast and allowed to nurse. This will also stimulate the uterus to contract and help to deliver the placenta.

Some bleeding, usually less than 250 cc, occurs before the placenta delivers. Once the placenta delivers, bleeding, except for a few drops, should stop. If any of the following three emergency situations occurs during the third stage of labor, the mother should be transported promptly to the hospital.

1. If more than 30 minutes elapse and the placenta has not delivered.
2. If there is more than 250 cc of bleeding before delivery of the placenta.
3. If there is significant bleeding after the delivery of the placenta.

The baby should be brought with the mother. The EMT should place a sterile pad or sanitary napkin over the vagina, place the mother in the shock position and give oxygen, and monitor her vital signs closely. Never should anything be put into the vagina.

Once the placenta delivers, it should be carefully inspected. The normal placenta is round, measures about 7 inches in diameter, and is about 1 inch thick. One surface is smooth and covered with a shiny membrane; the other surface is rough and **lobulated** (Figure 38.12). The entire placenta and cord should be put in a plastic bag and brought to the hospital. Hospital personnel will examine the placenta to make certain that the entire placenta has been delivered and that no part has been retained. If a piece of the placenta has been retained, it could cause persistent bleeding or infection.

Before proceeding to the hospital, the EMT should place a sterile pad or sanitary napkin over the vagina and lower the mother's legs. Before taking her, the baby, and the placenta to the hospital, the EMT should take a minute to thank anyone who assisted, congratulate the mother, and record the time of birth on the record-of-live-birth form. The Apgar scores at one and five minutes should also be recorded.

ABNORMAL DELIVERIES AND COMPLICATIONS

Failure of the Amniotic Membrane to Rupture

Usually, rupture of the amniotic membranes is one of the first signs that labor is beginning. The membranes may also rupture during contractions, signaled by the resulting gush of fluid. On rare occasions, the membranes will not rupture at all, and the baby will be born still covered by the membranes. As the head presents, a saclike membrane will cover the head and face. This situation is serious, for the membranes will suffocate the baby if they are not removed. The membranes should be broken immediately, using fingers, a sterile clamp, or scissors. If an instrument is used, the EMT must be very careful not to cut the baby. The amniotic fluid will gush out when the membranes are ruptured. The baby's nose and mouth should be cleared immediately, using a bulb syringe and a gauze sponge.

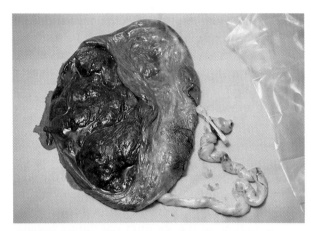

FIGURE 38.12 The normal placenta is round, measures about 7 inches in diameter, and is 1 inch thick. One side is smooth, and the other is rough and lobulated. The entire placenta should be placed in a plastic bag and brought to the hospital.

Resuscitation of the Newborn

A newborn baby will usually begin breathing spontaneously within 30 seconds after birth. If it does not breathe spontaneously, or if it is limp and its Apgar score is low, resuscitation should be instituted, following these steps:

1. Suction the airway again, as was done previously.
2. Place the baby on its side with the head lower than the rest of its body.
3. Stimulate the baby. This is best done by snapping an index finger against one of the baby's feet. If this is not successful and the baby still does not breathe spontaneously, begin mouth-to-mouth and nose resuscitation.
4. Cover the baby's *mouth and nose* with your mouth and breathe with the same force you would use to exhale a puff of cigarette smoke. This should be just enough force to make the baby's chest rise. Do not use a lot of pressure, and make sure that air is getting into the baby's nose. Babies are nose breathers rather than mouth breathers. Start the resuscitation with two breaths delivered slowly (1 to 1½ seconds each) and watch for inflation of the lungs and motion of the chest wall. If the baby starts to breathe spontaneously, place an infant oxygen mask over its nose and

mouth and let it breathe the oxygen until it becomes pink. If two minutes go by and the baby is still not breathing spontaneously, begin full cardiopulmonary resuscitation (CPR).

5. Cardiac compression is performed with the baby lying on a firm surface or cradled in one arm while the EMT applies cardiac compressions with the other hand. In the infant, the heart lies beneath the lower half of the sternum. Cardiac compression is done with the index and long fingers. Select a point in the midline of the sternum one finger breadth below the line between the nipples. Place the more superior finger at this point. The other finger will then lie on the lower part of the sternum. Press the two fingers gently against the lower half of the sternum. The sternum and rib cage of the newborn are flexible and easily compressed. Use only enough force to compress the sternum ½ to 1 inch. Compressions should be applied at the rate of 100 per minute. Recall that ventilation is absolutely vital in the neonate. For this reason mouth-to-mouth and nose ventilation should be given after every fifth cardiac compression (Figure 38.13).

6. Continue CPR while transporting the baby to the hospital. You will have to get help to transport the mother and baby since you must maintain continuous cardiopulmonary resuscitation. Continue your efforts at resuscitation until the baby breathes spontaneously or is pronounced dead by a physician. *Do not give up your efforts!* Many babies have survived, and developed without brain damage, even after long periods without spontaneous breathing if they have been given good cardiopulmonary resuscitation.

7. Keep the baby warm, but not hot, at all times. The baby is not yet able to regulate its body temperature well and must be kept in a warm environment.

8. If the baby is obviously dead when born, and is covered with blisters, has a foul smell, and the head is soft, then, and only then should you *not* attempt CPR. If there is any doubt in your mind that the baby has a chance for survival, you should start resuscitation.

Breech Delivery

Most babies are born with the head coming out first (**vertex presentation**). Occasionally, the buttocks come out first. This delivery is called a **breech presentation.** The occurrence of a breech presentation cannot be determined until the buttocks, rather

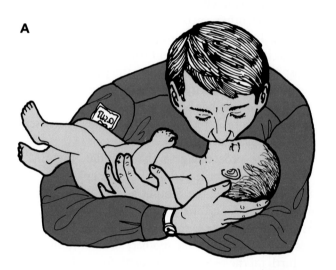

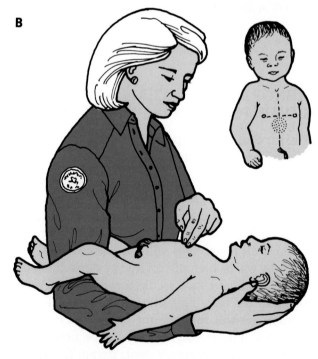

FIGURE 38.13 Cardiopulmonary resuscitation is different in a baby than in an adult. (a) Ventilation is through both the mouth and the nose with a very gentle force, just enough to make the chest expand. (b) Cardiac compression in the infant is done with the index and long fingers.

than the head, appear in the mother's vaginal opening. Breech deliveries are usually slow, so that there is time to get the mother to the hospital. However, if the buttocks have already passed through the vagina, delivery is underway and the emergency procedures just outlined should be carried out.

The preparations for a breech delivery are the same as for a vertex delivery. The EMTs should position the mother, unwrap the emergency delivery kit, and place themselves as for a normal delivery. The buttocks and legs should be allowed to deliver spontaneously. The EMT can support them with his hand to prevent rapid expulsion. The buttocks will usually come out easily. The legs will dangle on either side of the EMT's arm as the EMT supports the trunk and chest as they are born. The head is almost always face down and should be allowed to deliver spontaneously. As the head is delivering, the EMT should keep the baby's airway open by putting a gloved finger into the vagina and keeping the walls of the vagina from compressing the baby's airway. Note that this is one of only two circumstances when the EMT should put his or her fingers into the vagina.

During a breech delivery, the EMT should never try to pull the head out. If the head is stuck in the vagina and fails to deliver, the EMT should apply firm pressure to the uterus with the hand that is not supporting the infant. Pressure is applied to the lower abdomen, just above the pubic symphysis. The EMT

may be able to feel the head through the mother's abdominal wall. This maneuver will frequently enable the head to be delivered spontaneously. If the head delivers spontaneously, the delivery can continue as for a normal birth. If the head does not deliver spontaneously within three minutes, the mother and baby should be transported rapidly to the hospital, with the EMT holding the baby's airway open (Figure 38.14).

On very rare occasions, the presenting part of the baby is neither the head nor buttocks, but a single arm or leg or foot. This is called a **limb presentation.** An EMT cannot successfully deliver such a presentation; these babies must be delivered in a hospital. If faced with a limb presentation, the EMT must transport the mother to the hospital immediately. If a limb is protruding, it should be covered with a sterile towel. Never should it be pushed back in. The mother should be placed on her back and transported promptly.

Prolapsed Umbilical Cord

On rare occasions, the umbilical cord may come out of the vagina before the baby, a presentation called **prolapse of the umbilical cord.** This situation is very dangerous, as the baby's head will compress the cord during birth and cut off all circulation to the baby. Prolapse of the umbilical cord usually occurs early in labor, so there is time to get the mother to the hospital. The EMT should never

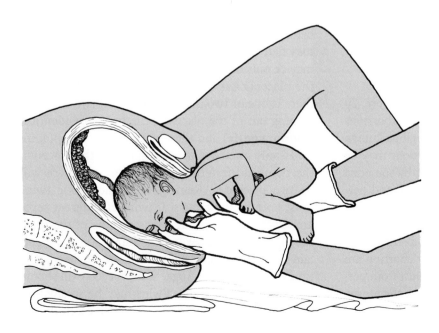

FIGURE 38.14 The infant who presents as a breech delivery has the legs and buttocks coming first. Usually they are easily delivered. The head, the largest part, comes last and may be difficult to deliver. An airway must be provided to the mouth and nose in the vagina, and the baby must be supported.

attempt to push the cord back into the vagina. This complication must be treated in the hospital. The EMT's job is to try to keep the baby's head from compressing the cord. The mother should be placed on a spine board in the shock (**Trendelenburg**) position, with her hips elevated on a pillow or folded sheet. The EMT should carefully insert his sterile gloved hand into the vagina and gently push the baby's head away from the umbilical cord. Note that this is the only other occasion that the EMT should actually place a hand into the vagina. A sterile towel moistened with saline should be wrapped around the exposed cord. The mother should be given oxygen and transported rapidly to the hospital.

Excessive Bleeding

Some bleeding always occurs with delivery. However, if there are more than five blood-soaked pads (approximately 250 cc) after delivery, this is considered excessive bleeding. There are several possible causes for excessive bleeding, all of which may be serious and require emergency care. The EMT should treat excessive bleeding by covering the vagina with a sterile pad, and changing the pad as often as necessary. The blood-soaked pads should not be discarded because the hospital personnel will use them to estimate the amount of blood that has been lost. Any tissue that may have passed from the vagina should be saved as well. The EMT should place the mother in the shock position, administer oxygen, monitor vital signs frequently, and transport her immediately to the hospital. The EMT should never hold the mother's legs together in an effort to stop the bleeding.

Abortion (Miscarriage)

Delivery of the fetus and placenta before 20 weeks is called miscarriage or abortion. Abortions may be **spontaneous** (without any obvious known cause) or **deliberate.** Deliberate abortions may be self-induced (by the mother herself) or by someone else. Deliberate abortions may be planned and performed in a hospital or clinic setting. Regardless of the reasons for the abortion, complications can occur that the EMT may be called on to treat.

The most serious complications of abortion are bleeding and infection. Bleeding may result from portions of the fetus or placenta being left in the uterus (**incomplete abortion**) or from damage to the wall of the uterus. Infection can result from the same causes. If the mother is in shock, she must be treated for shock and transported promptly to the hospital. Any tissue that passes through the vagina must be saved and brought to the hospital. The EMT should never try to pull any tissue out of the vagina; rather, it should be covered with a sterile pad. On rare instances, massive bleeding may occur from an abortion and cause severe hypovolemic shock. The use of the Pneumatic Anti-shock Garment should be considered in such a situation, just as it would be for a patient with severe intra-abdominal bleeding.

Twins

Twins occur about once in every 80 births. Sometimes there is family history of twins. The mother may suspect she is having twins because she has an unusually large abdomen. Twins are usually diagnosed early in pregnancy, but occasionally they manage to keep their existence a surprise until the time of delivery.

Twins are smaller than single babies, and the delivery is usually not difficult. Twins should be suspected if the baby is small or if the mother's abdomen remains fairly large after the birth. If twins are present, the second one will usually be born within 45 minutes of the first. About 10 minutes after the first birth, labor pains will begin again, and the birth process will repeat itself.

The procedure for delivering twins is the same as for single babies. The cord of the first baby should be clamped and cut as soon as it has been born and before the second baby is delivered. The second baby may deliver before or after the first placenta. There may be only one placenta or there may be two. When the placenta has been delivered, look at it to see if there is one or two umbilical cords. If two cords are coming out of the placenta, the twins are identical (**monozygotic**) and there will only be one placenta. If only one cord is coming out of the placenta, the twins are fraternal (**dizygotic**), and there will be two placentas. Remember, monozygotic twins must both be the same sex; twins of different sexes are dizygotic. Dizygotic twins may be of the same sex or of different sexes. It is important to be certain that both placentas, if present, are delivered. The time of birth and the Apgar score of each twin should be recorded separately. Twins may be so small as to be premature; they must be handled carefully and kept warm. The Apgar score should be used as a guide in the same way as it would for a single birth.

Delivery without Sterile Supplies

On rare occasions, an EMT may have to deliver a baby without a sterile emergency delivery pack. Clean sheets and towels that have not been used since they were laundered should be used. Without sterile gloves, the EMT should be very thorough with hand washing. The delivery should be carried out as if sterile supplies were on hand. As soon as the baby is born, the inside of its mouth should be wiped out with the EMT's finger to clear the mouth of blood and mucus. Without the delivery pack, the cord should not be cut and tied. Instead, as soon as the placenta is born, it should be wrapped in a clean towel and transported together with the baby. The placenta and the baby should remain at the same level so blood does not drain from the baby into the placenta. The baby should be kept warm, and mother, baby, and placenta should be transported to the hospital promptly (Figure 38.15).

Premature Infant

The usual period for the development of a baby (**gestation period**) is nine calendar months. A normal, single baby will weigh around 7 pounds at birth. Any baby that delivers before 8 months gestation or weighs less than 5½ pounds at birth is considered premature. Often, the exact gestation time cannot

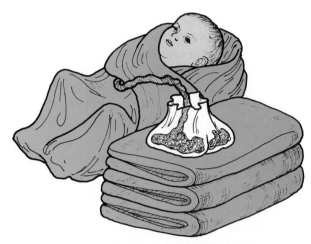

FIGURE 38.15 When sterile supplies are not available and the umbilical cord cannot be cut, the placenta, attached to the cord, should be kept at the same level as the baby during transport to the hospital.

be determined; nor will there be a scale to weigh the baby. A **premature baby** is smaller, thinner, and redder, and its head is proportionately larger in comparison to the rest of its body than a full-term baby (Figure 38.16)

Premature babies need special care to survive. With such care, even babies as small as one pound have survived and developed into normal children. Certain procedures should be followed when handling a premature infant:

FIGURE 38.16 A premature infant (right) is smaller, thinner, and redder than a full-term baby (left). In addition, the premature baby's head is larger in comparison to the rest of its body than in the full-term infant.

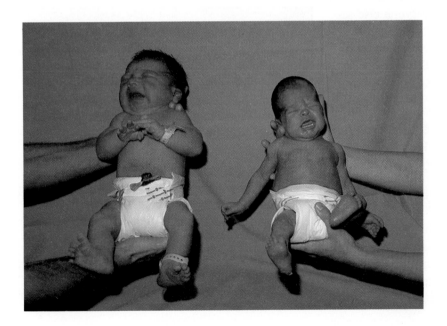

1. Keep the baby warm. Wrap it in a warm blanket as soon as it is born. Keep the face exposed, but keep the head covered. Keep the baby in a place where the temperature is between 90 and 95 degrees Fahrenheit.
2. Keep the mouth and nose clear of mucus. Like all babies, premature ones are nose breathers, and the small nasal passages can be obstructed easily. Use the bulb syringe to suction the mouth and nostrils frequently. Handle the baby and all its parts very gently.
3. Carefully observe the cut end of the cord attached to the baby and be sure that it is not bleeding. The loss of even a few drops of blood can be very serious.
4. Give oxygen. Open the valve on your oxygen cylinder slowly to give a steady stream of oxygen (about 70 to 100 bubbles per minute through the water bottle that is attached to the oxygen tank). Do not direct the stream of oxygen directly into the baby's mouth, but make a small tent over the baby's head using a blanket or a piece of aluminum foil, and direct the oxygen into the tent. While there may be some danger to a premature baby from receiving very high concentrations of oxygen, there is no danger if it is given over a short period of time in this manner.
5. Do not infect the baby. Premature babies are very susceptible to infection. Protect them from contamination. Do not breathe directly into the baby's face. Keep everyone else as far away from the baby as possible.
6. Notify the hospital. Do this before transporting the baby and mother. Bring a family member with you to the hospital.

Some large medical centers have mobile infant carriers for the transportation of high-risk infants. If such a vehicle is available, the hospital personnel may want to send it rather than have the EMT transport the baby in the ambulance. If such a vehicle is not available, the EMT should transport the baby in a special carrier (Figure 38.17). The premature infant carrier has supplies that can be used for the immediate care of the premature infant as well as for its transport. These items include a quilted pad, baby blanket, diaper, thermometer, suction tube and suction bulb, sterile Kelly clamp, and, most im-

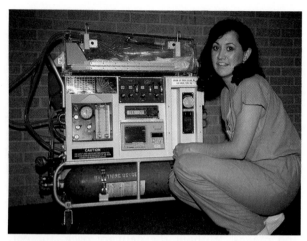

FIGURE 38.17 A mobile infant carrier is used by some large hospitals for transporting premature infants and other high-risk babies.

portant, hot water bottles and an oxygen cylinder with the necessary attachments. The hot water bottles should be filled and padded well so they don't come in direct contact with the infant's skin. They should be placed in the carrier so that one is on the bottom and one on each side of where the baby will lie. Once the baby is wrapped in a blanket and placed inside the carrier, the carrier should be secured inside the vehicle. The temperature of the vehicle should be kept at 90 to 95 degrees Fahrenheit while the baby and mother are being transported to the hospital.

YOU ARE THE EMT...

1. The patient tells you she is in labor and too far along to get to the hospital in time. How will you decide whether to take her in the ambulance or help her to deliver at home?
2. Should you cut the umbilical cord before or after the placenta delivers? Why?
3. You have just evaluated the baby you helped deliver. Its Apgar score is a perfect 10. Describe the areas of activity that are measured and what a 2 in each area means.
4. You arrived just in time to help a woman deliver an eight-week premature baby girl. Although tiny, her color is good and she is crying. What steps will you take in the care of this newborn that you wouldn't normally have to take with a healthy full-term baby?

SECTION 8

ENVIRONMENTAL EMERGENCIES

39 Burns

OVERVIEW

Burns are among the most serious and most painful of all injuries. They occur when the body receives more energy than it can absorb without injury. The sources of this energy are heat, toxic chemicals, electricity, and nuclear radiation. The severity of a burn is usually rated by the amount of injury to the skin. The actual depth of the burn and the surface involved are calculated together to determine the seriousness of the burn.

The EMT who has to treat a burn may be faced with other problems. The fire or substance that caused the burn may have to be extinguished or removed. The patient may be experiencing shock or respiratory arrest caused by the burn, especially in the case of a lightning strike. Or the person may have sustained fractures from falling, especially after electric shock. And not the least of the EMT's problems is avoiding the live wire, the toxic fumes, or the exposure to radioactivity that may have caused the burn.

Chapter 39 begins with a review of skin anatomy. It then describes how the most common type of burn — the thermal burn — is evaluated for degree of seriousness and how thermal burns should be treated. The chapter next addresses chemical and electrical burns. The last section of the chapter discusses nuclear radiation injuries. These include burns from solar radiation and injuries resulting from exposure to radioactivity.

OBJECTIVES

The objectives of Chapter 39 are to

- review the anatomy of the skin.
- identify the features of first-, second-, and third-degree burns and learn how to calculate the extent of a thermal burn using the Rule of Nines.
- learn how to determine the seriousness of a thermal burn and the management of thermal burns.
- identify the various types of chemical burns and learn how to treat them.
- understand how electrical energy, including lightning, enters and exits the body and how to treat electrical burns and injuries.
- describe the effects of exposure to solar radiation and nuclear radiation.
- learn the emergency medical care for exposure to radioactive materials.

ANATOMY OF SKIN: A REVIEW

Burns are primarily injuries to the skin. The anatomy of the skin has been presented in Chapter 13. To review, consider two layers of the skin: the epidermis and the dermis. The **epidermis** is the tough, impervious outer layer. The epidermal cells are constantly being worn away and replaced as new cells are produced by the germinal layer. The **dermis,** the layer just below the epidermis, contains the structures that give the skin its characteristic appearance. These are the hair follicles, sweat glands, sebaceous glands that secrete the oil which lubricates the skin, blood vessels, and nerve endings. Even deeper than the dermis is the **subcutaneous tissue,** the fatty layer that varies in thickness in different parts of the body and from person to person. The final and deepest layer, below the subcutaneous layer, is the **fascia,** which covers the muscles (Figure 39.1). A burn may extend through some or all of these layers.

The skin is an organ, not merely a tissue. The skin serves many functions. For example, it keeps bacteria out of the body. It maintains the water content of the body. It serves as insulation and helps control the body's temperature. And through the nerve endings, the skin is the organ that reports to

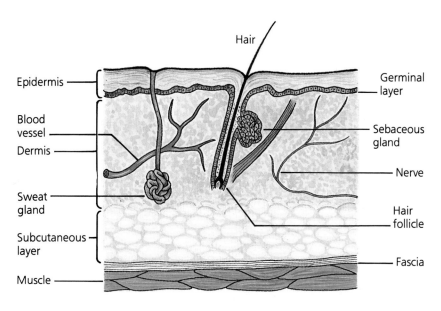

FIGURE 39.1 Layers of the skin. A burn may extend through some or all of these layers.

the brain on the body's environment and on the many sensations with which the body comes in contact. Any break in the skin destroys this protective envelope and allows bacterial invasion and infection, fluid loss, and loss of temperature control, any of which may cause death.

THERMAL BURNS

The EMT frequently must evaluate or treat burn injuries. Burns are responsible for a large number of accidental deaths, particularly in children. The most common type of burn is the **thermal burn,** also called a heat burn. The seriousness of the burn may be determined by observing the damage to the skin and calculating the extent of the body surface area that has been burned. The terms *first-, second-,* and *third-degree burns* are used as a measure of the depth of the burn to the skin (Figure 39.2).

First-degree burns are those in which only the superficial part of the epidermis has been injured. The skin turns red (**erythematous**) but does not blister or actually burn through (Figure 39.3). A sunburn is a good example of a first-degree burn.

FIGURE 39.2 Three common degrees of thermal burn injury. (a) A first-degree burn causes epidermal injury with redness of the skin. (b) A second-degree burn causes partial destruction of the dermis and is characterized by blisters. (c) A third-degree burn causes complete epidermal and dermal destruction, and may extend even deeper.

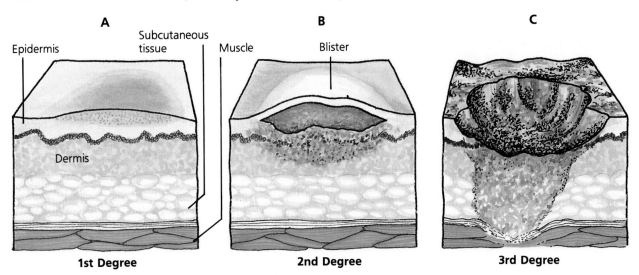

1st Degree   **2nd Degree**   **3rd Degree**

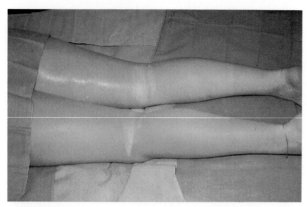

FIGURE 39.3   In a first-degree burn only the superficial part of the epidermis is injured. The skin will be red and very painful, as is often the case after a day at the beach.

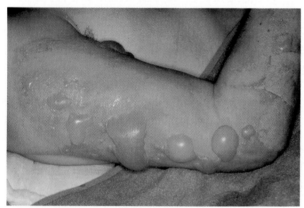

FIGURE 39.4   In a second-degree burn the epidermis and part of the dermis are injured. Blister formation characterizes the second-degree burn.

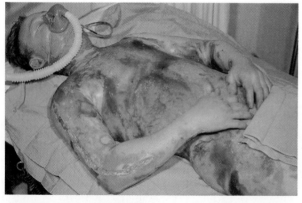

FIGURE 39.5   In a third-degree burn, the epidermis and the dermis are injured. Because superficial nerve endings are destroyed, the burned area may not have feeling. The surrounding areas, however, are extremely painful.

Second-degree burns are those in which the epidermis and a varying extent of the dermis are burned, but the entire thickness of the dermis is not destroyed and the subcutaneous layer is not injured. The second-degree burn is characterized by blister formation (Figure 39.4).

Third-degree burns extend through the dermis and into, or beyond, the subcutaneous fat. The area becomes dry, leathery, and discolored (charred, brown, or white). Clotted blood vessels may be visible under the burned skin, or the subcutaneous fat may be visible. Superficial nerve endings and blood vessels will have been destroyed in this severe injury, and the burned area may be without feeling (**anesthetic**), although the surrounding, less severely burned areas will remain extremely painful (Figure 39.5).

The extent of the burn, or the amount of surface area involved, may be calculated using the **Rule of Nines.** This system divides the surface of the body into sections, each of which is approximately 9 percent of the total body surface area. In infants and toddlers, the head makes up a larger portion of the body, and the legs a smaller portion, so that the rule is modified in younger children. Using the Rule of Nines, the EMT can make a rough estimate of the surface area that has been burned (Figure 39.6).

Seriousness of Thermal Burns

Five factors determine the seriousness of a thermal burn:

1. The depth (first-, second-, or third-degree)
2. The amount of surface area (Rule of Nines)
3. Involvement of critical areas (hands, feet, face, or genitalia)
4. The patient's age (very young or very old)
5. The patient's general health (are other injuries or illnesses present?)

These five factors will enable the EMT to determine if the burn is critical, moderate, or minor.

Critical burns are the most serious. All burns that are complicated by fractures or any degree of respiratory injury are considered critical burns. In addition, they include any third-degree burns that involve the hands, feet, genitalia, or face, or any third-degree burns that involve more than 10 percent of the body surface. They also include any second-degree burns that involve more than 25 percent of

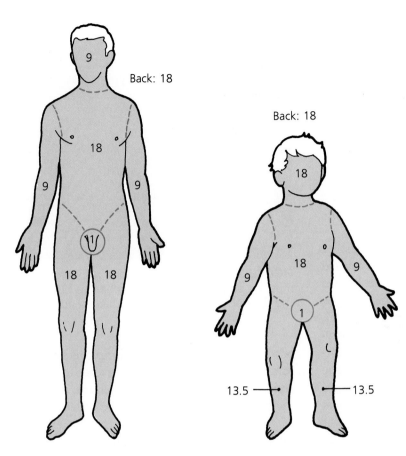

FIGURE 39.6 In the adult, most areas of the body can be divided roughly into portions of 9 percent, or multiples of 9. This division, called the Rule of Nines, is used to estimate the percentage of body surface damage sustained in a burn. In the small child, relatively more area is taken up by the head and less by the lower extremities. Accordingly, the Rule of Nines is modified.

the body surface. Finally, they include any otherwise moderate burn in an elderly or critically ill patient.

Moderate burns are less serious than critical burns but are still serious injuries. They include third-degree burns that involve 2 percent to 10 percent of the body area (excluding the hands, feet, face, or genitalia). They also include second-degree burns that involve 15 to 25 percent of the body surface area and first-degree burns that involve 50 to 75 percent of the body surface area.

Minor burns include third-degree burns that involve less than 2 percent of the body surface area or second-degree burns that involve less than 15 percent of the body surface area.

A different system is used to determine critical burns in children. A second-degree burn of more than 20 percent of the body surface is considered a critical burn in a child. A second-degree burn of 10 to 20 percent of the body surface area would be a moderate burn, and any first-degree burn in a child would be considered a moderate burn. Finally, any third-degree burn in a child is considered a critical burn.

Management of Thermal Burns

The EMT should direct the emergency care of a thermal burn toward four goals:

1. Stop the burning process and prevent further injury.
2. Cover the burned area with a dry, sterile dressing to decrease heat loss and decrease the risk of infection.
3. Support the patient's vital functions.
4. Transport the patient promptly to a hospital that has the ability to treat burn injuries.

The EMT's first responsibility when responding to a burned patient is to stop any further burning from occurring — in other words, put out the fire. The patient should be moved away from a burning area to prevent further injury from the heat or from smoke inhalation. Any smoldering clothing should be removed. If the skin and clothing are still hot, they should be immersed in cold water or covered with a wet, cool dressing. This will relieve pain and stop any further burning. The burned area should not be immersed for more than 10 minutes, however. Prolonged immersion in cold water, particularly of an extensive burn, can result in body heat loss (**hypothermia**). If the burning has stopped before the EMT gets to the patient, then immersing the burned part in cold water will not help. If the burn appears to be a third-degree burn, it should only be immersed if it is still burning. The greatest danger with a third-degree burn is infection. Immersing it in water (other than to stop it from burning) may increase the risk of infection. Clean dressings and clear water should always be used to minimize the risk of infection.

The extent and severity of the burn must be rapidly estimated. The burned area should be covered with a dry dressing. Sterile gauze is best if the burned area is not too extensive. A clean sheet may also be used if there is not enough sterile dressing material. The most important instruction is not to put anything else on the burned area. The emergency treatment of a burn calls for application of a dry, sterile dressing — ointments, lotions, or antiseptics should never be used. If the patient has sustained a critical burn, oxygen should be given as well. The patient may also need to be treated for shock before being promptly transported.

The patient who has sustained burns about the face or has inhaled smoke or fumes may develop respiratory distress. This patient will need oxygen and prompt transport (Figure 39.7).

Patients who have sustained critical burns should be treated in a burn center. The EMT should alert medical control that a patient with a critical burn is being brought in so that prompt and appropriate triage can be carried out. EMTs should know the location of the nearest burn center in their area.

CHEMICAL BURNS

Chemical burns may occur from any toxic substance that comes in contact with the skin. Most chemical burns are caused by strong acids or strong alkalis that get on the skin or clothing. Sometimes the fumes of strong chemicals can cause burns, especially to the respiratory tract. The eyes are particularly vulnerable to chemical burns.

Most chemical burns occur in industry — in factories or laboratories. Places where such chemicals are used usually have some facilities for treatment

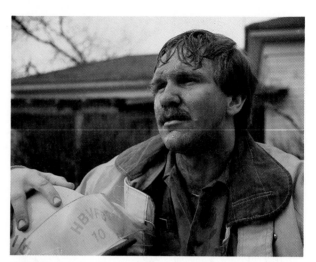

FIGURE 39.7 Burn injury to the respiratory system must be suspected in anyone who has burns about the face or who has inhaled smoke or fumes.

of accidental chemical burns. Employees often have some training in emergency measures to be used in accidental chemical burns; however, this is not always the case. The EMT may well be called to a scene of a chemical burn and find that no emergency measures have been carried out.

The emergency care of a chemical burn is basically the same as for a thermal burn. To stop the burning process, the chemical itself must be removed from contact with the patient. With very few exceptions, this means the area must be flooded with water. ("The solution to pollution is dilution" is the best rule to follow in most instances of chemical burns.) Most industrial plants have special showers or hoses for this purpose (Figure 39.8). The area of burn should be flooded with water. A forceful stream of water from a hose should not be used because extreme water pressure may add mechanical injury to the skin. Clothing should be removed from the affected area while the skin is being flushed. Often the patient will announce that the burning pain has stopped once the flooding begins. The flooding, however, should continue for 10 minutes after the burning pain has stopped. Many chemicals have a delayed reaction and will continue to cause injury even though the patient feels no further pain. Once the flooding is completed, the burned part should be covered with a dry, sterile dressing as would be done with a thermal burn. Then the patient should be transported to the hospital.

kinds of fires. Carbon monoxide inhalation is different from smoke inhalation. Because carbon monoxide gas is odorless and tasteless, victims may not realize they have inhaled carbon monoxide.

Anyone who has been trapped inside a burning building or room and has been breathing air from that room may be suffering from carbon monoxide poisoning. Very few symptoms other than mild dyspnea may be present until the patient suddenly develops respiratory arrest. An EMT who suspects that a victim may have inhaled carbon monoxide should administer 100 percent oxygen through a nonrebreathing mask. The EMT should be alert for respiratory arrest and be ready to begin basic life support immediately.

Chemical Injuries of the Skin

Chemical (acid and alkali) burns may cause severe skin injury. Strong alkalis, such as concentrated sodium hydroxide or potassium hydroxide, may cause more severe burns than strong acids because alkalis penetrate the skin more deeply. The treatment for liquid acid or alkali burns is to flood the area with water. If a solid substance such as lime has been spilled on the patient, it should be brushed off before flushing. A dry chemical is activated by contact with water and will cause more damage to the skin than when it is dry (Figure 39.9). The patient's clothing should be removed because residual

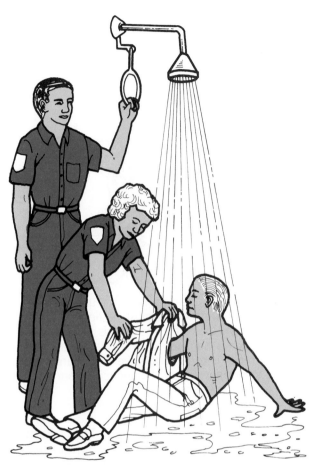

FIGURE 39.8 Chemical burns are treated by flooding the affected area with water. Clothing should be removed as the flooding is taking place. The flooding should continue for 10 minutes after the burning pain has stopped.

Inhalation Injuries

Inhalation injuries from chemical fumes (often incorrectly called respiratory burns) are particularly serious. If the patient complains of **dyspnea** (difficult breathing), or if there are obvious fumes in the air, or if the patient says he has inhaled fumes, then the EMT can assume that some respiratory injury has occurred. Oxygen should be given and the patient promptly transported to the hospital. Even if the patient has no obvious signs of respiratory distress, significant respiratory difficulty may occur later.

A particularly dangerous form of inhalation injury comes from inhaling **carbon monoxide.** This can happen when someone is trapped in a burning building without fresh air. Carbon monoxide is a deadly poison that is given off from many different

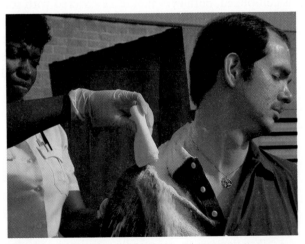

FIGURE 39.9 Dry chemicals must be brushed off the skin and clothing before the area is flooded. Dry chemicals are activated when they mix with water and can cause a more severe burn than when they are dry.

amounts of chemicals are retained in the creases of the clothes. Shoes, stockings, and gloves should be removed for the same reason.

If the burn has been caused by phenol (carbolic acid), it should first be washed off with water as would be done for any other chemical burn. However, phenol is not very soluble in water; therefore, the skin should be washed off with a phenol solvent, such as polyethylene glycol, propylene glycol, or glycerol. Controversy exists about the emergency treatment of a phenol burn. EMTs who work in an area where this chemical is widely used should consult the local medical authorities as to how to proceed if called to the scene of a phenol burn.

Chemical Injuries of the Eyes

Chemical burns of the eye are particularly serious. Permanent blindness can result from these injuries, even after a very brief exposure to the chemical. The basic principle in the emergency management of these injuries is the same: flood the area with water. The normal reaction of the eye to any injury is to close tightly. The eyelids must be held open while flooding the eye. A gentle stream of water should be used, with care being taken not to wash the chemicals into the uninjured eye. Flooding should continue for at least 5 minutes for an acid burn and 10 to 20 minutes for an alkali burn. The EMT may have to support the patient's head under a faucet during the flushing process. When flushing is completed, both eyes should be covered with soft pads and the patient transported promptly to the hospital. No substances other than water should be put into the eyes, regardless of the chemical that has caused the burn. Any chemical added to the eye will cause further injury (Figure 39.10).

ELECTRICAL BURNS

Electrical burns may occur as a result of contact with high- or low-voltage electricity. Ordinary household current is powerful enough to cause severe burns. High-voltage burns may occur in electrical utility workers, or from direct contact with a power line.

Two dangers are specifically associated with electrical burns. First, the amount of tissue injury is usually far more extensive than what is expected from the appearance of the skin wound. Despite the small size of the skin burn wounds, severe damage may

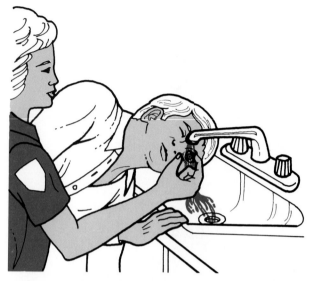

FIGURE 39.10 Chemical burns to the eyes are serious. The affected eye must be flooded with a gentle stream of water. The eyelids must be held open, which is hard to do because the patient's natural reflex is to keep the eye shut. Care must be taken to prevent any of the chemical from getting into the other eye during flushing.

occur to deeper tissues. Second, the burn may be accompanied by cardiac arrest, which further complicates the patient's injury. Electrical energy is capable of producing severe tissue injury. In order to cause a burn, the electricity must enter the body at one point and exit at another point. There is always a wound (a burn) where the electricity went into the body, and another at the point of exit. The entrance wound may be quite small, but the exit wound may be extensive and deep (Figure 39.11). High-voltage electrical energy can destroy muscles and skin to such an extent that amputation may become necessary.

Electric Shock Injuries

The energy from a high-voltage electrical current passing through the body may disrupt the normal electrical rhythm of the heart and cause cardiac arrest. Also, the electrical current may cause violent muscle contractions that could result in fracture or dislocation. Furthermore, the electrical shock will cause the patient to fall to the ground, often resulting in further injury. Therefore, when called to the scene of an electrical accident, the EMT must be prepared to evaluate and treat a patient in cardiac arrest, with multiple injuries, and severe burns.

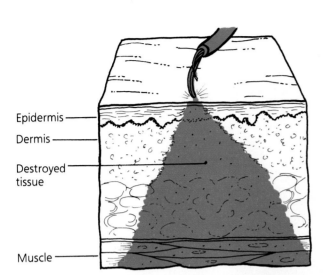

Epidermis
Dermis
Destroyed tissue
Muscle

FIGURE 39.11 Electrical burns can cause severe tissue damage. Although the surface burn at the point of entry may be very small, the exit wound may be extensive and deep.

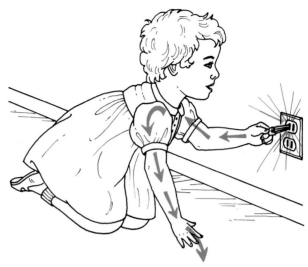

FIGURE 39.12 The human body is a good conductor of electricity. An electrical burn usually occurs when the body, acting as a conductor, completes a circuit connecting the power source with the ground.

Treatment of an electrical injury calls for instituting cardiorespiratory resuscitation if needed, placing dry sterile dressings on all burn wounds, and splinting suspected fractures. All electrical burns are potentially severe injuries that require further treatment in the hospital.

The EMT may sometime be called to an accident involving a downed power line. Any downed power line should always be assumed to be live unless the power company has shut it off. Power lines may have anywhere from 115 to 50,000 volts running through them. Telephone lines have a much lower voltage but still enough to cause a shock. Unless absolutely certain that a downed line is a low-voltage line, the EMT should assume that it is a live, high-voltage line and not touch it.

If an electrical line has fallen across a car and there are people inside, they are safe as long as they stay inside the car. The rubber tires of the car will insulate them. In order for electricity to flow, a circuit must be completed from the source of the electricity to the ground. Any substance that prevents an electrical circuit from being completed is an **insulator.** Rubber, for example, is an insulator. Any substance that allows a current to flow through it is a **conductor.** Water and most metals are conductors. The human body is also a good conductor. Electrical burns occur when the body, or a part of it, completes a circuit connecting the power source with the ground (Figure 39.12).

Most electrical burns in the home occur from faulty electrical equipment or the careless use of appliances. Small children can suffer electrical burns from putting an electrical cord into their mouth. Electrical burns outside the home often occur from accidental contact with a downed power line or from accidental contact with a power line by a construction worker doing excavation work. The power must be turned off before the EMT approaches anyone who may still be in contact with an electrical wire or appliance. If there are people in a car with a power line fallen across it, they should be instructed to stay in the car until the power company can shut the power off (Figure 39.13). In very rare instances this situation is compounded by a danger from fire. If their lives are threatened by fire, the passengers should be instructed to jump clear of the car, making certain that they do not touch the car and the ground at the same time. Small children should be tossed out of the car to the EMT first. The wire should never be moved unless the EMT is absolutely certain that it is not live, or unless the EMT has had special training and has the necessary special equipment to handle it. EMTs have been fatally injured from accidental contact with electrical wires while answering an emergency call.

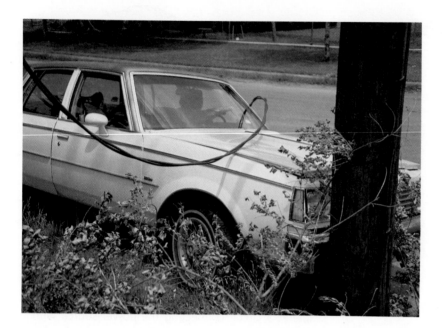

FIGURE 39.13 A downed power line should not be touched until the utility company has shut off the power. If a live wire has fallen across a car, the passengers should be warned to stay inside. If they have to escape because of fire, they must jump clear of the car, without touching the ground while touching the car.

Lightning Injuries

Lightning injuries are a specific form of electrical burn. Lightning strikes with a force of many thousands of volts, but only for a fraction of a second. Not everyone who is struck by lightning is killed. Frequently, people survive lightning injuries. An EMT may be called to the scene of a lightning injury and find one or several people who need treatment.

Lightning is a high-voltage, total body exposure. Many systems of the body are involved, principally the nervous and cardiovascular systems. A characteristic superficial skin burn occurs with lightning, but deep burns rarely occur. The major problems with lightning are nervous system injuries and cardiac arrhythmias.

Most people struck by lightning are rendered unconscious for a period of time and have no recollection of being struck. A patient may complain of numbness, tingling, partial or complete paralysis, blindness, loss of hearing, **dysphasia** (difficulty in speaking), or may be completely **aphasic** (unable to speak). These symptoms are usually temporary. Of greater concern is cardiac arrhythmia. Patients may have a severely disrupted heart rhythm, have ventricular fibrillation or full cardiac arrest. However, the EMT should never assume that a patient who has been struck by lightning and has no obvious heartbeat is dead. Such patients may often be successfully resuscitated if basic life support is ad-

ministered promptly. It is safe to handle a patient who has been struck by lightning. There is no danger of being electrocuted by touching the patient. A patient struck by lightning may have sustained skeletal or other injuries as well; spine fracture is particularly common. All patients should be transported to the hospital on a spine board.

NUCLEAR RADIATION INJURIES

The energy produced from nuclear reactions can cause injury in several ways. Burns similar to thermal burns can occur from exposure to **solar radiation** (the sun) or from the heat of an atomic explosion. In addition, exposure to radioactive chemicals and materials can cause a wide spectrum of problems ranging from acute burns to chronic illness and even death.

Radiation Burns

Atomic reactions continually take place on the sun to produce both heat and ionizing radiation. Some of the ionizing radiation passes through the protective ozone layer of the atmosphere and can cause a burn injury. Solar burns are usually not serious. Occasionally, a person may be exposed to too much sun without realizing it. The pigment in the skin (**melanin**) protects it from some of the solar radiation. Therefore, darker-skinned people have less risk for solar burns. Solar burns are very similar to thermal burns and rarely are more than first degree. However, if a large percentage of the skin is involved, such a burn may cause significant discomfort and occasional systemic symptoms due to mild hypotension. When these symptoms are present, the patient should be transported to the hospital.

Nuclear radiation burns can occur from the heat of an atomic explosion. The type of injury will depend on the proximity of the injured person to the explosion. Persons within a few miles of the nuclear explosion will sustain thermal burns of the skin and, in addition, severe internal injuries as a result of the penetration of ionizing radiation. Persons at a greater distance from the nuclear explosion will not sustain thermal burns but will still sustain radiation injury of the deeper tissues. Without doubt, a nuclear explosion is a catastrophic event to which hopefully the EMT will never be exposed. Currently, the major concern with regard to nuclear radiation injury occurs from exposure to nuclear chemicals and leaks from nuclear energy plants.

Nuclear Radiation Exposure

Humans have always been exposed to small amounts of nuclear radiation through cosmic rays and naturally occurring radioactive materials. Since the discovery of x-rays and the refining of radium almost 100 years ago, the risk of accidental overexposure to nuclear radiation has increased greatly. With the development of nuclear power, many people now work with highly radioactive materials. The processing, fabrication, and transportation of nuclear fuels and the disposal of used radioactive material provide increasing sources of accidental exposure or contamination. While many safety systems are in place for managing nuclear emergencies and preventing nuclear exposure, these systems can become disabled or misused. There is a chance that the EMT may be called to the scene of a nuclear accident. For that reason, EMTs should have some knowledge of nuclear radiation and its effects on the body.

Nuclear radiation is the result of energy produced by **radioactivity,** the spontaneous release of energy by particles that make up **atoms.** Atoms were once thought to be the smallest parts of all matter. However, atoms are themselves made up of smaller particles: protons, neutrons, and electrons (Figure 39.14). Protons and electrons are electrically charged;

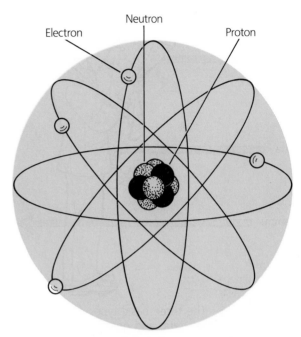

FIGURE 39.14 Atoms are made up of protons, neutrons, and electrons. The release of energy and subatomic particles from excited atoms is called radioactivity.

neutrons are not. If an atom is excited by some form of energy brought into contact with it, it will become unstable and then will return to its original, stable condition. During this conversion from an unstable to a stable state, energy and subatomic particles are released. This release of energy and subatomic particles is called radioactivity, and the products released by radioactivity are called **nuclear radiation.** Nuclear radiation that has the ability to alter body cells is called **ionizing radiation.** Nuclear radiation and ionizing radiation are both forms of energy transmission.

There are three types of ionizing radiation: **alpha radiation, beta radiation,** and **gamma radiation.** Alpha rays possess very low energy. They are easily stopped by paper, a few inches of air, or light clothing. Thus, they pose little danger. Beta rays are commonly emitted from laboratory chemicals and are widely used in biomedical research and in industry. Beta rays can penetrate to a greater depth than alpha rays but are effectively stopped by clothing, glass, or a thin metal shielding. The great danger from beta rays is accidental ingestion of beta-radioactive chemicals that can be absorbed into the bloodstream and then emit radioactivity into the body

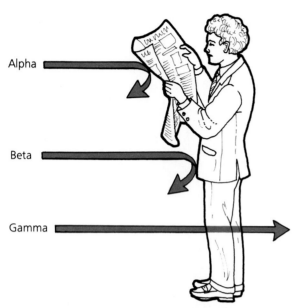

Alpha

Beta

Gamma

FIGURE 39.15 The three basic types of ionizing radiation are alpha, beta, and gamma. Alpha rays are easily stopped by paper. Beta rays are stopped by clothing. Gamma rays are very powerful and can penetrate through the body. They can be stopped only by heavy shielding such as lead or concrete.

for a prolonged time. Gamma rays are very similar to x-rays and are much more powerful than alpha or beta rays. Gamma rays can penetrate through the human body. Heavy shielding such as lead or concrete is necessary to protect against these rays (Figure 39.15).

The energy produced by ionizing radiation decreases rapidly as the distance from the source of the radiation increases. A person 4 feet away from an x-ray machine will receive one-quarter the radiation he would receive if he were 2 feet away. Other variables that affect the amount of radiation exposure include the strength of the radiation source, the duration of the exposure, the extent of area exposed, and the amount of shielding between the person and the source.

Measurement of Nuclear Radiation

Gamma and x-ray radiation are measured in **roentgens** or **rads.** While the definitions of these two terms differ, the differences are very slight. The EMT may encounter situations in which the radiation has been measured in either roentgens or rads. Radiation from beta particles is measured in **Curies,** or, since the amounts of radiation are usually very

small, **millicuries** or **microcuries.** These terms may be encountered by an EMT who is called to a laboratory where a radiation accident has taken place. A **Geiger counter** or similar instrument is used to measure the level of radioactivity in the environment. These instruments are generally designed to detect gamma radiation. A Geiger counter displays the rate of radiation in roentgens or milliroentgens per hour.

The Effect of Nuclear Radiation on the Body

Life is dependent on billions of individual cells that have specific functions and the capacity to reproduce themselves. The ability of these cells to reproduce and to perform their specific functions may be changed or destroyed by nuclear radiation, which disrupts the structure of individual atoms within the cells. Exposure to exceedingly large doses of radiation over a short time span will produce nuclear burns as described earlier in this chapter. More commonly, exposure to low doses of radiation over a long period of time occurs. The biological effects of this type of radiation are delayed for periods of from a few days to many years, depending on the dose, the type of radiation received, and whether part or all of the body has been exposed.

When an overexposure is detected through its biological effects, there has already been serious tissue damage. The most striking, long-term effects of overexposure are as follows:

Decrease in the number of white blood cells
Loss of hair **(alopecia)**
Sterility
Mutation (altered heredity of offspring)
Cancer
Destruction and death of bone
Cataracts of the eyes
Leukemia

With short-duration overexposure, some of these effects occur within a matter of minutes, days, or weeks. These are called the acute effects (Table 39.1). When a low grade of exposure occurs over a prolonged period of time, the accumulated effect of exposure can produce some or all of these same problems. There is no effective treatment for most problems of radiation exposure; therefore, prevention of exposure must be of primary concern.

TABLE 39.1   Acute Effects Caused by Short-Term Radiation Exposure

Dose Rads	Response
20–100	Changes in relative numbers of circulating white blood cells; chromosome changes in a few blood cells
200–400	Severe reduction in white blood cells; nausea and vomiting; loss of hair; some deaths within 60 days due to increased susceptibility to infection
600	Fifty percent of those exposed die within 30 days; bone marrow, a source of white blood cells, is destroyed; some dysentery or diarrhea; sterility
1,000–2,000	Lining of intestine destroyed; diarrhea severe; death within two weeks
2,000 and more	Central nervous system severely damaged; death within hours

Accidents Involving Radiation Hazards

The vast majority of accidents involving radioactive materials occur in facilities that use these materials daily. The EMT should seek and follow the professional advice that is readily available in these centers. Accidents occasionally happen where professional guidance is not available. In these cases, the EMT should be able to do the following:

1. Recognize indications of radioactivity.
2. Obtain the necessary assistance.
3. Initiate appropriate emergency medical care, while exercising caution.
4. Minimize self-exposure to the radiation.
5. Avoid spreading possible radioactive contamination.

All radioactive substances are kept in labeled and shielded containers when not in use. Radioactive materials shipped by interstate commerce must be packaged with a label indicating the maximum amount of external radiation. Vehicles used to transport radioactive materials must be marked with a placard indicating a radioactive shipment (Figure 39.16).

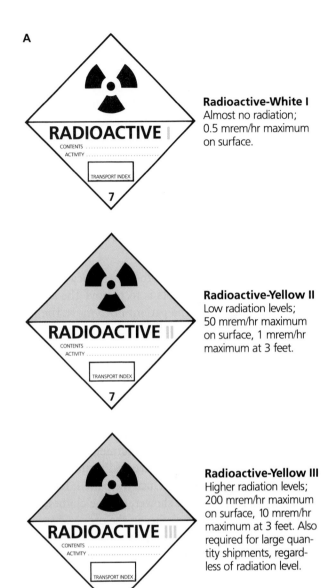

Radioactive-White I
Almost no radiation; 0.5 mrem/hr maximum on surface.

Radioactive-Yellow II
Low radiation levels; 50 mrem/hr maximum on surface, 1 mrem/hr maximum at 3 feet.

Radioactive-Yellow III
Higher radiation levels; 200 mrem/hr maximum on surface, 10 mrem/hr maximum at 3 feet. Also required for large quantity shipments, regardless of radiation level.

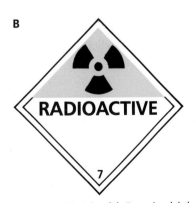

FIGURE 39.16 (a) Required labels for packages containing radioactive materials. (b) Typical warning placard required on any vehicle that transports radioactive materials.

To provide professional guidance and assistance as necessary, a national plan has been developed. Called the **Interagency Radiological Assistance Plan (IRAP),** it may be activated by a telephone call to the appropriate regional coordinating office in an EMT's area. Assistance can range from expert technical advice on the telephone to the dispatch of an emergency team or expert to the scene. The EMT's dispatch center should become familiar with the location and telephone number of the regional coordinating offices of IRAP in its area.

Emergency Medical Care for Radiation Accidents

The primary concern in the emergency management of radiation accidents is to remove the source of the radiation from the patient or to move the patient away from the source of radiation. If radioactive material has been spilled onto the patient's clothes, the clothes should be removed and stored in a special container. The patient should then shower. EMTs must be very careful in treating such patients not to get any of the radioactive material on themselves. Obviously, if the patient has sustained another injury that requires treatment, the EMT must provide the necessary care and assume that he has become contaminated. Once the patient has been treated, the EMT should shower, change clothes, and place the contaminated clothes in the proper disposal containers. Facilities that handle radioactive materials are required to have special disposal containers for this purpose.

If an accident involves gamma radiation and the patient is still being exposed to the radiation, the person must be removed from the area, even if this means violating some basic principles of emergency care. This situation must be handled as if the pa-tient were in the path of a fire and had to be moved immediately for safety's sake. Once the patient is removed from the radiation exposure, the basic rules of emergency care should be followed. Patients who have been exposed to gamma or x-rays are not themselves radioactive and will not contaminate the EMT or their environment. On the other hand, persons who have had radioactive materials spilled on them remain radioactive as long as the material is still present on their body.

After a patient who has been contaminated by contact with radioactive materials has been transported to the hospital, the EMT must decontaminate the vehicle as well as himself. Most hospitals have a radiation safety officer who will be able to provide guidance as to the specific techniques for proper decontamination.

YOU ARE THE EMT...

1. Which is more severe — a first- or a third-degree burn? How would you determine whether a patient was suffering from a first-, second-, or third-degree burn?
2. Your patient is a two-year-old youngster who spilled his mother's hot tea over himself. Clad only in a diaper, he received second-degree burns on his chest, stomach, and thighs. Would this be a critical, moderate, or minor burn? What factors did you use to determine the degree of severity?
3. What two dangers are associated with electrical burns? How should you treat an electrical burn?
4. Explain the difference between nuclear radiation and ionizing radiation. What are gamma rays?

Hazardous Materials

40

OVERVIEW

A great variety of hazardous materials pass through the streets and over the railways of any city every day. The exact extent of this traffic is not known, but accidents involving vehicles carrying hazardous materials are not uncommon. Hazardous materials may be of many different types, including chemicals, radioactive materials, and poisons, in the form of solids, liquids, or gas. They are appropriately named because they represent a hazard to everyone exposed — rescue personnel and the public, as well as persons injured in the accident.

When responding to a hazardous materials incident, the EMT cannot follow those "move-fast-take-action-save-lives" instincts that are an EMT's trademark. Instead, time must be taken to assess the scene. That means identifying the size of the hazard area, finding a safe location to which patients can be removed, and taking self-protective measures against contamination. Safety is the EMT's prime consideration. The patient certainly needs help, but if a hazardous materials accident is not carefully handled, a lot of people, including rescue personnel themselves, can become casualties.

Chapter 40 stresses the safety precautions an EMT must take when responding to a hazardous materials incident. The chapter begins with a description of the assessment process that must be carried out. Assessment includes identifying the hazardous material and establishing a hazard zone. The chapter next addresses decontamination — for the patient and rescue personnel. The last portion of Chapter 40 deals with triage in a hazardous materials accident — that is, sorting casualties when the number of casualties is greater than what emergency facilities can handle.

OBJECTIVES

The objectives of Chapter 40 are to

- stress the importance of assessing the scene of a hazardous materials incident, which includes identifying the hazardous material and establishing a hazard zone before instituting emergency treatment.
- describe the process of decontamination — for the EMT as well as the patient.
- explain how triage works in a major hazardous materials accident.

PRELIMINARY ASSESSMENT OF A HAZARDOUS MATERIALS INCIDENT

Sometimes when dealing with hazardous materials, the hazard is obvious; other times it is not. Sometimes the dangerous nature of the situation is not recognized until many people have been needlessly exposed. Rescuers have lost their lives or become permanently disabled because of a lack of understanding and appreciation of the potential dangers of hazardous materials.

EMTs and rescue personnel are generally taught that rapid response at the scene of an accident can be life-saving and is of paramount importance. They pride themselves on their ability to make quick decisions. Even so, they are sometimes criticized for taking too much time at the scene of an accident. However, when called to the scene of an accident where hazardous materials may be present, the EMT must first step back and assess the situation. Safety — for the EMT, for the patient, and for the public — is of primary concern. The necessary emergency care can only be carried out after the EMT puts on the necessary protective equipment. The EMT must not become a casualty!

425

Only those people trained in the management of hazardous materials should come near the hazard zone. Some hazardous materials accidents involve small quantities of toxic materials; others, however, involve barrels, boxes, tanks, or even carloads of harmful substances. An important first step in controlling the scene is to identify the danger zone, where exposure to the toxic substances may occur.

The **Hazmat Rule of Thumb** is one way to determine the size of the danger zone. In this method, the EMT's arm is held out straight, with thumb pointing up. The EMT then centers his thumb over the hazardous area. The thumb should cover all the hazardous area from view. If the hazardous material can still be seen, the EMT is too close. Special precautions should be taken when toxic fumes are present. The safe area will be upwind from the site of the spill. But remember, wind direction can change quickly.

Identifying Hazardous Materials

The single most important step in any hazardous materials incident or accident is to identify the substance(s) involved. Accurate identification of the materials is critical. Such information should be prominently displayed on all boxes or cartons that contain a hazardous material, on all vehicles that transport it, and in all factories that produce it. Manufacturers and transporters are required by law to display a four-digit identification number on the ends of a tank, vehicle, or rail car used to carry hazardous substances (Figure 40.1). This same four-digit identification number (some are preceded by the letters UN or NA) can also be found on the shipping paper or packaging of the material (Figure 40.2).

Upon arriving at the scene of a hazardous materials incident, the EMT should read labels and identification numbers using binoculars. Never should the EMT risk personal exposure to the hazardous materials. Information should be relayed to the dispatch center where it can be used to identify the hazardous material.

The U.S. Department of Transportation publishes *Hazardous Materials: The Emergency Response Guidebook* (DOT P 5800.2, 1980), which lists all hazardous materials and the proper emergency action to take with regard to control of the scene and emergency care of ill or injured patients. Some state and local government agencies may also have pertinent information regarding hazardous materials found frequently in their areas. A copy of the guidebook and other information relevant to a local area should be readily available in the dispatch center so that proper emergency management may be undertaken as soon as the hazardous material is identified.

In addition, the Chemical Manufacturers Association has established the **Chemical Transportation Emergency Center (CHEMTREC)** in Washington, D.C. This center operates 24 hours a day, seven days a week. It accepts toll-free calls

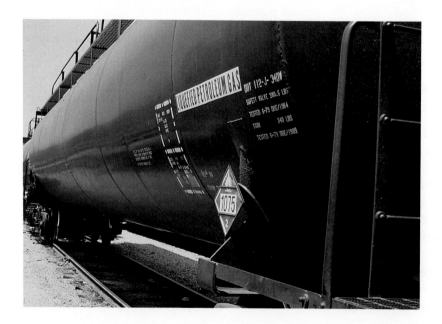

FIGURE 40.1 Any tank, vehicle, or rail car that carries hazardous materials is required by law to display a four-digit identification number on the end of the vehicle. In case of accident, these numbers can be matched against a list of toxic substances so that the hazardous material can be quickly identified.

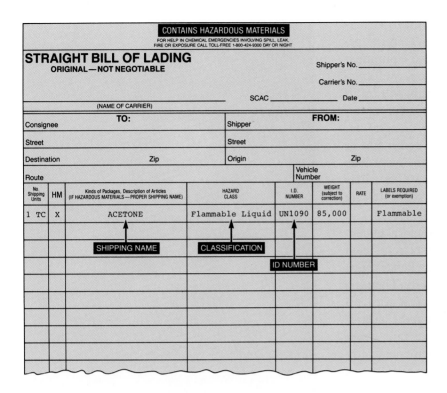

FIGURE 40.2 A typical shipping label identifying a hazardous material by name, classification, and identification number. The identification number is matched against a list of hazardous materials so that the properties of the substance can be determined and appropriate cleanup measures taken.

(1-800-424-9300) from anywhere within the continental United States. CHEMTREC will provide hazardous information warning and guidance for proper emergency management if the DOT identification number, the chemical name, or the product name of the hazardous material is given. The information must be accurate, however, if CHEMTREC is to help. CHEMTREC cannot identify an "unknown" substance.

Establishing a Hazard Zone

While the process of identifying the hazardous material is going on, a hazard zone should be established. Using the Hazmat Rule of Thumb, the danger area should be isolated. The EMT should remain upwind of the area and avoid low areas where toxic fumes may tend to settle. Bystanders should be kept away. Often, well-meaning people try to help. Unless specifically trained for such situations, they should be kept away. On the other hand, experienced, knowledgeable people such as company safety officers may be able to offer valuable assistance. These experts should take charge of the scene, and the EMT should follow their directions.

If an accident has resulted in injury to one or more people, the injured must be removed from the area to avoid further exposure. This is the most dangerous time in any hazardous materials accident — dangerous to the injured people and dangerous to the rescuers. Very little information about the nature of the hazardous materials or the extent of the danger may be available. Therefore, these situations must be considered extremely unstable and dangerous until proven otherwise.

The EMT should not enter the area until fully protected. Full turnouts are recommended. A **self-contained breathing apparatus (SCAB)** is a must. This step is particularly important if the injury has taken place in a closed space, such as in a tank or building. The EMT should avoid entering any closed space until clothed in adequate protective gear and assured of a safe escape route. The EMT who fails to do so endangers other rescuers and risks becoming a casualty as well. And not much is gained if the EMT succumbs.

DECONTAMINATION

Once the patient has been removed to a safe area, basic life support should be carried out, dressings applied, and fractures splinted as indicated. The EMT must avoid coming in contact with any of the hazardous material. However, if it happens — perhaps from contact with the patient — then the patient, the EMT, and any contaminated equipment will have to undergo **decontamination.** Failure to decontaminate adequately and promptly will result in prolonged exposure to the hazardous substance, which may cause more serious injury. In addition, inadequate decontamination may expose other EMTs and rescue and hospital personnel to the hazardous materials. The result will be many more casualties and a reduced number of available personnel to care for them.

Decontamination starts with the removal of contaminated clothing. All clothing should be considered contaminated, including shoes, socks, and underwear. Therefore, all clothing must be removed. Then the skin must be flushed with water for at least 15 minutes. The EMT should assume that the hazardous material has burned the skin and thus avoid forceful flushing. Rather, the skin should be gently flooded with water, just as would be done for a chemical burn. Many factories and laboratories have showers for this purpose. However, a garden hose can be used if special showers are not available. It is important that the entire body surface be flushed, including body creases and hair. When the flushing is completed, the patient should be covered with a sheet or blanket and transported to the hospital. Although flushing may be painful, particularly if there are burns, abrasions, or scrapes, decontamination of the skin is extremely important.

Decontamination of the EMT's clothing and equipment is important as well. Any contaminated clothing should be isolated and placed in a special container so that it does not come into contact with anyone or any part of the equipment (Figure 40.3).

TRIAGE IN A HAZARDOUS MATERIALS ACCIDENT

Triage is a term that means the sorting of casualties when the number of casualties is greater than what the emergency facilities can handle. Triage is frequently discussed in the context of mass casualties and disaster planning. Most disaster drills have focused on such mass casualty situations as an airline crash, which results in large numbers of killed and seriously injured people. In real life, however, hazardous materials incidents occur every day, ex-

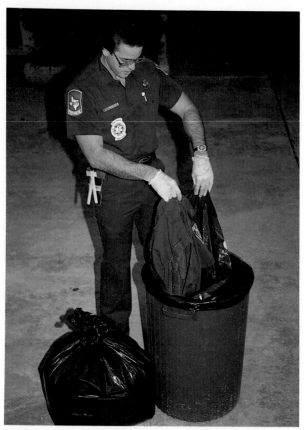

FIGURE 40.3 All clothing exposed to hazardous materials must be placed in special sealed containers to avoid further spread of the hazardous substance.

posing many people to possible injury or contamination (Figure 40.4). In addition, hazardous materials accidents cause concern and even hysteria among the public. This means the EMT has to sort out the truly injured from those who may have been contaminated and those who are anxious and worried. In such cases, triage should have one major function: to identify those victims who truly have an acute injury from the hazardous materials exposure. These patients should be removed from the area, decontaminated as necessary, given the necessary emergency care, and transported to the hospital. People who have had a "possible exposure" should be sent to a separate area for observation. If delayed symptoms of exposure do occur, these patients can then be transported to the hospital after the more seriously injured have been taken care of. In most cases, patients who do not develop symptoms do not require evaluation at a medical facility.

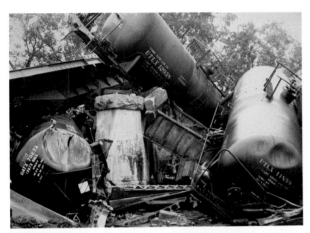

FIGURE 40.4 Hazardous materials spills occur frequently and in any community. The EMS system must be prepared to respond to these situations.

Emergency treatment of exposure to hazardous materials is primarily aimed at supportive care. There are very few specific antidotes or treatments for most injuries due to hazardous materials. Fortunately, most patients do not require anything more than supportive care. Because most fatalities and serious injuries from hazardous materials result from problems with the airway and breathing, respirations should be closely monitored. The airway should be maintained and oxygen given as needed. The patient may also have to be treated for shock.

Transporting patients who have been injured in a hazardous materials incident may pose many problems. The number of injured may be far greater than the transportation system can handle. The initial triage decisions will usually determine the priority of transportation. Constant reevaluation of patients awaiting transportation is necessary so that a patient whose clinical condition worsens can be moved to a higher priority for transport. Prior to transport, it is extremely important that adequate decontamination has taken place. It is very dangerous to the patient and the rescue personnel to place a poorly decontaminated patient inside an ambulance or helicopter and then close the doors. Any toxic fumes given off by the patient or by the patient's clothing can contaminate the inside of the transport vehicle, perhaps causing injury to the EMT, other attendants, the driver, or the pilot. Bags of contaminated clothing and other personal effects must be properly sealed

if they are going with the patient. Receiving hospitals should be notified of the impending arrival of patients who have been involved in a hazardous materials accident. This will alert hospital triage teams so that appropriate precautions can be taken once the patients begin to arrive.

Cleanup of equipment and personnel takes place after the hazardous materials incident has been completely controlled and all patients treated and transported. Trained disposal crews should be available to clean the site. The EMT crews need to thoroughly evaluate their own needs. Equipment, protective gear, and clothing, as well as the personnel, must be decontaminated. This not only minimizes the risk to the personnel but protects their families and friends as well from any hazardous materials that may be accidentally carried from the scene to their homes or elsewhere. Any rescue personnel who develop symptoms should be promptly transported to the hospital for evaluation since the rescuers may have the most prolonged exposures, even with protective gear. Finally, rescue personnel should take time to critique the incident soon after the job is done. This kind of evaluation will go a long way toward providing a more effective, and safer, response next time.

YOU ARE THE EMT...

1. You have been warned on countless occasions not to rush into the area of a hazardous materials accident until you have assessed the situation. What exactly should this assessment consist of?
2. You have to enter an established hazard zone to treat and rescue injured persons. What kind of self-protective measures should you take before entering the area?
3. Describe three hazardous materials accidents that could require triage procedures. Briefly describe the steps you would take if you were the triage officer at one of these accidents.
4. Decontamination is an important part of any hazardous materials incident. How will you prevent contamination from spreading to you, the ambulance, and other rescue and hospital personnel? What decontamination procedures will you follow after you have transported the patient to the hospital?

41

Heat and Cold Exposure

Environmental emergencies due to heat or cold exposure may be encountered in any part of the country, in urban or rural areas. Proper care of patients who are suffering from the effects of heat or cold exposure will help to minimize their injuries and speed their recovery. On the other hand, improper treatment of these emergencies can result in serious consequences, even death. Therefore, it is important to have a thorough understanding of the effects of heat and cold on the body, as well as the emergency management of these injuries.

The first half of Chapter 41 is about heat exposure. The chapter begins with an explanation of what happens when the body becomes overwhelmed by heat. Next, the three forms of heat exposure — heat cramps, heat exhaustion, and heat stroke — are discussed. The second half of Chapter 41 is about cold exposure. Again, this section begins with an explanation of how the body reacts to cold temperatures. The chapter describes the five stages of hypothermia and the treatment for hypothermia. In addition to hypothermia, cold exposure can cause local cold injuries such as frostnip and frostbite. These conditions are also described. The chapter concludes with a warning to EMTs about avoiding cold exposure themselves.

OBJECTIVES

The objectives of Chapter 41 are to

- describe the three forms of heat exposure: heat cramps, heat exhaustion, and heat stroke.
- identify the five ways the body can lose heat.
- describe the stages, symptoms, and treatment of hypothermia.
- learn how to treat local cold injuries, specifically frostnip and frostbite.
- understand the importance of self-protection against cold exposure.

HEAT EXPOSURE

Illness will result when the body is exposed to more heat energy than it can deal with. The normal body temperature of 98.6 degrees **Fahrenheit (F)** or 37.0 degrees **centigrade** or **Celsius (C)** is maintained by complicated mechanisms. This internal temperature remains constant, regardless of the temperature of the environment. When the body is in a hot environment, or when excessive body heat is produced by vigorous physical activity, the body will attempt to rid itself of the excess heat. As described in Chapter 13, several mechanisms can be used to decrease body heat. The most efficient mechanisms are sweating (and evaporation of the sweat) and dilation of skin blood vessels, which brings blood to the skin surface to increase the rate of radiation of heat from the body. In addition, the person who becomes overheated will remove clothing and attempt to move to a cooler environment. Ordinarily, the heat-regulating mechanisms of the body work very well, and people are able to tolerate significant temperature changes quite well. Illness from heat exposure occurs when the normal regulatory mechanisms are overwhelmed and the body is no longer able to tolerate the excessive heat. Illness from heat exposure can take three forms: heat cramps, heat exhaustion, and heat stroke.

Heat Cramps

Heat cramps are painful muscle spasms, usually of the leg muscles, that occur after vigorous exercise. They do not occur just in hot environments. Factory workers or even well-conditioned athletes sometimes are afflicted with them. The exact cause of heat cramps is not understood. It is known that sweat produced during strenuous exercise, particularly in a warm environment, causes a change in the body's salt (electrolyte) balance and may result in the loss of essential **electrolytes** from the cells. If the muscles are working vigorously, their cells will be vulnerable to this electrolyte loss. However, as of yet there is no proof that the muscles which develop cramps are actually depleted of electrolytes. **Dehydration** may also play a role in the development of muscle cramps. Large amounts of water can be lost from the body from excessive sweating. This loss of water may affect muscles that are being stressed and cause them to go into spasm.

The EMT can treat heat cramps by following these steps:

1. Rest the cramping muscles by having the patient sit or lie down until the cramps subside.
2. Give water by mouth. A diluted (half-strength) balanced electrolyte solution may be used. Several solutions such as Gatorade® are available commercially.
3. Remove the patient from the hot environment. These patients should not be given salt tablets or fluids with high concentrations of salts. Patients with heat cramps have an adequate amount of electrolytes in their system. The electrolytes are just not distributed properly. With adequate rest, the body will adjust the distribution of salts, and the cramps will resolve. No long-term problems result from heat cramps. For example, an athlete with heat cramps can return to play once the cramps have disappeared. However, the cramps could recur with continued vigorous activity.

Heat Exhaustion

Heat exhaustion, also called **heat prostration** or **heat collapse,** is the most common illness caused by heat. Heat exhaustion occurs when the body loses so much water and electrolytes through very heavy sweating that fluid depletion (**hypovolemia**) occurs. For sweating to be an effective cooling mechanism, the sweat must be able to evaporate from the body. If evaporation does not occur, cooling will not take place. Persons standing in the hot sun with several layers of clothing on (football fans or parade watchers, for example) may sweat profusely but experience little body cooling. High environmental humidity will also decrease the amount of evaporation that can occur. Thus, persons who exercise vigorously and those who wear heavy clothing in a warm, humid environment are particularly prone to heat exhaustion.

Patients who have developed heat exhaustion are in mild **hypovolemic shock.** The signs and symptoms of heat exhaustion are those of hypovolemia. Patients will often admit they were working hard or exercising in a hot, humid environment and sweating heavily. Their skin is usually cold and clammy and their faces gray. They may also complain of feeling dizzy, weak, or faint, with accompanying nausea or headache. Their vital signs may be normal, although the pulse may be rapid. Oral or rectal temperatures are usually normal, or slightly elevated, but on rare occasions they may be as high as 104 degrees F (40 degrees C).

The patient should be treated for mild, hypovolemic shock and removed promptly from the hot environment. Any tight clothing should be loosened and excessive layers of clothing removed. The patient should be urged to lie down. If fully alert, the patient should be encouraged to drink up to a liter of water or a diluted, commercially available balanced salt solution. The EMT who is treating a patient who is not fully alert should not force fluids by mouth for fear the fluid could be aspirated into the patient's lungs. In most cases these measures will reverse the patient's symptoms, and the person will feel better within 30 minutes (Figure 41.1). If the symptoms

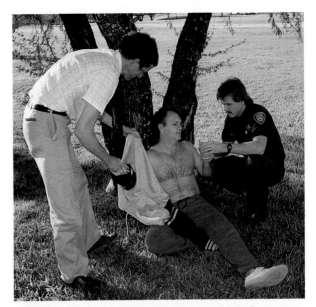

FIGURE 41.1 The patient suffering from heat exhaustion should be removed to a cool environment, allowed to lie down, and, if fully alert, given water or a diluted balanced salt solution to drink.

do not clear promptly, the level of consciousness decreases, or the temperature remains elevated, the patient should be transported to the hospital promptly for more vigorous treatment, such as intravenous fluid therapy and close monitoring.

Heat Stroke

Heat stroke is the least common but most serious illness caused by heat exposure. Untreated heat stroke will result in death. Heat stroke occurs when the body is subjected to more heat than it can handle. The normal mechanisms for getting rid of the excess heat are overwhelmed. The body temperature then rises rapidly to the level where tissues are destroyed and death results. Heat stroke will occur during vigorous physical activity, particularly in a closed, poorly ventilated, humid environment. Heat stroke is likely to occur during heat waves among people (particularly the elderly) who live in non-air-conditioned buildings without good ventilation. It is also the cause of death in children left unattended in a locked car on a hot summer day. The symptoms of heat exhaustion often precede heat stroke; if not treated, heat exhaustion can develop into heat stroke. A patient with heat exhaustion whose temperature is elevated may be developing heat stroke.

Heat-stroke patients have hot, dry, flushed skin; they do not sweat because the sweating mechanism has been overwhelmed. While these physical signs contrast significantly with heat exhaustion (sweaty, clammy skin), remember that patients who are progressing from heat exhaustion to heat stroke may retain some moisture on the skin. The body temperature rises rapidly in heat-stroke patients. As the body core temperature rises — and temperatures as high as 106 degrees F (41 degrees C) have been recorded — the patient's level of consciousness falls and the person becomes unresponsive very quickly. The pulse is usually rapid and strong at first, but as the patient becomes more and more unresponsive, the pulse becomes weaker and the blood pressure falls.

Heat stroke is a life-threatening emergency; untreated heat stroke will always result in death. Recovery of the patient depends on the speed and vigor with which treatment is administered. The entire body must be cooled by any means that are available. The patient must be removed from the hot environment and placed in the ambulance with the air conditioning set to maximum cooling.

The patient's clothing must be removed. Then, the EMT should place wet towels or sheets on the patient and direct a fan on the person. The patient must be transported rapidly to the hospital. The hospital should be given advance notice of the problem so that an ice-water bath can be prepared for immediate use upon the patient's arrival.

COLD EXPOSURE

Cold exposure may cause injury to individual parts of the body and to the body as a whole. Normal body temperature (98.6 degrees F or 37 degrees C) must be maintained within a very narrow range to allow chemical reactions in the body to work efficiently. The mechanisms that regulate body temperature can maintain it in hot or cold weather. However, in situations where the body is exposed to freezing or near freezing temperatures, these mechanisms may be overwhelmed and the body temperature will fall. This condition is called **hypothermia.** Sometimes only parts of the body such as the feet, hands, ears, or nose may be exposed to the cold and injured as a result. This condition is called **frostbite.**

While normal body temperature is 98.6 degrees F, the ambient (surrounding) temperature of the environment is rarely this high. Heat always tends to travel from a place where it is greater to a place where it is less. Since the body is usually warmer than its surroundings, the body will tend to lose heat. The body generates heat through the metabolism of food as it uses the food to do work. In this way the body can usually replace heat that is lost to the surrounding environment.

The body can lose heat in the following five ways:

1. Conduction. **Conduction** is the direct transfer of heat from a part of the body to a colder object. Conduction occurs when a warm hand touches a cold piece of metal or comes into contact with ice or snow. Conduction heat loss occurs when the body or a part of it is immersed in water with a temperature of less than 98 degrees F (37 degrees C). Heat passes directly from the body to the colder substance.

2. Convection. **Convection** occurs when heat is transferred through air moving across the

body surface to a cooler area. A person wearing light clothing who is standing outside when the temperature drops will lose heat by convection.

3. Evaporation. The conversion of any liquid to a gas is called **evaporation.** This conversion requires energy (heat). When sweat or water evaporates from the skin surface, the heat necessary for this process is taken from the body. Swimmers coming out of the water will feel a sensation of cold from the removal of body heat as the water evaporates from their skin.

4. Respiration. With normal breathing, the warm air in the lungs is exhaled into the atmosphere during **respiration** and body heat is lost.

5. Radiation. Heat always travels from a warm object to a cooler one, even if the objects are not in contact with each other. Warmer objects give off (radiate) heat to a cooler environment. A person standing in a cold room will lose heat by **radiation.**

The rate and amount of heat loss by the body can be modified in a variety of ways. One way is for the body to increase the rate of metabolism of its cells. This increased activity, which occurs most obviously in muscles as shivering, generates more body heat. Moving out of a cold environment and seeking shelter from winds is another way to decrease heat loss from radiation and convection.

Protective clothing serves in several ways to decrease heat loss. Materials which do not conduct heat are called **insulators.** Dry, still air is an excellent insulator. Thus, layers of clothing that trap air, or wool, down, or synthetic foams which have small pockets of entrapped air, are good insulators. Protective clothing also traps perspiration and does not allow evaporation. Sweating without evaporation will not result in cooling. Covering the head is also important in decreasing radiation. Heat radiates rapidly from the uncovered head. Thus, covering the head will minimize heat loss significantly.

Hypothermia

Generalized, progressive cooling of the body results in hypothermia. It can develop quickly as when someone is immersed in cold water, or more gradually as when a lost hunter is exposed to the cold environment for several hours or more. Hypothermia does not always occur in rural or remote areas; it is a problem in the cities as well. Nor does the temperature have to be below freezing for it to occur. In winter, homeless persons and those who lack heating for their homes may develop hypothermia. It is also more common among elderly and ill individuals.

The body can tolerate a drop of a few degrees of internal body temperature. However, when the temperature of the heart, lungs, brain, and other vital organs — the **core temperature** — falls below 95 degrees F (35 degrees C), symptoms of hypothermia will occur; the body loses its ability to regulate the body temperature and to generate body heat. Progressive loss of body heat then begins to occur.

Symptoms of Hypothermia

The symptoms of hypothermia become progressively more severe as the core temperature falls. Hypothermia progresses through five general stages (Table 41.1). While there is no clear distinction between the stages, the EMT will be able to estimate the severity of the problem by knowing the signs and symptoms present in each stage.

Shivering occurs in the first stage. Shivering is a subconscious attempt to generate more heat through muscular activity. In addition, jumping up and down and foot stamping will occur as the patient tries to produce more heat. Body temperature in this stage ranges from 90 degrees to 95 degrees F (32 degrees C to 35 degrees C). Below 90 degrees F, shivering stops. The second stage is characterized by decreased muscular function. It occurs when the core temperature is about 90 degrees F (32 degrees C). At first small, fine muscle activity — for example, coordinated finger motion — ceases. Eventually, as the temperature falls, all muscle activity stops.

In the third stage, when the core temperature is about 85 degrees F (29 degrees C), the patient becomes lethargic and loses interest in combatting the cold environment. In the fourth phase, about 80 degrees F (27 degrees C), decreased vital signs become apparent. The pulse slows and becomes weaker. Respiration slows and cardiac arrythmias may occur.

Apparent death characterizes the fifth and final stage when all cardiorespiratory activity may be completely absent. The word "apparent" is used because

TABLE 41.1 Systemic Hypothermia

Core temperature	95°F	90°F	85°F	80°F	78°F and below
Degree of hypothermia	Mild		Moderate	Severe	
Signs and Symptoms	Shivering; foot stamping	Loss of coordination	Lethargy	Coma	Apparent death
Cardiorespiratory Response			Slow pulse	Weak pulse; arrhythmias; slow respirations	Ventricular fibrillation; cardiac arrest
Level of Consciousness	Withdrawn	Confused	Sleepy	Irrational	Unconscious

patients who have appeared dead have been revived. There is an old saying: "No one is dead unless he is warm dead." Thus, the EMT should never assume that a cold, pulseless patient is dead. The person may be in a "metabolic ice box," and, if further heat loss can be prevented, may be successfully resuscitated.

Treatment of Hypothermia

Even mild degrees of hypothermia can have serious consequences and complications. All patients must be evaluated and treated in the hospital. Management of the patient in the field, regardless of the degree of exposure, consists of two steps: stabilizing the vital functions and preventing further heat loss.

Full rewarming of the hypothermic patient should not be attempted in the field. Rewarming can produce very serious cardiac arrythmias, which are especially difficult to correct, even in the hospital setting. They cannot be corrected in the field. Therefore, complete rewarming should only be done in the hospital where the patient can be monitored closely and maximum resuscitation can be provided when necessary. In all hypothermic patients, even when no vital signs are present, the EMT should begin basic life support and transport the patient rapidly to the hospital. As mentioned previously, patients can be hypothermic for long periods of time and still recover.

Although formal rewarming procedures are not carried out in the field, the EMT should strive to prevent further heat loss from the body. The patient should be removed immediately from the cold environment and placed in the ambulance warmed to

room temperature of about 70 degrees F. If the patient requires oxygen, it must be warm; an oxygen tank that has been sitting in the cold environment should not be used. The patient should be covered with dry, warm blankets after any wet clothing has been removed.

Rapid transportation of the hypothermic patient to the hospital is essential. If a medical facility is less than 15 minutes away, then the EMT should transport the patient immediately. When the hospital is more than 15 minutes away, the EMT should attempt to stabilize heat loss as described above. The receiving hospital should be notified of the patient's condition so that preparations can be made for rewarming to begin as soon as the patient arrives.

Management of Cold Exposure in a Sick or Injured Person

Frequently, an EMT will encounter a sick or injured person who has been trapped in a cold environment. This patient may develop hypothermia or already have problems related to the cold exposure. Remember, an injured person is more likely to be affected adversely by the cold. The following steps should be taken promptly to prevent further cold injury:

1. Remove wet clothing and keep the patient dry.
2. Prevent conduction heat loss. Do not allow the patient to lie against any wet or cold surfaces (such as a car frame).
3. Insulate all exposed body parts (especially the head) by wrapping with a blanket or any other dry, bulky material that is available.

4. Prevent convection loss by erecting a wind barrier around the patient.

5. Remove the patient from the cold environment as promptly as possible.

Local Cold Injuries

Most injuries from the cold are localized to exposed parts of the body. The extremities, particularly the feet, are especially vulnerable to cold injury. When exposed parts of the body become very cold but not frozen, the condition is called **frostnip, chilblains,** or **immersion foot (trench foot).** When the parts become frozen, the injury is called **frostbite.** The three most important factors that determine the severity of a local cold injury are (1) the duration of the exposure, (2) the temperature to which the body part was exposed, and (3) the wind velocity during exposure.

The following six factors may make a person more susceptible to local cold injury:

1. Inadequate insulation from cold or wind
2. Restricted circulation from tight clothing or shoes or from circulatory disease
3. Fatigue
4. Poor nutrition
5. Alcohol or drug abuse
6. Hypothermia

In hypothermia, blood is shunted away from the extremities in an attempt to maintain the temperature of the body core. This shunting of blood increases the risk of local cold injury to the extremities. Thus, the patient with hypothermia may also develop frostbite or other local cold injury. The reverse is also true, and the EMT must remember that both local and systemic cold exposure problems can occur in the same patient.

Frostnip and Immersion Foot

Frostnip (chilblains) occurs after prolonged exposure to the cold, but freezing of the skin and deeper tissues has not occurred. Because this condition is usually not painful, the patient often is not aware that a cold injury has occurred. The skin becomes pale (**blanched**). Exposed parts of the body, particularly the ears and nose, are commonly affected. Immersion foot, also called trench foot, occurs after prolonged exposure to cold water. It is particularly common in hikers or hunters who stand for a long time in cold water. The skin of the foot is wrinkled, pale, and cold to the touch.

The emergency treatment of these less severe local cold injuries includes removing the patient from the cold, wet environment and rewarming the part. With frostnip, contact with a warm object such as the EMT's hands or the patient's body, or blowing warm breath onto the part may be all that is needed. During rewarming, tingling and redness of the affected part will occur. With immersion foot, wet shoes, boots, and socks should be removed and the foot gradually rewarmed and protected from further cold exposure.

Frostbite

Frostbite is the most serious local cold injury. The tissues are actually frozen. Freezing permanently damages cells, although the exact mechanism by which the damage occurs is not known. The presence of ice crystals within the cells may cause physical damage to the cells. This change in the structure of the water in the cells may also cause changes in the concentration of critical electrolytes, which produce permanent changes in the chemistry of the cell. When the ice thaws, further chemical changes occur in the cell. As a result, the damaged cells die (**gangrene**) or become permanently damaged. If gangrene occurs, the dead tissue has to be amputated. If less severe damage occurs, there will still be permanent changes in the injured part. It becomes reddened, tender to touch, and cannot tolerate further exposure to cold.

Frostbite can be identified by the hard frozen feel of the affected tissues. Much like a burn, the depth of damage to the skin will vary. Frostbite may be superficial or deep. With superficial frostbite only the skin is frozen, and with deep frostbite the deeper tissues are frozen as well. Estimating the depth of a freezing injury is very difficult on examination. Only with time can the extent of an injury be determined. Most frostbitten parts are white, yellow-white, or blue-white. They are hard and cold to the touch (Figure 41.2).

Treatment of frostbite should include the following steps:

1. Remove the patient from further exposure to the cold.
2. Protect the frostbitten part from further injury. *Never rub frostbitten tissue.* Rubbing the

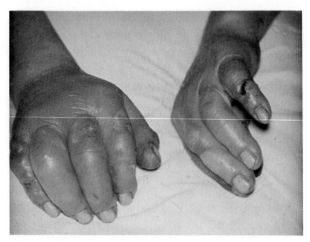

FIGURE 41.2 Frostbitten tissue is white, yellow-white, or blue-white and is hard and cold to the touch. Frostbite is much like a burn in that the depth of damage to the skin varies. Only with time can the extent of damage be determined.

injured tissues just causes further damage to the cells from the sharp ice crystals. Similarly, the patient should not be allowed to stand or walk on a frostbitten foot. Always protect the part by gentle handling.

3. Remove any wet or restricting clothing and cover the injured part loosely with a dry, sterile dressing.
4. Evaluate the patient's general condition for signs or symptoms of systemic hypothermia.
5. Support the patient's vital functions as necessary and transport the patient promptly to the hospital.

Rewarming of the frostbitten extremity is rarely done in the field. Heating it with something warm such as the exhaust from the ambulance engine or, even worse, an open flame will only cause further damage to the fragile tissues. Rewarming is best accomplished under controlled circumstances in the emergency department. If hospital care is not available and the EMT is instructed to institute rewarming in the field, it is best accomplished in a warm-water bath. The frostbitten part should be immersed in water at a temperature of between 100 degrees and 112 degrees F (38 degrees and 44.5 degrees C). The water temperature should be checked with a thermometer before the limb is immersed. The water should *never* exceed 112 degrees F (44.5 degrees C). The frostbitten part should be kept in the water bath until it feels

warm and the color (redness) has returned. Rewarming should never be done if there is any chance that the part may freeze again before the patient reaches the hospital. Some of the most severe consequences of frostbite (gangrene and amputation) have occurred in parts that were thawed and then refrozen.

Cold Exposure and the EMT

When working in a cold environment, the EMT is also at risk from becoming a victim of hypothermia. Specific survival training and precautions should be given to EMTs who work in regions where cold-weather search-and-rescue operations may be needed. EMTs must be thoroughly familiar with the specific conditions in their assigned areas, be cognizant of existing weather conditions, and stay tuned to forecasts of predicted weather changes. Proper clothing should be available and worn at all times (Figure 41.3). The vehicle must be properly equipped and maintained for a cold environment. As with many other hazards, the EMT must be concerned with self-protection in order to remain capable of helping others.

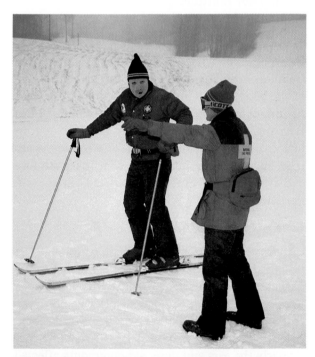

FIGURE 41.3 An EMT who works in a cold environment must wear proper clothing to protect against hypothermia, especially during search and rescue operations.

YOU ARE THE EMT...

1. What causes heat cramps? Why shouldn't you give salt tablets to patients who are suffering from the muscle spasms of heat cramps?

2. It's the end of August and football practice has just started. You are called to treat a 16-year-old boy who has collapsed in the 80-degree heat. After ruling out medical problems and injuries, you realize he has collapsed from the heat. How will you decide whether he has heat exhaustion or heat stroke? How should each condition be treated?

3. Why shouldn't you attempt to rewarm a hypothermic patient in the field? What measures should you take in the field?

4. What is the difference between frostnip and frostbite?

42 Water Hazards

OVERVIEW

Each year 8,000 Americans die as a result of water accidents. Many of these people could be saved by proper emergency care. Such care may be as simple as removing the person from the water and clearing the airway. Or, high-technology equipment may be necessary to rescue someone who has had a diving accident at a lake.

Drowning and near drowning account for only 5 percent of water accidents. Serious injuries from diving, scuba, or boating accidents account for another 5 percent. The remaining 90 percent are much less serious. In any water hazard emergency, the victim has a much better chance of being revived if the EMT knows how to start artificial ventilation in the water; prevent further injury, especially to the spine in diving accidents; and begin cardiopulmonary resuscitation once the patient is out of the water.

Chapter 42 begins with an explanation of how submersion in water affects the lungs. Then the chapter discusses the emergency care of near-drowning victims, including victims who have suffered spinal injuries. The chapter next describes diving problems, especially the problems of scuba divers. These include ruptured eardrums, air embolism, and decompression sickness. The last section of Chapter 42 briefly touches on other water hazards.

OBJECTIVES

The objectives of Chapter 42 are to

- understand why drowning or near drowning occurs after submersion in water.
- learn the emergency care for near-drowning victims.
- learn how to identify and treat potential spinal injuries associated with near-drowning accidents.
- become familiar with problems associated with diving, especially air embolism and decompression sickness (the "bends").
- recognize other water hazards, including hypothermia and breath-holding blackout.

DROWNING AND NEAR DROWNING

Drowning is defined as death by suffocation after being submerged in water. **Near drowning** means at least temporary survival after submersion in water. Drowning may result from a cycle of events that result in panic in the water (Figure 42.1).

The mechanism of death by drowning is different in people drowning in fresh water, such as in a pool or a lake, and in salt water, such as the ocean. Records show that in most drownings (85 to 90 percent) significant amounts of water enter the lungs. Fresh water is quickly absorbed across the walls of alveoli of the lung into the bloodstream. The water then dilutes the body electrolytes and causes red blood cells to rupture. Also, the alveoli rupture and lung tissue receives irreversible damage. Salt water, if inhaled into the lungs, will cause injury by a different mechanism. The highly concentrated sea water will literally pull the body water out of the cells and into the lungs, causing **pulmonary edema.** As a result, it is difficult to transport oxygen across the wall of the alveolus into the blood. Contaminants in the water such as bacteria or chemicals will cause additional injury to the lungs.

Inhaling even very small amounts of either fresh or salt water causes severe irritation of the larynx. The extremely sensitive muscles of the larynx will go into spasm. This phenomenon is called **laryngospasm.** Its purpose is to prevent any more water from entering the lungs. However, the patient's lungs cannot be ventilated when laryngospasm is present. Progressive hypoxia occurs until the patient eventually becomes unconscious. At this point the laryngospasm relaxes.

Emergency Care in Drowning Accidents

The emergency care of a near-drowning victim begins with immediate ventilation. Full cardiopulmonary resuscitation (CPR) should be started if no pulse is present. A patient who has not inhaled large

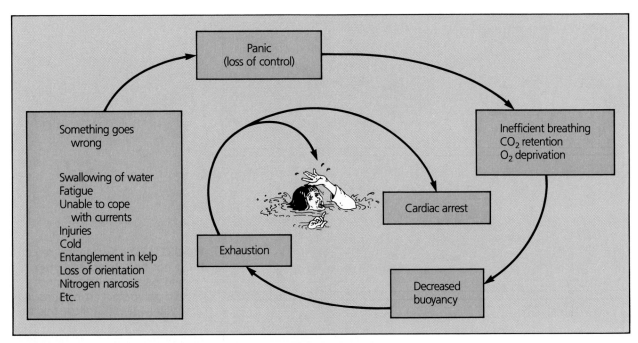

FIGURE 42.1 A schematic drawing shows the effect of panic in water accidents where it can contribute to the death of the person who loses self-control.

amounts of water may rapidly revive as the effects of hypoxia are reversed by adequate ventilation with oxygen. A victim who has inhaled large amounts of water requires the same emergency treatment, although revival may not be as rapid. The EMT should establish the airway, ventilate the patient, administer oxygen, and transport the person as quickly as possible to the hospital.

If the patient is conscious and still in the water, a water rescue is necessary. A rope, life preserver, or anything that will float should be thrown to the person. A swimming rescue should not be attempted unless the EMT has been trained and is experienced. Well-meaning but inexperienced people have themselves become drowning victims while attempting a swimming rescue. Many items can be floated out to the victim. For example, an inflated spare tire, rim and all, will float well enough to support two people in the water. The basic rule of water rescue can be remembered by this old saying: "Throw, tow, row, and *only then* go" (Figure 42.2).

The EMT who works in a recreation area near a lake, river, or ocean front must have a prearranged plan for water rescue. That includes having access to local personnel who are trained and skilled in water rescue and who can help develop a preplanned pro-

tocol for water rescue. Knowing how to obtain and use life jackets and other rescue equipment is also vitally important because the success of a rescue depends on how rapidly the victim can be removed from the water and given proper ventilation.

Spinal Injuries in Drowning Accidents

Spine fractures and spinal cord injuries frequently complicate drowning accidents. The EMT must assume that spinal injury exists if the drowning has resulted from a diving accident, if the patient is unconscious, or if the patient is conscious but complains of weakness, paralysis, or numbness in the arms or legs. When a spinal injury is suspected, the neck must be protected from further injury, and cardiac compression cannot be started until the spine is stabilized. Most spinal injuries in diving accidents occur in the cervical spine. The injured spine must be stabilized while the patient is in the water.

When a spinal injury is suspected and the patient is face down in the water, the following procedure should be carried out:

1. Turn the patient face up. Two rescuers are required to turn the patient safely. The entire upper half of the patient's body must be

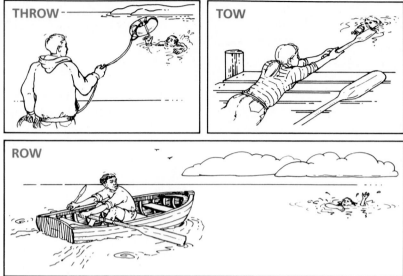

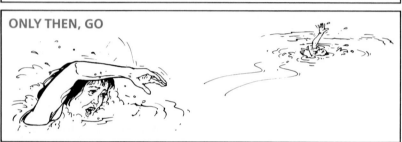

FIGURE 42.2 Swimming rescues must not be attempted by untrained personnel who cannot handle panic-stricken persons in the water. Always follow this sequence: Throw a floatable object, or tow the swimmer in by pole or rope. If these approaches fail, try to use a boat. Only when these courses have been exhausted, and only if the EMT is capable of doing it, should a swimming rescue be attempted.

turned as a unit. Twisting only the head will aggravate any injury to the cervical spine.

2. Restore the airway and begin ventilation, by the mouth-to-mouth technique or with available adjunctive equipment, as soon as the patient is face up in the water. The head and trunk should be supported as a unit by one rescuer while the other rescuer opens the airway and begins artificial ventilation. Immediate ventilation is the primary treatment of all drowning and near-drowning patients (Figure 42.3).

3. Float a wooden spine board under the patient. The head and trunk should be secured to the spine board to eliminate motion of the cervical spine. Do not remove the patient from the water until he or she is secured to the spine board.

4. Remove the patient from the water on the spine board and begin cardiac resuscitation. Effective cardiac compression for full cardiopulmonary resuscitation cannot be carried out in the water.

Recovery Techniques

On occasion, the EMT may be called to the scene of a drowning where the victim is not floating or visible in the water. An organized recovery effort must be made by personnel experienced with the equipment (scuba gear, snorkels, and goggles) and techniques of recovery. As a last resort when standard recovery techniques do not work, a grappling iron or large hook may be used to drag the bottom for the victim. The hook may seriously wound the patient, but it may be the only effective method of bringing the patient to the surface for resuscitation.

Resuscitation Efforts

Never should the EMT give up on resuscitating a drowning victim. When a person is submerged in water colder than body temperature, heat will be conducted from the body to the water, lowering the body temperature. Particularly in water colder than 70 degrees F (21 degrees C), hypothermia will occur and protect the vital organs from the lack of oxygen. Furthermore, in some circumstances exposure to cold

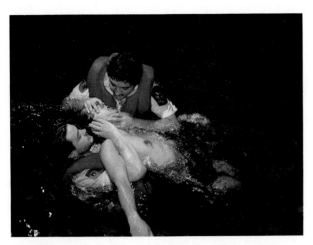

FIGURE 42.3 Artificial ventilation, the primary treatment of all drowning and near-drowning patients, should be started as soon as the patient is face up in the water.

water will induce certain reflexes, which may preserve basic body functions for prolonged periods. The hypothermia and protective reflexes may significantly prolong the patient's tolerance for hypoxia. Some people have been resuscitated successfully with little or no permanent injury. So full resuscitation efforts should be maintained until the victim recovers or is pronounced dead by a physician at the scene or in the hospital.

DIVING PROBLEMS

Most serious water-related problems are associated with dives, either with or without scuba gear. Some of these problems are related to the nature of the dive; others result from panic. Panic is not restricted to the person who is unfamiliar and frightened by water; it happens to the experienced diver or swimmer as well. Panic can set up a cycle that will result in death, and it can affect someone who is submerged or immersed in water for even a short period of time. The person will struggle to reach the surface or the shore and become fatigued or exhausted. Such panic-driven efforts will only cause the person to sink even deeper into the water.

The **diving reflex** can occur in people who dive or jump into very cold water. A sudden reflex involving the vagus nerves may cause immediate cardiac arrest or **bradycardia** (reflex slowing of the heart rhythm); the person may lose consciousness and

drown. However, because of the hypothermia and related slowed metabolic rate, the victim may be able to survive for long periods of time under water. Full resuscitation efforts should be undertaken, regardless of the length of submersion.

There are over 3 million sport divers in the United States, and medical problems relating to diving techniques and equipment are becoming increasingly common. These problems can be separated into three phases of the dive: descent, bottom, and ascent.

Descent Problems

Descent problems are usually due to the sudden increase in pressure on the body as the person dives deeper into the water. Some body cavities cannot adjust to the increased external pressure of the water. Severe pain results. The usual areas affected are the lungs, the sinus cavities, the middle ear, and the area of the face surrounded by the diving mask. Usually, the pain caused by these "squeeze problems" forces the diver to return to the surface to equalize the pressures, and the problem goes away by itself. A diver who continues to complain of pain after returning to the surface, particularly in the ear, should be transported to the hospital.

A person with a ruptured eardrum may develop a problem while diving. If cold water enters the middle ear through a **perforated tympanic membrane** (ruptured eardrum), the diver may lose his or her balance and orientation. The diver may shoot suddenly to the surface and sustain ascent problems.

Bottom Problems

Problems related to the bottom of the dive are rarely seen. Most of them are due to faulty connections in the diving gear and result either from inadequate mixing of oxygen and carbon dioxide in the air the diver breathes, or from poisonous carbon monoxide being accidentally fed into the breathing apparatus. All of these situations can cause drowning or rapid ascent, and all require emergency resuscitation and transport.

Ascent Problems

Most of the serious emergencies associated with diving are related to ascending from the bottom and are referred to as ascent problems. These emergencies usually require vigorous resuscitation. Two particularly dangerous problems are **air embolism** and **decompression sickness,** also called the **bends.**

Air Embolism

The most common, most dangerous, and yet least recognized emergency in scuba diving is air embolism. It may occur in a dive as shallow as 6 feet. Air embolism results from the diver holding his or her breath during a rapid ascent. The air pressure in the lungs remains at a high level, while the external pressure on the chest decreases. As a result, the air inside the lungs expands rapidly. This rapid expansion causes the alveoli in the lungs to rupture. The air released can cause injury in several areas. Air may enter the pleural space and create a **pneumothorax** (air in the pleural space that compresses the lung). It can also enter the **mediastinum** (the space within the thorax that contains the heart and great vessels) causing a condition called **pneumomediastinum.** Or it may enter the bloodstream and create bubbles of air in the vessels called **air emboli.**

Pneumothorax and pneumomediastinum both result in severe dyspnea. A bubble of air in the bloodstream (air embolus) will act as a plug and pre-vent the normal flow of blood and oxygen to a specific part of the body. The brain is the organ most severely affected by air embolism because it requires a constant supply of oxygen (Figure 42.4).

The following are signs and symptoms of air embolism:

1. Blotching (mottling of the skin)
2. Froth (often pink or bloody) at the nose and mouth
3. Severe pain in muscles, joints, or abdomen
4. Dyspnea and/or chest pain
5. Dizziness, nausea, and vomiting
6. Dysphasia (difficulty in speaking)
7. Difficulty with vision
8. Paralysis and/or coma

Decompression Sickness (the Bends)

Decompression sickness ("the bends") also results from too rapid an ascent from a dive, although the mechanism of injury is different. In decompression sickness, bubbles of nitrogen form in the blood vessels when the diver ascends rapidly. During the dive, nitrogen that is being breathed dissolves in the blood because it is under pressure. When the diver ascends rapidly, the external pressure is decreased, and the dissolved nitrogen forms small bubbles

FIGURE 42.4   Air embolism occurs as air in the lungs rapidly expands when compression on the chest is suddenly released. The resulting outward pressure can rupture alveoli and bronchioles and create the conditions shown here.

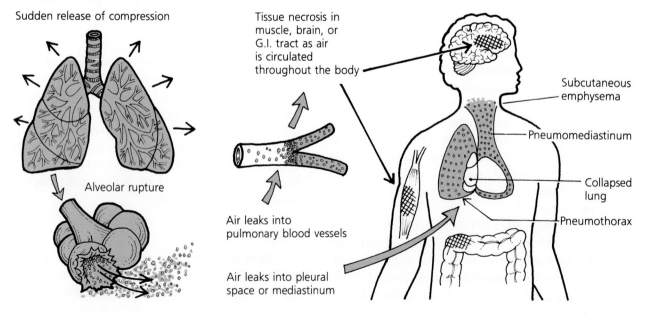

Sudden release of compression

Alveolar rupture

Tissue necrosis in muscle, brain, or G.I. tract as air is circulated throughout the body

Air leaks into pulmonary blood vessels

Air leaks into pleural space or mediastinum

Subcutaneous emphysema

Pneumomediastinum

Collapsed lung

Pneumothorax

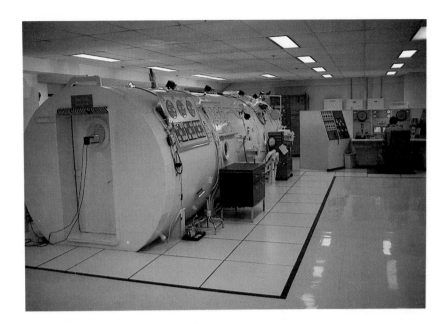

FIGURE 42.5 Treatment in a recompression chamber may be lifesaving for a patient with air embolism or decompression sickness.

within the blood vessels. These bubbles of nitrogen cause the same problem that occurs in air embolism — blockage of the blood vessels, which deprives parts of the body of their normal blood supply.

The signs and symptoms of decompression sickness are similar to those of air embolism. The most striking symptom is severe abdominal and/or joint pain — so severe that the patient literally doubles up or "bends." This characteristic posture gives the name "the bends" to this problem. Dive tables are available to show the proper rate of ascent from a dive, including the number and length of pauses that a diver should make on the way up from a deep, long dive. If these tables are followed, decompression sickness should not occur.

Decompression sickness can also occur from flying in an unpressurized airplane that climbs too rapidly to a great height. The problem is exactly the same as ascent from a deep dive — a sudden decrease of the external pressure on the body and the release of dissolved nitrogen from the blood that forms bubbles of nitrogen gas within the blood vessels.

Often it is difficult to distinguish between air embolism and decompression sickness. As a general rule, air embolism occurs immediately upon return to the surface, while the symptoms of decompression sickness may not occur for several hours. The emergency treatment is the same for both: basic life support followed by **recompression** in a recompression chamber. In treating patients suspected of hav-

ing air embolism or decompression sickness, the EMT should follow these steps:

1. Remove the patient from the water. Try to keep the person calm.
2. Begin basic life support and administer oxygen.
3. Place the patient on his or her left side, with the patient's head lower than the feet (the Trendelenburg position). This position will decrease the chance of an air embolus traveling to the brain.
4. Listen to the chest carefully for absent or decreased breath sounds that would indicate a pneumothorax.
5. Transport the patient promptly to the nearest recompression chamber for treatment. Know the location of and the best means of access to the recompression chamber in your area. Most of these chambers (also known as Hyperbaric Oxygen Chambers) can easily be reached by modern air transport, even if they are many miles away (Figure 42.5). Transport the patient at or near sea level, or in an aircraft pressurized to sea-level pressure.
6. Continue to administer oxygen while transporting the patient to the chamber.
7. Obtain a history of the duration and depth of the dive. If facilities are available, the patient's scuba tank should be analyzed for the

amount of air remaining in it, and its carbon monoxide content.

8. Assess and monitor the patient's level of consciousness using the AVPU scale. This information will help the personnel at the chamber select the correct treatment program.

The aim of recompression treatment is to restore the body to a high-pressure environment so that the bubbles of gas (air or nitrogen) can be redissolved into the blood and the pressures inside and outside the lungs can be equalized. Once the pressures are equalized, gradual decompression can be accomplished under controlled conditions.

Injury from decompression sickness is usually reversible with proper treatment. However, if the bubbles plug up critical blood vessels that supply the brain or spinal cord, permanent brain injury or paraplegia may result. Therefore, the key in the emergency management of these serious ascent problems is to recognize that an emergency exists. The EMT should begin basic life support, administer oxygen, and arrange for recompression as rapidly as possible.

OTHER WATER HAZARDS

Hypothermia is often seen in patients who have been immersed in cold water. The progressive lowering of the body temperature makes it more difficult for these victims to help themselves. After removal from the water, the patient will continue to lose heat through evaporation. The EMT must pay close attention to the temperature of a person who is rescued from cold water. The same rules that are used for treating hypothermia caused by cold exposure apply to hypothermia from immersion in cold water: the body temperature should be stabilized and the patient transported promptly.

Breath-holding blackout sometimes occurs in shallow water swimmers who are trying to prolong their capacity to stay underwater. The swimmer breathes in and out rapidly and deeply before entering the water. This hyperventilation lowers the carbon dioxide level in the bloodstream while it increases the oxygen level. Swimming under water, the per-

son consumes the oxygen but does not build up a high level of carbon dioxide since so much of it has been blown off by hyperventilation. An elevated level of carbon dioxide in the blood is the strongest stimulus for breathing. Without this stimulus, the swimmer will not feel the need to breathe even though all of the oxygen in the swimmer's lungs has been consumed. The person will then lose consciousness and may drown. The emergency care of a breath-holding blackout is the same as that for a drowning or near drowning.

Associated injuries may occur in the water. For example, contact with boat propellers, sharp rocks, water skis, or dangerous marine life can result in injury complicated by the problem of water immersion. The patient should be removed from the water (taking care to protect the spine from further injury) and given basic life support as needed. Dressings and splints should be applied as indicated, and the patient should be monitored closely for any signs of immersion or cold injury.

Another associated injury that may occur in water is child abuse. The EMT must be aware that a child involved in a drowning or near drowning may be the victim of child abuse. While it may be difficult to prove, such instances should be handled according to the rules that apply to cases of suspected child abuse (see Chapter 37).

YOU ARE THE EMT...

1. You have responded to a swimming pool diving accident. The victim's friends have pulled him to the surface, and he is floating face up when you arrive. He is unconscious but alive. Should you remove him from the pool or start ventilation in the water? Why will this patient need CPR? When will you start CPR?
2. How can hypothermia increase the chances of resuscitation from near drowning?
3. Describe the diving reflex. What other condition can it cause?
4. How does air embolism differ from the bends? What do these two problems have in common?

PSYCHOLOGICAL ASPECTS OF EMERGENCY CARE

43 Interacting with Patients

PRINCIPLES OF EFFECTIVE COMMUNICATION

Effective communication will come more easily to the EMT who realizes that the sick or injured patient is frightened and may be misinterpreting the EMT's gestures, body movements, and attitude. The following guidelines will help the EMT relate to a patient and keep the patient in a calm state:

1. Make and keep eye contact with the patient at all times. Give the patient your undivided attention, and let him know that he is your main interest. Look the patient "straight in the eye" to establish rapport and communicate your concern with his problem.

2. Tell the truth. Never knowingly tell the patient something that isn't true. Even if what you have to say is something very unpleasant, that is better than lying. Telling an untruth destroys the patient's trust in you and decreases your own confidence. You may not always tell the patient everything, but, in general, if the patient or family asks a specific question, answer truthfully. A straightforward question deserves a straightforward answer.

3. Communicate at a level that the patient can understand. Don't "talk up" or "talk down" or be in any way patronizing. Do not assume that an elderly person is deaf or otherwise unable to understand you. And never use "baby talk" with elderly people.

4. Be aware of your own body language. Patients may misinterpret gestures that you may make. Be specifically careful not to assume a threatening posture; instead maintain yourself in a calm, professional stance. Nonverbal communication is extremely important in dealing with patients.

5. Always speak slowly, clearly, and distinctly.

6. Use a patient's proper name. Do not use terms such as "pops" or "lady" or "kid." Try

to avoid using first names. Rather, use the patient's surname, preceded by the proper qualifier (Mr., Mrs., or Ms.).

7. If a patient is hard of hearing, speak clearly so that the person can read your lips. Be very careful not to shout at a hearing-impaired person. Shouting will not make it any easier for the patient to understand you, and shouting may frighten the person.

8. Allow time for the patient to answer or respond to your questions. Do not rush the patient unless there is immediate danger. Sick and injured people may not be thinking clearly and will need time to answer even simple questions.

9. Try to make the patient comfortable and relaxed whenever possible. Is the patient more comfortable sitting or lying down? Is she cold or hot? Does she want a friend or relative to be with her?

SPECIFIC COMMUNICATION PROBLEMS

Geriatric Patients

Most elderly patients, often called **geriatric patients,** are rational and can give a clear medical history. An older patient is not necessarily senile or confused. The EMT should approach an elderly patient slowly and calmly, allowing plenty of time for the patient to respond to the EMT's questions. The EMT should be alert for signs of confusion, anxiety, or impaired hearing or vision. The patient should feel confident that the EMT is in charge and that everything possible is being done to provide assistance.

Often, an elderly patient's spouse will also need attention. Seeing a person whom one has loved or been married to for many years taken away in an ambulance can be a particularly frightening and anxiety-producing experience. The EMT should take a few minutes to speak with the patient's spouse or family, telling them what is being done and why such action is being taken.

Pediatric Patients

All persons in an emergency situation experience some degree of fright, but fear is accentuated in children. The EMT should assume that all children will be frightened about what is happening to them, by the EMT's uniform, and especially by the ambulance. Even the child who says little is very much aware of all that is going on. Familiar objects and faces will help to lessen the fear. Letting the child keep a favorite toy, doll, or "security blanket" will give the child some sense of security and a lot of comfort. So will having a relative or friend nearby, but this person must be emotionally stable. Sometimes adults become too upset by what has happened to the child to be of assistance. The EMT must be careful about selecting the proper adult for this role.

Children can easily see through lies or deceptions, so the EMT must always be honest with them. The EMT must constantly explain to the child what is happening and why certain procedures are taking place. If the treatment is going to cause pain (such as applying a splint), the child should be warned ahead of time. The EMT can explain that it will not hurt for long and, most importantly, that it will help "make it better."

EMTs must respect a child's modesty. Little girls and boys are embarrassed if they have to undress or be undressed in front of strangers. When a wound or site of injury has to be exposed, the EMT should try to do so out of sight of strangers.

An EMT's tone of voice is also important: It should be professional yet friendly. The child should feel reassured that the EMT is going to help in every way possible. Maintaining eye contact with the child will let the child know that the EMT is helping and can be trusted.

Hearing-Impaired (Deaf) Patients

Deaf patients are rarely ashamed or embarrassed by their deafness. They have learned to deal with it long ago. It is those around the deaf person — in this case, the emergency medical service personnel — who may have a problem dealing with a hearing-impaired person. The EMT should first assume that a hearing-impaired person has normal intelligence and is able to understand what is going on *if* the EMT can successfully communicate with the person. Most deaf people can read lips, so the EMT should be positioned such that the patient can see his lips. The following reminders will also help the EMT to communicate successfully with the hearing-impaired person:

1. Don't cover your mouth or mumble. Speak slowly, clearly, and distinctly.
2. Don't shout!
3. Know some of the simple phrases used in sign language, including those for "sick," "hurt," and "help" (Figure 43.1).
4. Have a clipboard handy to write down questions and for the patient to write down answers if necessary.
5. Write legibly and use short questions and answers. Remember that many hearing-impaired people can speak distinctly, even though others cannot.

Blind Patients

Like hearing-impaired patients, blind patients have usually accepted their disability long ago and learned to deal with it. Most blind people have usually developed very sharp and acute senses of hearing and touch. Therefore, the EMT should assume that a blind person has normal hearing and normal intelligence. Everything the EMT is doing should be explained in great detail. The EMT should also keep in physical contact with the patient with a hand lightly held on the patient's shoulder or arm. When it is time to move the blind patient — if he can walk — the EMT should lead him with a hand on his arm, and not push the person. Any mobility aids (such as a cane) should be transported with the patient to the hospital.

A blind person may have a Seeing Eye dog. The dog can be identified by its special harness. Seeing Eye dogs are trained not to leave their masters and not to respond to strangers. The blind patient who is conscious can tell the EMT about the dog and give instructions for its care. Seeing Eye dogs are often allowed into places where ordinary dogs are forbidden. If circumstances permit, the dog may be brought to the hospital with the patient. If the dog has to be left behind, the EMT should make arrangements for its care.

Non-English-Speaking Patients

After the primary survey is completed and the patient's vital functions are stabilized, it is essential that the EMT obtain a medical history from the patient. This task is the responsibility of all medical personnel and cannot be omitted simply because the patient does not speak English. Many patients who

A

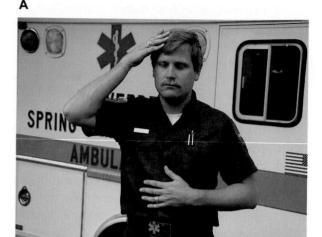

B

C

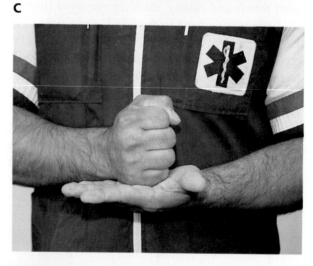

FIGURE 43.1 Some common hand sign language expressions to be used when communicating with hearing-impaired patients: (a) "sick"; (b) "hurt"; (c) "help."

do not speak English fluently will know certain important words or phrases.

Initially, the EMT should determine how much English the patient can speak. If communication is impossible, the EMT should seek out a family member or friend as an interpreter. Simple questions and lay terms should be used whenever possible. Medical jargon should especially be avoided. Questions can be supplemented with visual clues by using appropriate gestures and pointing to specific parts of the body. EMTs who work in areas with a large non-English-speaking population should become familiar with their language, especially the common medical terms and phrases. EMTs can carry cards that show the pronunciation of these terms.

Confused Patients

Patients may be confused for a variety of reasons. The stress of the emergency situation may be sufficient to confuse persons who in routine circumstances can function normally. Occasionally, illness or injury may cause confusion. Finally, some people appear constantly confused and are unable to cope with normal daily routines, much less emergency situations. In communicating with a confused patient, the EMT should assume that the confusion is only temporary and that the patient has normal intelligence. The EMT should speak slowly and distinctly, being certain that the patient understands what is being said. Sometimes a confused patient's response time is quite long. This person needs and should be allowed plenty of time to respond to the EMT's questions and requests. Certain procedures may have to be explained more than once. It is important that every effort be made to communicate fully despite the patient's confused state. One final point is that the EMT must remember that confusion may be a sign of significant injury or illness that will require medical care.

Mentally Retarded Patients

At times, severely mentally disturbed or retarded patients can be very difficult to communicate with. From the family, the EMT should try to determine the patient's normal level of communication. The presence of a physical impairment does not necessarily mean that the patient cannot communicate. Even more important, many patients with physical impairments have normal intelligence and are able to understand the spoken word quite well. Once certain that the patient is truly retarded, the EMT should speak slowly, using short and simple words. As with the confused patient, these patients sometimes need to have things repeated to them more than once before they understand what is happening. These patients should be handled with an especially caring concern to minimize their fear and confusion.

DISRUPTIVE BEHAVIOR

Disruptive behavior is defined as behavior that presents a danger to the patient or others or causes a delay in treatment. The standard communication techniques outlined in the first part of this chapter are ineffective in altering disruptive behavior. Therefore, special techniques are required for dealing with such patients. Although there are many causes of disruptive behavior, it is important to remember that for some people it is simply a normal reaction to stress.

Possible Causes of Disruptive Behavior

Certain physical and medical conditions can result in disturbed behavior as well. One or more of these conditions may be present in an unruly patient.

Alcohol or drug abuse is discussed extensively in Chapter 35. The presence of drug paraphernalia or an empty liquor bottle may point to this cause of disruptive behavior. The EMT must bear in mind that other causes of such behavior may be present in a patient who has been drinking or taking drugs. Special care must be taken not to write off the unruly or abusive patient as "just another drunk."

Head injury may be a cause of disruptive behavior. The abnormal behavior may occur immediately after injury (from a concussion) or may be delayed for as long as two to three weeks after the injury (from a chronic subdural hematoma). When the family reports that the patient has had a significant change in personality, the diagnosis of head injury must be considered.

Certain metabolic disorders can cause disruptive behavior. Both insulin shock and diabetic coma can result in abnormal patterns of behavior. Other endocrine disorders (especially thyroid disease) can produce wide ranges of abnormal behavior from extreme agitation to marked lethargy. An attempt should be made to determine if the patient has a history of such a metabolic disorder. (Have similar reactions occurred before? Is the patient taking any prescription medication?)

Neurological diseases may cause very disruptive or irrational behavior. Many different terms are used to describe these diseases. The general descriptive term is **organic brain syndrome.** The vast majority of patients with organic brain syndrome are elderly and have experienced a gradual loss of function. Frequently, the first sign of organic brain syndrome is a change in personality. The family, and sometimes even the patient, will be aware of the personality change. Patients with organic brain syndrome are often disoriented. The do not know where they are; they may not know the date or they may not be able to answer a simple question such as "Who is the President of the United States?"

Many different forms of psychiatric illness will also cause disruptive behavior. Psychiatric disorders may produce a wide range of behavioral problems, among them the following:

Paranoia. A person may believe that people (including the EMT) are plotting against him, planning to hurt or kill him.

Mania. The patient may be severely agitated (manic) — moving around frantically, speaking rapidly but never finishing a sentence or a complete thought.

Depression. The patient may not want to do anything, even move, and will not cooperate or answer questions.

Suicidal act. The patient may be threatening to kill himself or have already made a suicide attempt.

These are just a sample of the common presentations of psychiatric illness. Psychiatric patients may show great variations in their behavior over a short period of time. They often experience wide mood swings, appearing calm one minute and violent the next.

Management of the Disruptive Patient

The following steps should be taken in the management of any patient who is exhibiting disruptive behavior:

1. Assess the situation. Try to find out the cause of the patient's disruptive behavior. Unless the patient is in danger and must be moved immediately, you should spend some time assessing the situation. There is usually no rush to hurry off to the hospital, and spending some extra time with the patient can often make the job of transporting much easier. Look for a possible cause of a head injury or for drug or alcohol use. Try to obtain a history of the behavior. Did it come on suddenly or gradually? Does the patient have diabetes or other medical problems? Has the patient been ill recently? Does the patient have a history of similar previous behavior or psychiatric illness?

2. Protect the patient and yourself. Do not take your eyes off of the patient and be alert for any obviously aggressive behavior. Even small people can be dangerous if they are severely agitated. Never turn your back on the disturbed patient or leave him alone. If the patient has a knife or gun, stay clear: You do not want to become a casualty yourself. Do not attempt to deal with the disturbed, armed patient until he has been disarmed. Do not try to disarm the patient unless you have been trained to do so. This is a job for the police.

3. Take charge. Establish yourself as the health care professional who is responsible for helping the patient. Act confidently and decisively. Your mood, your spoken *and nonspoken* communication to the patient, will go a long way toward beginning effective treatment.

4. Provide proper emergency medical care. If the patient has sustained an injury, self-inflicted or otherwise, carry out the appropriate emergency medical care as soon as your personal risk has been minimized. Explain what you are doing to the patient.

5. Describe the patient's behavior as accurately as possible. Is the patient alert and oriented (lucid)? Calm or agitated? Frightened? Is there evidence of alcohol or drug use? Report these observations to medical control. Rarely will you be able to make a specific diagnosis. It is often difficult to distinguish between such diseases as organic brain syndrome and psychiatric illness. One important exception to

this point is the diabetic patient in insulin shock. You must determine promptly if the disruptive patient has diabetes or another metabolic disease that may be causing the abnormal behavior. These patients require prompt medical treatment.

6. Avoid expressing accusations and anger at a disruptive patient. These patients are frightened, and, to them, their fright is a real concern and has a real basis. Do not try to judge the patient's actions or lecture the person on the evils of alcohol or drugs. Remember, this frightened patient is ill, and your responsibility is to provide emergency care and transport to a treatment facility.

7. Be careful about "labeling" a disturbed, disruptive patient. Do not use terms like "crazy" or "drunk," or, if the patient's symptoms seem minor, "a crock." Be very careful about labeling a patient as someone who is faking illness or **malingering.** That determination is often very difficult to make, even by experienced people. It is far better to be "taken in" by someone who, for whatever reason, fakes an illness than it is to deny treatment to someone who actually has a legitimate complaint but appears to be faking or malingering. Assume that the patient's complaints are genuine. True malingering is a very rare condition.

There may be times when a patient simply cannot be approached — the person won't let anyone near him or touch him, and refuses to go to the hospital, despite all efforts to convince him that he can be helped, that the EMT wants to help him, and that no one is going to hurt him. Sometimes family, neighbors, or friends will insist that a disturbed patient be taken to the hospital. However, unless ordered to by the police or another law enforcement agency, the EMT cannot do this. Furthermore, a patient cannot be physically restrained, in most areas, without police direction. EMTs must know their local laws regarding restraints. If someone has to be restrained, the EMT should get help. Frightened, agitated, disruptive patients may be capable of causing serious injury to the EMT, bystanders, or themselves. Soft, wide leather or cloth restraints, not police-type handcuffs, should be used when necessary (Figure 43.2).

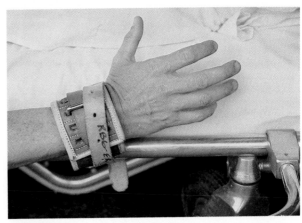

FIGURE 43.2 Soft, wide leather or padded cloth restraints — not police-type handcuffs — should be used when disruptive patients have to be restrained.

YOU ARE THE EMT...

1. Give an example of how you might sound patronizing to a patient. Rewrite that example so it is no longer in patronizing language.
2. Your patient is a woman in her sixties who is deaf. She fainted while standing in line at the local supermarket. Write out ten questions you would ask her. Keep the questions as short as possible and write them so that she can answer in one or two words.
3. Your patient is a six-year-old boy who was struck by a car while chasing a ball into the street. He was not severely injured but has lacerations on his face and arms that are bleeding. You need to transport him, but his parents are not home. He is hysterical because of all the blood and because you have told him you have to take him to the hospital. How will you reassure him and how will you select someone from the neighborhood to ride in the ambulance if you feel that is necessary?
4. You have been called to treat a man who is exhibiting disruptive behavior. Identify three causes other than alcohol or drugs that might cause disruptive behavior and indicate how you might determine if this patient is suffering from any of these problems.

44

Crisis Intervention

SUDDEN DEATH CRISIS

Responding to Sudden Death

Frequently, the EMT is called to the scene of sudden and unexpected death. The causes of sudden death are many: Trauma, heart attack, stroke, sudden infant death syndrome (SIDS), suicide, and homicide are a few. Often, the patient will not have been previously ill or in any danger, and the death will come as a great shock to everyone.

Upon arriving at the scene of sudden death, the EMT must be prepared for a number of reactions if the patient's family is present. A wide range of responses to sudden death will occur, especially from severely anxious and agitated family members. Remarks such as "He was never sick a day in his life" or "I warned him not to go out today" are a family's way of coping with something that they do not understand.

Common, general emotional responses to sudden death include denial ("It can't be happening; I know he's going to be all right"); guilt ("It's my fault that I bought him that motorcycle" or "I knew I should have stayed home with her today"); obvious grief (hysterical sobbing, wringing of hands); and hostility — to others, to the dead person, to the EMT ("Why did he have to go and do this?" or "If you had gotten here sooner, he wouldn't be dead," or "It's her fault; she drove him to it").

Sometimes the responses come in sequence, one after another, and various people will demonstrate different types of responses. Occasionally, a person will withdraw and not show any response. This person might experience a delayed response, however, particularly someone who appears unusually calm. Responses to sudden death are sometimes physical — that is, a person may feel faint, dizzy, or nauseated, and even have to vomit. The important thing to remember is that some type of emotional or physical response is a normal part of the grief that follows sudden and unexpected death.

EMTs and other medical personnel may experience some of these responses as well. The EMT may feel helpless or frustrated because providing further medical care will not do any good. The EMT may experience guilt ("Maybe if I had driven the ambulance faster..."). Anger is another common response ("What a stupid thing to do, driving his motorcycle into that truck. Now, I have to deal with his family"). Avoidance or denial is sometimes used to cope with these situations, and the EMT may have the urge to leave the scene quickly, hoping that the memory will go away.

In an attempt to avoid the emotional impact of the situation, some EMTs may become "hyperclinical," discussing in great detail the medical and technical aspects of the problem with other medical personnel. A few may even respond by making "sick jokes" about the situation or even about the people involved. Sometimes EMTs experience recurring memories of the tragic events surrounding sudden death and have nightmares or difficulty sleeping. All of these responses are normal and should lessen and eventually end with time. The EMT must acknowledge that these responses do accompany sudden death and then be prepared to cope with them.

Management of Sudden Death

Only a licensed physician can pronounce someone dead — an EMT cannot. The conclusive signs of death are **lividity, rigor mortis,** decapitation, or decomposition (see Chapter 4). If there is *any* question that the person is dead, full resuscitation should be carried out. Even if the EMT is certain the person is death but the family feels "something has to be done," resuscitation should be instituted. Once begun, resuscitation efforts should not stop until a physician so directs or the patient recovers.

When the person is obviously dead, support should be given to the family and friends. Once again, the EMT must be aware of and prepared for the many and various responses these people may demonstrate. The EMT should keep the family informed of what is being done. Close relatives or friends should be allowed to see the body if they desire, but the obvious mutilated areas should be covered up. Never should the EMT raise false hopes. For example, if resuscitation is started on someone who is almost certainly dead, the EMT should not tell the family that everything is going to be all right.

When confronted with a sudden death crisis, the EMT should communicate with the family in the following manner:

1. Answer questions as truthfully as possible. If you do not know the answer to a question, say so.
2. Give straightforward answers to all questions. Do not hide unpleasant facts.
3. Report all information that you know to be true.
4. Do not speculate or guess about the unknown.
5. Respect the family's need for sympathy. If they want to be near the victim, or if they want to be alone, try to follow their wishes.
6. Maintain a professional attitude at all times. Control your own feelings, demonstrate caring and concern for the victim and the family, and go about your business calmly and efficiently.

TERMINAL DISEASE CRISIS

Responding to Terminal Disease

When called to a scene where someone is dying after a long illness, the EMT must be prepared for the emotional and psychological responses of the patient and the patient's family. Although not always as emotionally charged as the scene of a sudden unexpected death, impending death from **terminal disease** can present the EMT with a difficult challenge.

Often the patient has been suffering from cancer or some other chronic, fatal disease. Usually the patient is elderly, although younger patients can also die from cancer or some congenital abnormality or defect. Usually, terminally ill patients know or strongly suspect that they are about to die. Most experience these four phases of emotional response to their impending death:

1. Denial: often the first response to the news of a fatal illness. Refusing to believe the doctors or assuming that "I'm going to beat this thing" is a common reaction.
2. Anger: often follows denial. The patient wonders and asks, "Why is this happening to me?" "What have I done to deserve this?" or "Why did you have to tell me?" A dying patient often has a hostile, angry attitude.

3. Depression: perhaps the most obvious and a very common response to the situation. The patient has no further interest in anything. The patient "turns to the wall" and refuses to participate in the activities of life.
4. Acceptance: ultimately the response of most terminally ill patients. They will come to accept the condition and try to go on as best they can for as long as they can.

The family usually goes through the same responses of denial, anger, depression, and acceptance. The EMT must realize that the family may be extremely hostile and demanding ("Do something! He's going to die!") or so accepting that they do not want any efforts at all to change the inevitable ("Let her die in peace").

The EMT is likely to experience the same feelings of helplessness and inadequacy that accompany the sudden death crisis. The sadness of the situation may be overwhelming, particularly if the dying patient is a young person. Or, again, defense mechanisms may take over, and the EMT may resent being called to see a patient for whom little or nothing can be done.

Management of Terminal Disease

There may be little to do for the terminally ill patient other than to be certain that the person is as comfortable as possible. The EMT should try to determine if the patient and the family are aware that death is approaching and if they are prepared for it. If death seems near, the family should be told. The EMT should point out to the family the signs (hypotension, unconsciousness, bradycardia) that indicate the gravity of the patient's condition. If the patient's status cannot be determined, the EMT must advise the family.

The patient should not be separated from the family. The EMT should keep familiar faces and voices around the patient and allow the family to be close in the last moments. The family and patient should be encouraged to talk about the imminent death and all allowed to maintain their dignity. In general, the patient should not die alone if there are family or friends nearby. If the patient is going to be transported to the hospital, the EMT should let one or two family members ride in the ambulance with the patient. The family may or may not want

to take the patient to the hospital. Transport to the hospital should be encouraged but, remember, patients cannot be transported to the hospital against their will. If the family strongly opposes transport, their wishes should be respected as well. If the patient is not going to be transported, the EMT should contact medical control for further specific directions in the care of the patient.

If cardiac arrest occurs, the EMT should institute resuscitation efforts unless a specific state or local protocol directs otherwise. In general, only a written order by a physician will permit an EMT *not* to resuscitate someone who has undergone a witnessed cardiac arrest.

Patients may have **living wills.** These are legal documents with specific instructions that the patient does not want to be resuscitated or to be kept alive by mechanical life support systems. The patient's wishes expressed in a living will should be respected. On occasion, a family member may disagree with the will's intent ("Grandpa was senile when he wrote that — go ahead and give him mouth-to-mouth respiration"). In such situations, medical control should be contacted for advice. States and communities have different laws for handling this situation. In general, the EMT will be directed to follow the patient's wishes. The patient should be allowed to make any statements, and the EMT should write them down. The laws in most states recognize that a statement by someone who knows he is dying may be accepted as a sworn statement in a court of law (a dying declaration). Sometimes patients who know they are dying want to relieve themselves of some long-held secret or other important information. The EMT should listen to these statements carefully and write them down word for word, as they may become very important to someone in the future.

To summarize, the dying patient should be made as physically comfortable as possible. Any wishes and concerns should be fully addressed so that the patient's last minutes can be passed in peace and dignity.

ABUSE CRISIS

Responding to Abuse

Abuse is one of the more unpleasant crises that the EMT will encounter. The exact incidence of abuse as a cause of injury is not known, but it is more frequent than commonly thought. Abuse is a crime. Thus, law enforcement agencies must and will become involved with the problem. Part of the EMT's responsibility, in addition to providing emergency care and transportation, is to cooperate with the law enforcement agencies. Many individuals who are responsible for a serious injury from abuse go free because there is not enough evidence to convict them of the crime. Sometimes evidence was present but was destroyed during the emergency care of the victim. The EMT should always bear in mind that abuse is a criminal act, and that some day testimony may be required in a court of law. That testimony may be an important factor in deciding that a criminal is convicted, *or* that an innocent person goes free.

Abuse may take many forms — beatings, burns, rape, or even attempted murder. Anyone may be the victim of abuse, although it is seen most often among family members. Patients who have been the victims of abuse may demonstrate any or all of several responses: Anger or outrage is often the first and most obvious reaction of an abuse victim. Sometimes this anger is directed at the EMT, the police, the government, or anyone else, including the person who caused the abuse. The abused person should be allowed to talk as a way to "ventilate" some of this anger. The EMT must not take personally any statements the abused patient makes. Anger is part of the natural reaction to this particularly stressful situation.

Disbelief often follows abuse, just as it often follows sudden death or the realization that someone is dying. It is also a natural reaction. The EMT must be careful not to get into an argument with the victim regarding the specific circumstances of the event. When questioned, the EMT should always be truthful: A straight question deserves a straight answer.

Withdrawal may be particularly apparent following rape or child abuse. The victim may say little, appear not to care, or not want anyone near. This patient needs to be convinced that the EMT is there to help. The EMT who in a calm, professional manner can convey a genuine desire to provide support is often successful in getting the victim to communicate. If an accurate or complete history cannot be obtained from the patient, the EMT should obtain information about the event from relatives, friends, or witnesses.

Hysteria may also occur in a victim following abuse. The patient may be screaming, crying, talk-

ing in unintelligible sentences, running up and down, and refusing all attempts of help. The EMT should try to calm the patient and "talk the patient down," as when dealing with someone with a drug overdose (see Chapter 35). Often the right friend or family member can assist in calming the patient. An EMT cannot forcibly transport or restrain anyone without a police order. Medical care cannot be forced on an abused patient who refuses treatment.

Depression often follows abuse. The victim becomes withdrawn and may show some of the same characteristics as with drug withdrawal. The depressed victim will give a sketchy history, will permit minimal examination and treatment, but will usually consent to transport to the hospital.

Management of Abuse

Regardless of the cause of abuse, the EMT's responsibilities are to provide proper emergency care, transport the victim to the hospital, and make sure the police can obtain the pertinent evidence about the case. If the victim is unconscious, the airway should be restored and the patient placed on a spine board. Particular attention should be directed at the airway in people who have been beaten about the head or face. The EMT should also look carefully for rib fractures and blunt abdominal injuries. Once all wounds are dressed and splinted, the patient should be transported promptly.

Obtaining pertinent evidence is an important responsibility of the EMT in cases of suspected abuse. Physical evidence of injury will be very critical to effective prosecution if legal remedies are sought at some later date. Although law enforcement agencies are responsible for collecting the physical evidence, the EMT can be of significant assistance. The EMT's efforts are directed toward maintaining the **chain of evidence,** which means carrying out the following protocol:

1. Do not move or touch anything at the scene unless it is necessary to do so for medical reasons.
2. Avoid touching or disturbing any item that might have been used as a weapon (knife, gun, broken bottle, or other implement).
3. Note if the patient's clothing has been torn, especially if it is necessary to cut away clothing to provide care for an injury.

4. Carefully note all injury sites.
5. Record a specific list of injuries when more than one is present.

The written record of the EMT's observations and treatment may be used in court at some future date to document the extent of injuries. Therefore, the EMT should carefully record all observations, the results of the patient examination, and a specific description of the treatment administered. Any statements made by the patient should be recorded word for word and in quotation marks. A detailed, accurate written record will be of far greater value in court than vague recollections of the incident months or years after it occurred. EMTs should always cooperate to the full extent with law enforcement officials at the scene. While their first priority is to provide medical care, EMTs also have a responsibility to maintain the chain of evidence and to remain aware of the legal implications in the case of abuse.

Victims of rape require significant emotional support in addition to the kind of care that abused patients receive. The EMT should look for and carefully record any objective evidence of abuse such as torn clothing, bruises, and other injuries. Often, evidence of beating will be seen about the patient's head and face. The patient's genitalia should not be examined unless there is obvious bleeding that will require a sterile dressing.

The EMT should enroll the assistance of a female EMT or police officer to help console the female rape patient. She should be treated gently and professionally. Never should the EMT criticize or condemn the rape victim, especially with comments such as "Don't you know that's a tough area?" or "Everyone knows the people you meet there are weird."

Some rape victims are withdrawn and others are hysterical. Medical control or a professional rape counseling service is a good source of advice on how best to manage these common reactions.

Most EMS systems have an established protocol for treating the rape victim. This protocol will include preserving the necessary evidence to prove that a rape took place. The EMT must work closely with local law enforcement agencies to maintain the chain of evidence. To do so, the EMT must make sure that the rape victim does not bathe, urinate, or douche before being examined at the hospital. If the vaginal

area is not cleaned, the chance of recovering sperm is increased. The recovered sperm can be analyzed and used later as evidence of rape in a court of law.

All patients who have been raped or claim to have been raped should be evaluated by a qualified physician in the emergency department. During transport, the EMT should provide comfort and emotional support.

CHILD ABUSE CRISIS

Responding to Child Abuse

Child abuse was once believed to occur rarely and then only in lower-income families and broken homes. Now, estimates are that 10 percent of all pediatric patients seen in emergency rooms are victims of child abuse. Over 15,000 cases are reported yearly in the United States, and some 5,000 children die each year from child abuse. Researchers do know a lot more about child abuse. For example, they know it occurs at all social and economic levels; some children come from good homes, some from broken homes. They know child abuse may be caused by a parent, an older brother or sister, a baby-sitter, or an acquaintance of a parent, particularly a single parent. They know that some cases of child abuse are obvious, and some are not. Finally, researchers know that child abuse is often progressive; the child is abused with greater and greater severity over a period of time and ultimately can die from the injuries.

Child abuse takes many different forms. Physical abuse includes beating, burning (often with a lighted cigarette), and immersion in hot water. Sexual abuse (**child molestation**) can occur in boys and girls. Emotional abuse, although more difficult to recognize, is another form of child abuse. Neglect (abandonment) may occur through inadequate provision of food or clothing. A combination of these abuses can prevent a child from gaining weight or growing properly, a condition described in medical terminology as the **failure to thrive.**

The EMT should suspect child abuse if any of the following circumstances exist:

1. If the history given does not fit the injury. For example, a fall from a chair will usually not be enough of an injury to cause a fracture of a femur in an otherwise normal child.

Nor will that same "fall" produce multiple contusions on a child's body.

2. If the history is vague or the person or persons who give the history say they didn't see the accident.
3. If the child is obviously malnourished.
4. If the child admits to having been beaten.
5. If the child is withdrawn or refuses to tell what happened.
6. If the child has multiple injuries that have occurred at different times, such as old bruises or healing burns in a child with a fresh injury (Figure 44.1).
7. If the child has unusual wounds, such as cigarette burns, particularly about the genitalia.
8. If you or one of your partners has been called to the same address before for injuries to the same child.

Management of Child Abuse

The EMT who suspects child abuse should try to convince the parent (or whoever called the emergency medical service) that the child should be taken to the hospital. The parent or caretaker can be told that a more thorough examination is necessary to provide better care for the child. It can be suggested that the child may have a severe injury that can only be diagnosed in the hospital. Never should the EMT accuse anyone of child abuse. A calm and professional approach must be maintained at all times.

With a case of suspected child abuse, the child should be transported to the hospital regardless of the apparent severity of the injuries. The first step in the treatment of child abuse is to remove the child from the environment that is producing the abuse. Hospital personnel can, if necessary, get a court order to admit the child. Of course, the EMT cannot transport the child to the hospital without the consent of the parent or legal guardian, regardless of how serious the injuries may be or how convinced the EMT is that the child is a victim of child abuse. Again, if the parent or guardian refuses to allow transport of the child, the EMT should stress the need for hospital evaluation. By emphasizing the need for x-rays, "blood tests," and other hospital studies to rule out serious injury, an alert EMT will frequently convince a responsible adult to consent to transport.

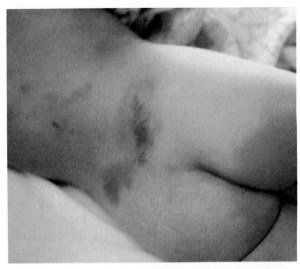

FIGURE 44.1 Old skin burns and multiple bruises that are apparent at the time of a fresh injury are signs that the patient may be an abused child.

All cases of suspected child abuse, whether the child was transported to the hospital or not, must be reported to the proper authorities. Any suspicion of abuse should always be reported to medical control. The law in every state requires all health care professionals to report suspected child abuse. The law also protects those who do report suspected child abuse from being sued by the person(s) whom they report. When transport to the hospital is denied, the hospital personnel will contact the police or the local department of human services to investigate. Child abuse is a very serious crime that could result in the child's being placed in a foster home if the judge believes that child abuse has occurred. People convicted of child abuse face severe punishment.

Dealing with suspected child abuse can be a very difficult emotional experience for the EMT. Perhaps the hardest part is keeping a calm, professional manner and refraining from judging or accusing anyone of child abuse. Such accusations must come from the law enforcement agencies and the courts.

SUICIDE CRISIS

Responding to Suicide

Not all suicide attempts are fatal; nevertheless, **suicide** is a significant cause of death in the United States. The EMT may be called to the scene of a suicide attempt by a family member, a friend, or even by the patient. As with other crises, the EMT's first responsibility is to provide the necessary emergency care. In addition, several special problems and considerations must be dealt with.

All suicide attempts must be taken seriously. There is always the possibility that the patient's efforts to commit suicide will be successful. Even if the call for help has come from the patient, the EMT should not assume the threat has passed and that the patient has given up on the idea. Statistics support the fact that the patient who attempts suicide once will attempt it again. Upon arriving at the scene of an attempted suicide, the EMT must never turn away from the patient or leave the patient alone, even for a few seconds.

Most patients who attempt suicide have a severe psychiatric illness. Many are suffering from alcoholism or depression. Some people will attempt suicide while under the influence of drugs. For many people, the underlying disease is treatable, and with proper treatment the patient will no longer be suicidal. However, until that treatment is carried out, the suicidal patient must be considered suicidal at all times. Most EMTs are not able to distinguish between a "gesture" for help and a serious suicide attempt that has failed. Therefore, all suicide attempts should be considered serious attempts. Anyone who has tried suicide will try it again if given the chance. The EMT must not provide that opportunity.

Management of Suicide

Patients may attempt suicide by ingesting poison, shooting themselves, jumping from a height, jumping in front of a speeding car or train, cutting their wrists or neck, or hanging, to name a few of the more common methods. When called to the scene of a suicide attempt, the EMT must first find out how it was attempted. If the person swallowed a bottle of pills, the bottle should be examined. Most of the time, it will contain a narcotic, a sedative, or a tranquilizer, which may have been prescribed by a physician or bought over the counter.

The EMT must be prepared to begin cardiopulmonary resuscitation, administer oxygen, and maintain the airway. The person may have serious injuries. For example, jumping from a height may have caused a spine fracture that will require moving the patient on a spine board. Obvious fractures should be splinted, and obvious wounds dressed.

Another problem occurs if the patient attempted suicide by more than one means — maybe swallowing a bottle of sedatives and then jumping out the window. Unconsciousness may be from a head injury or the sedatives *or both.* Patients who cut their wrists rarely bleed to death (**exsanguinate**) because the vessels involved are not that large. Often, however, they will have severely injured the median or ulnar nerves. And victims of self-inflicted gunshot wounds to the head may not have suffered fatal brain injury, but instead have sustained massive facial bleeding and airway obstruction.

The family of a suicide patient may need emotional support. Many ethnic groups consider suicide a sacrilege — something evil and against the will of God. The EMT must be careful not to judge the victim, the family, or the victim's lifestyle. A suicide attempt is often considered a "cry for help." The EMT should reassure the family that suicide results from psychiatric illness — that it is not the fault of the family or friends.

SUDDEN INFANT DEATH SYNDROME (SIDS)

Sudden infant death syndrome (SIDS) is one of the most severe and difficult crises to manage. It is often said that a family never fully recovers from the death of a child. SIDS occurs without warning in a healthy baby. The usual history is that the parents put the infant into the crib at night, and then found the baby unresponsive either later that night or the next morning. Approximately 7,000 infants, usually between the ages of 2 and 4 months of age, die each year this way.

The EMT who is called to the scene of a SIDS crisis will find *very* upset parents. However, the EMT must focus on the infant. Often it is a good idea for the EMT to begin resuscitation and transport the infant rapidly to the hospital, even if the infant appears to be dead. This response will assure the parents that everything possible has been done. If the baby is cold and stiff and has obviously been dead for several hours, resuscitation should not be undertaken. However, if there is any doubt, *or* if the parents insist, the EMT should go ahead with resuscitation efforts.

The EMT must be careful not to raise the hopes of the parents; instead, they should be kept informed and reassured that everything possible is being done to revive the infant. The EMT may be tempted to reassure the family that everything will be all right, but if the infant is surely dead, then, sadly, everything will *not* be all right. Therefore, any reassurance must be aimed at convincing the family that everything possible is being done and that they will have to wait until hospital personnel can give a more definite statement. The parents usually want to ride in the ambulance with their baby, and they should be allowed to do so.

Sometimes the EMT is not sure if the problem is SIDS or child abuse. There are several clues to distinguish these two problems. SIDS almost always occurs in infants between 2 and 4 months old, while child abuse can occur at any age. The characteristic feature of SIDS is that there are no marks on the infant, while an abused baby will usually have scars, bruises, or obvious deformities. A dead SIDS baby may have frothy sputum on the nose and mouth and **dependent lividity** (blood settling in the skin of the back or abdomen). In other words, the SIDS baby will show evidence of a quiet death, not a violent one. Any siblings are likely to be healthy appearing. An infant who has died from child abuse will look malnourished; so will the siblings. The typical history of SIDS is that the baby was perfectly healthy when put to bed. The initial examination will support this: The baby looks like a normal, well-fed baby. On the other hand, the abused baby's family will often give a confused, unclear history that does not fit the infant's injuries.

Even if suspicious of child abuse, the EMT should never accuse the parents. Instead, sympathy for their tragedy should be extended. The EMT must do all that is possible for the infant and the family. After bringing them to the hospital, however, the EMT should report any suspicion of child abuse to the emergency department personnel. (SIDS and child abuse are also discussed in Chapter 37.)

THE EMT'S RESPONSE TO STRESS

As a health care professional, the EMT has chosen a most stressful career. Life and death crises occur almost daily, and sometimes there is little to do to alter the effects of serious illness or injury. One of the most common problems in the health care field is excessive emotional involvement with patients and their problems. It is natural and appropriate for EMTs to care about the people they are helping, but excessive emotional involvement may hinder their ability to carry out emergency care effectively and objectively. EMTs must strive at all times to keep a balance between sympathetic concern and emotional involvement. Another potential problem for EMTs following a life and death crisis is that they may be criticized unfairly by a patient, the family, the community, or even by co-workers. It is very frustrating to hear criticism that is based on inaccurate information or sensationalism.

EMTs are vulnerable to the stresses of this professional life; therefore, they must learn to recognize the symptoms of stress so that it does not interfere with their work or life away from work, including family life. The signs and symptoms of chronic stress may not be obvious at first, as they may be subtle and not present all of the time. The following may indicate the presence of excessive stress:

1. Irritability
2. Lack of enthusiasm (apathy)
3. Chronic fatigue
4. Feelings of not being appreciated
5. Difficulty sleeping
6. Excessive drinking
7. Drug usage
8. Decreased social activities
9. Change in appetite
10. Desire to quit work
11. Physical complaints (headache, gastrointestinal upset)
12. Rigid thinking

Any of these symptoms may indicate chronic stress. EMTs should recognize them as such and take steps to relieve their cause. Concerns should be discussed with co-workers, many of whom will have had similar experiences. Such discussions may be enough to resolve the problem once the EMT realizes how common are some of these symptoms. Persistent and severe symptoms may require professional guidance from a counselor within the EMS system, a physician, or a member of the clergy. Early recognition of chronic stress problems is most important because a solution is much easier to achieve with early recognition. Persistent problems tend to increase in scope and complexity, making a solution much more difficult.

YOU ARE THE EMT...

1. You are at the home of a terminally ill elderly woman. She is unconscious and is experiencing hypotension and bradycardia. Her husband wants to let her die in peace, in her own home. Her two daughters want their mother transported immediately. How will you proceed?

2. You are treating a woman who has been badly beaten by her husband or boyfriend — you are not sure what their relationship is. Prepare a written report of what you might have observed. Include what is necessary to maintain the chain of evidence.

3. You suspect you are dealing with a serious child abuse case, and even though the toddler does not have life-threatening injuries, you want to transport him to the hospital. The parents "know you know" and are saying their child is fine and that you can go now. Write down what you will say to convince them to let you transport the boy.

4. Review the signs and symptoms of chronic stress on page 459. Choose one or two that you recognize as accompanying stressful situations in your life and describe how you know they relate to stress and what you do to alleviate the problem.

PATIENT HANDLING AND EXTRICATION

45

Patient Handling and Triage

OVERVIEW

The safe handling and extrication of patients, whether they are found on the highway, at home, or in the workplace, presents the EMT with a broad spectrum of challenges. The handling of patients falls into two broad categories. The first is patients who are found in a readily accessible location. No matter how serious their injuries, they can be moved rather routinely from the home, building site, sidewalk, street, or wherever they are located. The second category is patients who must be extricated, or removed, from a location of difficult access, with possible danger to the rescuer as well as to the patient. The patient's injuries may or may not be serious, but removing such patients from their precarious situations may require special techniques and tools of extrication (see Chapter 46).

Chapter 45 begins with the basics of handling patients with communicable diseases, pediatric patients, geriatric patients, and handicapped patients. Then, the techniques of lifting and moving patients, transferring them to a stretcher, and utilizing specialized packaging techniques are described. The next section discusses ancillary patient-handling equipment, including spine boards and scoop stretchers. The last section of Chapter 45 is about triage — the concept of sorting patients and allocating resources in a disaster.

OBJECTIVES

The objectives of Chapter 45 are to

- understand the basics of patient handling and the specifics of handling patients with communicable diseases, pediatric patients, geriatric patients, and handicapped patients.
- learn how to lift and move patients safely from one location to another.
- learn how to use a standard ambulance stretcher.
- become familiar with special patient packaging techniques and ancillary patient-handling equipment.
- understand the concept of triage and the duties of a triage officer.

BASIC PATIENT HANDLING

After the safety of the patient and rescuer has been assured and the scene is "secured," attention must be directed toward immediate life-threatening medical conditions. The patient's airway must be opened, breathing ensured, and major bleeding controlled. While the procedures and protocols for the actual techniques of patient extrication and transfer have been relatively well defined (see Chapter 46), less attention has been paid to the medical aspects of entrapment and extrication. In the zeal to free, treat, and transport the patient, the ABCs of basic life support must not be forgotten once the safety of all concerned has been assured. If advanced life support personnel are available, intravenous lines sometimes need to be placed prior to beginning extrication and transfer procedures. Carrying out emergency medical management procedures may be very difficult and sometimes impossible. It is in these situations that EMTs have to be creative in rendering emergency medical care, keeping in mind their duty to do no further harm. After on-scene emergency medical care has been completed, the ill or injured patient must be transferred to a stretcher or other carrying device, positioned properly, covered as necessary, and securely strapped to the stretcher. This whole process is called **packaging** the patient. The stretcher or carrying device should be placed as close as possible to the patient before the transfer, to keep the distance the patient needs to be moved as short as possible. Every attempt should be made to minimize patient movement during transfer to the stretcher. Placing the patient on a long spine board or a scoop stretcher will allow the easiest transfer to the ambulance stretcher, the emergency department stretcher, or an x-ray table, with minimal movement or risk of aggravating the patient's condition.

Except during the infrequent situation in which the life of the EMT or patient is in danger, movement of the ill and injured patient should be orderly, planned, and unhurried. This approach will protect the patient from further injury and reduce the risk of aggravating the original condition. For the most part, such movement will consist of transferring the patient from a bed, the floor, or the ground to an ambulance stretcher. The transfer should be carried out by at least two EMTs, with bystanders used for assistance as necessary. These recruits must be instructed simply, but in detail, as to their role before actual patient movement is carried out. Such movement involves lifting, lowering, pulling, and supporting both patient and equipment. If any of these tasks is conducted improperly, discomfort and additional injury may result to both the patient and rescuers. One of the main goals in planning the transfer should be to eliminate or reduce the need for additional movement of the patient after the transfer is completed. The trauma patient should be placed on a long board or scoop stretcher with an antishock garment in place, ready to be applied if necessary (Figure 45.1).

The only time the patient should be moved prior to completion of the initial care, assessment, stabilization, and treatment is when the patient's or EMT's life is in immediate danger. This would be the case if the victim was in a burning building, if toxic fumes were present, or if the EMT was unable to administer the needed emergency medical care due to the location or position of the patient. The objective of every patient-handling situation is to ensure that the victim and the rescuer do not sustain additional injury during the rescue.

Patient packaging and handling are technical skills that are learned and perfected through practice and training. The only way EMTs can be sure of utilizing the best technique for a particular situation is to practice continually the various skills listed in the text. After each patient transfer has been completed, the EMTs should evaluate the appropriateness of the actual techniques used as well as their technical skills in completing the techniques.

The overriding objective for each rescue/transfer is to complete it as safely and as efficiently as possi-

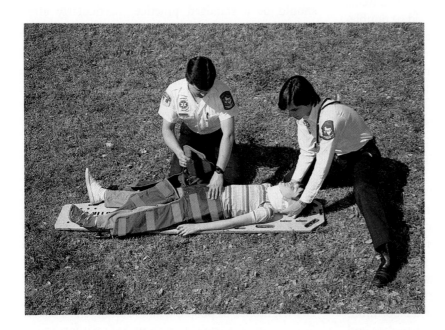

FIGURE 45.1 All seriously injured patients should be transported on a spine board with an antishock garment in place ready for prompt application and inflation should the patient develop hypotension.

ble. As rescuers, EMTs must consider the use of their body and their skills. The outcome of a rescue is frequently determined by an EMT's ability to provide the needed care. Therefore, it is important that the rescuer utilize good body mechanics, practice size-up and patient-packaging and transportation skills, and understand safe versus risky patient transfer/transport techniques.

Handling Patients with Communicable Diseases

For emphasis, and to dispel concerns due to lack of knowledge, some points in the handling of patients with communicable diseases previously covered in Chapter 34 will be repeated here. Several guidelines can be used when caring for potentially infected patients. The following guidelines should decrease the risk to the EMT and to other patients who are cared for by the EMT on separate, subsequent rescue incidents:

1. Use disposable, one-time-only equipment and supplies. Reusable equipment must be cleaned and disinfected after use by each patient.
2. Thoroughly wash hands between each patient. Friction and an antibacterial soap, such as a hexachlorophene soap, are excellent tools in decreasing the spread of germs.
3. Dispose of all infected or contaminated items properly. Disposable items should be double-bagged and thrown away in an appropriate waste container. Wash reusable equipment, such as a bag-valve mask, airway, scissors, splints, cervical collars, and cots, with a clean cloth and a disinfectant soap. Small equipment, such as the bag-valve itself, should be autoclaved. If mattresses or cots become contaminated, follow the washing with air/sun drying.
4. Bathe and launder all clothing after exposure to patients with a known communicable disease. At the end of each day, bathe and change clothes even if exposure has not knowingly occurred. Clothing should be washed in hot, soapy water and dried in a warm dryer. A clean uniform should be worn each day.
5. Maintain your own health at an optimum level, keeping immunizations up to date and participating regularly in an individualized exercise program.

When it is known in advance that a patient has a communicable disease, preventive measures can, to a great extent, protect the EMT and the ambulance from contamination. Precautions that can be taken include the following:

1. Wear clean coveralls set aside for the purpose of handling patients with known infections.
2. Wear a surgical mask and, better still, place one on the patient.
3. Remove all but the needed basic equipment from the ambulance prior to the run.
4. Use disposable equipment whenever possible (for example, gloves and bed linen).
5. Isolate the patient by wrapping wounds in clean/sterile bandages and sheets.
6. On termination of the run, double-bag the coveralls and turn them in for decontamination. Clean and disinfect the ambulance. Shower immediately.

In view of the prevalence of some communicable diseases in the general population and in the patient groups often cared for by prehospital personnel, EMTs are well advised to wear disposable gloves when there is a risk of coming in contact with the patient's body fluids and secretions, particularly blood, vomitus, and feces. Frequent hand washing should be a standard practice, particularly after handling any patient or equipment that has been used on or by a patient. All EMS systems should have medical policies and procedures relating to the protection of field personnel against disease. These should include recommended immunization levels and booster (reimmunization) intervals and postexposure precautions and treatment recommendations for all EMTs who might have come in contact with an infected patient.

Handling Pediatric Patients

Children who require transport come in all sizes and shapes. Most are lighter than a typical adult, and most have smaller body parts. They are generally easier to move. Few are able to tell you much about how they feel or where they hurt, and most are usually frightened of people who are strangers. For this last reason, it is important to include parents in the

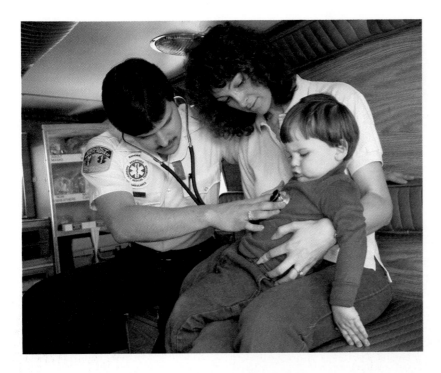

FIGURE 45.2 When evaluating children, it is sometimes necessary to change the assessment routine because of the child's fear. Here the EMT is listening for breath sounds, leaving the child's shirt in place.

care and transportation of children. The reassurance of a familiar face does wonders for increasing cooperation and safety when dealing with the pediatric patient. Sometimes the assessment routine must be changed slightly until the EMT has gained the confidence of the child (Figure 45.2).

Because most transport equipment is designed for the adult-sized body, children need to be securely strapped on the stretcher and observed continuously, so that their safety is not compromised (Figure 45.3). Another important factor in handling children is the tendency for them to lose body heat rapidly due to their relatively larger body surface area. This means that the younger the child, the more rapidly the EMT should cover the child as a protection against the elements. If it is extremely cold, putting a hat or cover on the child's head will help decrease loss of body heat.

Handling Geriatric Patients

The older patient often has special needs when being transported. For example, many older persons are very slow and deliberate in their movements. They may have decreased vision and hearing, along with slower general body movement. They are at greater risk for secondary injury. Older patients, especially women, frequently have a condition called osteoporosis, which causes their bones to be very brittle and easily fractured. The EMT needs to be aware of these limitations when providing care and assistance. In addition, the EMT must remember to speak clearly and directly to the older patient, carefully explaining everything that is being done. By maintaining a reassuring and calm attitude rather than abruptness and impatience, the EMT can care for the geriatric patient successfully.

Handling Handicapped Patients

Increasingly, more and more people with physical handicaps are living in the community. These people may be at increased risk for injury due to their decreased mobility. They must be handled with special care and all the protection available. Some may be at increased risk for pathologic fractures due to the handicap. The person who has muscle contractures or fused joints must be moved and stabilized in a position that suits and supports these deformities. This patient must be adequately restrained on the stretcher or in the wheelchair before being moved. The EMT who has a patient with an expressive communication disorder accompanying some neurologic conditions should try communicating using written messages, a word board, or signaling with pantomime. Talking slowly, simply, and

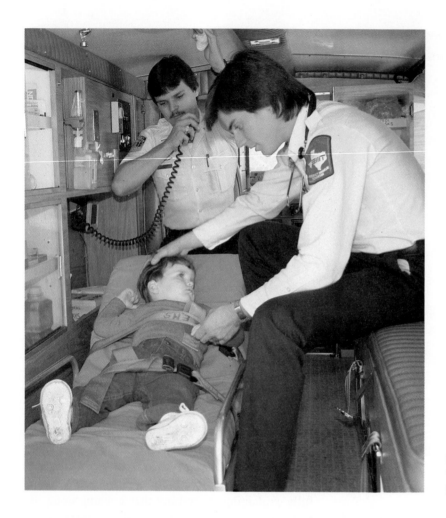

FIGURE 45.3 Children must be well secured to the stretcher designed to transport larger patients.

directly toward this patient may also help. Handicapped patients deserve all the care and respect of any other injured patient, plus some special assistance.

LIFTING AND MOVING PATIENTS

Body Mechanics

Moving a patient from one location to another requires a definite plan. Just as one mentally organizes for work each day, the EMT needs to have a strategy, thought out ahead of time, for packaging and transporting the patient. Part of the planning includes knowledge of the EMT's limitations and the availability of resources. Assistive devices and equipment such as stretchers, blankets, straps, splints, and so forth should be used whenever possible. The rescue should be accomplished without undue risk or compromise to the EMT's health. Dead or injured EMTs cannot save lives. Among several elements that need to be considered when planning for the packaging and transfer of a patient are the following:

1. The patient's problem, including the actual and potential threats to the person's health and safety.
2. The environmental risks and limitations that may compromise the safety of the patient, you, or your fellow EMTs.
3. The availability of assistive equipment and/or manpower at the scene.
4. Your own physical and technical capabilities and limitations, as well as those of your colleagues. If you have a weak or injured wrist, do not overstress the wrist and risk additional injury that could compromise the patient's safety.

When actually performing a patient transfer, the following principles of good lifting mechanics should be used:

1. Only lift a patient whom you cannot roll, push, or pull.
2. Work with your limbs close to your body so that your center of gravity is not malaligned and your muscles are not overstressed.
3. Use the longest and strongest available muscle groups (biceps, quadriceps, and gluteals) when moving patients. Maximum efficiency of contraction occurs when the muscle smoothly contracts at a moderate rate.
4. Flex your body at the knees and hips to keep your back straight when working below knuckle height. Try to avoid bending at the waist to lift.
5. Establish a firm support base by placing both feet flat on the ground, with one foot slightly in front of the other.
6. Distribute the patient's weight evenly over both of your feet.
7. Straighten your knees as you lift to help ensure that the major lifting forces will be provided by the thigh and buttocks muscles.
8. Hold your abdomen firm when you lift and tuck in the buttocks, keeping the shoulders aligned over the spine and pelvis.
9. Use pivoting movements rather than rotating or twisting actions when changing direction. Keep your shoulders square over your pelvis if possible.
10. Keep your head erect and move in a smooth, coordinated manner. Sudden, jerky movements tend to overstress muscles, resulting in injury.
11. Only lift weights you can comfortably handle. Weight maximums are individualized, based on age, sex, muscle mass, and condition.
12. Walk slowly, using coordinated movements. Steps should not be longer or wider than shoulder width when carrying a patient or stretcher.
13. Whenever possible, move forward rather than backward to facilitate normal balance and smoothness of movement.
14. Use assistive equipment whenever it is available. Use it properly, making sure that it is in good working order before using it during a rescue.

The patient's transfer and transportation are not complete until the patient is safely delivered to the hospital. Restraining straps must be used and appropriately placed whenever the patient is being moved. All those helping to move the patient must know how the transfer is planned and what their specific duties are. This coordination of movements will aid in a rapid, efficient patient transfer.

After the patient is safely delivered to the emergency department, the EMTs must begin preparing for their next rescue effort. They should review the positive points that occurred during the transport. Then they should discuss adaptations or changes that would improve the management of the next patient. This review and evaluation process helps clarify procedures that need revision, identifies equipment that needs repair, and demonstrates skills that are in need of review or retraining. Most important, a critical review assists in the development of more confident and better skilled EMTs.

Emergency One-Person Rescue Techniques

When prompt patient movement is necessary because of a life-threatening hazard and only one EMT is on the scene, one-person rescue techniques for moving patients to a safe area must be utilized. For example, an EMT might have to act alone to remove a patient from a fire, a smoke-filled or contaminated area, or a building in danger of collapse. It must be emphasized that these are emergency transfer methods only. They are difficult and should not be used if there is time to obtain adequate assistance. The EMT must also be aware that entrance to a hazardous environment such as a smoke-contaminated area requires protective equipment, including a self-contained breathing unit. EMTs should *not* attempt any rescue that poses a danger to themselves without proper training in the use of a self-contained breathing apparatus and protective equipment. Likewise, an incident scene is *not* the time or the place for such training. The drag, carry, and lift techniques for one-person rescue are illustrated in Figures 45.4 through 45.10.

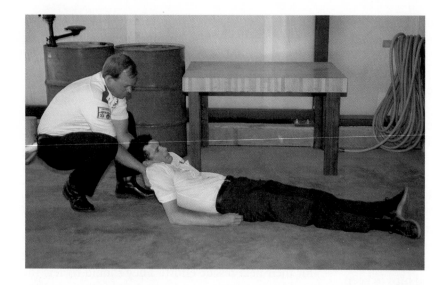

FIGURE 45.4   The fireman's drag. The rescuer supports the patient's upper body weight on his shoulders and upper arms. Balance and weight transfer is best achieved by the rescuer keeping his head up and arms straight.

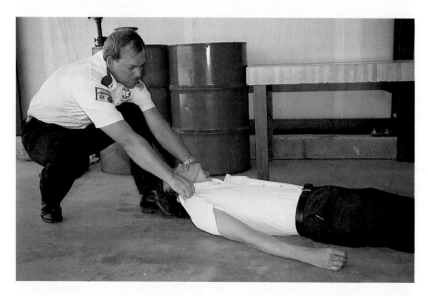

FIGURE 45.5   The clothes drag. The rescuer must pull with the long axis of the patient's body. The rescuer can achieve the strongest pull using his leg and back muscles and keeping his arms straight.

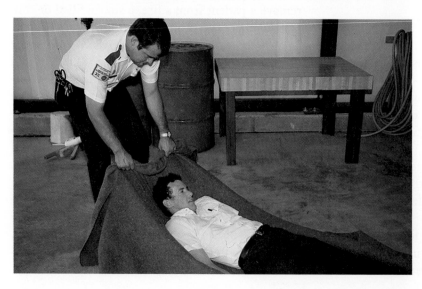

FIGURE 45.6   The blanket drag. The rescuer can reduce friction by using a blanket to drag the patient. The strongest pull is achieved using the leg and back muscles while keeping the arms straight. The blanket should encompass the body. It will provide some protection and support for the head, neck, and extremities.

A

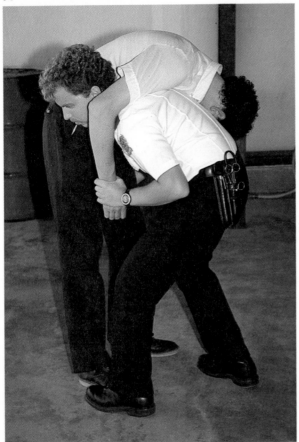

B

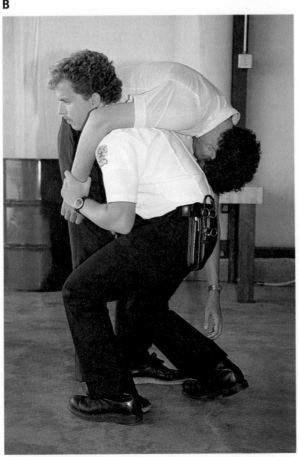

C

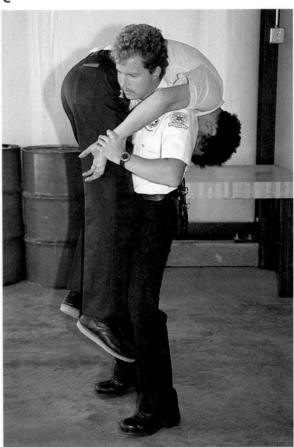

FIGURE 45.7 The fireman's carry. (a) Balance and weight transfer are best achieved by drawing the patient's upper torso across the rescuer's shoulders. (b) At the same time, the rescuer bends at his knees, to bring his hips under the patient's hips. (c) The rescuer should lift with his legs, keeping his feet apart for stability. Be alert to loss of balance due to sudden weight shifts.

FIGURE 45.8 (photo right) The front cradle. The rescuer bears considerable weight on his arms, shoulders, and back. The best balance and weight transfer is achieved by the rescuer bending at the hips and knees, using the legs for lifting. Leaning the patient's upper torso slightly back against the rescuer's arm may be helpful. Because the forward centered weight of the patient is in his arms, the EMT must be careful to maintain his balance while moving with the patient.

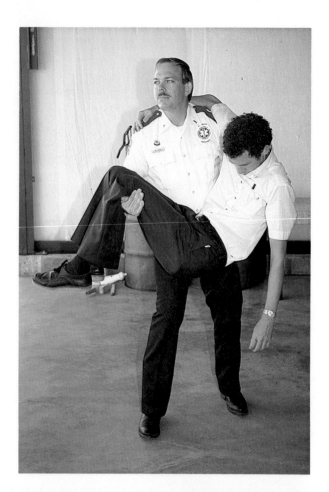

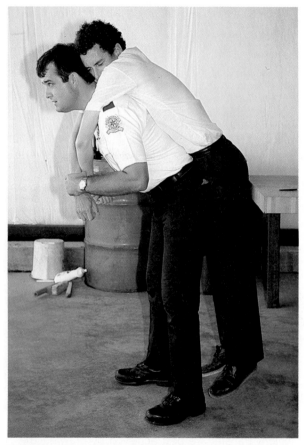

FIGURE 45.9 The pack strap. The rescuer bears the majority of the patient's weight along his spine, into his legs. Weight transfer is best achieved by the rescuer bending at his knees and hips and lifting with his legs. The rescuer must be alert to the position of the patient's legs to protect against tripping.

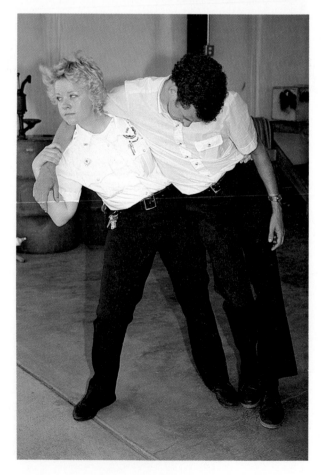

FIGURE 45.10 (photo right) The side crutch support. The patient bears most of his own body weight. The rescuer supports a portion of the patient's weight only on demand. The rescuer must be alert to the patient's loss of balance and subsequent sudden weight shift. The rescuer should stand on the side opposite the injury.

A

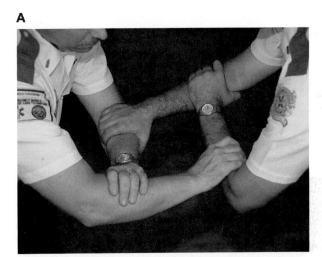

B

Emergency Two-Person Rescue Techniques

When two rescuers are available, both should work to remove the patient from danger using one of the techniques illustrated in Figures 45.11 through 45.13.

A

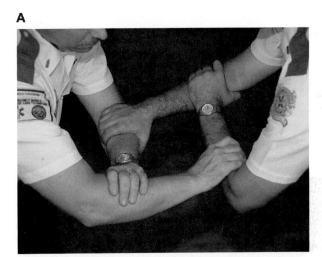

B

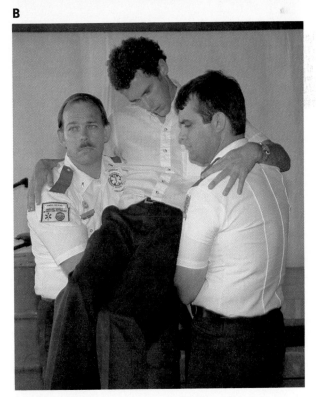

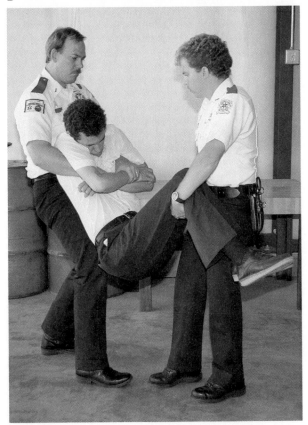

FIGURE 45.11 The extremity lift and carry. (a) Both rescuers must coordinate their movements through direct, verbal commands. The patient's hands should be crossed over his chest and grasped by the rescuer's arms coming through the axillae. (b) Balance and lifting are best achieved by the rescuers bending at their hips and knees, using their legs for lifting. The patient may experience a degree of discomfort in this position due to increased pressure against the thoracic cavity.

FIGURE 45.12 The seat (chair) lift and carry. (a) Two EMTs grasp each others forearms as illustrated. (b) Balance and lifting are accomplished by both rescuers bending at the hips and knees to use their legs for lifting.

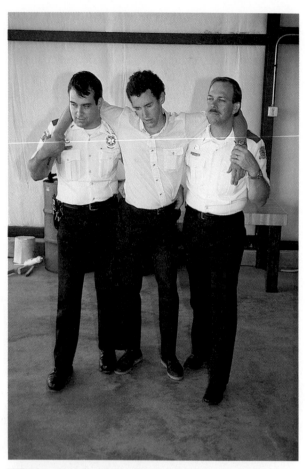

FIGURE 45.13 The side crutch support. The patient will bear a substantial portion of his own weight. The rescuers support a portion of the patient's weight on demand. The rescuers must be alert to the patient's loss of balance and sudden weight shift.

Patient Movement Under Stable Conditions

Figures 45.14 and 45.15 illustrate methods of moving patients when conditions are stable and adequate manpower can be recruited.

A

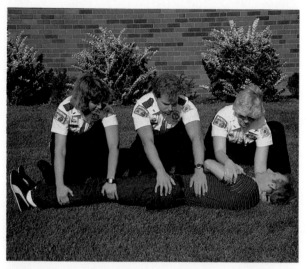

B

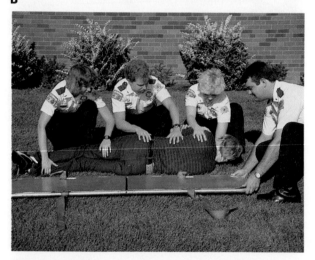

FIGURE 45.14 Log roll with no cervical injury. (a) Coordination of movement during the log roll is achieved through direct, verbal commands. Positioning the hands on the far side of the patient increases leverage for the three rescuers. (b) Weight control is best achieved through a smooth, coordinated pull using the rescuers' body weight and shoulder and back muscles to pull. The rescuers should concentrate their pull on the heavier portions of the patient's body.

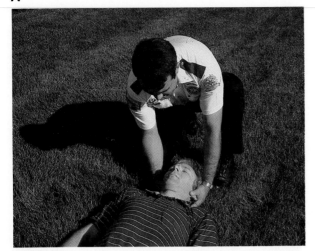

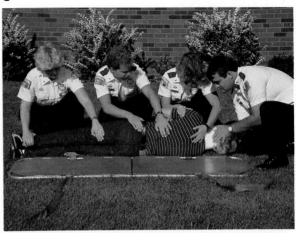

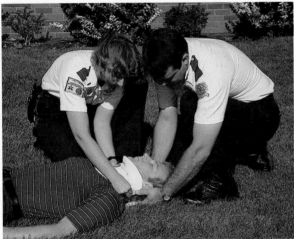

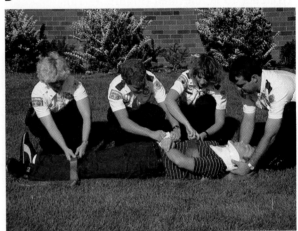

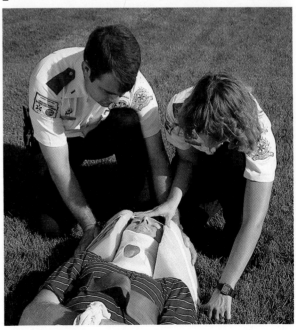

FIGURE 45.15   Log roll when cervical support is required. (a) In cases of suspected spine injuries, immediate gentle longitudinal support is applied to the cervical spine. (b) A cervical or extrication collar should be applied before the patient is moved. Cervical support must be maintained until the patient is secured on a spine board or equivalent, and the head and neck are stabilized and secured. (c) The rescuer supporting the head and cervical spine is responsible for coordinating the log-roll procedure through direct, verbal commands. Positioning the hands on the far side of the patient increases leverage for the rescuers. Weight control is best achieved through a smooth, coordinated pull using the rescuers' body weight and shoulder and back muscles. The rescuers should concentrate pull on the heavier portions of the patient's body. The spine board is positioned as close as possible to the patient's body. (d) The patient is then slowly and gently rolled back onto the spine board and secured. (e) A small pad is placed behind the occiput to prevent hyperextension of the cervical spine. The head and neck are then secured to the spine board using foam blocks, sand bags, or a blanket roll. Straps may be placed over the forehead, but should never be placed around the chin to avoid airway management difficulties.

STRETCHERS

The standard ambulance stretcher has wheels and either a fixed or adjustable height. Attached handles are used for lifting and rolling. Side bars and restraint straps secure the patient. The stretcher should have a reasonably comfortable mattress. A good way to carry the short spine board is to place it beneath the mattress at the head of the stretcher. The board is then immediately available for extrication or for providing a firm surface on which to perform external cardiac compressions (when placed between the patient and the mattress). In medical emergencies such as angina or dyspnea, the short board generally will not have to be removed to allow the head of the stretcher to be elevated (Figure 45.16).

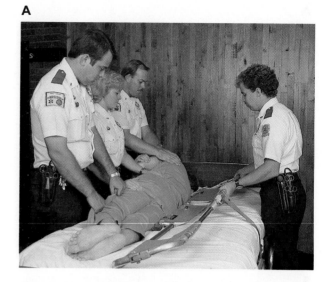

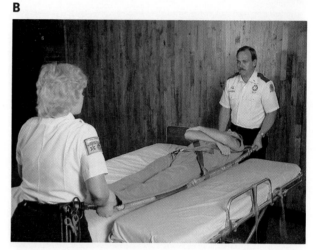

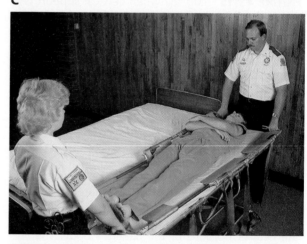

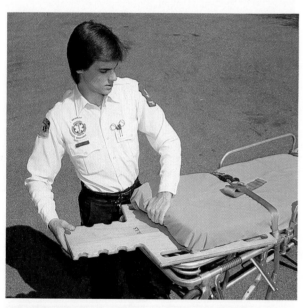

FIGURE 45.16 A short spine board should be placed beneath the mattress at the head of the stretcher to facilitate CPR.

The techniques for transferring and lifting patients to the stretcher are illustrated in Figures 45.17 through 45.21. A chair-to-wheelchair transfer is described in Figure 45.22. The proper methods of lifting, moving, and loading stretchers are shown in Figures 45.23 through 45.27.

FIGURE 45.17 Bed-to-stretcher transfers. (a) The patient is log-rolled onto the break-away stretcher. The stretcher is then positioned parallel to the bed and locked or held in position. (b) The patient is then transferred from the bed onto the stretcher. (c) The break-away stretcher may then be removed if desired. The weight transfer is best achieved by the rescuers keeping their arms extended close to their bodies, while keeping their heads up and backs straight.

A

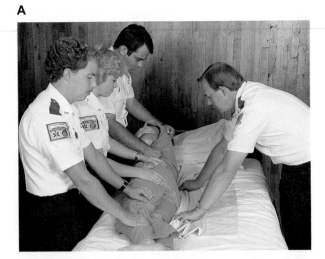

B

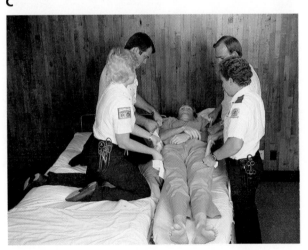

C

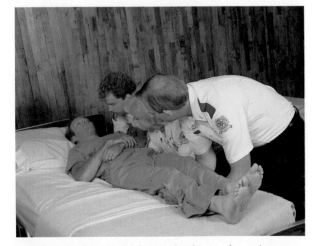

FIGURE 45.18 Bed-to-stretcher transfer using a drawsheet. (a) The patient is log-rolled onto a fan folded draw sheet. (b) The stretcher is brought in parallel to the bed and secured. The patient is pulled gently to the edge of the bed. (c) The patient is then transferred to the stretcher. Weight transfer is best achieved by the rescuers using their shoulders, upper body weight, and back muscles to pull. The stretcher may roll if it is not secured during the patient transfer.

A

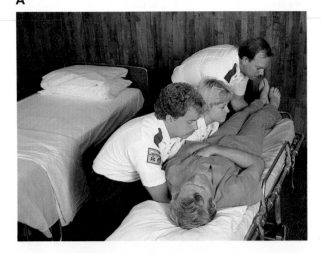

B

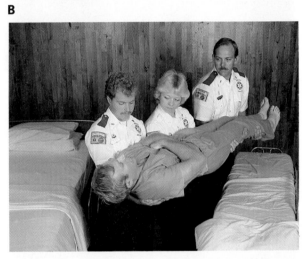

C

FIGURE 45.19 Stretcher-to-bed transfer using a three-person lift. (a) The stretcher is brought in parallel to the bed with the patient's feet facing toward the head of the bed. The stretcher should be secured to keep it from rolling. The patient is then lifted from the stretcher in a smooth, coordinated fashion. (b) The patient is slowly "walked around" into the appropriate position over the bed. (c) The patient is slowly and gently lowered into the bed.

475

A

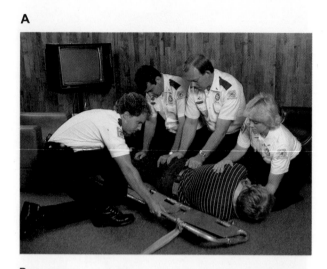

A

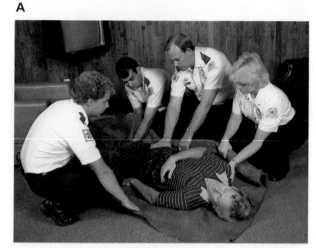

B

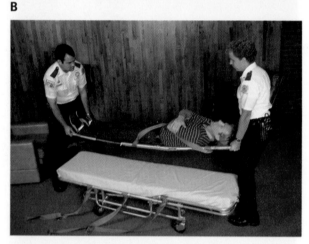

B

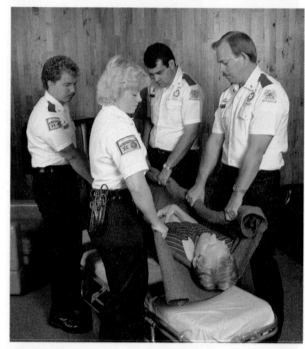

C

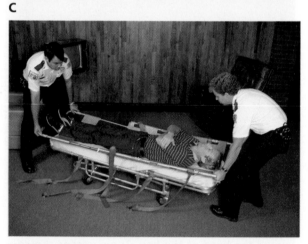

FIGURE 45.21 Floor-to-stretcher transfer using a blanket. (a) The patient is log-rolled onto a blanket. (b) Using the blanket, the rescuers gently lift the patient from the floor onto the stretcher. The stretcher should be secured so that it does not roll during the transfer.

FIGURE 45.20 Floor-to-stretcher transfer. (a) The patient is log-rolled onto a long spine board or a scoop stretcher. (b) Then the patient is transferred to the stretcher. The best weight transfer is achieved by the rescuers bending at the hips and knees and using their legs to lift. (c) The scoop stretcher may then be removed if desired.

A

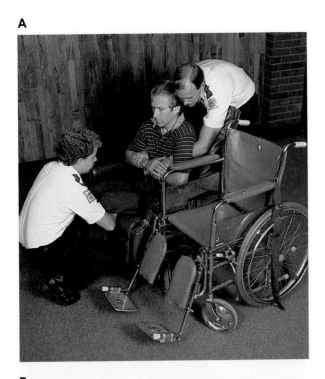

B

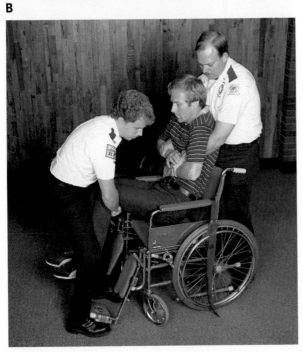

A

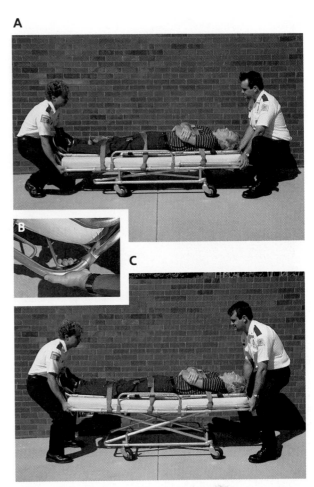

D

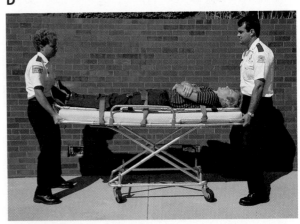

FIGURE 45.22 Chair-to-wheelchair transfer. (a) The EMT who is positioned behind the patient brings his arms through the patient's axillae and grasps the patient's crossed arms. The second EMT grasps the patient's legs at the knees. (b) The patient is then gently lifted into the wheelchair, which must be secured to prevent it from rolling away. Transfers from a wheelchair to a chair or stretcher can be made in a similar fashion.

FIGURE 45.23 Raising the stretcher with a patient. (a) The rescuers must coordinate the lift with direct, verbal commands. Hips and knees should be bent and the arms held extended, with the back as straight as possible. (b) The release mechanism at the foot of the bed is activated. (c) The lift should be a smooth straightening of the legs. (d) The rescuers may lift both ends or both sides of the stretcher simultaneously.

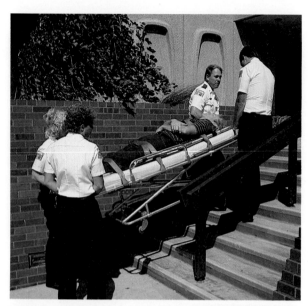

FIGURE 45.24 Ascending or descending stairs with a loaded stretcher. The rescuers must coordinate their moves with direct, verbal commands. The patient must be *well secured* with straps and other immobilizing devices. If the stretcher must be tipped on end, the patient's hips must be secured to keep him from slipping downward. The stretcher should be kept as level as possible. If there is a single rescuer on the lower end, he should be backed up by a watcher with a steadying hand.

A

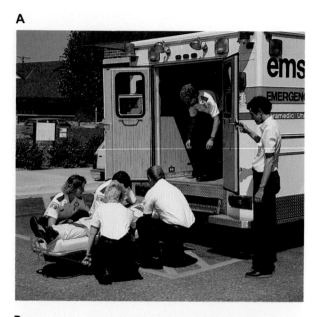

B

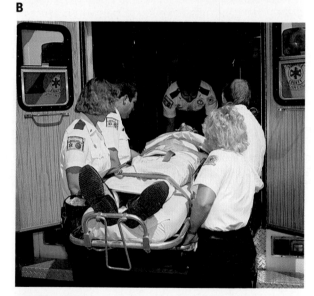

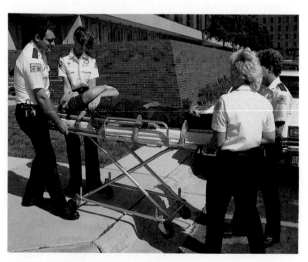

FIGURE 45.25 Moving the stretcher over obstacles. On firm surfaces, it is usually easiest to maneuver the stretcher in the elevated position. When an obstacle such as a curb or firehose is encountered, the stretcher should be lifted over the obstacle while keeping it as level as possible.

FIGURE 45.26 Loading a multi-level stretcher into the ambulance. (a) The rescuers must coordinate their moves with direct, verbal commands. The stretcher must be locked into its lowest position. There must be an open pathway to the ambulance, and the ambulance doors must be secured in the open position. The rescuers should position themselves around the sides of the stretcher, with their feet sufficiently apart to give a stable base.
(b) Bending at the hip and knees with their backs and arms straight, the rescuers smoothly complete the lift using the legs and stop. On a second command, the stretcher is moved into the ambulance. If sufficient manpower is available, it is best to have at least two rescuers on each side of the stretcher and another inside the ambulance to guide the stretcher into position.

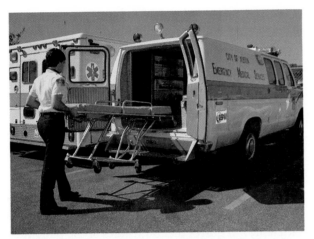

FIGURE 45.27 Loading a "Knockdown" stretcher into the ambulance. The stretcher is brought up to the rear entrance to the ambulance. With the wheels in the ambulance, the stretcher is allowed to collapse as it is pushed into the patient compartment of the ambulance and secured. A second attendant should lift the undercarriage up to meet the bed frame.

SPECIAL PATIENT-PACKAGING TECHNIQUES

Certain unusual circumstances will necessitate specialized packaging of the patient. Some of these techniques are illustrated in Figures 45.28 through 45.32.

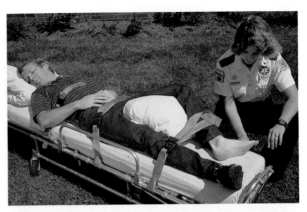

FIGURE 45.29 Packaging techniques for the patient with a dislocated hip. The patient is placed in a position of comfort, and pillows or rolled blankets are added as needed to support the injured extremity.

A

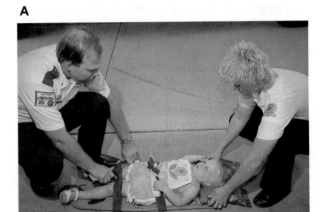

B

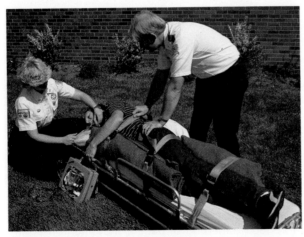

FIGURE 45.28 Packaging techniques for the unconscious patient, lateral position. The patient is placed on his side. The base of support is broadened using pillows or rolled blankets to support the flexed extremities, the head, and the back.

FIGURE 45.30 Packaging techniques for pediatric patients. (a) The standard ambulance stretcher and equipment are often not appropriately sized for children and must be adapted for the pediatric patient — for example, a short spine board can be used as a long board. (b) Equipment sized for pediatric patients should be used when available.

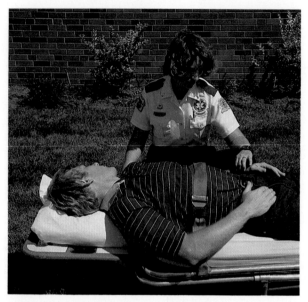

FIGURE 45.31 Packaging techniques for the too-tall patient (or overhanging equipment). Extending the standard ambulance stretcher with a short spine board may prove effective for the extra-tall patient. Place the spine board at the head end of the stretcher to allow rear doors of the ambulance to close.

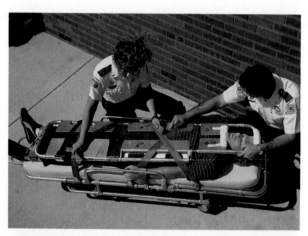

FIGURE 45.32 Packaging techniques for the combative patient. A scoop stretcher secured over the combative patient is one option to protect both the patient and the EMT.

ANCILLARY PATIENT-HANDLING EQUIPMENT

Special skills are required to use the equipment described in this section. All of this equipment will be very useful to the EMT in stabilizing and transporting patients. EMTs must master the skills necessary for its use. A stair chair is illustrated in Figure 45.33. Figure 45.34 illustrates management of the wheelchair patient.

Another important piece of ancillary patient-handling equipment is the **split-frame** or **scoop stretcher** (Robinson, Green, Sarole, etc.). Although efficient, it requires that both sides of the patient be accessible. Unlike a long spine board, it cannot be slipped under the patient in the long axis of the body. Scoop stretchers are narrow, well constructed, compact for storage, and have excellent body support

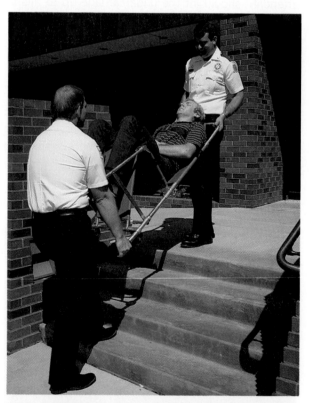

FIGURE 45.33 A stair chair. Sturdy straight-back chairs or a commercial stair chair may be used as an effective method of patient movement in a narrow corridor, small elevator, or a steep stairwell where other methods are not available. The patient must be *well secured* to the chair. The EMTs must communicate with each other and the patient continuously to coordinate movements.

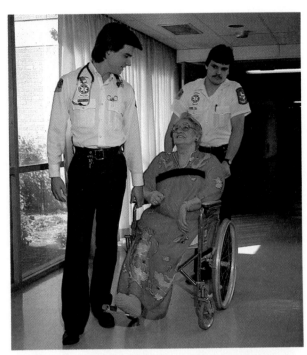

FIGURE 45.34 Wheelchairs, when available, provide easy management of the patient. The patient should be *well secured* in the wheelchair. At least two EMTs should manage the wheelchair patient — one in front and one behind. Movement should be as smooth as possible without sudden jerks or maneuvers.

features; however, they are insufficient for spinal injury immobilization. Considerable practice is required to maintain proficiency in the use of scoop stretchers. The EMT must be careful if using a scoop stretcher in cold environments, as heat conduction from the body is significantly greater than on a regular stretcher because the patient's back is exposed.

"Scooping" a patient requires special attention to the closure area beneath the patient. The stretcher may trap clothing, body tissue, or other objects. As with the long spine board, complete, full body stabilization and securing of the patient are essential for good patient care. Scoop stretchers are illustrated in Figure 45.35 on page 482.

TRIAGE

So far, this chapter on patient handling has limited itself to situations involving only one patient. The EMT will frequently encounter situations in which there are two or more patients. The circumstances may range from an auto accident with two victims to a natural disaster such as a tornado with dozens of injured or dying patients. A disaster cannot be defined simply by the number of injured. It is best defined as any incident that will overload the capabilities and resources of the local medical community. In such situations, the concept of triage comes into play. **Triage** is a French word meaning to pick, sort, or choose. With multiple patients, it describes the process of sorting patients and allocating resources according to a system of priorities. Triage is a continuing process that is directed by the most highly trained medical individual at the scene of the incident or disaster.

The first EMT on the scene is responsible for beginning the triage process and contacting the dispatch center for additional equipment and personnel. It is better to overmobilize and later cancel responding units than to come up short-handed. This EMT then surveys the scene by making the first triage round and determining the number of victims who require priority medical treatment based on the familiar "ABCs." The EMT also notifies the dispatch center of the number of victims so that area hospitals can be alerted. Having assumed the initial duties of the triage officer, this first EMT should not become involved in patient care, but rather assign assistants to handle such duties.

Patients who are obviously dead or have such devastating injuries that they are unlikely to survive are bypassed during the initial round of triage. Although it seems cruel and uncaring, these patients must be left untended if there are limited personnel and resources to treat the people who can be saved. A trauma scoring system similar to the modified **CRAMS** (circulation, respiratory, abdomen, motor, speech) **scale** of Clemmer (Table 45.1) can be used to determine the probability of survival. The cardinal rule of triage is to do the *greatest good for the greatest number*. Patients whose injuries are not an immediate threat to their airway, breathing, or circulation are also bypassed on the first round of triage.

In the meantime, other rescuers should have arrived and will be unloading equipment and supplies and establishing a triage area. The triage officer will continue triage rounds in the triage area. As more experienced medical personnel arrive, the initial triage officer may relinquish his or her duties, but

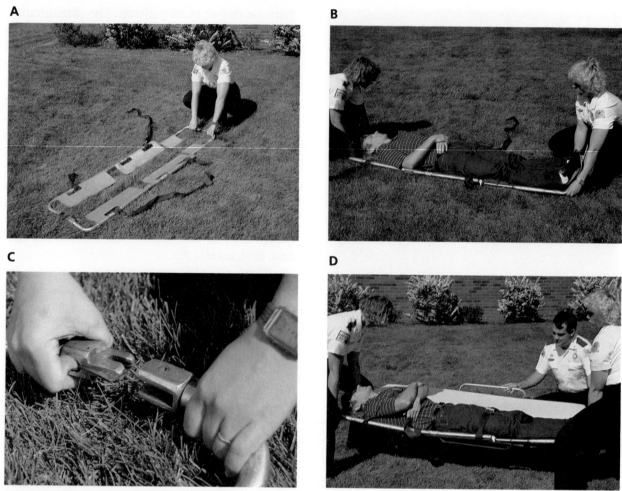

FIGURE 45.35 The split-frame or scoop stretcher. (a) To apply a scoop stretcher, it is first separated lengthwise. (b) The two halves are then slid under the patient from each side. Pinching of the patient or catching clothing between the stretcher's halves may be prevented if the patient is gently lifted by his clothes as the halves are closed. (c) The locking brackets or knobs are latched and checked to make sure they are secure. (d) The patient is now loaded on the scoop stretcher and is ready to be transferred to the wheeled litter. Once the scoop stretcher is beneath the patient and he is secured by straps, the patient may be picked up in the same position in which he was found. He may be moved down narrow stairs without fear of slipping, even if the stretcher must be tipped sideways or tilted as much as 10 to 15 degrees. If the stretcher must be tipped on end, the patient's hips should be secured to prevent him from slipping downward.

not before giving an oral briefing to the party assuming the duties of the triage officer. The briefing should be brief and succinct. It must include the number of injured and a rough estimate of the severity of their injuries. The steps that have been taken regarding triage and treatment must be reported, and requests for additional personnel and supplies made.

If any patients have been transported, the new triage officer must know their number, the severity of their injuries, and to what medical facilities they were transported.

During the second round of triage, those patients who require more definitive care for airway, breathing, and/or circulation problems are identified, and

TABLE 45.1   CRAMS Scale

Circulation 2—Normal cap. refill and BP > 100 mm Hg systolic 1—Delayed cap. refill or BP 85–99 mm Hg systolic 0—No cap. refill or BP < 85 mm Hg systolic
Respiration 2—Normal 1—Abnormal (labored, shallow, or rate > 35) 0—Absent
Abdomen 2—Abdomen and thorax not tender 1—Abdomen or thorax tender 0—Abdomen rigid, thorax flail, or deep penetrating 　　injury to either chest or abdomen
Motor 2—Normal (obeys commands) 1—Responds only to pain—no posturing 0—Postures or no response
Speech 2—Normal (oriented) 1—Confused or inappropriate 0—No or unintelligible sounds
＿＿＿ Total CRAMS score (add the five areas)

Note: The CRAMS Score for trauma patients is determined by adding the scores from the five body areas. A score of 6 or less indicates a critically injured patient. (Clemmer, et al., *J. Trauma* 25(3): 188–191, Mar. 1985.)

preparations are begun for priority transport. The second rule of triage is that *preservation of life takes precedence over preservation of limbs.* The third round of triage begins after immediate life-threatening conditions have been controlled. Secondary injuries such as spine injuries, major or open fractures, burns, and abdominal trauma are identified and stabilized. This round of triage is similar to the secondary assessment phase of the patient examination.

Triage rounds continue until all patients have been treated and transported. Patients must be evaluated during these continuing rounds of triage for any deterioration in their condition that might elevate their priority for treatment and transportation. The triage officer must maintain a record of all patients, their medical priority status, and to which medical facility they have been taken. The triage officer should try to allocate patients, based on number and severity, among local medical facilities to mini-

mize the overload on any one facility. These record-keeping and allocation duties may be delegated, but the ultimate responsibility comes back to the triage officer. If the magnitude of the situation warrants, the triage officer may designate a communications officer to control and direct radio traffic to free the triage officer for other duties. In a major disaster, a medical triage officer may be responsible for patient care and an incident commander may be responsible for all support services.

A variety of systems are used to identify patients and treatment priorities. EMTs must become familiar with the system used in their locale. All the systems are based on the four following basic categories of patient treatment priority and injury severity. Patients with certain conditions or injuries are granted priority for treatment and transportation over others:

1. Lowest priority: dead or impending death. These are patients who are deceased or have such devastating injuries that they have little chance for survival. If resources are limited, these patients must be ignored to enable the resources to be used on "salvageable" patients.

2. Highest priority: immediate care and transportation. These patients must be treated first at the scene and then transported as soon as possible. They will have one or more of the following problems:

   airway and breathing difficulties
   cardiac arrest
   exsanguinating hemorrhage
   open chest or abdominal wounds
   severe head injuries or head injuries with
   　　decreasing levels of consciousness
   major or complicated burns
   tension pneumothorax
   pericardial tamponade
   impending shock
   complicating severe medical problems: poisonings, diabetes with complications, cardiac disease, pregnancy

3. Intermediate priority: treatment and transportation can be delayed temporarily. These patients are likely to have injuries such as the following:

burns without complications
back injuries with or without spinal injuries
major, open, or multiple fractures
eye injuries
stable abdominal injuries

4. Delayed or low priority ("the walking wounded"): treatment and transportation can be delayed until last. These patients will have fractures and sprains, lacerations, soft tissue injuries, and other lesser injuries.

There is a separate category of triage for patients who have suffered radiation contamination and who are themselves carrying radiation particles. This category supersedes all others. Contaminated patients *must* be segregated immediately as an initial step. They must not be allowed to contaminate other patients, the EMTs, ambulances, or hospitals. A discussion of radiation injury management is found in Chapter 39.

Triage, like other EMT skills, must be practiced to maintain proficiency. Disaster drills should be run at least yearly, preferably in conjunction with local hospitals and other public safety and rescue units. Disaster plans must be developed and practiced in advance of need. The mass confusion of a disaster site is no time to experiment with organization.

YOU ARE THE EMT...

1. In what ways is handling a geriatric patient the same as handling a pediatric patient? In what ways is it different?
2. What are some of the factors you must consider before attempting a one-person rescue?
3. Describe the differences between a standard stretcher and a scoop stretcher. Under what conditions are each best utilized?
4. Identify the resources available in your community that could be utilized in a disaster. Divide these resources into those who would respond to the scene and facilities that would receive the injured.

Extrication and Rescue

46

OVERVIEW

Rescue, by definition, means to free from the danger of death or destruction by prompt, vigorous action. One aspect of rescue is extrication, a method of freeing patients from that which binds or restrains them, by means of force, ingenuity, or both. Extrication may range from simply opening a car door to gain access to the patient to a complex situation involving multiple patients such as a passenger train derailment or the collapse of a building. In between are many emergency situations, such as fires, cave-ins, water accidents, farm machine injuries, and snowmobiling accidents, that require the use of extrication skills.

Because of the specialized skills and equipment needed for complex extrication work, the EMT is not supposed to be an expert in every aspect of rescue and extrication; nor will this chapter attempt to cover the total field. Furthermore, in many areas of the country, the extrication phase of a rescue is under the control of specialized rescue units, usually attached to the local fire department.

Chapter 46 begins with an explanation of how rescue operations are classified. Then the eight principles of extrication are presented. Next, extrication techniques and tools are described, with a focus on vehicle entrapment, the most common extrication problem the EMT will encounter. Preparing the patient for transfer to an ambulance follows. The last section of Chapter 46 is on specialized rescue, which includes rescue in rough terrain, water, cold weather, and ice, and urban rescue.

OBJECTIVES

The objectives of Chapter 46 are to

- see how rescue operations are classified.
- identify the eight principles of extrication.
- become familiar with extrication techniques and tools.
- learn how to prepare and package a patient for removal to an ambulance.
- know what is required of specialized rescue in rough terrain, water, cold weather, ice, and in an urban setting.

CLASSIFICATION OF RESCUE OPERATIONS

Light rescue involves the transfer of injured patients from uncomplicated motor vehicle accidents and from stable buildings. Light rescue is the simplest to carry out and generally is handled with a minimum of equipment. For the most part, the EMT will be involved in rescue and extrication activities that fall in the category of light rescue.

Even if a rescue vehicle accompanies the ambulance on every accident run, light (basic) rescue tools should be standard equipment on all ambulances, whether in rural, suburban, or urban service. Every EMT must be trained in the use of this extrication equipment. Multiple vehicle accidents that

require simultaneous patient access or delay of the rescue vehicle by traffic or a breakdown are sufficient reasons to require light rescue equipment to be carried on all ambulances. The element of time is so critical in life-threatening situations that waiting for the arrival of basic extrication tools and equipment cannot be tolerated. But even in such situations, EMTs must not attempt extrications beyond their training and expertise.

Medium rescue involves specialized equipment normally found on a rescue vehicle. Medium rescue implies the use of rigging, A-frames, and tripods for patient access and transport. Medium rescue also involves the use of extrication tools for disentanglement of the patient.

Heavy rescue may include complicated rigging, patient handling under extremely difficult or adverse conditions, breaching of walls, disimpaction of vehicles, and all types of rescue involving buildings with major structural damage.

Incidents involving medium and heavy rescue usually involve the fire department rescue squad, and the fire department will receive the initial call. Under protocol in many areas of the country, the EMT uses light extrication skills and equipment to gain access to the patient to provide emergency medical care, while the rescue squad provides the extrication capabilities for disimpaction and disentanglement of the patient.

In disaster situations with multiple patients, the following four phases of rescue operations should be established. These phases are distinct and different from the usual medical triage priorities and apply only to the extrication operations.

1. Remove lightly pinned casualties — those who can be freed by lifting a beam or removing a small amount of debris.
2. Remove those patients who are trapped in more difficult circumstances but who can still be rescued by use of the equipment at hand in a minimum amount of time.
3. Remove those patients who require an extended time commitment for a difficult extraction. Such rescue may involve cutting through floors, breaching walls, removing large amounts of debris, or cutting through an expanse of metal. An example would be removing a worker from under a large piece of machinery.
4. Locate and remove those who have died.

During all phases of rescue and extrication operations, the primary responsibilities of the EMT are to provide emergency medical care to the patient and to prevent further injury to the patient or others. Although occasionally there are too few personnel to begin the routine of patient care immediately, this is the exception rather than the rule. Usually, far too many people are involved in the extrication process; some are of little use, and others may be dangerous to themselves and others when placed in such uncontrolled and anxiety-provoking situations.

The most evident problem in rescue situations involving several medical and rescue units is the lack of identifiable leadership at the scene and the accompanying disorganized provision of care. It is essential that one person be in charge of the overall rescue operation. This person must be medically trained and qualified to judge the priorities of patient care. This person has to assume responsibility for the overall management of the extrication process, as well as the details of patient care. It is best to reach an agreement on the protocol of assigning this responsibility in advance.

PRINCIPLES OF EXTRICATION

Although no two accident situations will be identical, the following basic principles of extrication apply to all rescue situations:

1. Evaluate the situation (size-up).
2. Provide for the safety of rescue personnel and the patient.
3. Secure the scene.
4. Gain access to the patient.
5. Provide emergency medical care.
6. Disentangle the patient.
7. Prepare the patient for transfer.
8. Transfer the patient.

Ingenuity, common sense, and a basic knowledge of mechanics will solve most extrication problems. All EMTs should enhance their basic training through additional workshops and courses, as well as with practice sessions on wrecked vehicles at the local junk yard.

Evaluation of the Situation (Size-up)

Size-up is a term used by firefighters that means to gather rapidly the facts about the situation, analyze the problem, and decide how to handle it. Size-up differs from triage in that it involves all aspects of the situation, including the type, severity, and location of the incident, the environmental conditions and hazards, the equipment and manpower resources, and the number of victims and their medical condition. Selection of the extrication procedures is based on decisions made during size-up. Size-up must be a continuing evaluation of the situation throughout extrication, since new problems may arise that demand alterations in the extrication process.

A few of the frequently conflicting factors the EMT must anticipate and evaluate during size-up are provided in order to stimulate thought and discussion. The list is not complete; nor is it meant to serve as a checklist.

1. Is the patient located in a building with stairwells that will require a special litter? Is there an elevator in the building? Will the ambulance stretcher fit in the elevator?

2. Is there a fire involved? The presence of a fire complicates the extrication process by altering the available methods of patient removal and provision of emergency medical care.

3. If a vehicle is involved, is it stable? All unstable vehicles must be stabilized before entry is attempted. This is one of the reasons why shoring blocks and ropes are standard ambulance equipment. Some services have installed towing hooks on their vehicles to provide a rapid method of securing an unstable vehicle.

4. Is the vehicle right-side up, upside down, or lying on its side?

5. Is the patient hanging from a seatbelt, or lying crammed under the dash and up against the firewall?

6. Are there objects protruding from the vehicle that must be removed before entry can be accomplished?

7. Is the equipment necessary for extrication available on the ambulance? Will specialized equipment and personnel be required?

8. Are all patients accounted for? A "head count" must be routine in the questioning of patients. Ideally, such questions should be directed at the least injured patients.

9. Are there hazards present, such as spilled gas, downed electrical wires, or hazardous materials, that could endanger the patient or the rescue personnel?

Safety of Rescue Personnel and the Patient

EMTs are frequently called on to undertake rescue and extrication activities at dangerous locations. A prime consideration for the EMT should be the avoidance of personal injury and prevention of further injury to the patient. To be successful in this endeavor, the EMT must be properly prepared and equipped before the call comes in. Special equipment should be worn or be available for the protection of the EMT.

Safety of Rescue Personnel

All EMTs should wear sturdy shoes or workboots while on duty. Glass and sharp metal are frequently encountered at accident scenes. A rescuer with a lacerated foot only complicates the whole incident.

In cool environments, polypropylene long underwear provides warmth even when it is wet or when the EMT is perspiring. During the cooler months, EMTs may be uncomfortable sitting around in "longies" waiting for a call, but at an accident scene, they can cool down very rapidly, especially if they have to stay in one position for an extended period during a prolonged extrication. A stocking cap or other hat will significantly decrease the loss of body heat. Hypothermia is as dangerous for the rescuer as for the patient.

A pair of leather gloves should be worn by all rescue personnel to protect their hands during the rescue and extrication process. Handling ropes, broken glass, hot or cold objects, or sharp metal can be dangerous to the unprotected rescuer.

A **hard hat** or protective helmet is very useful, both for identification of rescue personnel and personal safety (Figure 46.1). The hard hat is designed to

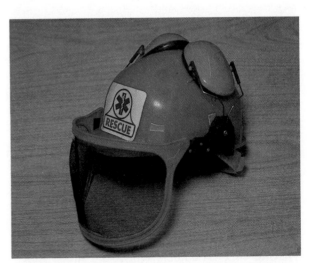

FIGURE 46.1 A hard hat is an essential piece of protective equipment during any rescue activity.

protect against fixed objects, as well as light missiles such as falling rock or flying glass. Some services like the hard hat used by lumberjacks and tree trimmers because it has a fine metal mesh face guard to protect the face from branches or small flying objects. Because the face mask is mesh rather than plexiglass, it does not fog up in cold weather and seems to provide good visibility in the rain. The helmet also has ear protectors that provide some protection from the high decibel sound levels of portable power units that are used for the extrication equipment or machines found in a heavy industrial environment.

A hand-held **strobe light** may help the EMTs keep track of each other in a crowd or in rural or wilderness locations (Figure 46.2). When working along the highway, the EMTs can hook these lights to their belts or attach them to their upper arm to provide additional visibility to oncoming vehicles. Strobe lights are lightweight, quite durable, and readily visible at night at a distance of approximately 1 mile.

Safety of the Patient

While gaining access to the patient and during disentanglement, great care must be exercised to avoid further injury to the patient. This is the time when extrication tools and equipment are closest to the patient. The EMT should cover the patient with a heavy, nonflammable blanket to protect against flying glass or other missiles (Figure 46.3). The EMT

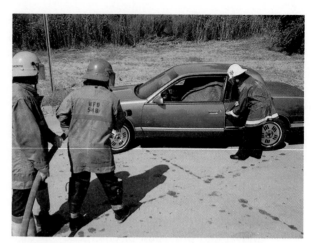

FIGURE 46.3 During extrication, the patient should always be covered with a heavy, nonflammable blanket to protect from further injury.

who is maintaining traction or providing other care during the extrication should be covered with the blanket as well. A short spine board may also be used as a protective shield. Heat, noise, and force should be kept to the minimum required to extricate the patient safely.

Securing the Scene

One of the most common environmental hazards is spilled gasoline, which must be washed down at the scene of an incident. If gasoline or other flammable material is present, a fire crew with charged hoses should be standing by during the rescue and extrication process. The EMT should make sure that the vehicle ignition is turned off and the key removed at any accident scene.

Hazardous materials, sometimes in tremendous quantities, are transported over our highways and railways each year. The release of these agents by an accident may endanger the lives of all those nearby. Vehicles transporting such material are usually marked with warning signs. When responding to such incidents, the EMTs who can identify the hazardous cargo from outside the danger zone may save their own lives as well as the lives of other EMTs and rescue personnel. Carrying a pair of binoculars in the ambulance may allow the EMT to observe the scene from a distance (see Chapter 40).

Downed electrical wires are another significant potential danger to the EMT and the patient. The utility company must be notified of any downed or

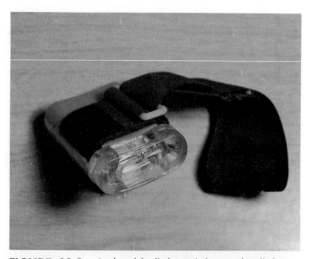

FIGURE 46.2 A durable lightweight strobe light provides increased visibility of the EMT in many situations.

sagging wires at once. When informed that an accident involves a utility pole, the dispatcher should inquire about downed or dangling wires and notify the utility company if wires are damaged. *EMTs must not attempt to deal with downed power lines.* EMTs must also be extremely alert to the lethal potential of standing in water in the area of downed power lines.

Environmental hazards include adverse conditions such as collapsed buildings or mine shafts, temperature extremes with risk of hypothermia or hyperthermia, and dangerous locales, such as a freeway off-ramp at rush hour. Ingenuity and resourcefulness are the only recommendations for handling such situations.

Poor visibility at the rescue scene can be a serious problem. It is impossible to work in the dark or with inadequate lighting. However, there is no excuse for inadequate lighting. Each ambulance must be equipped with sufficient stand-up flashlights, as well as sufficient floodlights, to provide adequate lighting at a distance from the ambulance.

Finally, bystanders, relatives, and others can pose significant hazards to themselves and the overall management of the incident. They must be controlled by the police or other personnel at the scene. Occasionally, a bystander, particularly one with some medical credentials, may be difficult to manage. This situation is always challenging. All services are advised to have a protocol for dealing with this potential problem. Many states provide wallet-sized copies of licensure to physicians for use as identification, although, unfortunately, not all physicians are as well versed in field emergency medical care as is desirable. Communication between medical control and the doctor at the scene may eliminate some of these problems. The EMT may also find it helpful to assign the individual particular duties that provide minimal actual involvement in the rescue process, yet occupy the eager volunteer. This will reduce the potential of confrontation and tension which direct attention away from the primary goal of patient management.

Gaining Access to the Patient

Gaining access to the patient depends on the type of incident — for example, the location and position of the vehicle, the damage to the vehicle, and the position of the patient. The means of gaining access to the patient must take into account the patient's injuries and their severity. The chosen means of access may have to be changed during the course of the extrication as the nature or severity of the patient's injuries becomes apparent.

Occasionally, it is necessary to extricate an injured patient rapidly from a threatening environment, or to position the patient in an environment more conducive to performing CPR and other basic life support measures. The technique illustrated in Figure 46.4 will allow adequate manual immobilization of the injured spine, thorax, and extremities as long as a sufficient number of hands are available to support the injured body parts. The use of this technique is indicated only in those instances when there is a fire or high probability of fire; when the patient has rapidly deteriorating or no vital signs, requiring the rapid initiation of resuscitation techniques such as airway management, ventilation, CPR, or the management of shock with pneumatic antishock trousers; or when the position of the vehicle poses a significant hazard to the life of the EMT or the patient. This technique should not be used if there is enough time to stabilize the patient with appropriate immobilization devices. There are two key elements to the successful use of this emergency extrication technique: (1) an adequate number of people must be available to stabilize all of the patient's injuries, and (2) the lead EMT must coordinate the activities of all rescuers to ensure that the patient moves as a unit.

Figure 46.5 illustrates the technique of rapidly removing a patient, if there is no danger of a cervical injury, using a special rope sling. Again, this procedure is for emergency removal only.

Providing Emergency Medical Care

Providing emergency care is the same for the entrapped patient as for any other. Initial priority goes to the ABCs, followed by more definitive care as required. The EMT must remember that for cardiopulmonary resuscitation to be effective, the patient must be supine on a hard, flat surface. The patient should be placed on a long or short spine board and external cardiac compression begun as soon as the patient is removed from the vehicle. External cardiac compression is not effective when the patient is in a sitting position or on the soft seat of an automobile.

FIGURE 46.4 Emergency patient removal. (a) With the patient seated, EMT A gets behind the patient and positions the head in a neutral, in-line position, with gentle longitudinal traction. (b) EMT B performs a rapid primary assessment. An extrication collar is applied to help stabilize the cervical spine. (c) Meanwhile, EMT C has placed a long spine board on the stretcher. With the door opened as wide as possible, the stretcher is positioned as close to the seat as possible. Stretcher height is adjusted if necessary. (If there is a possibility that the pneumatic antishock trousers will be needed, they should be laid out on the spine board at this point so that the patient may be transferred directly from the car into the trousers.) (d) EMTs B and C then slide the spine board onto the car seat. The edge of the spine board should be just under the patient's buttocks and thigh. (e) EMT B stands as close to the rear of the door opening as possible, with arms extended and hands perpendicular to the arms. (f) EMT B reaches into the door opening and places one hand on each side of the patient's head, maintaining the neutral position and longitudinal traction on the cervical spine. (g) EMT A then moves into position alongside the patient, placing his arms under the patient's legs just above the knees. (h) While another rescuer stabilizes the stretcher and the spine board to prevent movement, EMT C places one hand in the patient's armpit. (i) EMT C places his other hand behind the patient's back to provide support in the mid-thorax. (It is best if EMT C can stand on the side of the stretcher opposite EMT B as illustrated. If there is inadequate room, EMT C may stand behind EMT B and reach between EMT B and the car to stabilize the mid-thorax.) (j) While EMT B maintains neutral, longitudinal traction, EMT A, controlling the patient's legs, and EMT C, controlling the patient's back, rotate the patient in a sitting position as a unit until lined up with the spine board. (k) Moving the patient as a unit, EMT A lifts the patient's legs, as EMTs B and C lower the patient onto the backboard, maintaining the sitting position. EMT B must continue to maintain neutral, longitudinal traction during this movement. (l) The patient is then gently slid up the spine board as a unit 6 to 12 inches at a time, as EMT B maintains neutral, longitudinal traction.

(Procedure continued on page 492.)

A

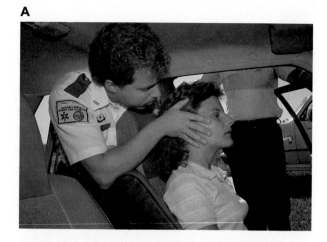

B

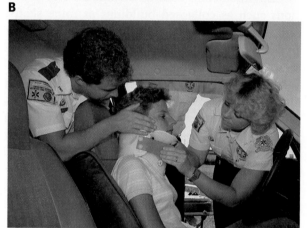

C

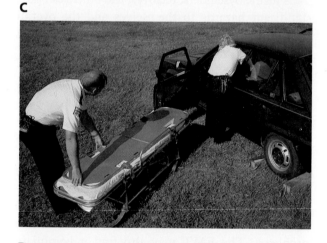

D

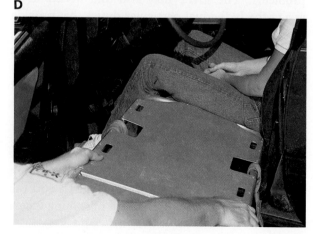

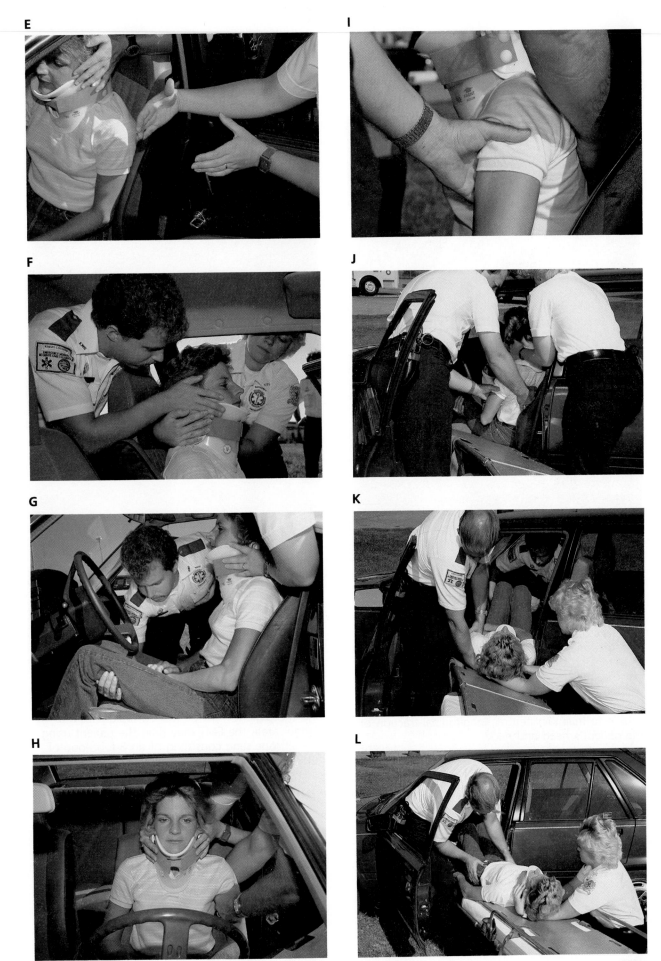

E

F

G

H

I

J

K

L

491

M

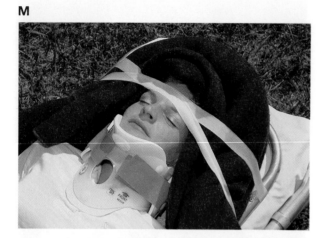

N

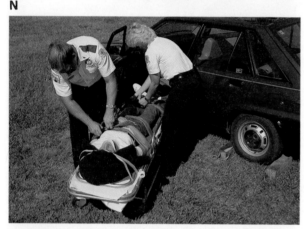

A

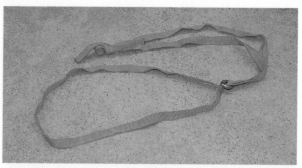

B

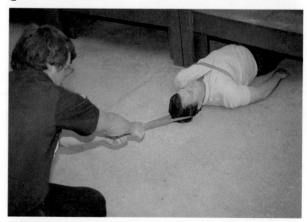

C

FIGURE 46.4 *(continued)* (m) The head and cervical spine are then stabilized with a blanket roll, foam blocks, or sandbags. (n) The patient is secured to the stretcher and may be moved to a less hazardous area where basic life support measures may be instituted. If the patient cannot be extricated through his door, he may be rotated out through the door on the opposite side. This will require that the spine board be placed across the seat. EMT B will also have to get inside the vehicle to maintain neutral, longitudinal traction on the patient's head and neck.

FIGURE 46.5 Emergency removal using a rope sling. (a) If there is no danger of a cervical injury and the patient must be moved rapidly from a danger area, the EMT may drag the patient using a special rope sling consisting of an 8-foot loop of tubular nylon or a 1-inch rope with a metal ring sliding connector. (b) The traction loop must not be used without the sliding connector. The slide is placed on the loop before the loop is spliced. The loops should be placed below the nipple line in a male or below the breasts in a female. The "slide" is forced down between the shoulders at the base of the neck before traction is exerted on the loop. These precautions must be taken so that there is no danger of the loop pressing against the axillae of the patient and injuring the nerves and vessels to the arm. (c) The patient then may be dragged from the area of danger.

Disentanglement of the Patient

Disentanglement of the patient requires medium to heavy extrication skills, which for the most part are beyond the scope of this text. The technique section of this chapter will show only some light extrication techniques for disentanglement of the patient.

Preparation of the Patient for Transfer

Preparing the patient for transfer means maintaining continued control of all life-threatening problems, dressing all wounds, splinting all suspected spinal injuries, and immobilizing all suspected fractures. The use of standard splints in confined areas is difficult and frequently impossible, but stabilization of the arms to the patient's trunk and of the legs to each other will often be adequate until the patient is positioned on a long spine board, which may serve as the ultimate splint for the whole body.

Packaging — that is, preparing the patient for movement as a unit — is best accomplished by means of a spine board or similar device. Such packaging converts difficult situations into easier ones. The boards are essential in moving patients with potential or actual spine injuries; they are helpful in other cases as well.

Transfer of the Patient

Transfer of the patient from the injury site to the ambulance is usually accomplished using a long spine board, or equivalent, as described later in this chapter.

EXTRICATION TECHNIQUES AND TOOLS

The most common extrication problem the EMT will encounter is the entrapped patient following a motor vehicle accident. The basic principles, skills, and tools used in the extrication of a patient from an automobile may be used in many other rescue situations involving entrapped patients. Commonly used vehicle extrication equipment is illustrated in Figures 46.6 through 46.12.

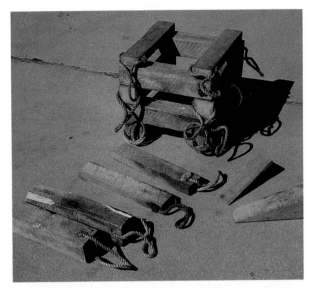

FIGURE 46.6 Shoring (cribbing) normally consists of pieces of hardwood, cut in standard, easy-to-carry lengths, with draw cord attached.

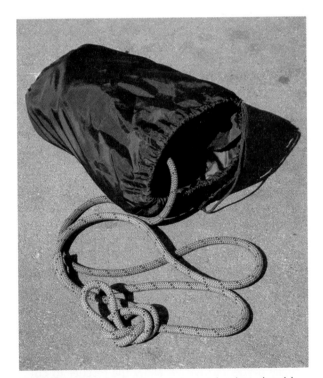

FIGURE 46.7 Rope for use in extrication should be a low-stretch, high-strength rope. It must be maintained in good condition. Each rope segment should be carried in a bag for easy deployment and storage. Manila ropes should not be used for rescue, extrication, or stabilization. They lose 20 percent of their strength each time they get wet.

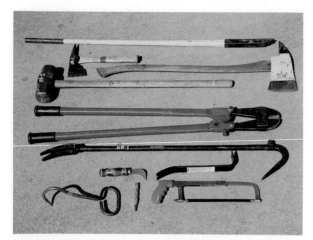

FIGURE 46.8 Hand tools. Light extrication tools should be carried on every ambulance. They allow prying of lightly damaged doors and sheet metal. They also may allow limited access to the patient through cutting of some sheet metal components on the vehicle or breakage of the glass.

FIGURE 46.9 (photos right) Cutting tools. (a) Air chisels may be used to cut sheet metal and supporting columns. They require an air compressor or a compressed air cylinder at the scene. (b) Hydraulic shears allow fast cuts of supporting columns using the hydraulic power from pumps that may be manually activated, or powered by a gasoline or electric motor. Extreme caution must be used to protect the patient and the rescuers from exposure to the hydraulic fluid, which is extremely corrosive. Goggles or a full face shield must be used to protect the eyes whenever hydraulic equipment is being used. Gloves must be worn to protect the skin from exposure. The patient should be covered with a protective blanket. (c) The electric saw-all may be used to cut sheet metal and supporting columns. It requires an electric generator on the scene. There is a potential fire hazard from sparking. (d) High-speed saws, normally powered by a gasoline engine, are capable of cutting sheet metal and heavier supporting components. The risk of fire and explosion from the sparks created must be considered when using this tool. (e) Cutting torches, usually oxygen/acetylene, allow the rescuer to cut through heavy metal components, including vehicle frames. In addition to the considerable risk of fire and explosion which must be considered, there is the potential for burning the patient from the heat generated during the cutting process. Cutting torches should be used only when no other alternative exists.

A

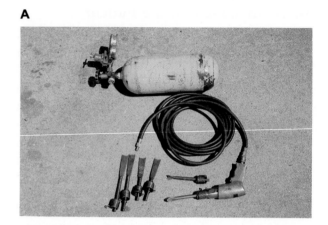

B

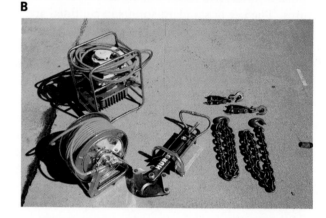

C

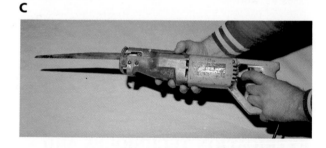

D

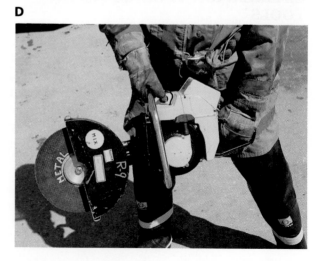

E

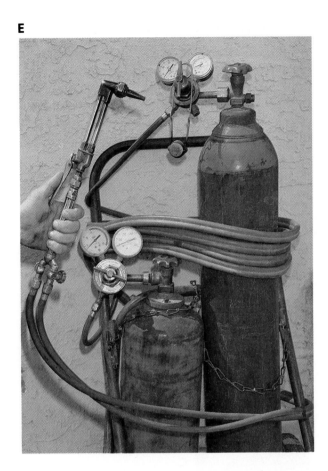

A

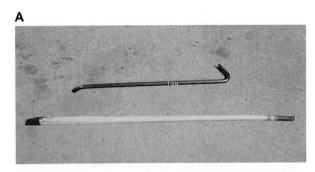

B

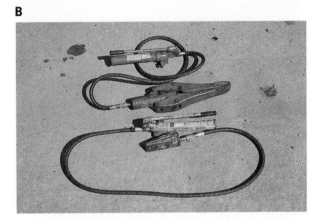

C

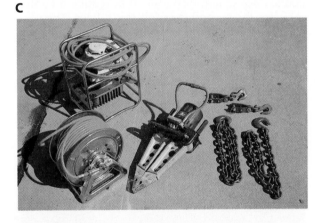

D

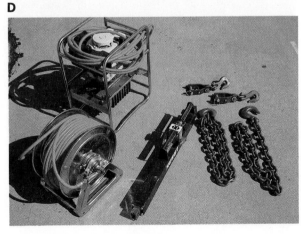

FIGURE 46.10 (photos right) Spreading tools. (a) The pry bar and crowbar are hand tools commonly used to expose door-locking mechanisms and to bend sheet metal components. (b) Normally powered by hand pumps, Porta-power spreaders use hydraulic fluid as a power transfer medium to develop spreading forces in excess of 2,000 ft/lb. As with all hydraulic equipment, exposure to the corrosive hydraulic fluid must be carefully avoided. (c) Hydraulic spreaders ("jaws") require manual, electric, or gasoline-powered hydraulic pumps to develop spreading forces from 10,000 to 16,000 ft/lb. They may also be used for lifting. (d) Hydraulic rams require manual, electric, or gasoline-powered hydraulic pumps to develop spreading forces ranging from 8,000 to greater than 20,000 ft/lb. They may also be used for lifting and pulling.

A

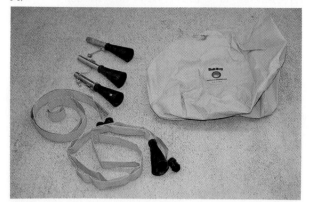

B

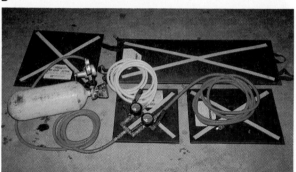

FIGURE 46.11 Lifting tools. (a) Low-pressure air bags are inflated with a compressor, compressed gas cylinders, or exhaust from a running vehicle. Pressure must be regulated to a maximum of 7 pounds per square inch (psi). They require a control valve for raising and lowering single bags. They have the capability to lift in the range of 7,000 to 10,000 lbs. (b) High-pressure air bags use a compressor or compressed gas cylinder regulated to a maximum of 110 psi. They require a control valve for raising or lowering. Single bags have lifting capabilities in the range of 14,000 to 40,000 lbs.

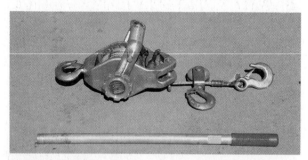

FIGURE 46.12 Pulling tools. A come-along is a manually powered tool with continuous pulling capability. It normally has a cable, a pulley, and a break-away handle. It requires chains or other devices to anchor it to the vehicle. Most will generate 4,000 lbs of pulling force. Hydraulic-powered rams and spreaders, normally used with chains for attachment, may also be used as tools for pulling, as demonstrated later in this chapter.

Passenger Vehicle Stabilization

Before extrication can begin, rescue personnel must stabilize the vehicle. The overall goal of stabilization is to broaden the vehicle's base of support and/or restrict the vehicle's movement. If the transmission has not already been put in park and the ignition key removed, these steps should be done as soon as possible. The parking brake should also be set. Figure 46.13 illustrates the technique of vehicle stabilization.

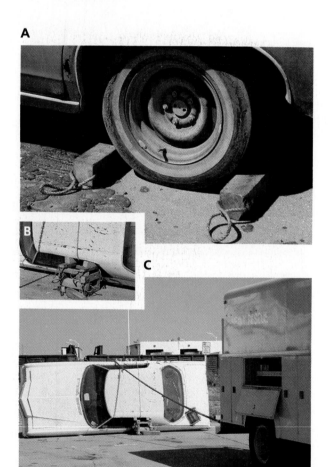

FIGURE 46.13 Vehicle stabilization. (a) If there is a danger of the vehicle rolling, wooden cribbing should be placed to block the wheels. (b) Wooden cribbing is used to extend the base of support of the vehicle if it is unstable or on uneven ground. Cribbing may also be used to build a force point against which a ram or spreader may apply its force. (c) Ropes, cables, and chains are used to restrict movement of the vehicle and broaden the base. Some services have special hooks attached to their rescue vehicles to allow rapid attachment of such stabilizers.

Passenger Vehicle Extrication

Automobiles have a structural framework that gives strength, stability, and passenger protection, as well as providing the overall shape of the vehicle. Rescuers may use the vehicle framework as anchors or push/lift points for extrication equipment.

The exterior "skin" of most passenger vehicles is made up of sheet metal and/or plastic or fiberglass components. Rescuers can easily cut through this skin with a variety of extrication tools if necessary to gain access to the patient. Figures 46.14 and 46.15 illustrate methods of opening a vehicle door to gain access to trapped victims.

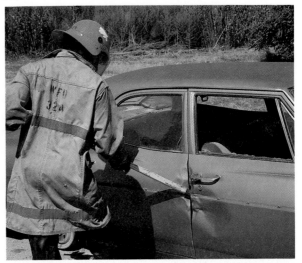

A

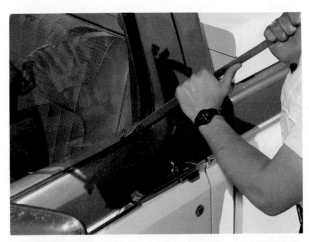

FIGURE 46.14 Opening a door with no structural damage. An attempt should first be made to access and release the lock in order to activate the normal latch. The metal safety lock on newer cars may prevent the usual methods of opening doors. A thin metal strip with a slot in the end (thief's bar) is a handy tool for rapidly unlocking a door to access a patient. It is inserted between the window and the rubber seal of the door until it can be hooked on the lever controlling the lock bolt.

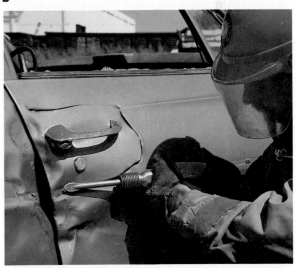

B

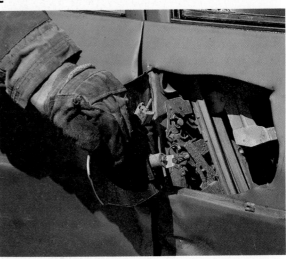

C

FIGURE 46.15 (photos right) Opening a door with structural deformity. (a) If the door is lightly damaged and cannot be unlocked, a pry bar may be used to attempt to spring the door and unjam the lock bolt. (b) Another method is to insert a "can opener" or air chisel into the door and cut a flap of sheet metal around the door handle. (c) The flap is turned back to expose the lock. The door jamb is then struck a heavy blow at the lock, which relieves the tension on the tempered bolt and allows the door to be opened.

If these relatively easy methods fail to gain rapid access to the patient, it may become necessary to break out a window to get at the door locks or to access the patient while heavier extrication equipment is used to disentangle the patient.

Glass in automobiles is usually either tempered, which means it shatters into small pieces when struck with a sharp, pointed object, or a laminate of two pieces of glass with a binding layer of plastic between the glass sheets. Side and rear windows commonly have tempered glass, while the windshield is usually laminated. Figure 46.16 illustrates removal of tempered glass windows. Figure 46.17 shows how to remove the laminated glass of a windshield.

If a door is sufficiently damaged so that it cannot be opened in the standard fashion or with a pry bar, hydraulic devices may be required. Figures 46.18 and 46.19 illustrate the use of hydraulic equipment to open a vehicle door. Sometimes it may be necessary to access the patient through the roof of the vehicle. Figures 46.20 and 46.21 illustrate vehicle access through the roof. Sometimes the patient is trapped beneath the steering wheel. Figures 46.22 through 46.24 illustrate the techniques of pulling a steering wheel with a jack, a come-along, and a ram. Figure 46.25 shows how to remove a brake pedal that may be entrapping a patient's foot. The same technique can be used to free a patient caught between bars or to free a foot caught in a tree (Figure 46.26). Figures 46.27 and 46.28 illustrate lifting equipment.

FIGURE 46.16 (photos right) Removal of tempered glass. (a) A tempered glass window is removed by taping it with masking or adhesive tape to cut down on the risk of flying glass. (b) A center punch is then applied to one corner. (c) The center punch is fired to shatter the glass. An alternate method is to strike the window a sharp blow with the point of a fire axe or head of a small hammer in one corner. (d) The glass is then removed to allow access to the interior of the car. To avoid additional injuries from the glass, it is a good idea to kick the removed glass out of the way under the vehicle.

A
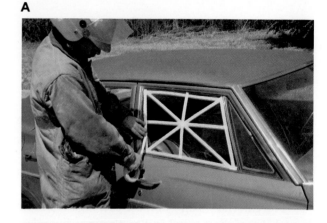

B
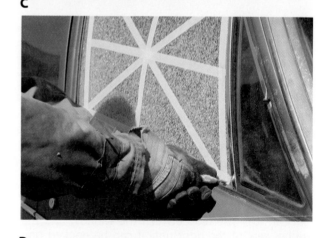

C

D
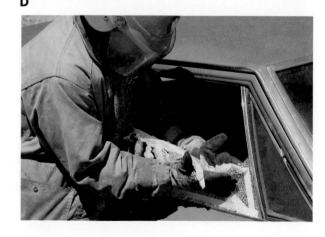

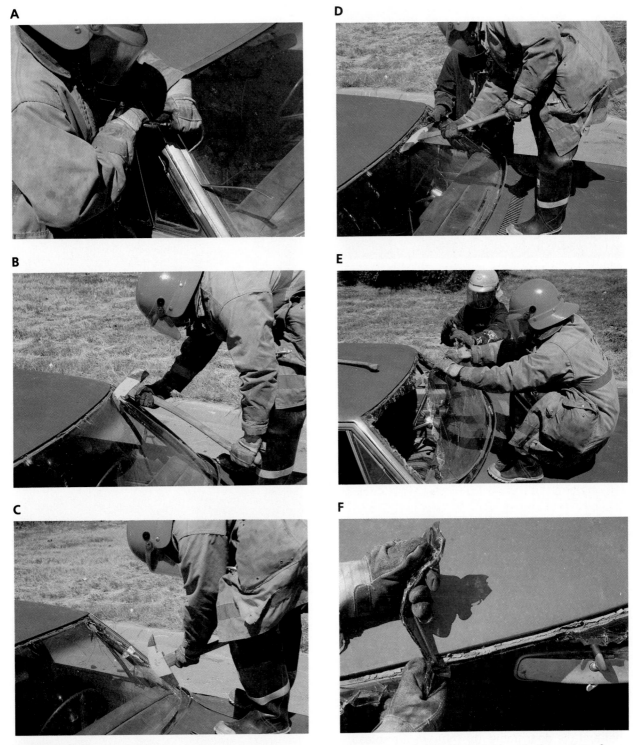

FIGURE 46.17 Removal of laminated glass. (a) Removal of the laminated glass of a windshield requires a different technique. First, all chrome trim strips should be removed. A baling hook will facilitate the removal. It is a good idea to kick the removed trim strips under the car to avoid additional injuries. (b) A hole is then made in one of the upper corners of the windshield with the point of a fire axe. (c) Both sides of the windshield are then cut with a fire axe. (d) With another rescuer supporting the windshield, the upper edge of the windshield is cut with a fire axe. (e) The windshield is then pulled out and lifted free. (f) Any remaining fragments of glass must be removed.

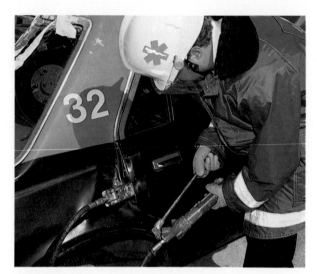

FIGURE 46.18   A Porta-power spreader may be used for doors with mild to moderate structural damage. The spreader jaws are inserted between the door and frame and pumped up to open the door by springing the lock bolt. Caution should be used with the longer spreader blades, as they may shatter if excessive force is generated.

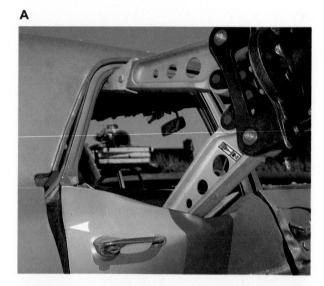

A

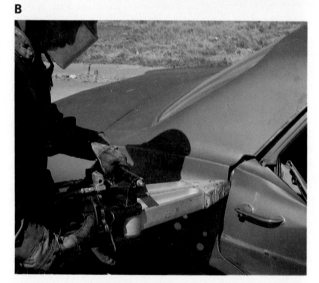

B

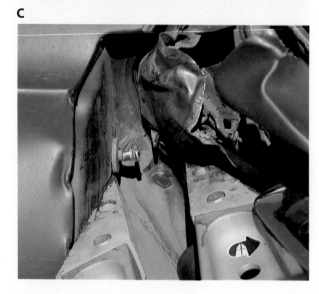

C

FIGURE 46.19   (photos right) To open a door with major structural damage, the hydraulic spreader tool is frequently used. (a) An insertion point for the jaws (see arrow) must be developed between the door and the frame at about the level of the lock bolt. This insertion point may be developed by placing the hydraulic spreader jaws between the roof and the door frame. (b) The jaws are spread until the door is sufficiently deformed to allow the jaws to be reinserted at the level of the lock bolt. The Porta-power spreader may also be used to develop this insertion point. (c) The jaws are inserted at the level of the lock bolt and spread until the lock mechanism has been popped free of the lock bolt. The door can then be opened on its hinges.

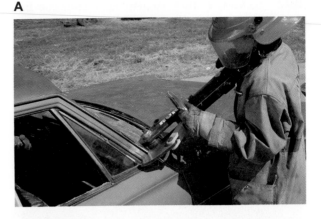

A

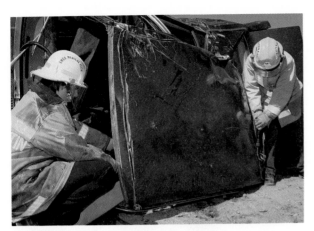

FIGURE 46.20 Rapid cutting of sheet metal is possible with a pneumatic air chisel. The T-type chisel should be replaced with the flat chisel to cut supporting members. The cuts are made in a "U" shape, and the roof is rolled back like a sardine can. If possible, cover, protect, and support the patient before cutting through the top.

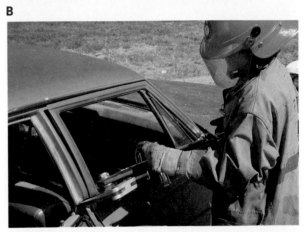

B

FIGURE 46.21 (photos right) Sometimes it is necessary to completely remove the roof to access the patient. (a) Initially, the windshield should be removed, and the side windows rolled down or removed. A hydraulic shear is then used to cut the front pillars at their bases. (b) The center door posts are cut at their bases. (c) The shears are then used to cut the curve of the roof just in front of the rear pillars. If necessary, the roof is creased with a sledge hammer along the line between the rearmost cuts. (d) The roof is then lifted from both sides and bent backwards out of the way.

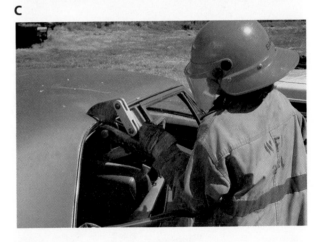

C

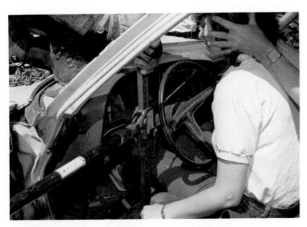

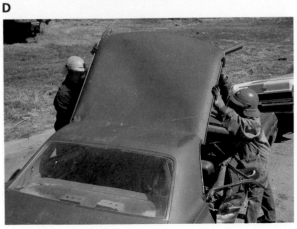

D

FIGURE 46.22 If a patient is trapped beneath the steering wheel, a standard automotive jack may be used between the floor and the steering wheel to free the patient.

A

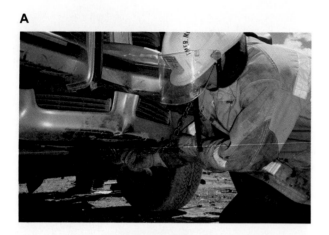

B

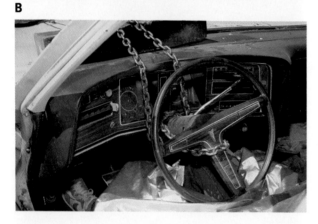

C

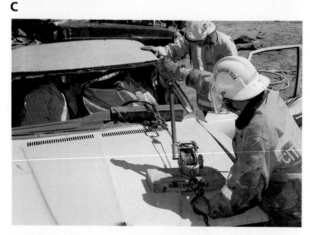

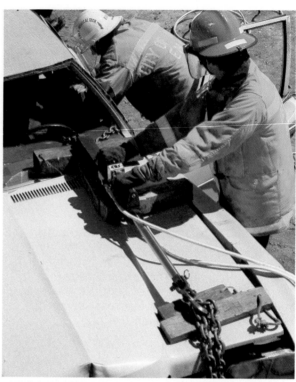

FIGURE 46.24   A steering wheel can also be pulled with a ram. A suitable anchor point is located in line with the required direction of pull on the steering wheel. The ram is secured to the anchoring point using chains or webbing. The patient is kept covered and informed. A second chain is attached around the steering wheel as low as possible. Cribbing should be placed at points where the chains and equipment contact the vehicle.

FIGURE 46.23   A steering wheel may be pulled away with a come-along. (a) A suitable anchor point is located on the vehicle, and the come-along is attached using chains or webbing. (b) Keeping the patient covered and informed, the rescuer attaches a second chain to the steering wheel, positioned so that it will pull upward on the outer end of the steering wheel shaft. (c) Cribbing should be placed wherever the chains, come-along, and cable touch the vehicle. A stack of cribbing in front of the steering wheel provides excellent leverage.

A

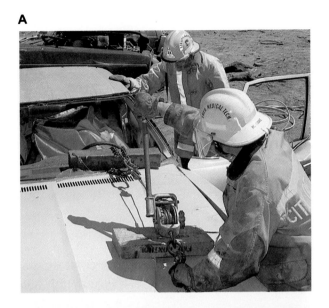

B

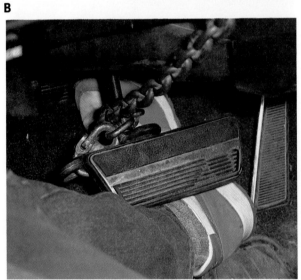

FIGURE 46.25 A brake pedal can be moved with a come-along and a deflector. (a) After locating an anchor point at the front of the vehicle, the rescuer anchors the come-along with chains or webbing. The pin-line pulley should be located at an angle in the direction of pull, and the pulley should be anchored. (b) Using chains or webbing around the pedal, the loose end of the come-along is attached to the cable hook. Cribbing should be utilized at all points of contact between the cable and the vehicle.

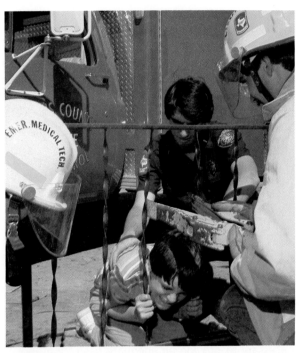

FIGURE 46.26 The hydraulic spreader is placed between the parts of the entrapping object, and the jaws are expanded until there is sufficient deformation that the entrapped body part can be removed.

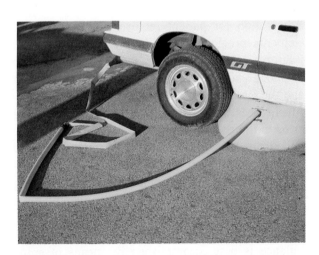

FIGURE 46.27 Lifting a vehicle with low-pressure air bags. The low-pressure air bags provide a wide base of support for lifting. Additional puncture protection should be added where necessary. Box cribbing must be used during the lift to protect the patient and the rescuers. Again, it is advisable to stabilize the vehicle to avoid slippage.

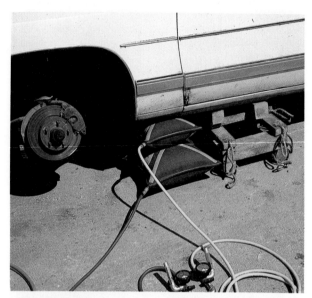

FIGURE 46.28   Lifting a vehicle with high-pressure air bags. High-pressure air bags provide a fairly wide base of support. Additional cribbing may be necessary to provide an adequate base for lifting. Once again, the vehicle should be secured to prevent rollover or slippage. Wide box cribbing must be used to maintain the position of the vehicle to prevent further injury to the patient or rescuer.

PREPARING AND ''PACKAGING'' THE PATIENT

Preparation for patient removal entails the basic elements previously described. Immobilization of fractures and the dressing of wounds should be balanced against the overall condition of the patient and the feasibility of carrying out such tasks in confined spaces. Stabilizing the legs to each other or the arms to the body will suffice if movement is gentle and planned. Some patients may have to be removed quickly because their general condition is deteriorating, and time will not permit meticulous splinting and dressing procedures. Clinical judgment must determine priorities in such cases.

Packaging the patient for removal to the ambulance is best accomplished by means of spine boards or similar devices. Such packaging will convert difficult situations to easier ones. The long spine board is essential in moving patients with potential or actual spine injuries. They are very helpful in other cases as well. Figure 46.29 illustrates packaging techniques using a spine board.

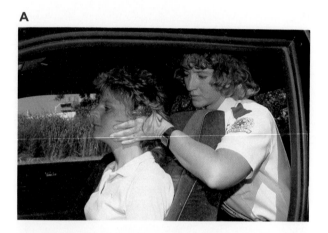

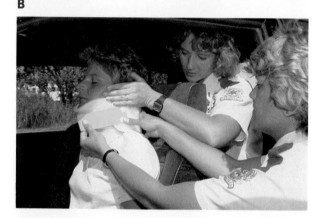

FIGURE 46.29   (photos above and right) Packaging techniques using a spine board. (a) The short spine board (or equivalent) is used most frequently for stabilization of the sitting patient. The patient's head is supported by an EMT who applies neutral longitudinal traction. (b) The neck is stabilized by means of an extrication collar applied by a second EMT. (c) The short board is then positioned behind the patient while gentle support is provided to the thoracic spine. (d) The patient is secured to the body of the board by the attached straps. There are several satisfactory methods for securing the straps. (e) An occipital pad is placed behind the head to prevent hyperextension of the neck. This pad must not be placed down in the curve of the neck, as it might increase neck extension in that position. (f) The patient's head is secured to the board with tape or Velcro straps. Chin straps are not used because of the danger of vomiting and difficulty with airway management. (g) The long spine board is moved in under the patient's hips. (h) The patient is rotated/lifted by the EMTs onto the long spine board. (i) The patient is positioned on the long spine board and secured. (j) The long board and patient are then slid onto the stretcher and secured. If the patient's injuries demand, she can then easily be positioned on her side.

C

G

D

H

E

I

F

J

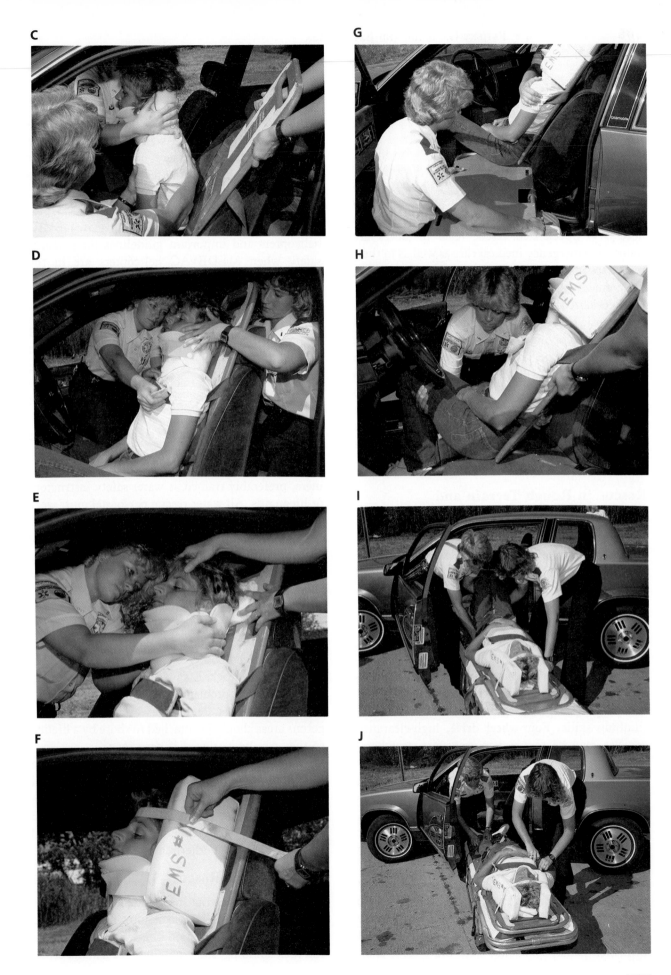

SPECIALIZED RESCUE

In certain situations or disasters, specialized rescue teams are necessary. If the situation warrants, and the dispatcher has not already done so, the EMTs must request a specialized rescue team. The EMTs must then stand ready to provide all assistance necessary. Specialized rescue team members are trained in emergency medical care as well as in their rescue specialty. They must be capable of providing basic emergency medical care to the patient.

Specialized rescue requires many skills not taught in the basic EMT training programs. A few general principles involving rough terrain and inaccessible areas, water rescue, snow and ice rescue, and urban rescue are all that will be covered here. Those who have an interest in specialized rescue are urged to contact the rescue team in their community. Most rescue services are anxious for additional volunteers and will assist in providing the additional training needed to become a member of the team.

Rescue in Rough Terrain and Inaccessible Areas

Rescue in rough terrain includes hilly or mountainous regions, flooded areas, or places where travel by road is impossible. Conditions may be aggravated by snow, ice, or rain. The main considerations in rough terrain rescue are locating the patient, providing emergency medical care as necessary, and using appropriate equipment to transport the patient to medical care.

Rough terrain rescues may involve such techniques as multiple-person stretcher passes up and over rough terrain, fording streams, or technical rock-climbing skills. Four-wheel drive, high-clearance vehicles may be required to transport stretchers. Rescues in rough terrain often require great ingenuity to suspend or pad a stretcher so that the patient is provided a reasonably comfortable ride. Padding such as inflated inner tubes, 4- to 5-inch foam padding, or loosely rolled blankets may be used and is superior to "slinging" the stretcher on straps, which may allow excessive swaying and bouncing.

Helicopters are increasingly being used for quick evacuation from remote areas. Additionally, they are used to transport EMTs to the scene of an emergency in a remote area. The EMT who is frequently faced with such situations should learn the various standard hand signals used for ground-to-air communication with the helicopter. As a rule, the crew of the helicopter is trained in emergency medical care, but the EMT should learn the techniques of boarding and off-loading helicopters. The methods of opening a landing area should also be learned. Chapter 47 contains more information regarding MEDEVAC helicopters and important guidelines for personal safety when MEDEVAC helicopters are in the vicinity.

Water Rescue

Water rescue involves rescue from a body of water, from boats, from marine structures, or from areas flooded by excessive rain or by overflowing dams and reservoirs. The extent of the EMT's involvement in water rescue depends on the local protocol.

To be effective in water rescue, the EMT must have a basic knowledge of water safety. All personnel involved in water rescue should be strong swimmers, preferably trained as water safety instructors or lifeguards. All water rescue personnel must wear an approved personal flotation device *at all times*. No EMT should ever enter a boat without *wearing* (not carrying) an approved personal flotation device. Prior to entering the water, excessive clothing and shoes should be removed if weather permits.

There is a great difference between simply wading out into a calm pond to rescue a person already hanging onto a flotation device and attempting to cross a river at flood crest to rescue a person off a bridge, pier, or rock. Likewise, the ocean front may create additional problems such as tides, large waves, and undercurrents. Personnel working in such dangerous areas should be attached to shore by a lifeline so they can be retrieved if necessary.

In water rescue situations, the rescuer must be alert to hypothermia in the patient as well as in all exposed personnel. Hypothermia may have some protective effect on the drowning victim, making delayed resuscitation possible. Chapter 41 contains additional information on hypothermia.

Cold Weather Rescue

Incidents involving snow and ice rescue are frequently encountered in association with recreational activities such as mountain climbing, technical ice and rock climbing, snowmobiling, ice fishing, cross-country and alpine skiing, snowshoeing, and skating. Incidents may also occur as a result of employment, particularly in occupations such as snowplow drivers, farmers, mail carriers, and foresters.

The most common source of injury in the cold, snowy, icy environment is the motor vehicle accident. Management of a motor vehicle accident is complicated by winter conditions. Response times are frequently longer in winter months because of additional clothing requirements for the EMT, prolonged warm-up time for the response vehicle, and hazardous driving conditions. Frequently, the environment will be both cold and dark. There will be rapid cooling of the accident vehicle, as the automobile has exceptionally poor insulating qualities. This will result in rapid cooling of the occupants and significant risk of hypothermia. Therefore, in addition to the usual concerns for airway, breathing, circulatory stability, splinting of the injuries, and dressing of wounds, there is the concern for hypothermia.

Splinting techniques may have to be modified under these circumstances. Specifically, if a pneumatic antishock garment is indicated, the protocol that calls for removing all clothing has to be modified. Opening the pant legs up the front crease with a scissors, examining the leg, and then allowing the clothing to fall back over the leg to keep it warm is a reasonable alternative. Pneumatic antishock garments, when partially inflated, provide good insulation, minimizing further heat loss from the lower extremities and lower abdomen.

Anyone who as a child placed a moistened tongue against a very cold metal object will vividly recall the incident. Likewise, care must be taken to avoid contact between exposed skin and metal splints and stretchers, as freezing of the skin to the metal is possible.

Use of inflatable splints must be carefully monitored. Warm air from the EMT's lungs will cool rapidly once the splint is applied, resulting in loss of pressure in the splint and loss of immobilization. This can be prevented by frequent observation of the splint as the air cools and further inflation becomes necessary. When the patient is placed in the warm ambulance, the splint may develop excessive pressure as the contained air warms. This can be prevented through close observation and releasing some of the air from the splint as necessary.

Both the inflatable plastic splints and the new vacuum splints have a significant potential for cracking as they are handled under frigid conditions. Some services do not use the inflatable plastic splints during the winter months to avoid this high complication rate. Pneumatic antishock garments do not seem to be as significantly affected by cold weather.

An effective splint for cold weather situations is the cardboard box splint (Figure 46.30). It is inexpensive and readily stored in quantity. It may be used once and discarded. Ski patrol units have found that nylon straps with Velcro closures work well for securing these splints. Such straps are easily managed with mittens or gloves. The Velcro straps will not freeze together like metal buckles. The straps are easily exchanged for disposable ties before or during the patient's evacuation to the hospital.

In addition to the triangular bandage, the large safety pin or blanket pin is a versatile piece of equipment for winter management of extremity injuries, particularly of the upper extremity. They can be used to fashion a sling by simply pinning the arm of the outer garment to the chest of the garment (Figure 46.31). This provides secure immobilization of the upper extremity without sacrificing the warmth the garment provides. In addition, the extent to which the extremities can be examined at the scene depends to a considerable extent on the weather conditions and other circumstances. Safety pin immobilization of one pant leg to the other, and the sleeves to the

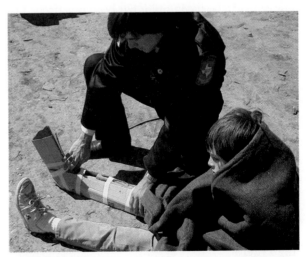

FIGURE 46.30 Cardboard box splints provide effective immobilization and are easy to work with in a cold environment.

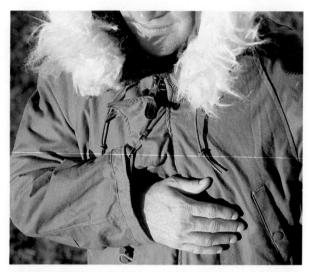

FIGURE 46.31 Preliminary immobilization of an injured upper extremity can be achieved with a large safety pin holding the injured arm against the chest wall.

chest of the jacket, can provide good temporary immobilization until a warm, dry shelter can be reached, and more definitive secondary evaluation accomplished. Also, the patient's head should be covered, if at all possible, after it has been examined. Fifteen percent of body heat can be dissipated through the exposed scalp.

Ice Rescue

As in all forms of technical rescue, ice rescue is not properly learned until it has been practiced. People who may be outstanding fire rescue or ambulance personnel may find themselves overwhelmed by the prospect of undertaking a difficult technical rescue. In areas where ponds, lakes, and rivers commonly freeze, practicing various forms of ice rescue procedures is of great benefit.

The toughest problem in ice rescue is timing. The cold water begins to affect the victim immediately. Setting up equipment for a safe rescue is time-consuming. Only through careful preparation and prior planning can the necessary equipment and personnel be gathered and put into service in time to save a life. Preplanning should include the following criteria:

1. The community should know how to access the proper dispatch center.

2. Dispatchers should alert, by protocol, those persons previously identified as having a specific role to play in the specialized rescue team (for example, scuba team, fire rescue, water rescue, drowning team). In areas where key personnel are not always on duty, locating them by beeper may be satisfactory.

3. Necessary equipment should be stored and dispatched by protocol, unless countermanded by the on-scene commander. Such equipment would include the air supply truck, ladder truck, rescue boat, and special rescue gear, including waterproof rope, harnesses, slings, belaying equipment, throwing lines, line gun, and a personal flotation device for each individual at the scene.

Keeping the victim located is a prime concern. If possible, two observers should be located a moderate distance apart from each other on the shore. They should be instructed to keep constant visual contact with the victim or the victim's last visible location using a stationary reference point. Throwing a rope or flotation device to the victim will stabilize the location, save the victim from having to waste energy swimming or treading water, and buy time to arrange a safe extrication.

Removing a victim over thin ice is a very dangerous procedure. It should only be accomplished by personnel who are prepared for immersion themselves — that is, they should be wearing wet or dry suits and flotation devices. They should be attached to shore with a lifeline. They may well use an inflatable rubber boat; the boat should be tethered ashore with a good rope.

Urban Rescue

For years technical rescue in an urban setting has been accomplished in admirable fashion by the local fire department. Rescue techniques using ladders and other equipment applicable to elevator shafts, building roofs, subway tunnels, and bridges have been developed. Recently, advances in the technology of mountaineering and technical climbing have fostered the production of new equipment that has been adapted to urban rescue. The use of figure-eight rapelling devices, the Russ Anderson "figure-eight with ears," belaying plates, bongs, shocks, nuts, and assorted mechanical jamming devices can all be of value in establishing **belays** (rescue lines) for rescuers and victims as well. Even if the fire department is going to use a direct ladder approach to a victim, the additional safety of a rope belay can be desirable when the belay is handled by *well-trained personnel.*

Experience must be gained in the use of such rescue techniques to recognize secure belaying points. A bong jammed under a door is only as strong as the door and door jamb. A sling around a pipe can be dangerous if the pipe is hot or rusty. Belaying to plumbing fixtures or furniture can lead to nasty surprises at the most inopportune times. Under all circumstances a secondary or backup belay point should be established. Before putting tension on a line, all belay points should be inspected by a second team member for security.

All patients suspected of spinal injuries should be evacuated in a horizontal position in a Stoke's stretcher or similar device. Patients with spinal injuries or major fractures may be evacuated from the upper levels of buildings without functioning elevators by a horizontal lowering in a Stoke's stretcher, either in an elevator shaft or stairwell, or perhaps outside the building. The use of an adjustable bridle on the Stoke's stretcher will allow some head-up positioning for head injuries, or head-down positioning for management of shock (Figure 46.32). Vertical evacuation is generally not advised for patients with suspected spinal injuries. Figures 46.33 and 46.34 illustrate the techniques of vertical extrication.

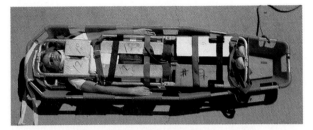

A

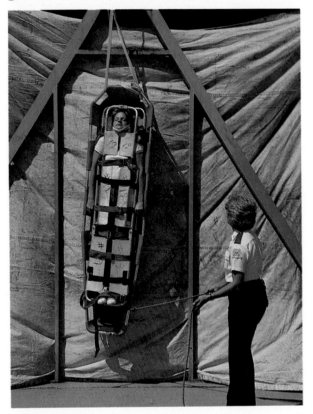

B

FIGURE 46.33 Vertical evacuation may be required under extreme circumstances such as recovery from a well, silo, or mine shaft. (a) The patient is sandwiched between two scoop stretchers placed on his anterior and posterior surfaces. The patient is immobilized and secured to the stretchers with appropriate strapping, including support for the hips. This combined unit is then secured into a Stoke's stretcher. (b) A bridle is then attached to the head of the Stoke's stretcher for raising or lowering. This system still allows some compression of the spinal cord to occur, but probably is as good as any system presently available. Using one of the spinal immobilization jackets may be of some help in immobilizing the spine during vertical evacuations. However, the manufacturer does not recommend the use of the handles on these jackets for lifting in this fashion.

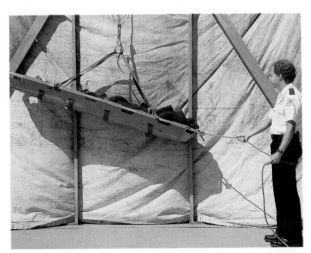

FIGURE 46.32 Patients may be evacuated from a building using a Stoke's stretcher or similar device.

A

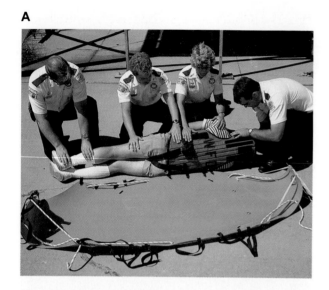

B

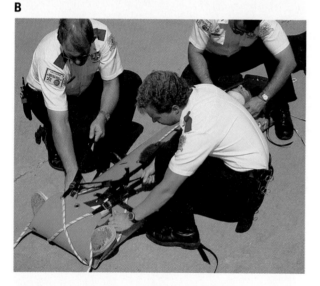

C

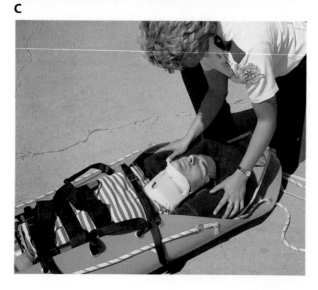

D

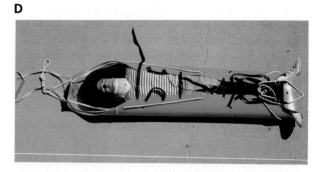

E

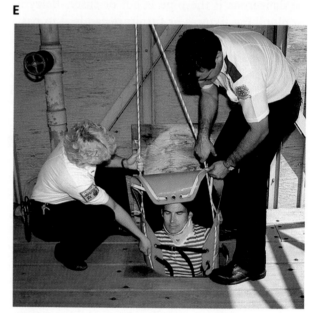

FIGURE 46.34 (a) An alternate method of vertical extrication using the SKED device. The patient is placed in a spinal immobilization jacket or on a short board to prevent forced flexion of the cervical spine during the extrication. He is then log-rolled onto the SKED. (b) The patient is then secured into the SKED. (c) The head is stabilized with foam blocks or a blanket roll. (d) With this kind of a protective packaging, the person can be lifted vertically without slipping out the bottom. (e) The packaged patient is compact enough to be removed through a standard manhole.

Careful thought should go into the selection of the ropes used in urban rescue as some are now quite use-specific. Rope is now specifically manufactured for water rescue that does not soak up or retain water or increase in weight. Nylon rope has a definite stretch factor that may be of value if it is required to withstand the shock of a fall. On the other hand, Dacron and some of the other synthetic ropes have very little stretch, which is much more suitable for tension lines. Obviously, it is very important that these ropes be handled with care; they should be inspected and tested frequently and discarded when they begin to show signs of heavy use. Ridge or hose rollers should be employed where necessary to prevent ropes from fraying.

The use of rescue pulleys with carabiners and various belaying equipment can greatly facilitate and enhance the safety of technical urban rescue. Gasoline, electric, and hand-powered winches are also available to assist with long lifts.

Training for the techniques, skills, and activities involved in technical urban rescue can be accomplished in a variety of ways, but adequate basic training, frequent practice sessions, and scheduled retraining are mandatory for those planning to use technical urban rescue. The use of an "Outward Bound" type of program, which involves training in the use of climbing skills, becoming familiar with belaying techniques, and relying upon one's partner for security, has been found beneficial to many rescue services.

YOU ARE THE EMT...

1. How does size-up differ from triage?
2. How does the glass in side and rear windows differ from the glass in windshields?
3. You have responded to an automobile accident in which two people have received injuries after their car skidded off the road and hit a telephone pole during a snow storm. How will you combat hypothermia during treatment?
4. Describe four rescue situations in which a rope belay would be an essential piece of equipment. Specify the type of rope that should be used in each example.

SECTION 11

AMBULANCE OPERATIONS

47 The Modern Emergency Vehicle

OVERVIEW

For many decades following the introduction of the first motor-driven ambulance in 1906, a hearse was the vehicle most frequently used as an ambulance because it could transport the patient in a recumbent position on a portable litter or stretcher. Few, if any, supplies were carried, and there was little space for the attendant in the back with the patient.

The dual-purpose hearse-ambulance has gone the way of its horse-drawn predecessor as better-equipped and better-designed emergency vehicles have become available. Ambulances are currently designed in accordance with government regulations based on suggestions from the ambulance services and the EMTs who use them. One of the most significant developments in ambulance design has been in the greater width, length, and height of the patient compartment.

Chapter 47 begins with an overview of ambulance design. This section discusses the definition of an ambulance, how a vehicle qualifies as an ambulance, standard external identification emblems and markings used on ambulances, and design specifications for an ambulance chassis and body. This section also describes ambulance speed and acceleration capabilities and warning devices. The chapter then lists the various types of equipment and supplies that an ambulance should carry, including equipment and supplies for patient care and equipment for personal safety and extrication. The next section of Chapter 47 talks about the increasing role of air ambulances and the safety issues that are so important to their success. The chapter concludes with a discussion of ambulance maintenance — another vital area of concern.

OBJECTIVES

The objectives of Chapter 47 are to

- become familiar with modern emergency vehicle design as it relates to national, state, and local standards.
- identify basic emergency vehicle equipment and supplies, including patient-care equipment and supplies, a jump kit, and equipment for personal safety and extrication.
- recognize the increasing role of air ambulances and learn how to approach a MEDEVAC helicopter safely and how to assist a MEDEVAC pilot in the sometimes difficult task of landing the aircraft.
- learn the procedures for inspecting the emergency vehicle after a daily shift change, after a run, and during periodic, scheduled maintenance checks.

EMERGENCY VEHICLE DESIGN

Manufacturers have enlarged and improved the ambulance in accordance with government-mandated design criteria and in response to the recommendations of those who use them — the EMTs and other emergency personnel. Thus, more working space in the patient compartment, including room for at least two litters, and storage facilities for the essential equipment as recommended by the Committee on Trauma of the American College of Surgeons, are among the additions that have resulted in greater width, length, and height of the patient compartment. In a highly competitive and limited-output industry, these medically necessary improvements have added significantly to the cost of the modern ambulance.

Manufacturers have welcomed the consolidated recommendations of EMTs, ambulance operators, physicians, and automobile design engineers who, through the National Academy of Sciences–National

Research Council (NAS-NRC) and the National Highway Traffic Safety Administration, established national standards. In addition to bringing about greater uniformity of design and equipment, these standards have provided not only for the needs of today, but also for adaptation for future medical advances without the necessity for radical changes in ambulance design.

The most pressing needs that modern ambulance design must meet are increased space for performing cardiopulmonary resuscitation, installed suction and oxygen devices, two-way radio communication equipment, storage room for required medical equipment and supplies, and facilities for safeguarding the patients and EMTs.

Regardless of whether ambulances are used in urban or rural areas, they must be standardized to carry the essential recommended equipment. The need for equipment for the personal safety of the patient and EMTs, for extrication, and for road clearance is just as necessary in the city as in rural areas.

Continued research and development of larger vehicles with more sophisticated equipment for EMT-paramedics will undoubtedly continue, but the presently recommended standard ambulance can provide storage for all the supplies as well as the space necessary for basic and advanced emergency medical care at the scene and during transport.

NAS-NRC Definition of an Ambulance

The NAS-NRC defines an ambulance as a vehicle for emergency medical care, designed to provide a driver's compartment and a patient compartment that can accommodate two EMTs and two litter patients. The patients must be positioned so that at least one can be given intensive lifesaving care — cardiopulmonary resuscitation (CPR) — during transit. This vehicle must carry equipment and supplies to provide emergency medical care at the scene and during transport, to safeguard personnel and patients from hazardous conditions, and to carry out light extrication procedures. It must have two-way radio communication between the ambulance and the dispatcher, the hospital, public safety authorities, and medical control. It must be designed and constructed to afford maximal safety and comfort so that transportation does not aggravate the patient's injury or illness.

Restrictions on Designation as an Ambulance

Each state establishes its own standards for ambulance licensure. In most states, to qualify as an ambulance, a vehicle must meet all of the NAS-NRC requirements just stated. Unless it is fully equipped and staffed to serve as an ambulance, no vehicle employed to transport nonemergency patients (litter, wheelchair, or seated) will be licensed as an ambulance. Specially designed mobile intensive care units may be licensed as ambulances, depending on the state in which they are registered.

Federal specifications (KKK-A-1822B, 1985) have been developed and are used by most states as the basis for their ambulance licensure requirements. Pertinent portions of these recommended specifications are discussed in this chapter. These specifications are for the following three types of basic ambulance designs:

Type I: conventional, truck cab-chassis with modular ambulance body (Figure 47.1a).
Type II: standard van, forward-control integral cab-body ambulance (Figure 47.1b).
Type III: specialty van, forward-control integral cab-body ambulance (Figure 47.1c).

External Identification

So that the ambulance will be universally distinguished from all other vehicles, the exterior color should be basically white, in combination with an orange stripe and blue lettering and emblems. The materials used for the emblems and markings should be reflectorized. The Star of Life® emblem should be on the sides, rear, and roof of the vehicle (Figure 47.2). State and local regulations specify the numbers, type, colors, and locations of the rotating beacons and warning lights. The siren should be capable of varying in pitch, "warbling," so that the drivers of other vehicles can recognize the sound. The word AMBULANCE should be in mirror image letters on the front of the vehicle for easy identification by drivers ahead who see an ambulance approaching in their rear-view mirror (Figure 47.3).

Ambulance Chassis

The chassis should provide optimal smooth-riding qualities. It should have a road clearance of at least 6 inches when loaded and be able to ford

A

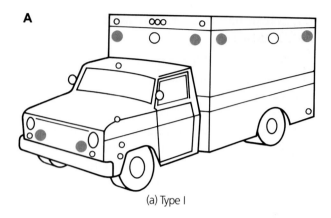

(a) Type I

B

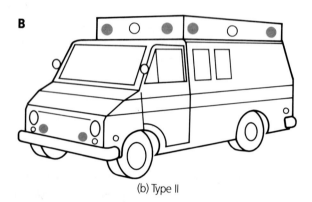

(b) Type II

C

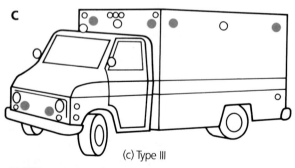

(c) Type III

FIGURE 47.1 Three ambulance designs that meet federal specifications: (a) Type I, conventional, truck cab-chassis with modular ambulance body; (b) Type II, standard van, forward-control integral cab-body ambulance; (c) Type III, specialty van, forward-control integral cab-body ambulance. (Redrawn from Federal Specification KKK-A-1822B, June 1985.)

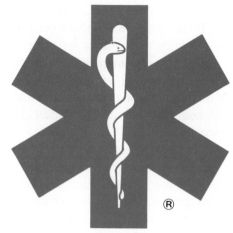

FIGURE 47.2 The Star of Life® emblem is displayed on the sides, rear, and roof of emergency vehicles that meet federal specifications as licensed ambulances.

water up to 12 inches deep. It must have a heavy-duty braking system and the highest-quality tires. A fuel range of at least 150 miles is suggested. Higher road clearance, dual rear wheels, and four-wheel-drive may be necessary where geographic location, climate,

or frequent off-highway operations are common. The ambulance body may be mounted on a passenger or truck chassis. Compliance should be made with general federal motor vehicle safety standards that are applicable to the chassis.

The overall length of the ambulance may vary according to whether the patient's and driver's compartment are constructed as a single unit or whether the driver's cab is mounted separately. In either case, the suggested minimum interior length of the patient compartment is 116 inches. The maximum overall length of the entire vehicle over the bumpers should not exceed 22 feet. The height at curbside should not exceed 110 inches, including roof-mounted equipment such as rotating beacons but excluding the flexible portion of radio antennas. It must be kept in mind that many hospitals were designed long before the modern ambulance. Therefore, if a service frequently transports to a hospital with an entrance lower than 110 inches, it might want to obtain a vehicle configured to the lower entrance. More than one ambulance has lost its expensive roof-mounted equipment on a low overhang or garage door.

Ambulance Body

The body must be crashworthy and free of interior protrusions and unsecured objects that could be dangerous to the patient or EMT. It should be climate-controlled, insulated, and easily cleaned. It

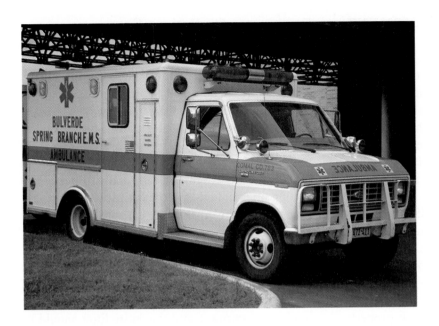

FIGURE 47.3 An ambulance with proper external identification. Notice that the word "ambulance" appears in mirror image letters so that drivers ahead can read the letters in their rear-view mirrors and pull over in time for the ambulance to pass safely.

must be large enough to accommodate two litter patients, two EMTs, and all installed and portable equipment and supplies necessary for optimal patient care. There should be no windows except in the front, rear, and curbside doors of the patient compartment (additional windows take up necessary storage space). Direct access between the driver and passenger compartments is desirable. If there is a passageway, a door should be provided that can be locked from the driver's side. In either case, there should be a window or intercom between the driver's and patient's compartments. The driver should be shielded from the light in the rear compartment when driving at night.

There should be a clear space of 25 inches at the head and 15 inches at the foot of a standard 76-inch litter in the patient compartment. Inside width should provide for two 23-inch-wide litters, with sufficient space between them to permit an EMT to kneel at the side of the primary patient and perform CPR. Thus, a free 25-inch working area is required, part of which can be unobstructed space for the lower legs and feet of the EMT beneath the second litter or squad bench. The minimum acceptable ceiling height is 60 inches, with no protrusions over the aisle between the litters nor over the head and chest of either litter patient.

All equipment necessary for patient care in transit must be permanently installed, secured, or stored in cabinets inside the patient compartment. Once again, eliminating side windows and extra doors frees up more space for needed storage. All items must be adequately secured so that in the event of an accident, equipment and supplies will not become potentially harmful missiles.

Speed and Acceleration

The fully loaded ambulance should be capable of speed and acceleration such that it is able to maintain its position in traffic on highways, as well as avoid hazardous situations in moving traffic. The criteria of speed and acceleration are designed to ensure safety of the ambulance in traffic on interstate highways. Training in defensive and high-speed driving, operational judgment, and a primary concern for the safety of the patient will determine the manner in which the driver responsibly uses the ambulance's high-performance capabilities.

Warning Devices

A siren and a public address system should be mounted on each ambulance. They may be a combined system. A noise-cancelling microphone and manual and automatic siren undulation and yelp should be part of the system. Two speakers are desirable. An air horn is a useful additional warning and signaling device. Rotating beacons and warning lights are specified by state or local regulation.

EMERGENCY VEHICLE EQUIPMENT AND SUPPLIES

In order to estimate the space requirements for installed, portable, and stored equipment and supplies, as well as locate them for easy accessibility, ambulance designers must be familiar with the size, weight, shape, and power requirements for each item. No new equipment or supplies should be ordered by EMTs without consultation with the medical director of the ambulance service.

Many items offered for use by EMS systems have never been rigorously tested and evaluated for effectiveness under field conditions. Therefore, purchase of such items may turn out to be expensive or perhaps even dangerous mistakes. As a general rule of thumb, the more complex a piece of equipment, the more difficult it is to learn how to use it properly, especially under adverse field conditions, and the more likely the equipment is to malfunction during a medical emergency.

Equipment and supplies should be located according to the relative importance of the item and its frequency of use. Priority should be given to items necessary to cope with life-threatening conditions. Equipment and supplies necessary for airway care, artificial ventilation, and oxygenation must be within easy reach of the EMT at the head of the primary litter. Equipment and supplies for cardiac resuscitation, control of external bleeding, and monitoring blood pressure must be easily available at the side of the litter.

To the greatest extent possible, equipment and supplies should be durable and standardized so that exchanges can be made between ambulances or between ambulances and emergency departments. Exchange is an important consideration for any ambulance service, as it decreases the delay in transfer of patients, prevents premature and possibly dangerous removal of required equipment from the patient, and decreases the time the EMTs and ambulance are detained at the hospital.

Storage cabinets and kits should open easily but must be fastened securely to keep them from opening during transit. The use of transparent construction materials for the fronts of cabinets and drawers allows rapid identification of their contents; otherwise, labeling of the contents on the cabinet fronts is recommended.

Equipment for Patient Care

Patient Transfer Litters

Each ambulance should have a wheeled litter, a folding litter, and a collapsible device that enables the EMTs to carry a patient in stairways and other narrow spaces where a full-length litter cannot be used because of its size. The collapsible and folding litters may be combined as one unit. Litters must be easy to move, store, clean, and disinfect. The folding litter should keep the patient elevated above floor level when in the flat, extended position.

The wheeled litter should be adjustable in height and designed so that when secured in the lowest position, the top is between 11 and 15 inches above the floor of the ambulance. The head of the litter should be capable of being tilted upward to a 60-degree semisitting position, and the entire litter should be capable of being tilted into 10 degrees of **Trendelenburg position** (head down) for airway care. So that patients can be full length in the supine, prone, or lateral position, litters must be at least 69 inches long and 20 inches wide. The frame or handles must be designed to permit up to four persons to carry the litter. Fasteners to secure the litter firmly to the floor or to the side of the vehicle during transport must be provided. The litter restraints should be capable of securing the litter to withstand a rollover of the ambulance. Restraining devices must be provided to prevent the patient from falling off the sides or sliding off the end of the litter.

Some ambulance services use an x-ray permeable, removable panel, such as the top of an emergency room cot or backboard, on top of the litter. This allows the patient to be moved easily through all the necessary diagnostic and treatment facilities, including surgery, without being removed from the panel until placed in a hospital bed (Figure 47.4). Such a panel decreases the discomfort for the patient during transfers, as well as the risk of further injury. The disadvantage of such a panel is that it prevents the patient from being placed in the semisitting position while the panel is in place on the litter.

Airways

Oropharyngeal airways for adults, children, and infants must be carried. Nasal airways for adults and children should also be available. Commercial bite blocks or those made from three tongue blades taped

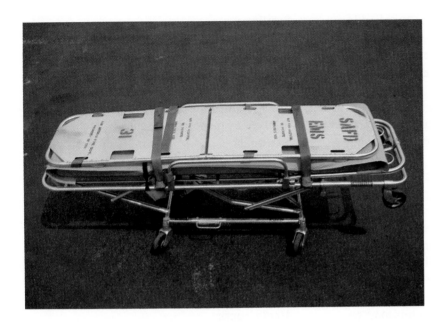

FIGURE 47.4 A wheeled ambulance litter with an x-ray permeable, removable panel from an emergency department cot or backboard placed on top. The patient can be moved easily from the ambulance to the emergency room to surgery without risk of further injury or discomfort.

together should be provided for possible use during convulsions to prevent injury to the patient's tongue.

Artificial Ventilation Devices

Portable artificial ventilation devices that operate independently of a supply of oxygen must be provided. Two units are desirable — one for use in the ambulance and the other for use outside the vehicle or as a spare. Portable artificial ventilation devices of the manually operated, self-filling, bag-valve-mask type that are capable of oxygen enrichment should also be carried. When attached to an oxygen supply, with the oxygen reservoir in place, the unit should be capable of supplying almost 100 percent oxygen to the patient. The unit must be easy to clean and decontaminate. The non-rebreathing valve must permit inhalation of oxygen during both artificial and spontaneous respirations. A pediatric-sized bag-valve-mask should also be carried.

Masks in a variety of sizes from infant to adult must be stocked. They should be transparent to permit the rapid recognition of color change in the patient and to detect vomiting or respiratory abnormalities. Adult and pediatric-sized bags should be used with the corresponding mask to deliver the proper volume of oxygen-enriched air to the patient.

Suction Equipment

Portable and installed suction equipment is very important. The suction units must be powerful enough to provide an airflow of 30 liters per minute at the end of the suction tube and a vacuum of 300 mm Hg (mercury) when the tube is clamped. The suction force must be adjusted for use on children and infants. It should be fitted with large-bore, nonkinking suction tubing with a semirigid pharyngeal tip. There should be an additional set of semirigid suction tips. On the installed unit, the suction yoke, unbreakable collection bottle, water for rinsing the suction tips, and suction tubing must be readily accessible to the EMT at the head of the litter. The tubing must reach the patient's airway, regardless of the patient's position. All suction apparatus must be of the type that is easily cleaned and decontaminated.

Oxygen Inhalation Equipment

An emergency vehicle must be equipped with two oxygen supply units — one portable and the other installed. The portable unit (300 liter capacity) should be located near a door for ready use outside the vehicle. It should be equipped with a yoke, pressure gauge, flowmeter (not gravity-dependent), delivery tubing, and oxygen mask. The unit must be capable of delivering oxygen at a flow rate of between 2 and 15 liters/minute (lpm). An extra portable 300 liter cylinder should be kept on the ambulance. Many services equip the back-up cylinder with its own yoke, gauge, regulator, and tubing so that it can be used for a second patient in an emergency.

The installed oxygen unit must be supplied by at least 3,000 liters of oxygen, delivered by a two-stage regulator under pressure of 50 psi (pounds per square inch). The unit must be fitted with yokes, reducing valves, and flowmeters (not gravity-dependent). The flowmeters must be visible and accessible to an EMT seated at the head of the litter. The system must be capable of delivering oxygen at a flow rate of between 2 and 15 liters/minute. Delivery tubes must reach the face of the patient who is being transported in a horizontal position. They should connect readily to oxygen masks and to bag-valve mask ventilation devices. Oxygen masks (with and without bags) should be semiopen, valveless, transparent, and disposable. Masks should be available in sizes for adults, children, and infants. Nasal cannulae should also be available.

Ambulance services that frequently transport patients on runs lasting longer than one hour should consider using a disposable, single-use humidifier for the installed oxygen system. For runs of less than one hour, humidification is rarely indicated and may actually lead to increased risk of infection in patients if the humidifiers are not scrupulously maintained.

Cardiac Compression Equipment

A spine board, when placed under the patient on the litter, provides the necessary resistance for effective external chest compression. A tightly rolled sheet on the board will raise the patient's shoulder 3 to 4 inches above the level of the board and keep the head in a position of maximum backward tilt, while maintaining the shoulders and thorax in a straight position without manual support. If a neck injury is suspected, such a roll for hyperextension of the neck must not be used.

Newer equipment for mechanical external cardiac compression is capable of providing adequate perfusion. Services that must provide CPR during prolonged transport may wish to consider the purchase of such devices after appropriate evaluation and consultation with their medical director.

Supplies for Patient Care

Basic Supplies

Ambulances should carry the following basic supplies:

2 pillows
2 pillow cases
2 spare sheets
4 blankets
4 towels
6 disposable emesis bags or basins
2 boxes of disposable tissue
1 bedpan
1 urinal
2 disposable thermometers
4 sandbags
1 blood pressure cuff
1 stethoscope
1 pair trauma shears
1 package of disposable drinking cups
1 unbreakable container of water
1 package of wet wipes
4 cold packs
6 ammonia inhalants
4 liters of irrigation fluid
2 restraining devices
1 package of plastic bags for waste or severed parts

Splinting Supplies

The following supplies should be on hand for splinting fractures and dislocations:

1. One half-ring, lower-extremity traction splint, with minimum 9-inch ring size and 43-inch length, with commercial limb-support slings, padded ankle hitch, traction strap with buckle, and a windlass. A telescoping splint may replace a rigid unit. A pediatric-sized splint should also be carried.
2. Splints for the upper and lower extremities, such as uncomplicated inflatable, cardboard, plastic, wire-ladder, canvas-slotted, lace-on, or padded boards. The number and types of splints should be determined by the local medical director or state law.
3. Triangular bandages and conforming roller bandages for fractures of the shoulder and upper arm and for fixation of rigid splints when necessary.
4. Short and long spine boards, cervical collars, and accessories for safe extrication, as well as splinting in case of suspected injuries of the spine.

5. A pneumatic antishock garment with inflation equipment to be used for the splinting of severe pelvic and upper-femur fractures as well as in the treatment of hemorrhagic shock.

Dressing Supplies

Supplies to be carried for the dressing of open wounds and for application and padding of splints include the following:

Sterile universal trauma dressing, approximately 10 × 36 inches, packaged folded to 9 × 10 inches
Self-adhering, soft roller bandages, 4 inches × 5 yards
Self-adhering, soft roller bandages, 2 inches × 5 yards
Sterile, nonporous, nonadherent dressing for occlusion of sucking chest wounds and eviscerations (aluminum foil sterilized in original package)
Adhesive tape in several widths
Safety pins, large
Sterile dressings, gauze, 4 × 4 inches
Sterile dressings, laparotomy, 6 × 9 inches

Childbirth Supplies

A sterile obstetrical delivery (OB) pack must be carried. It should contain the following supplies:

1 pair surgical scissors
3 cord clamps or umbilical tapes
5 towels
12 sponges, 4 × 4 inches
4 pairs sterile surgical gloves
1 baby blanket
2 large plastic bags
1 ear syringe, rubber-bulb type, for aspiration of baby's mouth and airway
1 box sanitary napkins, individually wrapped and sterilized

Each ambulance service must be able to obtain immediately, from a hospital or another source, a portable infant incubator that can either be fastened to the litter or stand alone for transporting newborn infants. The carrier should permit oxygen enrichment, humidification, control of body temperature, and accessibility to the baby's head for resuscitation. There must be artificial ventilation and sterile oro-

pharyngeal suction equipment in appropriate sizes for this purpose.

Acute Poisoning Supplies

Activated charcoal and syrup of ipecac in premeasured doses should be provided, as well as drinkable water and cups. A sufficient number of emesis basins or bags should be available. The phone number of the local poison control center should be prominently displayed on the "poisoning kit."

There should also be equipment and supplies for irrigation of the skin and eyes following exposure to toxic substances. A snakebite kit should be carried in those areas where a hazard of snake bite exists.

The Jump Kit

The ambulance should have a **jump kit** that will be used by the EMT who initially leaves the vehicle to tend to the patient while the EMT-driver parks the ambulance and secures the scene as necessary. Such a kit must be light, durable, waterproof, quick to open, and easy to secure (Figure 47.5). It should also have the phone number of the local poison control center prominently displayed on its side. The jump kit should contain the following supplies:

triangular bandages
trauma shears
adhesive tape in various widths
bite blocks
universal trauma dressings

(continued next page)

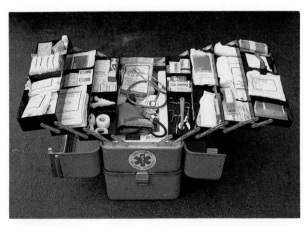

FIGURE 47.5 A typical jump kit. The kit must be light, durable, waterproof, quick to open, and easy to secure.

self-adhering soft roller bandages, 4 inches × 5 yards and 2 inches × 5 yards

oropharyngeal airways in adult, child, and infant sizes

bag-valve-mask artificial respiration unit with masks for adults, children, and infants

blood pressure cuff

stethoscope

penlight

portable suction with pharyngeal tips

sterile gauze pads, 4 × 4 inches

sterile "lap" pads, 6 × 9 inches

thermometer

Bandaids

sterile, nonporous, nonadherent dressing for occlusion of sucking chest wounds and eviscerations (aluminum foil sterilized in original package)

ammonia inhalants

abbreviated patient report form, "street form"

other supplies as determined by the local medical director

Equipment for Personal Safety

A weatherproof compartment that is accessible from outside the patient compartment should provide equipment to safeguard patients and EMTs, control traffic and bystanders, and illuminate work areas. These items would include:

reflectorized or intermittently flashing warning devices (replacing the formerly recommended flares, which have caused fires at the accident scene)

2 flashlights, battery powered, stand-up type

fire extinguisher, type BC, dry powder, size 5

hard hats with face shields or safety goggles

2 portable floodlights (if not easily and quickly available from other primary response vehicles)

Extrication Equipment

A weatherproof compartment outside the patient compartment should contain equipment needed for simple, light extrication, even if an extrication and rescue unit is readily available. The following items should be available:

wrench, 12-inch, adjustable, open-end

screwdriver, 12-inch, standard square bar

screwdriver, 8-inch, Phillips head

hacksaw with 12-inch carbide wire blades

vise-grip pliers, 10-inch

hammer, 5 pound, with 15-inch handle

fire ax, butt, 24-inch handle

wrecking bar, 24-inch handle (Hammer, ax, and wrecking bar may be one combination tool.)

crowbar, 51-inch, pinch point

bolt cutter with 1 to 1¼ inch jaw opening

shovel, folding, pointed blade

tin snips, double action, 8-inch minimum

gauntlets, reinforced, leather covering past mid-forearm (one pair per occupant)

rescue blanket

ropes, 5,400 pound tensile strength in 50-foot lengths in protective bags

mastic knife

bail hooks (2)

spring-load center punch

pruning saw

heavy duty 2 × 4 and 4 × 4 shoring (cribbing) blocks, various lengths

Additional extrication equipment may be required based on the needs of the area serviced. This would be especially true if rescue and extrication services were not easily and immediately available.

AIR AMBULANCES

Air ambulances are not the modern medical development they may seem. In 1870, 36 years before the first use of a motor-driven land ambulance, 160 wounded soldiers and civilians were safely evacuated by hot air balloon during the Prussian siege of Paris.

The EMT will be exposed to increasing use of air ambulances in the future. There are two basic types of air ambulances: fixed-wing and rotary-wing aircraft (Figure 47.6). Fixed-wing aircraft are generally used for interhospital patient transfers over distances of greater than 100 miles; for shorter distances, rotary-wing aircraft are more efficient. Specially trained medical flight crews accompany these flights. The EMT's involvement with fixed-wing aircraft transfers will probably be limited to providing ground transportation for the patient and medical flight crew between the hospital and airport.

Rotary-wing aircraft are increasingly becoming an important tool in providing emergency medical

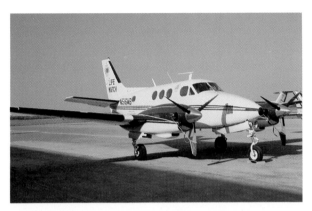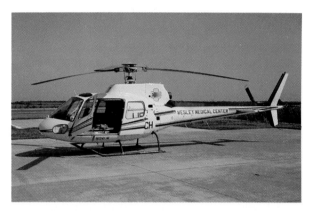

FIGURE 47.6 Air ambulances are playing an increasingly important role in the transportation of the sick and injured. The two basic types of air ambulances are (left) fixed-wing and (right) rotary-wing (helicopter) aircraft.

care. For example, in many areas, it is an everyday occurrence to see a **MEDEVAC helicopter** land at an accident scene and transport the victims to a trauma facility far distant from the accident. MEDEVAC helicopters have the potential to speed the delivery of appropriate lifesaving care to a patient, as well as speed the delivery of the patient to a lifesaving treatment facility. In order to use them safely and effectively, EMTs should be thoroughly familiar with the capabilities, protocols, and methods for accessing MEDEVAC helicopters available in their area.

Medical experiences in Korea and Vietnam proved that patient survival is directly related to the time that elapses between injury and definitive treatment. The speed and versatility of helicopters in transporting injured servicemen to military medical facilities have been adapted to emergency medical care in the civilian conflict that may be referred to as "the war on trauma." Most of the helicopters used for emergency medical operations fly well in excess of 100 mph in a straight line, without road or traffic hazards. The patient can receive varied degrees of medical care during the flight, based on the capabilities of the aircraft and the MEDEVAC flight crew; the crew may be made up of EMTs, paramedics, flight nurses, or physicians.

The types of helicopters used for MEDEVAC operations vary, but the dangers are the same. Helicopter safety is nothing more than good common sense, coupled with a constant awareness of the need for personal safety. If EMTs become familiar with the way helicopters operate and if they follow the instructions of the pilots, they should minimize any dangers involved in being part of a MEDEVAC operation. The most important rule is to stay a safe distance from the aircraft whenever it is on the ground and the rotors are spinning. Remember, the tips of the rotor blades are traveling near the speed of sound.

When accompanying a flight crew member of the aircraft, either to go on the mission or to assist in the loading of a patient, the EMT must follow the directions of the flight crew exactly. *Never* should the EMT attempt to open any aircraft door or move equipment unless instructed to do so by the flight crew member. Likewise, when directed to approach the aircraft, the EMT should do so with extreme caution, paying constant attention to the hazards present.

Another important safety rule is to *never approach the helicopter from the rear.* The approach area is between nine and three o'clock as the pilot faces forward (Figure 47.7). The approach area has been strictly defined because of the hazard of the tail rotor. In addition, the pilot may need to swing the tail boom to a different direction for takeoff.

The tail rotor is a spinning blade that is sometimes almost impossible to see because of its excessive speed of rotation. All ground personnel must stay away from the tail rotor. If it is necessary to move from one side of the helicopter to the other, the EMT should go around the front of the aircraft. No one should ever duck under the body, the boom, or the rear section of the helicopter. The pilot cannot see

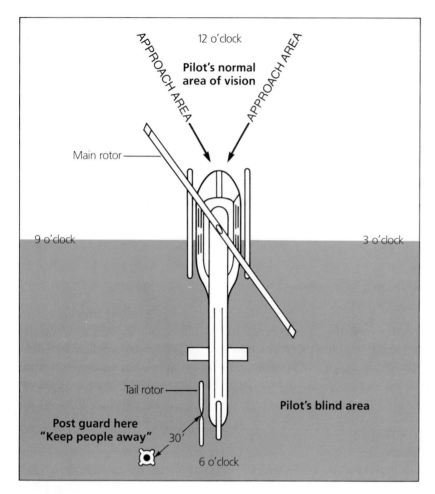

12 o'clock

Pilot's normal area of vision

APPROACH AREA

APPROACH AREA

Main rotor

9 o'clock

3 o'clock

Tail rotor

Pilot's blind area

Post guard here "Keep people away" 30'

6 o'clock

FIGURE 47.7 The EMT or any ground personnel should always approach a helicopter from the front. The tail rotor moves so fast that it is sometimes impossible to see. The pilot cannot see the area behind the helicopter or any people who might be standing there.

in these areas. An unseen rescuer could very quickly disable a helicopter by being struck by the tail rotor, probably at the expense of his own life. When enough personnel are available, someone should stand toward the rear of the aircraft, outside the arc of the rotor blades, to warn spectators and others away.

Another area of concern when approaching a helicopter is the height of the main rotor blade. Due to the flexibility of the blade, it may dip as low as 4 feet off the ground (Figure 47.8). When approaching the aircraft, the EMT should walk in a crouched position until at the helicopter. Wind gusts influence the blade height without warning. Special care must be used when IVs and equipment have to be carried under the blades. Air turbulence created by the rotor blades can blow off hats and loose equipment and cause them to become a danger to the aircraft and personnel in the area.

If no other site is available and the helicopter must land on a grade, further caution must be exer-

cised. The main rotor blade will be closer to the ground on the uphill side (Figure 47.9). Under these circumstances, the aircraft must be approached from the downhill side only. The patient should not be moved to the helicopter until the helicopter crew has signaled that they are ready to receive the EMTs. A flight crew member will direct and assist the EMTs with their duties in loading the patient.

The following information is presented to minimize the dangers associated with landing sites. While it is true that a helicopter can fly straight up and down, this is the most dangerous mode of operation. The safest and most effective way to land and take off is similar to that used by fixed-wing aircraft. Landing at a slight angle allows for safer operations. Takeoff is a reversal of this process, combining a gradual lift and forward motion to travel up and out on a slight angle.

Clearing a landing site is another important role that EMTs can perform. They should look for loose

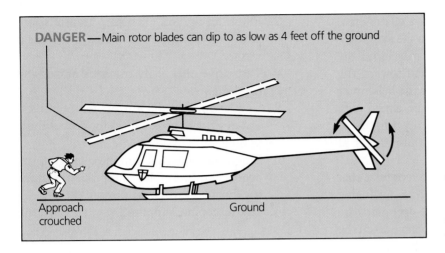

FIGURE 47.8 The EMT should always approach the front of a helicopter in a crouched position because the main rotor blade can dip to as low as 4 feet off the ground.

debris, electric or telephone wires, poles, or any other obstacles that might interfere with the safe operation of the helicopter. If any obstacles are noted, the pilot should be notified of them by radio or other signal. The pilot will usually "overfly" or make a reconnaissance of the landing site before final approach and landing to ensure that all potential dangers are identified. The pilot makes the final determination of the landing site. However, EMTs should designate suggested landing sites. If they are appropriate, the pilot will use them. Variables such as temperature, winds, and helicopter payload play a part in the pilot's final selection of a landing site. Local protocols will determine whether flags, lights, or other signaling devices should be used to mark the proposed landing site.

Nighttime operations are considerably more hazardous than daytime, because obstacles are not as visible to the pilot. Frequently, the pilot will fly over the area with the helicopter's lights on, not only to show obstacles, but also to have the lights reveal the shadows of overhead wires; while the wires may

FIGURE 47.9 The EMT must use extreme caution when approaching a helicopter that is on an incline. The main rotor blade will be closer to the ground on the uphill side, so the EMT must approach from the downhill side.

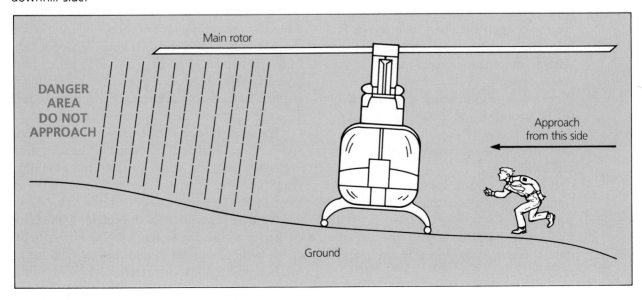

not be visible, the changing shadows are often noted. Rescuers should not shine spotlights in the air to help the pilot. These lights may temporarily blind the pilot. Light beams should be directed toward the ground at the landing site. Even after the helicopter is on the ground, lights should not be aimed anywhere near it. Of course, smoking, open lights or flames, and flares are prohibited within 50 feet of the aircraft at all times.

EMTs are increasingly coming to recognize that MEDEVAC operations are a welcome and valuable tool in emergency medical care. These operations are most effectively utilized by those who have taken the time to familiarize themselves with locally available MEDEVAC services. For further information on the subject of air ambulances, refer to DOT publication HS805-703, *Air Ambulance Guidelines*, February 1981, and DOT publication HS806-841, *Proceedings: National MEDEVAC Helicopter Conference*.

EMERGENCY VEHICLE MAINTENANCE

The EMT is responsible for the maintenance of the ambulance — it must be safe and available on a moment's notice. Routine inspections must be regularly scheduled, preferably using a written checklist that can also serve as a "squawk list" for equipment and supplies needing maintenance or replacement.

The first type of routine inspection is the daily/shift change inspection. The following items should be on the checklist:

1. Chassis systems: brakes; battery(s); engine cooling system, including fluid levels, fan belts, and water hoses; all lights, interior and exterior; warning equipment and sirens; and power systems.
2. Wheels and tires, including spare; check inflation pressures and unusual wear or any damage.
3. Doors for proper opening, closing, latching, and locking.
4. Temperature control systems.
5. Communications systems, vehicle and portable.
6. Fuel tank: should be at least one-half full unless local circumstances demand larger reserves.
7. Fluid levels: oil, coolant, transmission, power steering, power brakes, windshield washer.
8. Test drive once daily to check brakes and handling.
9. Check windows and mirrors for cleanliness and position; check wipers for proper functioning.
10. Emergency medical supplies: oxygen, on-board and portable; jump kits; splints; backboards; OB pack; poison kit; etc.
11. Housekeeping supplies.

The second type of inspection is the run inspection. After each trip, the interior of the ambulance should be cleaned and decontaminated as needed, in accordance with state and local health department regulations. Blood, vomitus, and other contaminants must be scrubbed from the floors, walls, and ceilings. The exterior of the vehicle should be cleaned as needed. Broken or damaged equipment should be replaced or repaired without delay. Supplies should be restocked as needed. If the fuel tank is below required reserves, the vehicle should be refueled. The oil level should be checked each time the vehicle is refueled.

The third type of inspection is carried out during periodic maintenance checks of the emergency vehicle. Ambulance chassis and engine components are subjected to significantly greater stresses than the typical automobile or truck. For this reason, the manufacturer's recommendations for periodic preventive maintenance must be strictly followed, especially regarding lubrication, oil and filter changes, transmission and differential service, brakes, wheel alignment, wheel bearings, and steering components. Many services are now using a Hobbs or engine hour meter in addition to the odometer to help determine periodic maintenance requirements.

Just as is the case with emergency medical care report forms, local and individual differences affect inspection routines. Ambulance services should develop their own inspection forms for at least the inspection time intervals just listed. These forms should include those items listed for inspection. They should be used as a checklist so that nothing is overlooked or omitted. The forms should then be filed for inspection and legal documentation.

YOU ARE THE EMT...

1. What kind of litter is needed in order to place a patient in the Trendelenburg position? What are the advantages and disadvantages of an x-ray permeable, removable litter panel?
2. In addition to containing certain supplies, what else should characterize a jump kit?
3. What is more dangerous—the main rotor or the tail rotor of a helicopter? How do you avoid both of these dangers?
4. You are on the ground helping a MEDEVAC pilot land the helicopter at night. What should you do?

48 Emergency Driving and Vehicle Operations

OVERVIEW

Many patients have said that the most frightening part of the experience of being suddenly ill or injured was not the problem itself but the ambulance ride to the hospital. The terrifying effect of a fast, swaying ride with a siren blaring overhead is not very reassuring to an already upset patient. While sometimes this kind of a ride is truly "lifesaving," most often excessive speed is unnecessary. What is necessary is that the patient be transported to a hospital safely in the shortest practical time. This takes common sense and defensive driving techniques on the part of the EMT, and speed should never be used to cover up a lack of these qualities.

Chapter 48 focuses on the techniques and judgment that an EMT has to learn in order to drive an emergency vehicle. The chapter begins with an explanation of why so many ambulance drivers are guilty of using excessive speed. The chapter next discusses emergency vehicle control and emergency vehicle operation. Both these topics are important factors in safe driving. The chapter then talks about the qualifications needed to be an ambulance driver. The last section of Chapter 48 focuses on emergency vehicles at the accident scene — where the ambulance should park and how the EMT should control traffic in the absence of police help.

OBJECTIVES

The objectives of Chapter 48 are to

- identify four factors that contribute to the problem of excessive speed in driving the emergency vehicle.
- become familiar with emergency vehicle control, including steering techniques, chassis set, fender judgment, road position, controlled acceleration and braking, and special driving situations.
- become familiar with emergency vehicle operation, including right-of-way privileges, use of the siren, planning alternate routes, intersection hazards, and safe driving guidelines.
- describe the qualifications needed to be an emergency vehicle driver.
- learn were the ambulance should be parked and how traffic should be controlled at the scene.

THE PROBLEM OF EXCESSIVE SPEED

EMTs who operate an ambulance assume great responsibility. They must employ the knowledge they have gained through training and experience to get the patient safely to the hospital in the shortest period of time. The "shortest period of time" does not necessarily correlate to rate of speed. In fact, only in extreme life-and-death emergencies is speed a factor. In most instances, if the patient is properly assessed and stabilized at the scene, speed during transport is unnecessary, undesirable, and dangerous.

Unfortunately, excessive use of vehicle speed during emergency calls is not uncommon. Four factors that contribute to this problem have been identified. The first is lack of expertise in the dispatcher. Dispatching is a job that requires a trained, experienced EMT. Only with a working knowledge of emergency calls can a dispatcher be in a position to help determine the urgency of the calls received. Dispatchers who are no more than switchboard operators cannot make such decisions properly. Even with EMT dispatchers, most services will respond to an incident with red lights and siren, mainly because it is very difficult to assess reliably the exact situation from an excited, distraught caller.

The second factor identified in the use of excessive speed is inadequate equipment in the ambulance. The EMT who does not have the equipment and supplies necessary to stabilize the patient may have little choice but to speed to the hospital to pass on the responsibility presented by the condition of the patient. The third factor is inadequate training of the EMT. The EMT who is inadequately trained or who lacks confidence in being able to care for the patient has little choice but to transport the patient rapidly to the hospital, in effect acting as a chauffeur rather than an EMT.

The fourth and final factor is inadequate driving ability. The EMT driver who has not received training in the safe operation of the ambulance will be unaware of the principles governing its proper use. This driver, lacking understanding of the added risks that excessive speed entails, may be inclined to select speed over safety.

EMERGENCY VEHICLE CONTROL

The EMT driver has only two means of controlling the vehicle: changing its direction or changing its speed. To accomplish either maneuver safely means maintaining a continuous rolling contact between the bottom surface of the tires and the surface of the road. Two factors are involved in this contact: the coefficient of friction (a measure of the "grip" of the tire on the road surface) and the "footprints" of the ambulance's tires through which the grip is applied. An ambulance tire's typical footprint is approximately 8 inches long and as wide as the tire.

The coefficient of friction may vary widely on different parts of the same road, depending on the condition of its surface, its age, and the weather. A driver must constantly evaluate the road surface with regard to the frictional force the tires can apply to the road surface at a given speed before a skid will begin. This observation is especially important in cornering, where additional centrifugal force is acting on the vehicle.

Steering Techniques

The method of holding the steering wheel, its movement, and the timing of movements are all factors in steering technique. The steering wheel should be held with the hands at the ten o'clock and the two o'clock positions. These positions allow the wheel to be turned without removing either hand. In moving the steering wheel, one hand pulls while

the other slides, paralleling the pulling hand's position on the wheel (Figure 48.1). When turning the vehicle, the hands should not pass the twelve o'clock or the six o'clock positions, since the hands will cross and become tangled. When these limits are reached, the opposite hand begins to grip the wheel, and the first hand slides. This technique will allow the wheel to be held firmly by at least one hand at all times.

Timing of steering wheel movement is proportional to the speed of the vehicle. All vehicles lag somewhat when responding to steering input. The faster a vehicle is traveling, the greater the lag becomes. The required steering input should anticipate the desired movement of the vehicle.

Chassis Set

Chassis set refers to the transfer of weight (center of mass) of the vehicle to different points on the chassis or frame. Basically, the weight of a vehicle is concentrated over one of three points on the chassis: in the front over the front wheels, in the rear over the rear wheels, or in the center between the front and rear wheels. The transfer of weight from one point to another is caused by acceleration or deceleration of the vehicle. When a vehicle accelerates, the weight is transferred to the rear; the front wheels lose some traction, which results in decreased ability to steer the vehicle — that is, the ambulance

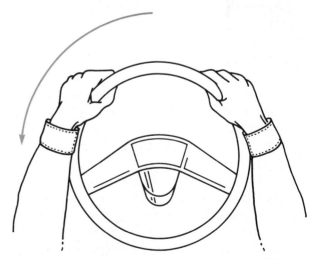

FIGURE 48.1 The hands of the driver should be at the 10 o'clock (left) and 2 o'clock (right) position on the steering wheel when driving straight ahead. A left turn is initiated by the left hand pulling the steering wheel in a counterclockwise direction while the right hand slides along the wheel. The driver's hands should never cross.

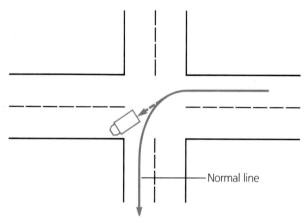

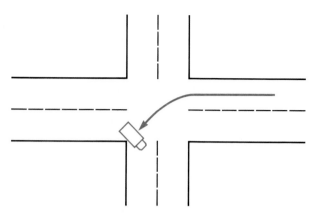

FIGURE 48.2 When a vehicle accelerates, the front wheels lose some traction. The vehicle becomes harder to steer because it has a tendency to travel in a straight line as the center of mass moves toward the rear of the vehicle.

FIGURE 48.3 When a vehicle decelerates, the rear of the vehicle tends to slide to the outside of a curve when cornering.

will have a tendency to travel in a straight line (Figure 48.2). When there is deceleration or braking, the opposite weight shift occurs and weight is transferred to the front of the vehicle; the rear end of the vehicle then tends to slide to the outside of a curve when cornering (Figure 48.3).

Fender Judgment

Fender judgment is knowing how much physical operating space a particular vehicle requires when traveling at a given speed. The ability of a vehicle to fit into a parking space or to pass between two objects depends on its size from fender to fender. While good fender judgment depends to a certain extent on visual ability, a more important factor is experience. Fender judgment will improve as the driver gains experience in parallel parking and practices other maneuvers. Even with excellent fender judgment, the experienced EMT will use an observer when backing to avoid unexpected surprises.

One important fact for the EMT to remember is that as speed increases, so too does the operating space required for the vehicle. This increase occurs because the distance traveled during the time taken for hazard recognition and reaction as well as the lag in vehicle response both increase as speed increases.

Road Position and Cornering

Road position describes the position of the vehicle on the roadway relative to the inside or outside edge of the paved surface and the interaction of this position with cornering efficiency. Knowing the vehicle's present position as well as its projected position is necessary in order to achieve efficient cornering.

Efficient cornering means negotiating a curve at the optimum speed to achieve good road position when exiting the curve. The vehicle's position is projected so that its path will apex at the desired point in the curve. The apex of a curve is the point at which the vehicle is closest to the inside edge of the roadway or traffic lane. The position of the apex depends on the desired road position at the exit point of the curve. An apex early in the curve will usually result in the vehicle's being forced toward the outside of the roadway when exiting the curve, while an apex late in the curve allows the vehicle to stay to the inside of the roadway, which helps keep the vehicle in the proper lane (Figure 48.4).

Controlled Acceleration

Controlled acceleration means the use of a controlled pressure on the accelerator and the use of acceleration to control the vehicle. Acceleration is most efficient when the vehicle is traveling in a straight line, because the force of acceleration is equally distributed to the rear wheels. Acceleration in a curve or during a turn results in a reduction of actual linear acceleration in the desired direction and an increase in acceleration to the outside of the curve. If the acceleration to the outside of the curve becomes excessive, the vehicle may drift out of control and into a skid or spin.

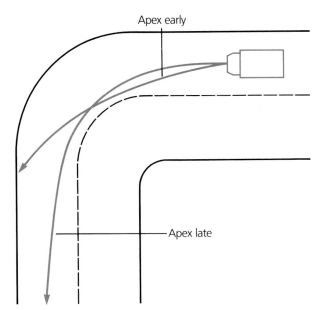

FIGURE 48.4 A vehicle will stay to the inside of the curve if the apex of the curve occurs late in the curve. An early apex will force the vehicle to the outside of the roadway.

Controlled Braking

Controlled braking refers both to the use of the brakes to control the vehicle and the controlled application of pressure to the brake pedal. Brakes not only control the movement of the vehicle, causing it to slow or stop; they also aid in directional control. Braking while the vehicle is traveling in a straight line is the safest and most efficient method. Braking in a turn causes a loss of efficiency that may be barely noticeable at low speed but becomes more apparent with increased vehicle speed. Applying the brakes while cornering has little effect on slowing the vehicle and may actually cause a skid or spin. The proper method for use of the brake during a turn or in a curve is to gradually ease off brake pressure and increase accelerator pressure to maintain the speed of the vehicle.

Getting the feel of proper brake pressure comes through experience and practice. The proper sequence in braking is to apply pressure intermittently. The brake pedal should not be jabbed; nor should the pressure be constant and complete. Either technique may result in wheel lockup, loss of directional control, sliding, or a spin. Some newer vehicles are equipped with an electronic antilocking brake system that automatically "pumps" the brakes by applying intermittent pressure to prevent brake lockup. In a vehicle so equipped, the EMT must be sure to understand the operational limitations of the system.

Special Driving Situations

Even the most conscientious driver occasionally will run into unexpected situations that may require special driving skills. Driving at a speed appropriate for the weather and road conditions will decrease the need to use these techniques.

Hydroplaning

On a wet road, a tire tends to displace the water on the surface and make direct contact with the road. As the vehicle's speed increases above 30 miles per hour, the tire may be lifted off the road surface by water piling up under it; there is not enough time for the water to be forced out from under the tire. This is known as **hydroplaning.** At higher speeds on wet roadways, the front wheels may thus be riding on a sheet of water, giving the driver no control over the vehicle. If hydroplaning occurs, the driver should gradually slow the vehicle without jamming on the brakes.

Water on the Roadway

If at all possible, driving through large pools of water should be avoided. If it cannot be avoided, the driver should slow down and turn on the windshield wipers. After exiting the pool, the driver should lightly tap the brakes several times until they are dry. Once the brakes are dry, they will slow the vehicle without pulling it to one side or the other.

Decreased Visibility

During periods of decreased visibility caused by fog, smog, snow, or heavy rain, common sense dictates that the driver carefully slow down after giving sufficient warning to following vehicles. At night, only low beams should be used to provide maximum visibility without reflection. EMT drivers should use their headlights during the day to increase their visibility to other drivers. EMT drivers should also watch carefully for stopped or slow-moving cars.

Ice and Slippery Surfaces

A light mist on an oily, dusty road can be just as slippery as a patch of ice. Good all-weather tires and an appropriate speed can help decrease traction problems significantly. Studded snow tires should be considered for vehicles frequently used in snow or icy conditions.

The EMT driver should be especially wary of bridges and overpasses when temperatures are close to freezing. These road surfaces will freeze much faster than surrounding road surfaces because they lack the warming effect of underlying ground.

EMERGENCY VEHICLE OPERATION

Safe driving during transportation is an important phase of the emergency care of the sick and injured. It requires training and judgment in the operation of the emergency vehicle. There is an old cliche that applies very well to emergency driving: "Practice makes perfect." The EMT can practice anytime, any place, and in any vehicle. No one is so proficient that additional practice will not be beneficial. And no one, EMTs included, can get too much practice.

The first rule in the safe operation of an emergency vehicle is that the EMT driver and all passengers wear seat belts and shoulder restraints at all times. Other EMTs should wear them enroute to the scene and when not actively engaged in direct patient care. Seat belts are without doubt the most important items of safety equipment on every ambulance.

EMT drivers have to become familiar with the characteristics of their vehicle with regard to acceleration, cornering, swaying, and stopping. For example, disc booster brakes improve braking efficiency but increase the sway. Drivers must also know exactly what the vehicle will do and how it will respond to steering, braking, and acceleration inputs under various conditions.

EMT drivers should be constantly alert to changing weather, road, and driving conditions. Warnings of ice or hazardous conditions must be taken seriously. Whether enroute to an emergency or returning to the hospital, drivers must modify their speed according to road conditions. While drivers should follow specified routes for most runs, they should have alternate routes available for contingencies. During a major disaster, it is especially important that all public safety and emergency services be coordinated, with all vehicles following assigned routes. A driver who encounters unexpected traffic congestion should notify the dispatcher so that other drivers can be advised of the congestion and delays and select alternate routes.

In most instances, on a multilane highway, the ambulance should keep to the extreme left-hand (fast) lane. Use of this lane offers the least amount of traffic under most conditions and allows other motorists to move over in a normal right-hand manner.

EMT drivers must always drive defensively. They should never rely on what another motorist will do unless a clear visual signal is received. Even then, a driver must be prepared to take defensive action in case of a misunderstanding, panic on the part of the other party, or careless driving.

Right-of-way Privilege

State laws vary regarding the right-of-way privileges of an ambulance. Some states allow an emergency vehicle to proceed through a red light or stop sign after stopping. Others, in effect, allow emergency vehicles to go through red lights or stop signs without stopping at all — a very dangerous practice. The EMT who is the driver must be familiar with the local right-of-way laws and should exercise this privilege only when it is absolutely necessary for the patient's well-being. The truth is very few emergencies require extremely rapid transportation of the patient.

Use of the Siren

Probably the most overused piece of equipment on an ambulance is the siren. In general, the siren does not help the EMT driver. The driver in a closed car, proceeding at the speed limit, with the radio playing and the air conditioner or heater fan going full blast, cannot hear even a penetrating electronic siren until the ambulance is only a short distance away. If the radio is particularly loud, such a driver may not hear the siren at all.

The use of a police escort is an extremely dangerous practice. The motorist, hearing a siren and seeing a police car passing, may assume that it was the only emergency vehicle and may begin to proceed, causing an accident with the ambulance that is being escorted.

Planning Alternate Routes

The EMT who plans and executes the necessary moves in proper sequence will gain time. Becoming familiar with the various routes in the town or city will allow the EMT to plan alternate ways to reach the destination. In fact, switching to alternate routes will save more time than increasing the speed of the ambulance. Knowing alternate routes around frequently opened bridges or blocked railroad crossings is especially important.

Intersection Hazards

The EMT driver often assumes that motorists and the public will do the "right thing" when an emergency vehicle is in the vicinity or is following a car. The EMT driver may believe that motorists will pull to the right-hand curb and stop or travel as close to the curb as possible. However, the motorist might stop suddenly in front of the ambulance. If the ambulance is not under control, a serious accident could occur.

Intersection accidents are the most frequent and usually the most serious. Intersections abound with hazards for which the EMT driver must be on the alert. If the call is so urgent that the ambulance cannot wait for red lights to change, the driver should still come to a momentary stop at the light and survey the intersection, looking for those drivers who will go around traffic and enter the intersection, usually at high speed. Another serious hazard at the intersection is the motorist who times the traffic lights and arrives just as the lights are changing, thereby avoiding a stop. This person is often an experienced truck driver who is hauling a heavy load that makes a quick stop impossible. Such a driver will arrive at the intersection knowing that the traffic light is about to change and expect to go through. If an ambulance arrives at the same time, with the green light in its favor but about to change, and the EMT driver also expects to proceed through the intersection, the stage has been set for a serious accident.

Still another intersection hazard is created when the driver of one emergency vehicle follows another emergency vehicle through an intersection without assessing the situation carefully. A motorist who has yielded the right-of-way to the first vehicle may proceed into the intersection not expecting a second emergency vehicle close behind. EMT drivers should never accept a police escort, and when following another emergency vehicle, EMT drivers must exercise extreme caution.

The driver of an emergency vehicle must also be alert for other emergency vehicles that might be approaching an intersection with their sirens on and expecting to proceed through without yielding. An open window and a "tuned" ear can significantly reduce this risk.

Driving through an intersection when vision is obstructed, without stopping to make sure that the passage is clear, is equivalent to driving blindfolded. Even more likely than the possibility of colliding with another vehicle is the possibility of striking a pedestrian who steps from behind an obstruction, such as a bus or truck.

Guidelines for Safe Driving

The following guidelines should help the EMT to operate the ambulance safely:

1. At the time of dispatch, select the shortest and, normally, the least congested route to the scene.
2. Avoid routes with heavy traffic congestion. Know alternate routes to each hospital destination during rush hours.
3. Avoid one-way streets. They may become clogged by the sound of your siren. Do not try to go against the flow of traffic on a one-way street.
4. When approaching the scene, be very careful and alert for pedestrians. Curiosity seekers rarely move out of the way.
5. At the scene, park in a safe place. If parked facing into traffic, turn off your headlights as they may blind oncoming traffic. Do keep warning lights on, however, to alert oncoming motorists.
6. When transporting the patient to the hospital, operate the ambulance within the stated speed limits for the area, except for the rare extreme emergency.
7. Go with the flow of traffic.
8. Use the siren as little as possible en route to the hospital. The patient is being cared for, and the duty of the driver is to reach the hospital safely. If you do have to use the siren, be sure to warn the patient before activating it.
9. If it is necessary to use the siren, still travel at a speed that will allow you to be able to stop the ambulance safely at all times if other drivers do not give way.

10. Never assume that warning lights and sirens will allow an ambulance to pass through a congested area.
11. Always assume that other drivers will have their car windows rolled up, their radios playing, conversation going on, and their heater or air conditioner fans going at full blast. They will not be looking for an ambulance and will not hear the siren, even though it is only a short distance away.
12. Always drive defensively.
13. Always maintain a safe following distance. Use the "two-second rule" of following at least 2 seconds behind another vehicle in the same lane.
14. Try to maintain an open space in an adjacent lane as an escape route if the vehicle in front should stop suddenly.

EMERGENCY VEHICLE DRIVERS

Not all persons who drive an automobile are qualified to drive an emergency vehicle. Drivers should be screened carefully. The same requirements for a person who is to perform as an EMT hold true for an EMT who is assigned to emergency driving duties.

One of the basic requirements is that the driver be physically fit. Experience has shown that many accidents can be attributed to a physical impairment. The EMT driver should not attempt to drive while taking medications such as cold remedies, analgesics, or tranquilizers that may induce sleep or slow reaction times. And of course, an EMT would never drive or provide medical care after drinking alcohol.

Another requirement is that the driver be emotionally fit. Emotions must be given much consideration. For example, the personality of an individual may change behind a steering wheel. Closely tied to emotional stability is the ability to operate under stress. The EMT driver must be capable of acting properly under the stresses of emergency conditions. In addition to knowing exactly what to do, the EMT must be able to do it under trying conditions.

The EMT who is serving as the driver must be aware of the important responsibilities of emergency driving and develop the proper attitude. Although an ambulance is usually granted right-of-way privileges, the laws are emphatic about the responsibil-

ity of the driver who exercises those privileges. Any idea that an emergency vehicle driver can do no wrong must be abandoned. Being able to drive to one's destination without interruption (as granted in right-of-way privileges) and being permitted to move from one lane of traffic into the opposite lane are valuable, timesaving privileges that must never be abused.

EMERGENCY VEHICLES AT THE ACCIDENT SCENE

Safe Parking

Emergency vehicles must be properly parked to maintain efficient traffic control and flow. The ambulance should not be parked beside the accident site, because it may block the movement of other emergency vehicles. The ambulance should instead pull in front of or behind the accident and park on the same side of the road. It is best to park uphill and/or upwind of the incident if smoke or hazardous material is present (Figure 48.5). If it becomes necessary to park on the backside of a hill or curve, the EMT driver must put out warning devices (Figure 48.6). All emergency vehicles should park well away from any collapsing structures, fires, explosive hazards, or downed wires.

An overall guideline is for the EMT driver to park as close to the accident as the immediate need for emergency medical care and personal safety indicates. If possible, on approaching the scene, the

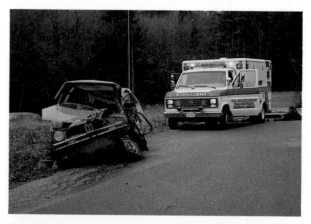

FIGURE 48.5   The EMT should park the ambulance uphill and/or upwind from smoke or hazardous substances such as gasoline.

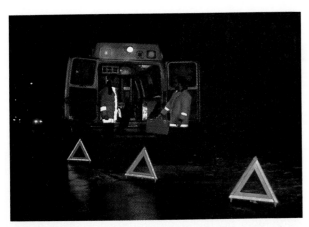

FIGURE 48.6 The EMT driver must place warning devices if it becomes necessary to park on the backside of a hill or curve.

driver should make a quick survey and choose the best place to park to unload equipment and to load patients. If necessary, the ambulance can be temporarily moved into a position to block traffic so that a patient can be moved safely and quickly. If this maneuver is required, it should be carried out as quickly as possible. Traffic should not be blocked any longer than is absolutely necessary. Of course, while traffic flow should continue with as little interruption as possible, the emergency medical care of the patient does take precedence over all else. Therefore, harassment over the obstruction of traffic should never affect the care the patient receives.

Traffic Control

The EMT's first responsibility at an accident scene is to care for the patients. If the authorities are not present when the ambulance arrives, the EMT may use bystanders to direct traffic. Only when all the patients have been treated and the emergency situation is under control should the EMT be con-

cerned with restoring the flow of traffic. If the police are delayed in arriving at the scene, the EMT may then be required to take action.

The purpose of traffic control is to ensure an orderly traffic flow and prevent another accident. Under ordinary circumstances, traffic control is difficult. Under the conditions that exist at the scene of an accident or disaster, traffic control presents serious additional problems. Passing motorists often try to observe the scene as they drive by, paying little attention to the roadway in front of them. Some curiosity seekers may park and return on foot, creating still other hazards. As soon as possible, appropriate warning devices, such as reflectors, should be placed at a sufficient distance on both sides of the accident. Volunteers should be recruited to slow and direct traffic. Ordinarily, the EMTs will need to concern themselves with traffic control for only a short time until the police arrive. Remember, the main objectives in directing traffic are to forewarn other drivers, prevent additional accidents, and keep vehicles moving in an orderly fashion so that continued care of the injured is not interrupted.

YOU ARE THE EMT...

1. An EMT driver controls the vehicle by changing what two factors? What role does friction play in vehicle control?
2. Explain what happens when a vehicle hydroplanes. What corrective action should a driver take?
3. Give five examples of how the EMT driver can drive defensively.
4. Research and report on the right-of-way privileges of ambulances in your state.

49 Communications

OVERVIEW

Radio and telephone communications are the framework that binds the components of an EMS system together. The communication system links one emergency health care provider with other members of the emergency health care team, thus permitting them to function effectively. It is imperative that all EMTs know the communication capabilities of their EMS delivery system. Especially important is knowing the equipment's limitations. EMTs must also become proficient in the effective and efficient use of the EMS communication system. They must be able to transmit concise, accurate reports relating to ambulance status, conditions at the emergency site, and the condition and treatment of the patient.

Being able to transmit concise, accurate information requires familiarity with communications terminology. Chapter 49 thus begins by presenting a glossary of key communications terms. Then the chapter discusses the skills that an EMT has to possess in order to be an effective communicator. Next the chapter looks at the capabilities that an EMS communications system must offer and how patients access that system. The alert and dispatch phase is examined next.

It emphasizes the crucial role of the dispatcher. The last section of Chapter 49 is about radio communication — what kinds of units are used, standard radio operating procedures, the medical communications capabilities possible, and the jurisdiction of the Federal Communications Commission over all radio communications.

OBJECTIVES

The objectives of Chapter 49 are to

- define key communications terminology.
- identify the training and skills an EMT needs for effective communication.
- describe the capabilities of EMS communications systems and how patients access the EMS system.
- recognize the essential role of the dispatcher in the alert and dispatch phase of EMS communications.
- become familiar with radio communications, including the type of units, standard operating procedures, medical communications capabilities, and the role of the Federal Communications Commission.

KEY COMMUNICATIONS TERMINOLOGY

In order to be an effective communicator on an emergency health care team, the EMT must have a rudimentary understanding of some of the key communications terms. The following is a glossary of such terms:

Base station: Any fixed radio hardware containing a transmitter and receiver. For EMS purposes, they will generally be within the class, land mobile service, as defined by the Federal Communications Commission (FCC).

Carrier: A basic radio signal (wave) generated by a transmitter without voice or other information imposed on it.

Channel: An assigned frequency or frequencies used to carry voice and/or data communications.

Control console: Typically, a desk-mounted, enclosed piece of equipment that contains the mechanical and electronic controls used to operate a radio base station either on or off the premises.

Coverage: The geographic area where reliable radio communications exist. It is usually based on the 90/90 standard — 90 percent reliable 90 percent of the time. Coverage is usually expressed as the radius in miles from a fixed base station.

Dedicated line: A special telephone circuit used for specific point-to-point communications purposes such as remote control of a base station or alerting EMS crew quarters.

Duplex: The ability to transmit and receive traffic simultaneously on a particular channel.

Frequency: The number of repetitive cycles/second completed by a radio wave. The basic unit of measurement is the Hertz (Hz), which is 1 cycle/second. A second important unit is the megahertz (MHz), which is 1,000,000 cycles/second.

Hot line: A dedicated telephone line between two specific points. It is always "open" or under the control of an individual at each end. The line is immediately available by lifting the receiver. Outside access cannot be obtained.

Interference: Any undesired radio signal on a radio frequency. It may come from another radio transmitter or other sources of electromagnetic radiation.

Land mobile service: Specified by the FCC; mobile communication service between a base station and mobile stations on land, or between two mobile stations on land.

Microwave: A term applied to radio waves in the frequency range of 1,000 MHz and upward. The signals are generated by special equipment that depends on line-of-sight placement to operate properly. Microwave channels have a wide band and thus can carry a large number of simultaneous transmissions.

Mobile relay station: A fixed base station established for the automatic retransmission of mobile or portable radio communications.

Mobile repeater station: A mobile radio station in land mobile service that is authorized to automatically retransmit any radio traffic originated by a hand-held portable, by other mobiles, or by base stations.

Multiplex: The ability to transmit simultaneously two or more different types of information in either or both directions over the same frequency.

Patch: A special connection between different communication systems — for example, the connection that allows a radio transmission to be carried over a telephone line.

Scanner: A radio receiver in which the frequency being received is automatically and instantaneously changed until a frequency carrying some message traffic is detected. At that time, the receiver locks on to that frequency until the message is completed. The process is then repeated.

Simplex: Single-frequency operating capability; radio transmissions can occur in either direction but not simultaneously in both; one party transmits, and the other receives.

Squelch: Several types of radio receiver circuits used for suppressing, though not eliminating, unwanted radio signals or radio noise.

Tone: An audio signal or carrier wave of controlled amplitude and frequency that is used for equipment control purposes or to selectively signal a receiver, such as activating a pager.

UHF (ultrahigh frequency): Those radio frequencies between 300 and 3,000 MHz.

VHF (very high frequency): Those radio frequencies between 30 and 300 MHz. The VHF spectrum is further divided into "high" and "low" bands.

THE EMT AS A COMMUNICATOR

Communications equipment, capabilities, and operating procedures vary among EMS systems, but all services rely on properly trained personnel to transmit concise, accurate reports. To achieve effective, efficient EMS communication, each EMT must be well trained in the following communications elements:

1. How to operate each piece of radio and telephone hardware.
2. The appropriate voice communication procedures.
3. The appropriate message to send and when to send it.
4. The current status of EMS unit readiness.
5. The relationships between EMS providers if a variety of providers or levels of service are available in the community.

6. The relationship of the EMS system to the community's health care system and other public safety services.

An EMT must also master many communications skills, including verbal communication, written reports, and radio skills. There are no substitutes for these skills. Efficiency and effectiveness in delivering patient care are directly related to how well the EMT can communicate with the rest of the emergency medical care team. The EMT must develop these traits of a good communicator:

1. Be able to use good judgment and common sense whenever operating equipment and communicating with other EMS personnel.
2. Be able to concentrate, listen, and follow instructions and protocols.
3. Be able to speak intelligibly.
4. Be familiar with all the communication tools available in the EMS system and how to use them. These include not only the radio and telephone, but also the vehicle lights, siren and PA system, hand signals, and written messages and reports.

Today, with the widespread public use of scanners, any EMS communication system can be readily evaluated. In fact, the community perception of the quality of the local EMS system may be greatly influenced by how efficiently and professionally its communications are conducted. That professionalism depends on the performance of the EMT.

THE EMS COMMUNICATION SYSTEM

Communication Capabilities

The EMS communication system must be operational 24 hours a day and must provide the following capabilities:

1. Public access for patient entry into the EMS system.
2. Assignment and dispatch of the appropriate EMS unit, with assistance in routing it to the scene as necessary.
3. Communications between EMS units at the scene.
4. Communications between other public safety units involved in the incident (police, highway patrol, fire, civil preparedness, Red Cross, mutual assistance EMS units).
5. Patient care communication between EMS field units and hospital emergency department personnel, including transmission of signs and symptoms, medical consultation, and medical control of treatment procedures at the scene.

The equipment and organization of EMS communication systems may vary significantly. But the key objective must be rapid mobilization and efficient coordination of EMS and public safety resources. Effective communication systems are configured to allow all local EMS services access to the system, as well as to provide compatible links to units from adjoining EMS services.

The heart of any EMS system is the communications control center (Figure 49.1). This may be a simple radio base station staffed by a single communications operator, or it may involve computers, sophisticated electronics, and a large staff of communication specialists. The control center's primary task is to monitor and coordinate the operation of the other communication components — base stations, repeaters, mobile units, hand-held portables, remote consoles, and telephone sets.

Patient Entry into the EMS System

The critical, though often overlooked, initial task of an EMS communication system is to promote rapid patient access to the EMS system. The telephone is the primary means of public access to the EMS system. Poorly publicized EMS numbers, with

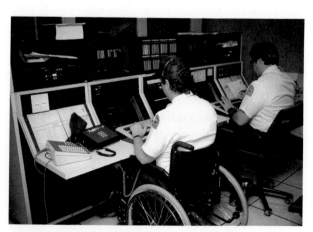

FIGURE 49.1 A communications control center.

too many digits to remember in an emergency, have for years been a common problem throughout the country. This creates confusion for callers, unnecessary delays, relaying of messages among public safety agencies, and delays in response by the appropriate EMS unit. An effective public access mechanism should:

1. Be easily remembered and used by all citizens.
2. Provide rapid, direct contact with the appropriate EMS dispatcher.
3. Have sufficient telephone line capacity and staff to handle anticipated ''peak'' call volume.
4. Offer reliable service with mechanisms to prevent calls from going unanswered, being lost, misunderstood, or waiting unnecessarily.

In the past few years, there has been a significant increase in the use of the 911 universal emergency telephone number to access all public safety services, including EMS. The **Enhanced 911 System, or E911,** is the most technologically advanced version of this telephone service. It is available to all communities in which the local telephone companies have installed electronic switching equipment. The key technical features of E911 for improved public access include automatic number identification (ANI), automatic call location identification (ALI), and automatic ringback. These features allow public safety dispatch personnel to view a digital display of the telephone number and the street address from which the call is being made. In addition, if the caller hangs up, the E911 equipment can prevent disconnection of the call, and automatically ''ring back'' the number (Figure 49.2).

There is little debate that E911 is technically effective for public access. All agree that 911 is a number that is easily remembered and dialed in an emergency. It provides the necessary reliability and capacity for busy situations. One of the chief obstacles to implementing 911, in addition to the expense of special telephone switching equipment, is the agreement required among public safety agencies and community leaders to determine the location for the 911 communication control center and to designate the group responsible for managing the center. Such agreements for a centralized public safety communication system have not been easy to achieve. EMS providers may sometimes become unwilling

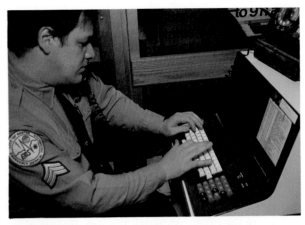

FIGURE 49.2 The 911 emergency telephone number and especially the Enhanced 911 System allow ready access of the patient to the EMS system.

participants in political controversies and interagency rivalries surrounding the planning of a centralized 911 system. By being well informed on the importance of easy, rapid public access for effective EMS and public safety services and on the capabilities of an E911 system, EMTs may make a positive contribution to the planning and implementation of such a central communication system in their community.

Despite the capabilities of 911 and E911 systems, most EMS systems still rely on a single, seven-digit telephone number for public access. In some areas, several numbers may be required simultaneously to summon a variety of EMS response units. In other areas, public access to EMS resources may be accomplished by other means. These include citizen band (CB) and other amateur radio networks (RACES, REACT, etc.), highway call boxes, and governmental or mutual-aid radio systems. Whatever the public access mechanism, the key elements of this initial phase of EMS communications are that the call be promptly received, properly screened, and efficiently acted upon by the EMS dispatcher.

ALERT AND DISPATCH PHASE

If the control center is the cornerstone of the EMS communication system, then the **dispatcher** is the key to the control center. The EMS communication system can perform only as well as the dispatcher performs. Thus, it is essential that the EMS dispatcher be trained to at least the EMT-basic level.

This will help the dispatcher understand the medical functions of the EMS system, including the roles, responsibilities, and capabilities of the EMTs who render patient care. The dispatcher must also be thoroughly familiar with the capabilities and limitations of the mobile and portable radio units in the ambulances and other EMS response units.

In addition, the dispatcher must be aware of the level of training of the EMTs in each EMS response unit, as well as the medical equipment carried on board. In appropriate emergencies, the dispatcher must be able to provide effective emergency self-help advice to the caller. Although the specific role of the dispatcher may differ from one EMS system to another, each dispatcher must have a working knowledge of the operation and limitations of each piece of radio and telephone hardware in the control center, know the applicable FCC rules regarding that center and its equipment, and understand the general operations, responsibilities, and interrelationships of the public safety service agencies in the area.

The alert and dispatch phase of EMS communications requires several important actions by the dispatcher. These include:

1. Properly screening and determining the priority of each call.
2. Selecting and alerting the appropriate EMS response unit(s).
3. Dispatching and directing the selected unit(s) to the correct incident location.
4. Coordinating the response of the EMS unit(s) with those of other public safety services until the conclusion of the incident.

After receiving the original call for assistance, the dispatcher must attempt to assess its relative importance in order to initiate the appropriate EMS response. The dispatcher must elicit the exact location of the patient needing help, the nature and severity of the emergency, some description of the surrounding scene (number of patients in a multiple injury situation, special environmental hazards, and so on), and, if possible, additional information such as the telephone number from which the call is being made, the patient's age and name, and other information determined by local protocol. From this information, the dispatcher will assign the appropriate EMS unit to respond based on the following criteria:

1. The dispatcher's perception of the severity of the problem (life-threatening or not).
2. Proximity of EMS units to the scene (response time).
3. Level of training (first responder, BLS, ALS) and experience of available EMS units.
4. The need for additional response units (EMS, fire department, hazardous materials handling team, MEDEVAC helicopter, additional police units, etc.)

Having made a decision, the dispatcher's next task is to alert and mobilize the appropriate unit(s). A variety of equipment may be used for the alerting function. The dispatch radio system may be used to alert those units already in service and monitoring the channel. Frequently, there will be a unit-specific tone generated to alert the selected unit of an incoming message. Special telephone circuits or "hot lines" may be used between the control center and the EMS crew station or "quarters." These circuits will ring without dialing whenever the dispatcher lifts the telephone handset. Another method is special tone-generating radio equipment that is activated by the dispatcher; it not only alerts the selected EMS crew, but also turns on the station lights and opens vehicle access doors at a distance of several miles from the communications center.

In EMS systems that rely on volunteer or part-time personnel not exclusively engaged in staffing EMS response units, paging is a common alerting system. **Paging** involves the use of a coded tone radio signal, and sometimes a voice message, transmitted to small individual radio receivers called "beepers." The paging signals may be sent selectively to alert only certain individuals, or a blanket signal can be sent that activates all of the pagers of that service. The alerted personnel must then contact the dispatcher, by radio or telephone, to acknowledge the message and receive details on the assignment.

Once the selected units have been alerted, all units must be properly dispatched and routed to the incident. Every EMS system should use a standard dispatching procedure. The dispatcher's instructions to the alerted units should be given by a distinct voice protocol that includes the following details:

1. The nature and severity of the injury, illness, or incident
2. The exact location of the incident

3. The number of patients
4. Responses by other public safety agencies
5. Special directions or advisories such as known adverse road or traffic conditions
6. The time at which the units are dispatched

All radio communications during the dispatch, as well as other phases of operations, must be brief and easily understood. Plain English transmissions, rather than elaborate codes, are generally preferred.

The dispatcher's job includes accurate tracking of EMS units and other public safety units throughout the incident. Personnel in responding units have the responsibility of keeping the dispatcher informed of their location and status.

An EMS system's dispatch protocol should designate the type of unit to respond to a particular situation. Many variations of such protocols are found. Based on the local situation, these may include the dispatch of a single emergency ambulance, a two-tiered response of basic life support (BLS) and advanced life support (ALS) units, with one unit providing transport capability, or a multi-tiered system in which first responders, such as fire or police units, are dispatched with BLS and/or ALS units to reduce response time. Whatever protocol is employed, the EMT dispatcher must maintain accurate status reports of all units being dispatched. To do so requires that the dispatcher concentrate, follow established procedures, and successfully employ any available status-keeping aids. These aids might range from a simple matrix board with flags or lights to indicate a unit's status and location to a sophisticated **computer-aided dispatch (CAD)** display (Figure 49.3).

The actions of the EMT dispatcher during the dispatch phase are aimed at mobilizing the appropriate resources quickly and ensuring the accurate exchange of information. The desired result is the shortest possible response time for the appropriate EMS unit. An effective EMS communication system will also mandate that its EMT dispatchers contribute their knowledge and training to the care being rendered. Instances of dispatchers providing emergency medical self-help information and advice to callers are increasing. In these medical self-help situations, the EMT-dispatcher gives callers information and instructions on effective actions to take for themselves or the patient until the EMS or first-

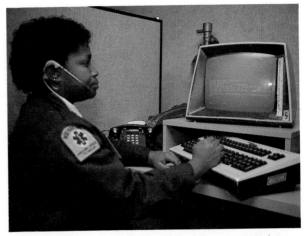

FIGURE 49.3 A sophisticated computer-aided dispatch (CAD) display.

responder unit arrives. This self-help information may include:

1. How to administer cardiopulmonary resuscitation.
2. How to control hemorrhage with direct pressure.
3. How to perform the abdominal thrust maneuver on a choking victim.
4. How to keep a victim of overexposure warm.
5. How to cool off a heat stroke victim.
6. How to prevent further injury to a victim with a neck injury or serious fractures.

This critical, medical self-help role of the EMT dispatcher may require calming a hysterical caller and remaining on the line for a considerable time, while simultaneously maintaining effective communication with EMS field units and other public safety agencies.

RADIO COMMUNICATIONS

Mobile and Portable EMS Communications

Every EMT who staffs an ambulance or other EMS response unit must be familiar with two-way radio communication. This means a thorough working knowledge of the vehicle's mobile radios and the hand-held portables. In addition, the EMT must know when to use them and what to say when transmitting.

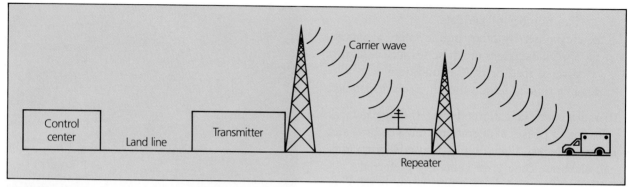

FIGURE 49.4 Two-way radio communication. The message is sent from the control center by a land line to the transmitter. The radio carrier wave is picked up by the repeater for rebroadcast to outlying units. Return radio traffic is picked up by the repeater and rebroadcast to the control center.

The EMT dispatcher usually communicates with field units by transmitting from a fixed radio base or repeater station controlled at the dispatch center (Figure 49.4). In a similar fashion, EMTs in an ambulance rely on their mobile and portable radios for communications. The portable radio is used to communicate with the dispatcher, hospital emergency department, medical control physician, or other EMS or public safety units at the scene. Portable radios are essential in helping coordinate EMS response at the scene of a multiple casualty incident. They are also effective in urban areas when searching for a patient in a multiple story building; one EMT has to stay with the unit until directed to the proper location by the other EMT after the patient has been found.

Ambulances are usually equipped with an external public address system, which may be a component of the mobile radio. Similarly, the intercom between the cab and patient compartment may also be a component of the mobile radio. EMS systems may employ a variety of two-way radio hardware. Some operate VHF equipment in the simplex (push-to-talk, release-to listen) mode, while others conduct duplex (simultaneous talk-listen) on UHF frequencies ("MED" channels). Some EMS radio systems are simply configured so that they require no off-site control links. Other systems rely on special telephone lines as control links for their remotely located base stations and antennae. Whatever equipment design is used, all EMS communications systems have some basic limitations. The field EMT must know the operational limitations of the communication equipment and understand how to cope effectively with and minimize them.

In any EMS radio system, the effectiveness and the extent of communication coverage are determined primarily by the "talk-back" capability of the weaker of either the mobile or portable units. Since the base and repeater stations normally have much greater power and higher antenna placement, their signal will generally be heard and understood at a much greater distance than the signal produced from a mobile unit. A portable or hand-held radio has an even shorter effective communication range, as it has the lowest power output and, frequently, the lowest antenna location. EMTs on field assignment must realize that although they can clearly receive the dispatcher or hospital on their radios, they themselves may not be heard or understood. Even small changes in the transmitting location of the portable or mobile unit can produce significant variations in the reception quality of the radio traffic.

EMTs must also be aware that the efficiency of the radio system's equipment greatly influences the success of communications. The antenna of an ambulance radio that has been loosened by a hospital overhang or a damaged microphone often prevents high-quality communications. The field EMT and the EMT dispatcher are responsible for checking the condition and status of the communication equipment they will be using at the start of each work assignment and correcting or replacing any deficiencies.

Standard Radio Operating Procedures

From the time they acknowledge receiving a call until completion of the run, EMTs must use their radio communication system effectively. Frequently, they must demonstrate their communications skills. To help all EMTs, dispatchers, and others in the EMS system communicate properly, EMS system directors should establish a standard radio communication protocol. This protocol should include the appropriate format for transmitting messages, a definition of key communications words and key phrases, and procedures for trouble-shooting common radio communication problems. For example, the "call-up" for establishing radio contact between two units is made by transmitting the identification of the called unit first, followed by the identification of the unit calling, as in "Dispatch, this is Medic One." Using the format, the EMT initiating the call gives the radio transmitter a chance to turn on and generate a suitable carrier wave for the voice message. This procedure alerts the unit being called to listen for the identity of the transmitting unit and helps eliminate the caller's clipping the first part of the message by speaking too soon.

Standard radio operating procedures are designed to reduce the number of misunderstood messages, to keep transmissions as brief as possible, thus making more "air time" available, and to develop effective radio discipline for use in critical situations. In addition to learning standard message formats, every EMT should practice these radio techniques:

1. Always monitor the channel before transmitting to avoid interfering with another unit's radio traffic.
2. Plan what you will say before pushing the transmit switch. This will help keep your transmissions brief and precise.
3. Speak distinctly and directly, but never shout, into the microphone. The microphone should be held about 2 inches from your mouth (Figure 49.5).
4. Always acknowledge a transmission promptly. If you are otherwise occupied and cannot immediately take a long incoming message, simply acknowledge the call-up with "Stand by."
5. Use standard English language. Avoid slang phrases or complex codes.

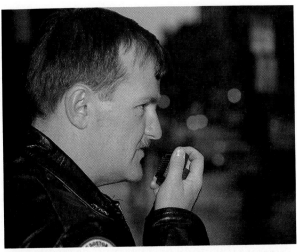

FIGURE 49.5 A radio microphone should be held about 2 inches from the EMT's mouth. Speak distinctly and directly; never shout.

6. Speak at a moderate, understandable rate.
7. Avoid showing negative emotions, such as anger or irritation, when transmitting. Your tone of voice should indicate courtesy, making it unnecessary to say "please" or "thank you," which wastes air time.

Becoming familiar with standard radio formats and techniques will help EMTs perform their jobs more effectively through proper use of the EMS communication system. From acknowledgment of the dispatch call until the EMT is cleared from the medical emergency, the mobile radio communications capability of the EMS system will be in use at several key points. The EMT must report at these intervals:

1. To acknowledge the dispatch information.
2. To estimate time of arrival (ETA) when actually responding to the scene.
3. To announce unit's arrival on the scene.
4. To announce unit's departure from the scene and the destination hospital. (Include number of patients transported if more than one.) Include estimated time of arrival (ETA).
5. To announce unit's arrival at the hospital or other facility.
6. To announce that unit is clear of the incident or hospital and is available for another assignment.
7. To announce unit's arrival back at quarters.

While en route to and from the scene, the EMT should also report to the dispatcher special road conditions that might affect other responding units. The EMT should report any unusual delays, such as road blockages, elevated bridges, etc. At the scene, the EMT may use the radio system to request additional EMS or other public safety assistance, and then help coordinate their response.

Medical Communication Capability

Every EMS system must have physician input and involvement. The physicians who provide medical consultation and control for the EMT must be familiar with the EMS communication system and protocols (Figure 49.6). They must be readily available to communicate on the radio equipment installed at the hospital or on a mobile or portable unit. It is essential that the EMS director, medical control officers, and providers develop standard medical treatment and radio communication protocols for use by the physicians and EMTs in EMS field operations. Such protocols will help decrease misunderstandings between physician and EMTs regarding patient reports and orders.

Ambulance-to-Hospital Communication

Field EMTs must have the capability of direct radio contact with hospital emergency department personnel. EMTs can utilize their vehicle or portable radios to request physician consultation and to transmit the patient assessment report. The patient report should follow the classical medical case presentation and briefly include these elements:

1. Patient's age and sex (name optional depending on local protocol).
2. Patient's chief complaint or EMT's perception of the problem and its severity.
3. Brief pertinent history of the patient's illness or injury, including medications, allergies, pertinent systemic problems such as diabetes, cardiac conditions, pregnancy.
4. Brief report of physical findings to include vital signs, level of consciousness, and general appearance and degree of distress.
5. Brief summary of emergency treatment provided the patient and patient's response, if any.
6. Estimated time of arrival at the hospital.

Where there are multiple patients at an incident, the EMT should carefully identify each patient with an appropriate number. This will decrease confusion at the hospital.

Medical control communication must be conducted on radio channels that are relatively free of other radio traffic and interference. EMS systems may employ a variety of means for controlling access on the ambulance-to-hospital channels. In some cases, the ambulance dispatcher also monitors and assigns appropriate clear medical control channels. Other systems rely on special communications operations, such as **CMEDs (centralized medical emergency dispatch)** or **Resource Coordination Centers,** to monitor and allocate the medical control channels among EMS providers. Still others use a scanning capability built into their radio system, such as a **RTSS (radio-telephone switch station)** base and its associated mobiles. This unit automatically selects a clear channel from among several UHF frequencies.

When communication personnel regularly monitor channels and assign clear ones to EMS providers as needed, they utilize the "real time" method of channel allocation. This method provides maximum flexibility for control and use of all EMS radio channels during busy radio traffic periods. An alternate method for allocating EMS radio channels may be used in some areas. This is the assignment of channels according to geographic sector. Only certain available channels are assigned to different providers

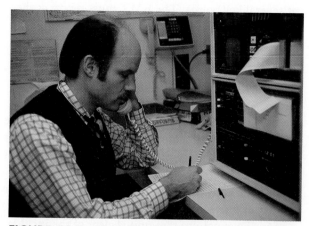

FIGURE 49.6 The physicians at the hospital must be familiar with the EMS communication system and protocols so they can provide medical consultation and control for EMTs in the field.

in any one geographic area. Each channel is then designated for "primary," "secondary," or other use by the appropriate EMS providers. This allocation method severely restricts the flexibility for using the radio frequencies, but it may be satisfactorily used in areas that have several providers operating in adjacent service sectors with relatively low radio traffic demands.

Hospital-to-Hospital Communications

Most day-to-day hospital communications rely on the commercial telephone system. Regular telephones, and even dedicated "hot lines," connect departments within the hospital or link closely related hospital facilities for a variety of everyday activities. In addition, hospitals are heavy users of paging systems to maintain contact with their own personnel within and outside the hospital's facilities.

In times of natural disasters, two-way radio communications may become important to the hospitals. During severe weather, or in incidents involving many sick or injured, the telephone network may fail or be overloaded with calls. Vital information may not be available to hospital personnel by routine means. In such situations, the EMS radio communications system may be utilized to send reports on bed availability, status of blood bank supplies, and other medical resource availability. Such interhospital communications should not interfere with EMS-to-hospital communications. EMS directors should make certain that their radio communication links among hospitals and the rest of the EMS system are tested regularly to ensure proper readiness. Most hospitals have their own base stations or are linked directly with the local EMS communication center via remote control receiving units.

The Federal Communications Commission (FCC)

All radio operations in the United States, including those used by EMS systems, are conducted according to regulations developed and enforced by the Federal Communications Commission. That agency also has jurisdiction over interstate and international telephone and telegraph services, which may occasionally involve EMS activity.

The FCC's main EMS-related responsibilities include:

1. Allocating specific radio frequencies for use by EMS providers. The "modern era" of EMS communication began in 1974, when the FCC created a block of ten UHF "MED" channels to be used by EMS providers. These were added to several VHF frequencies that were previously available for EMS systems, but were often simultaneously used by interfering non-EMS activities.
2. Licensing eligible individual base station operations and assigning appropriate radio call signs relating to those stations. An authorizing license is usually issued by the FCC to the operator for a five-year period, after which it must be renewed. Each FCC license is granted only for a specific operating group — for example, a specific base station control location on a specific frequency with specific antenna locations and for a specific number of associated mobile or portable units.
3. Establishing licensing standards and operating specifications for radio equipment to be used by EMS providers. Before it can be licensed, a particular item of radio equipment must be submitted, by its manufacturer, to the FCC for type-acceptance based on the established operating specifications and regulations.
4. Establishing limitations for transmitter power output. This principally involves base station hardware.
5. Monitoring radio operations, including making spot field checks to help ensure compliance with FCC rules and regulations.

FCC rules and regulations are available for purchase from the Government Printing Office in Washington, D.C. They are contained in many volumes of technical and legal language with only a very small section devoted to EMS communication issues (Part 90, subpart C). Most EMS systems have radio and telephone communication expertise available to them. Thus, EMTs need not wade through these government publications for appropriate guidance on technical issues; instead, they should rely on their EMS system supervisors.

One important element the FCC has largely relegated to EMS system providers and directors is proper and effective communication planning and coordination. The EMT should participate in this process at all available opportunities. The EMT can contribute knowledge of how communications will assist in providing emergency medical care in the field, what interference problems have traditionally occurred on particular frequencies, where the "dead" spots are located, and what needs exist for radio communications with other public safety, rescue, or adjacent EMS organizations. Although there are many possible solutions for hardware and system design problems, the planning process must first define the needs for a particular communication system in the form of answers to the following questions: Who needs to talk to whom from where and when?

YOU ARE THE EMT...

1. In addition to disagreeing over the location of a 911 communication control center, why do you think a lot of communities have not been able to implement an E911 system?

2. Why is it important that an EMS dispatcher have EMT training? What kind of problems could a dispatcher run into without such training?

3. You are a dispatcher and have received a call from a woman who says her two-year-old is choking and turning blue. What information must you obtain from her? What advice will you give her?

4. Research and report on the radio communication protocol in your community's EMS system.

Records and Reports

50

OVERVIEW

Paperwork is a pain. It is not the exciting, "save-a-life" part of the EMT's job that most people identify with. Yet it is such a vital part of providing emergency medical care. Adequate reporting and the keeping of accurate records ensure the continuity of patient care, guarantee proper transfer of responsibility, comply with the requirements of health departments and law enforcement agencies, and fulfill the administrative needs of the ambulance operator. While these reporting and record keeping duties are essential for the EMT, they must never come before patient care. With experience and alertness, the EMT will soon learn to obtain most of the necessary information from simple observation, listening, and quick questioning while rendering emergency care to the patient.

Chapter 50 begins with an overview of the general information requirements of ambulance report forms. Then the chapter describes the general procedures for filling out the forms, usually a preliminary street form, followed by a permanent ambulance run report. Throughout the chapter, the importance of accurate record keeping is stressed — these records are often consulted long after the incident has occurred.

OBJECTIVES

The objectives of Chapter 50 are to

- list the general information requirements of ambulance reports.
- describe the general procedures for record keeping, including how to fill out a preliminary street form and a permanent ambulance run report.

GENERAL INFORMATION REQUIREMENTS

Record keeping serves several important purposes. By delineating the nature of the patient's injuries or illness at the scene and the initial treatment provided by the EMT, ambulance report forms provide a mechanism for the efficient continuation of patient care. The forms should also be used in an ongoing program for evaluation of the quality of patient care. Additional data may be obtained from the forms to analyze causes, severity, and types of illness or injury requiring emergency medical care.

Records also provide administrative information for patient billing. In addition, they can be used to evaluate response times, equipment usage, and other areas of administrative interest.

The requirements on an ambulance report form are many and vary from jurisdiction to jurisdiction, mainly because so many agencies derive information from them. There is no universally accepted form, but the following information is typically obtained:

Patient Information

Patient's name, age, sex

Address

Nature of call

Mechanism of injury

Location of patient when first seen (specific details noted, especially if incident is vehicular accident or criminal activity is suspected)

Rescue and treatment measures by first responders

Signs and symptoms found during primary and secondary survey

Care and treatment given at site and during transport

Vital signs, patient condition, and changes in vital signs and condition during transport

Medications used by patient

Allergies

Hospital to which patient was taken

Disposition of patient's valuables

Signature of patient or relatives if medical care is refused

Procedures followed and disposition of body in the event of death

Dying statements

Circumstances involved if there are potential legal concerns such as homicide, suicide, or physical abuse

Statements made by patient or others that might serve as legal testimony

Administrative Information

Date of call

Time of call

Name and telephone number of caller

Time of dispatch

Time of arrival at scene

Time of arrival at hospital

Time of leaving hospital

Time of return to base

Patient's insurance identification

Dispatching agency

Names of EMTs responding to call

Type of run to scene, emergency/routine

Type of run to hospital, emergency/routine

GENERAL PROCEDURES FOR RECORD KEEPING

Specific procedures for collecting, reporting, and recording the information for each run will vary from community to community. The EMT must become familiar with local requirements, but general principles do apply.

Ambulance Street Forms

Initially, most EMTs make use of an **ambulance street form.** This is a compact form, frequently printed on a 3 × 5 index card, that allows the EMT to obtain and record the information needed to make a radio report to the emergency department (Figure 50.1). This information is also used to fill out the more detailed, permanent ambulance run record.

Reporting and record keeping begin with the dispatcher's notification of the need for the ambulance at the scene of an accident or illness. The first entry is the location to which the ambulance

is being sent. En route to the scene, the dispatcher may provide additional information on the patient or situation. Any unexpected delays in responding while en route to the scene should be reported to the dispatcher, especially traffic problems or road blockages that might affect other emergency vehicles. The dispatcher should be notified of arrival at the scene, the initial condition of the scene, and the need, if any, for additional units.

The EMT will then record the number of patients, if more than one, and begin recording pertinent information for each patient, such as name, age, injuries, signs, symptoms, vital signs, medications, and allergies as the primary and secondary surveys are performed. Following treatment of the patient, the dispatcher should be notified that the ambulance is en route to a specific hospital. During transport, the emergency department should be notified of the condition of the patient en route if it has not already been contacted by the EMTs. Any significant change in the condition of the patient needs to be reported to the emergency department as well as recorded on the run report. During transport to the hospital, the EMT may begin filling out the permanent run report if the patient is stable and not needing care or reassurance.

Run Reports

Upon arrival at the emergency department, the EMT should give a verbal report on the patient and the treatment provided to the physician or emergency department staff (Figure 50.2). Once the EMT's assistance in the emergency department is no longer needed, the permanent **ambulance run report** is completed (Figure 50.3). All parts of the report should be completed at this time and not left until later to be filled out. Appropriate copies of the permanent run report are left with the emergency department.

When completing the narrative portion of the run report, the following format will be helpful in organizing information. Each narrative report requires four basic components: (1) the patient's history, (2) the findings on physical examination, (3) the EMT's diagnostic impression, and (4) the treatment rendered.

The history section should contain information concerning the patient's chief complaint or problem. This includes a brief description of the patient's

AMBULANCE STREET FORM

Run number _____ Name _____ Age ___ Sex ___ Date _____

COMPLAINT _____

_____

_____

ASSESSMENT _____

_____

_____

	BLOOD PRESSURE	PULSE	RESP.	NEUROLOGICAL		
Time ___	___ ___	___	___	Time			

Time			
Talks	yes/no	yes/no	yes/no
Follows commands	yes/no	yes/no	yes/no
Pupil diameter	L R mm mm	L R mm mm	L R mm mm

Time ___ ___ ___ ___ ___ ___
Time ___ ___ ___ ___ ___ ___

SKIN
normal ___   warm, dry ___
pale ___   cold, clammy ___
cyanotic ___   warm, moist ___
flushed ___   cold, dry ___

BLOOD LOSS
None ___
Minor ___
Moderate ___
Severe ___

SITES OF INJURY

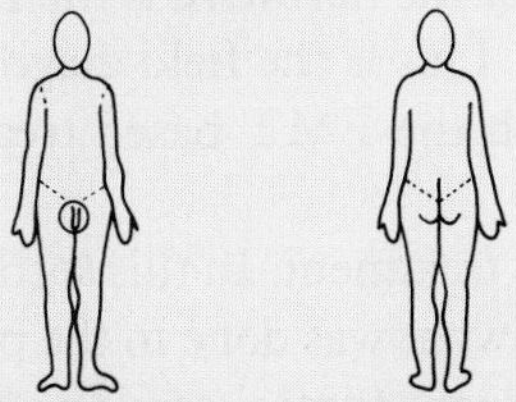

ANTERIOR   POSTERIOR

NEUROVASCULAR

	UPPER R or L		LOWER R or L		CHEST
Sensation					clear ___
Movement					rales ___
Pulse					wheezes ___
Capillary filling					other ___
Time					

EMERGENCY MEDICAL CARE RENDERED

_____

_____

TIME
Enroute _____
Arrival _____
Depart _____
Hospital _____

CREW

_____

_____

_____

FIGURE 50.1 Ambulance street form. This is a preliminary report to record the information that will later be entered on a permanent ambulance run record.

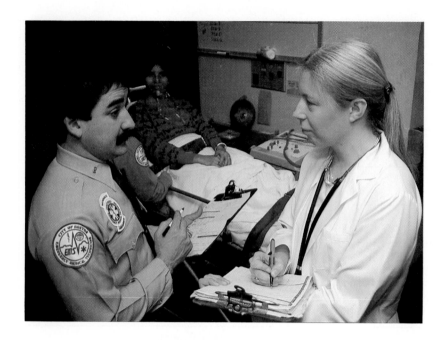

FIGURE 50.2 Upon arriving at the hospital, the EMT gives a verbal report to emergency department personnel on the patient's condition and the treatment provided.

present illness or injury, including mechanism of injury, position found, significant environmental findings, and so on. The **P–Q–R–S–T of pain** should be used to describe the patient's pain:

P — *Provokes:* What brought on the pain? What makes it better or worse?

Q — *Quality:* Sharp, dull, achy, burning, etc.?

R — *Region:* Where is the pain located?

S — *Severity:* Mild, moderate, severe?

T — *Time:* Onset, duration, recurrence?

The history section should also contain pertinent past medical history, including medications, allergies, and significant medical problems such as cardiac disease, diabetes, or pulmonary problems.

The next component of the narrative — findings on physical examination — contains information on the following:

1. Position in which the patient was found
2. Respiratory status (airway; respiratory rate, rhythm, and effort)
3. Cardiac status (pulse rate and character; perfusion)
4. Level of consciousness — **AVPU scale**
   A — *Alert:* oriented to time, person, place
   V — *Verbal:* responds to verbal stimuli
   P — *Pain:* responds to painful stimuli
   U — *Unresponsive*

5. Visual exam (wounds: location, type, severity; deformities: location, type, severity)
6. Secondary assessment findings (reported by body systems)

When writing the physical examination section, significant negative findings — for example, "The abdomen nontender on palpation" — should be recorded as well as the positive findings.

The third section of the narrative is the EMT's diagnostic impression. This is the field diagnosis of the patient upon which the EMT based treatment of injury or illness.

The final section is treatment. In this section the EMT briefly describes what was done to the patient, such as splinting, oxygen administration, and so forth. Changes in the patient's condition as a result of treatment are also included in this section.

Accurate recording of information on the ambulance run report form, especially in the narrative section, will answer many questions that might arise at a later date. In addition, such information provides a useful tool in a program for evaluating quality of patient care.

Ambulance records must be handled with care and stored in an appropriate manner once they have been completed. They are confidential documents of significant potential legal consequence and must be treated as such.

EMERGENCY MEDICAL SERVICE PATIENT FORM

_____ of _____

Date:_____

Unit No.:_____

Case No.:_____

Time:_____

Shift A B C D

Police/Sheriff:

on scene   requested

A Single Pt/Trans
B Multi Pt/Trans
C Multi Unit/Trans
D Aid Only/No Trans
E No Aid/No Trans
F Other _____

Location _____ Type of Call _____

Name _____ Age _____ Sex M F DOB _____

Address _____ City _____ State _____ Zip _____

Responsible Adult _____ Relationship _____ Phone _____

EMT-P _____ Badge No. _____ Pt's MD _____

EMT-P _____ Badge No. _____ Extra Attn. _____

Back-up   EMS/Fire _____ Authorizing M.D. _____

Chief Complaint: _____

Injury/Illness Description: _____

Remarks/Hx: _____

Medications: _____

Vital Signs   Lying   Sitting   Standing   BP _____ Pulse _____ Resp _____ Temp _____

PATIENT STATUS	DRUGS	AID

PATIENT STATUS

Repeat VS
2   3

BP _____ _____
P _____ _____
R _____ _____

Level of Consciousness
Initial

A —Alert
V —Responds to Verbal
P —Responds to Pain
U —Unresponsive

Repeat
A V P U

Pupils
left   right
size   size

●●●   ●●●
react   react
nr   nr

Skin
normal   cyanotic
pale   flushed
dry   moist

Respirations
normal   shallow
          labored

Breath Sounds
left   right
normal   normal
decreased   decreased
rales   rales
wheezes   wheezes
absent   absent

Bleeding
none
min mod sev

Pain
none
min mod sev

DRUGS

amt.   time   amt.   time

Atropine   **Dextrose**
1. _____ _____:_____   1. _____ _____:_____
2. _____ _____:_____   2. _____ _____:_____

Bicarb   **Epinephrine**
1. _____ _____:_____   1. _____ _____:_____
2. _____ _____:_____   2. _____ _____:_____
3. _____ _____:_____   3. _____ _____:_____

Bretylium   **Lidocaine**
1. _____ _____:_____   1. _____ _____:_____
2. _____ _____:_____   2. _____ _____:_____

Calcium   **Oxygen**
1. _____ _____:_____   nasal cannula
2. _____ _____:_____   face mask
                        L/min:_____
Naloxone   bag-mask
1. _____ _____:_____   demand valve
2. _____ _____:_____

Other: _____

Allergies: _____

AID

Antishock pants
Bandaging
Burn kit
CPR
C-Collar
Defibrillate/Cardiovert
    Joules:_____
Dextrostix:_____mg%
Extrication/KED
EDA
ET:_____mm
EKG
    Rhythm:_____
Ice pack
OB kit
Oral/Nasal Airway
Spine board
Splinting
Suction

IV   RL   D5W
      gauge   time
1. _____ _____:_____
2. _____ _____:_____

Response code to hospital:_____ Hospital: _____ Receiving M.D.: _____

I was offered aid by the City of _____ EMS, but chose not to accept emergency treatment and/or transportation.

Signature _____ Witness _____

FIGURE 50.3 Ambulance run report. This form is used by both EMTs and EMT-paramedics to document the four basic elements of prehospital care: patient identification and history, physical findings, the EMT's diagnostic impressions, and the treatment given.

Additional Records and Reports

In some instances, the EMT may be required to file special reports with appropriate authorities. These may include incidents involving gunshot wounds, dog bites, certain infectious diseases, suspected physical, sexual, or substance abuse, and so on. The EMT must be familiar with local requirements for reporting these incidents, as failure to report them may constitute a criminal act.

YOU ARE THE EMT...

1. What is the difference between an ambulance street form and an ambulance run report?
2. What kind of information on the street form can be transferred to the ambulance run report?
3. How can an EMS system use its ambulance run reports to review its performance and project future needs?
4. Research and report on the special reports that EMTs have to file in your community.

SECTION 12

APPENDICES

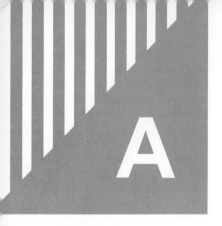

APPENDIX A
Intravenous Therapy

OVERVIEW

Intravenous therapy can be a valuable adjunct therapy for the EMT if allowed by state and local laws. This therapeutic modality requires extensive training in its use as well as an ongoing program of retraining to maintain the necessary skills level. In addition, the EMT must be aware of the indications for the use and maintenance of IV therapy as well as possible complications. Close medical control and supervision, as well as medical review, are absolutely mandatory if the EMT is to use IV therapy.

Appendix A begins with a definition of intravenous fluid therapy and the terms related to its use. Then the equipment and supplies needed to provide IV therapy are listed. Next the steps to start IV infusions are described, followed by a discussion of the importance of monitoring the patient and the IV. The last section of Appendix A warns of possible complications of IV therapy.

OBJECTIVES

The objectives of Appendix A are to

- define intravenous fluid therapy.
- identify the equipment and supplies needed to provide IV therapy.
- learn the steps to start an IV infusion.
- realize the importance of monitoring the patient and the IV.
- recognize the possible complications of IV therapy.

DEFINITION OF TERMS

Intravenous fluid therapy (IV therapy) is an intermediate or advanced EMT skill. The ability to use this skill is determined by state and local laws, ordinances, and standards of practice. Implementation of this level of care requires intensive training, clinical practice, and continuing education and skills practice. Additional requirements include mandatory medical control and medical quality assessment follow-up. As with any patient care procedure, meticulous documentation of indications for and patient response to the procedure are required. Additionally, EMT documentation of the physician's order for IV therapy is mandatory. Ongoing medical quality control is necessary to ensure appropriate and efficient patient care.

Intravenous fluid therapy is not a difficult skill to learn, although once learned, continuous practice is required to maintain it. This skill will be learned in a well-controlled environment, but generally will be practiced during stressful situations, under adverse environmental conditions and when time is a critical factor. In addition, potentially serious complications, of which the EMT must be aware, can accompany the use of IV therapy.

The EMT must understand the difference between transfusion and infusion. **Transfusion** is the introduction of whole blood or blood products into the vascular system. The EMT will probably never institute a field transfusion. Because a patient may be receiving a transfusion during interhospital transfers, however, the EMT must be familiar with the equipment and techniques used and the complications of transfusions.

Infusion is the introduction of fluid other than blood or blood products into the vascular system. The EMT will use this technique to establish and maintain direct access to the circulation or to provide fluids in order to maintain an adequate circulating blood volume. Fluids used for intravenous

TABLE A.1   Common Intravenous Fluids

Solution	Abbreviation	Component Electrolytes
5% dextrose	D5W	5% dextrose
10% dextrose	D10W	10% dextrose
Normal saline	NS	0.9% sodium chloride (NaCl)
Half-normal saline	½NS	0.45% NaCl
Quarter-normal saline	¼NS	0.2 NaCl
Lactated Ringer's	LR	NaCl, potassium chloride (KCl), calcium chloride (CaCl), sodium lactate

Note: All solutions may also be made containing dextrose, in which case they are abbreviated by adding D5 or D10 as a prefix. For example, Lactated Ringer's in 5% dextrose would be abbreviated D5LR.

infusion are frequently referred to as **electrolyte solutions** because the chemical components they contain are electrolytes. The most common solutions, their abbreviations, and components are listed in Table A.1.

Occasionally, the EMT may use another group of solutions called **plasma expanders** or **colloids.** They include Dextran (large molecules of dextrose that are not metabolized) and Plasmanate®. Although plasma expanders and electrolyte solutions may be used to replace up to two-thirds of the normal circulating blood volume, they have no oxygen-carrying capacity.

The appropriate fluid necessary for each patient situation will be determined by local medical control personnel or by protocol.

EQUIPMENT AND SUPPLIES

The following equipment and supplies are needed to provide intravenous infusion therapy:

Appropriate fluid (in an unbreakable container)
IV administration sets (tubing)
IV needles, various sizes (catheter and/or butterfly)
Prep swabs (povoiodine and/or alcohol)
Tape
Constricting band (Penrose or IV tourniquet)
Sterile pads (2 × 2 inch or 4 × 4 inch)
Bandaids
Immobilization boards
Cot-mounted IV pole
Contaminated needle container

Optional supplies may be added according to local preference:

Antiseptic ointment for dressing IV site
Tubes for the collection of blood samples
Syringes for the collection of blood samples

PROCEDURE TO START IV INFUSION

As with any procedure that the EMT performs, the patient must be prepared beforehand. The EMT should explain to the patient that an IV is going to be started, that it is medically necessary to do so, and that there may be some temporary discomfort.

Step 1: Preparing the Solution

The EMT first selects the solution — either ordered by medical control or appropriate for the particular situation — and checks the labeling on the container to see that it is the correct solution. Checking includes making sure that the expiration date on the container has not been exceeded, that the sterile seals on the container are intact, and that the solution is clear, without cloudiness or precipitates (particles).

Next, the EMT selects the **administration set** ordered by medical control or appropriate for the patient situation (Figure A.1). **Mini-drip sets** (with a needle in the drip chamber) are designed to keep an IV line "open" — that is, flowing with minimal volume infusion. These sets are generally used for medical emergencies; they are manufactured to deliver 60 drops/cc. They will generally keep an IV open while infusing less than 0.5cc (30 drops) per minute. **Solution sets** are capable of providing much

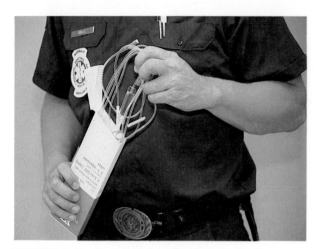

FIGURE A.1 An administration set for IV therapy.

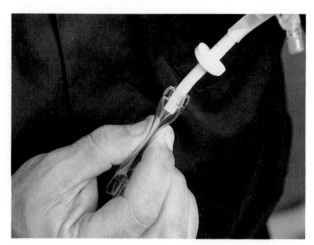

FIGURE A.2 The EMT holds the fluid container higher than the drip chamber while squeezing and releasing the drip chamber until it is about half full.

larger volumes in a shorter period of time. Designed without a needle in the drip chamber, they deliver 10 to 17 drops/cc. They are used for patients who require, or may require, large volumes of fluid to be infused over a short period of time, such as the adult trauma patient who is in hypovolemic shock.

After selecting the appropriate administration set, the EMT must check to see that the sterile seals are intact. The flow control clamp is moved to the desired position and closed. The sterile seal is removed from the end of the tubing closest to the drip chamber. After the sterile seal is removed from the fluid container, the tubing end is inserted into the fluid container. Care must be taken not to contaminate any of the sterile area.

While holding the fluid container higher than the drip chamber, the EMT squeezes the drip chamber and releases it until the chamber is approximately half full (Figure A.2). The flow control is opened, and the fluid is allowed to flush all remaining air from the administration set. While it may be necessary to loosen the sterile seal on the tubing to get the fluid to flow, it should not be removed. The EMT must be sure that there are no air bubbles in the administration tubing and that the drip chamber is still approximately half full. Next, the tape that will be used to secure the needle or catheter in place is laid out, along with the dressing and an antibiotic ointment if local practice permits. An arm board should be available for immobilization.

The IV needle or catheter to be used should be selected but not opened. EMTs generally use three types: the steel needle or "**butterfly**," the **catheter**

over the needle, and the **catheter through the needle** (Figure A.3). In most situations, the EMT will use the catheter over the needle because it is the easiest to use and immobilize and the least likely to cause problems. Needles and catheters are sized by gauge — the smaller the gauge number (i.e., 14, 16), the larger the internal diameter or bore. The larger the bore, the faster fluid can be infused. Thus, the EMT should use large-bore catheters (14, 16, 18) for situations that may require large volume infusions, and small-bore catheters when vascular access with minimal volume infusion is desired.

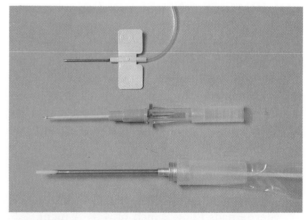

FIGURE A.3 The three types of IV needle assemblies most commonly used to administer IV fluids in the prehospital setting: (top) butterfly; (middle) catheter over the needle; (bottom) catheter through the needle.

Step 2: Selecting the Site

Next, the site for the **venipuncture** has to be selected (Figure A.4). When possible, an uninjured upper extremity should be used. The EMT should try to use the most distal upper extremity site compatible with the gauge of catheter to be used. The veins in the antecubital fossa are the largest but should be used only as a last resort or when severe circulatory collapse exists. Veins over other joints should also be avoided if possible, as they tend to be close to arteries, and also are difficult to immobilize.

The constricting band is placed about the extremity a few inches above the selected site (Figure A.5). The EMT should apply the band tightly

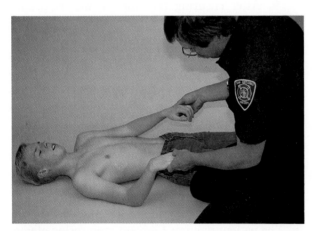

FIGURE A.4 The EMT selects the best site for the venipuncture.

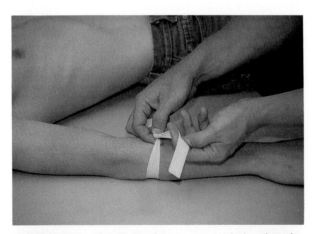

FIGURE A.5 The EMT places a constricting band about the extremity, just above the site for the venipuncture.

enough to restrict venous return but not arterial flow. The extremity is kept below the level of the heart, and the patient should be instructed to clench and unclench the fist several times to enhance venous distention and to make the veins easier to detect. Once a straight, easily accessible vein is identified, the EMT should palpate the vein to determine its location and degree of distention, and to be certain that the vein will not "roll away" from the needle.

Step 3: Preparation of the Site

Preparation of the site, the next step, is of utmost importance. The site must be thoroughly disinfected to prevent contaminants on the skin from being introduced directly into the bloodstream. This step is particularly important in the undesirable environments in which the EMT routinely works. A povoiodine swab is used for the initial cleansing. The EMT begins to wipe over the selected site, then moves in ever-widening circles outward from the site. Then the procedure is repeated using an alcohol swab to remove the povoiodine.

Step 4: Performing the Venipuncture

The EMT should now be ready mentally and physically to perform the venipuncture. Keeping the extremity at the level of the heart or lower, the EMT proceeds in the following manner:

1. With one finger, apply light traction to the skin and vein, distal and slightly to the side of the site selected, to keep the vein from moving.
2. Hold the needle at a 30 degree angle, with the bevel facing up.
3. Firmly and quickly perforate the skin 2 to 5 mm distal to the intended point of entry into the vein (Figure A.6).
4. Then, firmly and quickly enter the vein from above or from the side. You should feel resistance, then a "pop" as the needle enters the vein. If the vein is successfully entered, there should be a "flashback" of blood at the needle hub (Figure A.7).
5. When using steel needles, carefully thread the needle up the vein. For a catheter over the needle, insert the needle approximately 2 to 3 mm past the entry point in the vein and carefully slide the catheter off the needle into

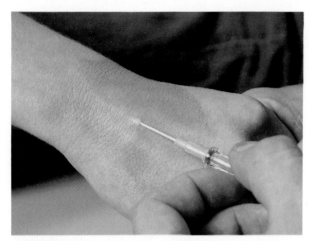

FIGURE A.6 Holding the needle at a 30-degree angle, the EMT quickly and firmly perforates the skin 2 to 5 mm distal to the vein.

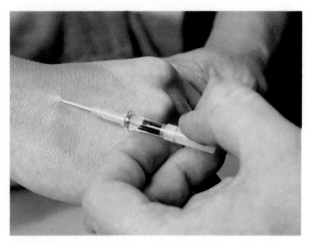

FIGURE A.7 When the vein has been entered, a small amount of blood will "flash back" at the needle hub.

the vein and remove the needle. (*Important note:* If a problem should arise in threading a catheter off of a needle, *do not* pull the catheter back onto the needle. The end of the catheter might be sheared off by the needle point and cause a **plastic catheter embolus**, which is a potentially serious complication for the patient.)

6. If blood samples are to be taken, the syringe should be attached to the needle hub at this time and the blood drawn up into the syringe.

7. Remove the sterile seal on the free end of the administration set tubing and attach it firm-

ly to the hub of the catheter, being careful not to contaminate any of the sterile areas (Figure A.8). To facilitate needle withdrawal and syringe or tubing attachment without unnecessary blood loss, place one finger over the vein at the end of the catheter and apply gentle pressure. When the administration set tubing is attached, remove the constricting band.

8. Slowly open the flow control clamp to allow fluid to infuse. Make sure that fluid is flowing into the vein and not infusing into the surrounding tissue. To confirm that the needle or catheter is inside the vein, place the fluid container below the level of the venipuncture site for a few seconds. If the needle or catheter is properly placed, blood will back up into the tubing of the administration set.

9. After ensuring that the IV line is patent, securely tape the catheter and tubing in place using an arm board if necessary (Figure A.9). When antiseptic dressings are used, they are applied as part of the securing process. Mark on the securing tape the catheter size, and date and time started. To ensure that the catheter stays in place, immobilize the extremity.

MONITORING THE PATIENT AND THE IV

The EMT must monitor the patient and the IV closely. The patient requires frequent monitoring of vital signs on a continuing basis. In addition, the patient

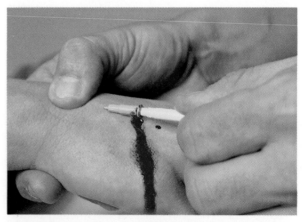

FIGURE A.8 The tubing from the administration set is attached firmly to the hub of the catheter.

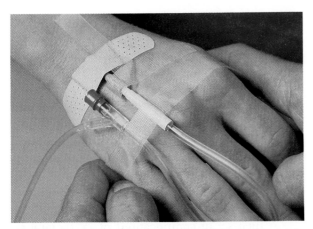

FIGURE A.9 The catheter and tubing are secured by tape, and the limb is immobilized using an arm board.

must be observed for signs of overhydration, such as distention of the neck veins, high blood pressure, rales in the chest, and dyspnea. If these signs appear, the flow rate must be decreased to the absolute minimum. The blood pressure should not be taken in the extremity in which the IV is running unless the other extremity is injured and unavailable.

In general, the EMT will be given a specific order for a flow rate by medical control such as TKO (*to keep open*, the minimum flow rate), wide open (maximum or full flow), or a specific number of cubic centimeters per hour (cc/hour). The flow rate in drops per minute is determined using the following formula:

$$\text{Flow rate in drops/min} \atop \text{(abbreviated, gtts/min)} = \frac{\text{cc/hr ordered} \times \text{drops/cc for drip chamber}}{\text{Time of infusion}}$$

As an example, assume the EMT was ordered to infuse a fluid at 100 cc/hr using a drip chamber manufactured to produce 10 drops/cc; the flow rate in drops per minute would be:

$$17 \text{ drops (gtts)/min} = \frac{100 \text{ cc/hr} \times 10 \text{ drops/cc}}{60 \text{ minutes}}$$

The IV must be checked periodically to ensure a proper flow rate. The flow rate must be checked each time the height of the fluid container changes in relation to the patient. If blood is "backflowing" into the tubing, the fluid container is too low in relation to the patient, and it must be raised or gently compressed. If the IV stops running or the flow rate slows, the tubing must be checked to make sure that it has not become kinked or compressed. Also, the IV site has to be checked to make sure that the catheter remains fixed in position, that the extremity is not flexed and impeding flow, and that the IV fluid is not infiltrating into the surrounding subcutaneous tissue. If **infiltration** is suspected, the surrounding area should be checked for swelling and tenderness. If the IV is infiltrating, the flow must be stopped immediately, and the IV discontinued.

If it becomes necessary to discontinue an IV due to infiltration or an IV malfunction, the EMT first closes the flow control clamp and gently removes the tape securing the catheter. The EMT places a small sterile dressing over the IV insertion site, firmly grasps the catheter hub, then quickly and smoothly withdraws the catheter. Pressure is maintained over the venipuncture site until bleeding stops to prevent the formation of a hematoma. After the bleeding has been controlled, the site is dressed with a Bandaid. Should an initial attempt at venipuncture to start an IV be unsuccessful, the technique for controlling bleeding is the same as just described.

The EMT who is ordered to start a new IV should try to use another extremity. If the same extremity must be used, a site proximal to the original site should be selected. The EMT should *never* start an IV at a site distal to a recently discontinued infusion.

Should a fluid container begin to "run dry," it must be exchanged for a full container before the drip chamber has emptied. The old container is removed from the tubing, care being taken to prevent contamination of the tubing end. The tubing end is inserted into the new container, as in preparing the IV initially, and the drip chamber is partially refilled.

COMPLICATIONS OF IV THERAPY

Complications may arise during or after IV therapy. Therefore, the EMT who is providing IV therapy must know how to manage them. Complications may be local, such as infiltration, or systemic, such as plastic catheter embolus. Certain complications may have grave consequences on the patient's condition.

Local Complications

Some pain from the needle stick is to be expected. The pain may continue as the infusion begins, but it should subside rapidly. Continued pain or burning is probably a sign of infiltration or local adverse reaction, and the IV should be discontinued.

Infection is another complication that may be caused by contaminants inadvertently introduced through the skin. Though not readily apparent at first, swelling, redness, and increased skin temperature at the site are possible indications of infection. The venipuncture site should be changed, preferably to another extremity if possible.

Accidental arterial puncture may also occur, especially if venipuncture is performed over a joint. If bright, red, pulsatile arterial bleeding should occur through or around a catheter, the catheter should be withdrawn immediately. Firm, direct pressure should be applied to the site for at least 5 minutes until the bleeding stops. Other possible local complications include nerve damage, tissue slough, and thrombophlebitis.

Systemic Complications

Systemic complications tend to be more serious than the local complications. Some complications may result in circulatory collapse. The EMT must be able to recognize these problems and be able to deal with them effectively.

Simple fainting may occur due to the emotional response of the patient to the venipuncture procedure. Supportive therapy may be required. All patients should be lying down when IV therapy is started. An **air embolism** may occur if air is allowed to leak into the IV line. The patient may rapidly lose consciousness and develop shock and cyanosis. The IV must be discontinued immediately and the patient transported as rapidly as possible in a head-down position with a high flow of oxygen. Careful attention to the details of IV administration will minimize the chances of this potentially fatal complication.

Circulatory overload (the administration of an excessive amount of IV fluids) should be a rare occurrence with proper monitoring of the patient and IV. Signs and symptoms of circulatory overload are the same as those of congestive heart failure (dyspnea, rales, and neck vein distention). The EMT must reduce the flow to the minimum rate and administer oxygen. **Anaphylaxis** is also rare. This condition usually occurs from medications added to the IV solution rather than from the solution itself. The EMT must discontinue the infusion and begin treatment for the anaphylaxis.

Environmental Complications

A final set of complications of IV therapy are related to the environment. In colder climates, the IV solutions may freeze in the tubing or container very rapidly. Under these circumstances, the EMT may prefer to start the IV in the ambulance or in a heated building rather than in the field. During transport between the ambulance and a building, the fluid container should be protected from exposure to the cold. Another effect of cold can occur in the patient who is receiving a large volume of fluids for hypovolemic shock; if the fluids being administered have not been kept warm, it is possible that the patient's core temperature will drop, which could lead to hypothermia.

YOU ARE THE EMT...

1. How does infusion differ from transfusion? Why must you be familiar with the equipment and techniques of transfusions even though you may never give one?
2. Describe the major difference between mini-drip sets and solution sets. Give an example of a medical emergency that would require the use of each of these types of administration sets.
3. What signs should you look for while monitoring the patient on an IV? What should you do if any of these signs appear?
4. How do you check the flow rate of an IV? What would cause blood to "backflow" into the tubing?

APPENDIX B
Advanced Airway Management

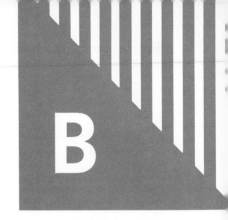

OVERVIEW

Advanced airway management means placing a tube into the airway to maintain an open airway, prevent aspiration of foreign bodies and stomach contents, and provide a pathway for the delivery of oxygen-enriched air. Two devices are used in advanced airway management to achieve these objectives: the endotracheal tube and the esophageal obturator airway. Both devices require considerable skill for proper insertion and use. Once the EMT develops these skills, either device can be used to maintain and protect the airway and provide effective ventilation.

Appendix B begins with a reminder of the importance of primary patient assessment and the need to establish and maintain an adequate airway. Then the chapter describes the two methods of advanced airway management and the contraindications and complications of each technique.

OBJECTIVES

The objectives of Appendix B are to

- emphasize the importance of patient assessment.
- describe advanced airway management using endotracheal intubation.
- describe advanced airway management using an esophageal obturator airway.

PATIENT ASSESSMENT

As always, the highest priority in the primary assessment of a patient must be the airway, breathing, and circulation. This rule applies to every patient. The obviously broken leg or amputated finger may be eye-catching, but the blocked airway must be cleared immediately or the patient will die. Always, the EMT must first think A, B, C. If a major problem is found during this primary survey, the EMT must correct it immediately.

The most important part of prehospital care is the ability to establish and maintain a clear airway. Most conscious patients will be able to maintain an adequate airway. The EMT will need only to provide oxygen and monitor these patients closely for any change. Semiconscious patients will need an oral or nasal airway and suctioning. Only those patients who cannot ventilate adequately and for whom the simpler, noninvasive airway management techniques described in Chapter 6 are found to be ineffective will require the advanced airway control that is described here.

ENDOTRACHEAL INTUBATION

Advanced airway management means **intubation** — the placement of a tube in the airway to improve ventilation. **Endotracheal intubation** is a method of intubation in which an **endotracheal tube (ETT)** is placed through a patient's mouth or nose and directly through the larynx between the vocal cords into the trachea (Figure B.1). The EMT uses a **laryngoscope** to view the vocal cords as the tube passes through (Figure B.2). A balloon near the end of the tube is then inflated with 5 to 10 cc of air to seal the trachea so that air can be blown into the lungs. The inflated balloon also prevents solids and liquids in the pharynx from leaking into the lungs. The ETT completely controls the airway and can be left in place for a long time if necessary.

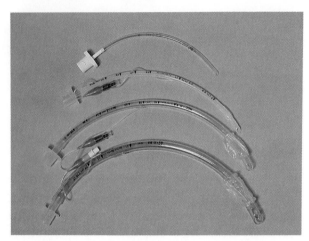

FIGURE B.1 Endotracheal tubes are available in several sizes. The inflatable balloon seals the airway when the tube is properly positioned.

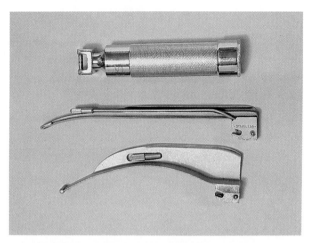

FIGURE B.2 A laryngoscope must be used to insert the endotracheal tube. The detachable laryngoscope blades are straight and curved.

The endotracheal tube is available in many sizes, and a complete selection of tube sizes must be carried. Most adult males will need a 7.5 or 8 mm diameter tube, while most adult females will accept a 7 or 7.5 mm diameter tube. For children, a rough

guide for the appropriately sized tube is to select one equal in size to the diameter of the patient's little finger across the nailbed (Figure B.3). After selecting a tube of proper size, the EMT should use a syringe to inflate the balloon to test for air leaks (Figure B.4). After testing, the balloon should be deflated, and the syringe left attached to the tube and filled with 10 cc of air.

A plastic-coated wire stylet (Figure B.5) may be inserted into the ETT. The stylet will give added rigidity to the tube, and it can be bent to maintain the desired curvature of the endotracheal tube during insertion. The tip of the stylet should be bent

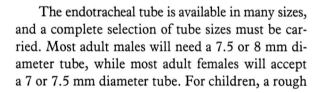

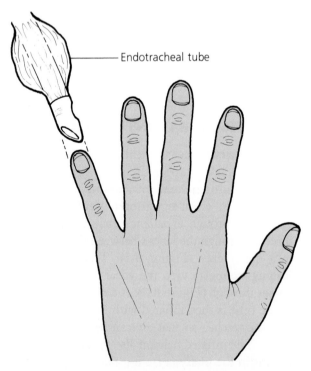

FIGURE B.3 The diameter of the patient's little finger at the nailbed can be used as a rough guide to ETT size selection for a child.

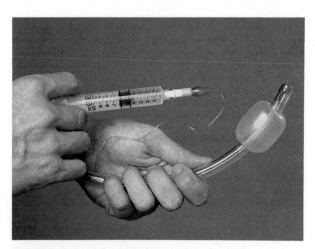

FIGURE B.4 Prior to placement, the balloon of the ETT must be tested for air leaks.

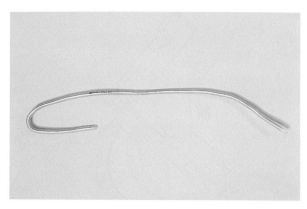

FIGURE B.5 A plastic-coated wire stylet can be used to hold the best shape of the flexible ETT during intubation. The tip of the stylet should be bent and must never protrude from the end of the tube.

to form a gentle curve. It must not stick out of the end of the tube, however, as it could puncture or lacerate the tissues of the airway.

The laryngoscope is used to give the EMT a direct view of the patient's vocal cords. The blade of the laryngoscope is detachable from the handle. Multiple blade sizes are available, all either curved or straight. Adequate lighting is essential for intubation. For this purpose, there is a light bulb near the tip of the blade. The light is activated by lifting the blade away from the handle until it locks at a right angle (Figure B.6). The light will not come on if the blade is not attached properly, if it is burned out, or if the batteries in the handle are dead. The EMT

must be certain that the light is working before trying to intubate the patient.

Inserting the ETT

Once the equipment is ready, the patient should be positioned properly. To simplify intubation, the three parts of the airway (the mouth, pharynx, and trachea) must be positioned in a straight line. First, the neck is flexed on the chest to align the pharynx and trachea (Figure B.7a). Then the head is extended on the neck, lining up the mouth and pharynx (Figure B.7b).

Once the airway is aligned, the mouth should be cleared of any loose or obstructing materials. Dentures or partial plates should be removed. Suction should be used to remove vomitus, blood clots, or other material blocking the upper airway.

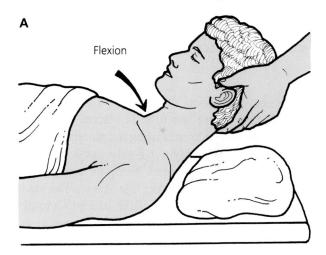

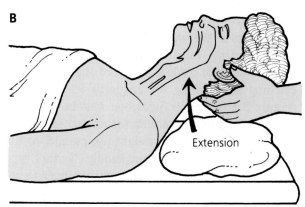

FIGURE B.7 To facilitate placement of the endotracheal tube, the pharynx should be aligned with the trachea by (a) first flexing the neck on the chest and then (b) extending the head on the neck.

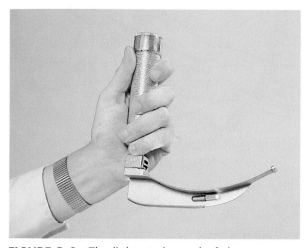

FIGURE B.6 The light at the end of the laryngoscope blade is activated by locking the blade at a right angle to the handle.

A

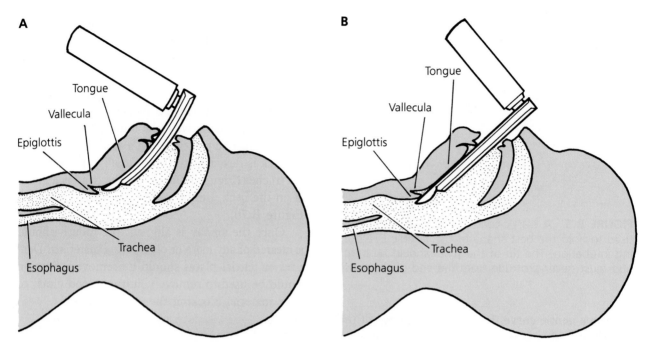

B

FIGURE B.8 To visualize the vocal cords, (a) a curved blade is advanced along the base of the tongue until its tip rests at the vallecula; (b) a straight blade is advanced slightly farther to lift the epiglottis forward.

Before intubation, the patient must be well ventilated. Just before the tube is placed, the EMT should give several breaths using the mouth-to-mouth technique or preferably a bag-valve-mask with 100 percent supplemental oxygen. Next, the laryngoscope handle is grasped in the EMT's left hand. The blade is placed on the right side of the patient's mouth, then moved to the center, pushing the tongue to the left. The final position of the blade will vary, depending on whether it is curved or straight. A curved blade is advanced along the base of the tongue until its tip rests at the **vallecula** — the space between the base of the tongue and the epiglottis (Figure B.8a). A straight blade is advanced slightly farther, catching and pulling the epiglottis itself forward (Figure B.8b). The laryngoscope must be lifted forward enough so the vocal cords can be seen. The lifting force is directed straight up, parallel to the long axis of the laryngoscope handle. Neither type of blade is used as a lever against the upper teeth. This maneuver will break teeth and will not allow visualization of the vocal cords (Figure B.9).

With the patient's vocal cords now in direct view, the EMT holds the ETT in the right hand and advances the tube from the right side of the patient's

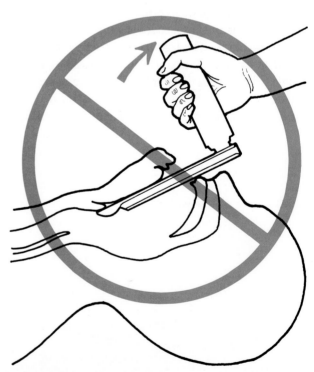

FIGURE B.9 The laryngoscope should *never* be pried or levered against the upper teeth. Visualization of the vocal cords should be achieved only by lifting the tongue forward.

mouth. The vocal cords and the tip of the tube must be kept in sight at all times. The tube should *not* be advanced down the center of the laryngoscope blade because the EMT will not be able to see its tip. The tip of the ETT must be watched as it passes through the vocal cords. The uninflated balloon is also watched as it passes through the vocal cords. The ETT is then advanced 1 inch beyond the upper edge of the balloon (Figure B.10). Once the tube has been placed through the vocal cords into the trachea, the stylet should be removed.

After placing the ETT into the trachea under direct vision, the EMT, using the syringe, inflates the balloon with 5 to 10 cc of air — just enough to block the passage of air around the tube. The syringe must then be detached or the air in the balloon will empty back into it. Proper tube position is checked by listening with a stethoscope over both lungs while ventilating the patient through the tube. Good breath sounds should be heard over both right and left lung fields. If good breath sounds cannot be heard on both sides, the balloon should be deflated and the ETT pulled back approximately 1 inch, the balloon reinflated, and the position checked again by listening for bilateral breath sounds.

Even with the balloon inflated, the endotracheal tube can migrate in the trachea. Therefore, it must be secured in the proper position. The EMT should never let go of the tube until it has been secured in place with tape. Adhesive tape can be used to secure the tube to the patient's mouth or a 30-inch length of umbilical tape can be wrapped around the tube and then around the patient's head to maintain its proper position.

Once the properly placed ETT is secured, an oropharyngeal airway or bite block should be placed between the patient's teeth to prevent the patient from biting on the tube (Figure B.11).

The placement of an endotracheal tube should be accomplished quickly and efficiently. No more than 30 seconds should be required to place the ETT in the proper position. If the ETT is not properly placed by then, it should be removed and positive pressure ventilation given for approximately 1 minute before a second intubation attempt is made.

The most frequent error made during endotracheal intubation is to advance the tube too far, placing it in the right mainstem bronchus where it will ventilate only the right lung. Good breath sounds

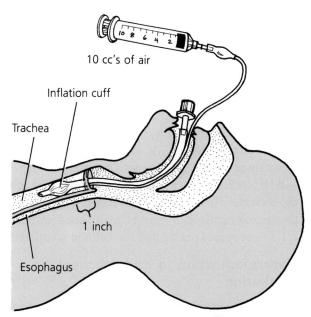

FIGURE B.10 When properly positioned, the upper edge of the balloon should lie approximately 1 inch below the level of the vocal cords.

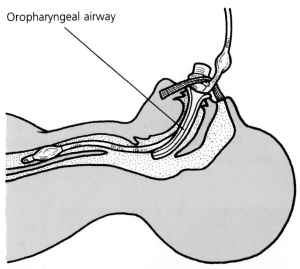

FIGURE B.11 Once proper position of the ETT is assured, it must be taped in place. An oropharyngeal airway should be inserted to prevent biting of the ETT.

must be heard on both sides of the chest to confirm proper tube placement. If breath sounds are heard only on the right, the balloon should be deflated, the tube withdrawn about 1 inch, the balloon reinflated, and both lungs rechecked for breath sounds.

The other common error occurs when intubation is forced without adequate visualization of the vocal cords. In this situation, the ETT usually ends up in the esophagus. In every patient, the EMT must see the vocal cords and must watch the tip of the tube as it passes between them. A second EMT can make it easier to see the vocal cords by pushing on the cricoid cartilage (Figure B.12). This is called "**Sellick's maneuver.**" While it may help to bring the vocal cords into view, it also may cause the patient to gag and vomit. As long as firm pressure is maintained on the cricoid cartilage, the esophagus will be blocked, preventing regurgitation of food into the airway. Therefore, once pressure is applied to the cricoid cartilage, it must be maintained until the ETT is properly placed and the balloon is inflated.

Contraindication to Endotracheal Intubation

The endotracheal tube provides the best means of ventilation for the unconscious patient. The only significant **contraindication** to its use — that is, when it should not be used — is injury to the cervical spine. Of course, airway and breathing still have the highest priority. However, the EMT must try to avoid further injury to a patient's spinal cord. For a patient in cardiac arrest that is not due to trauma, the patient should be intubated in the standard fashion just described, using laryngoscope, neck flexion, and head extension. The patient who is unconscious as a result of trauma presents a more difficult problem. In such a patient, an alternative means of controlling the airway (chin-lift or jaw-thrust,

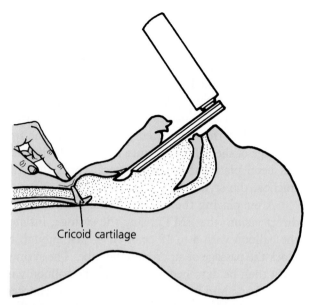

FIGURE B.12 Applying pressure on the cricoid cartilage will improve visualization of the vocal cords and block the esophagus.

oropharyngeal airway, and bag-valve-mask) will usually suffice. However, if the EMT must intubate the unconscious trauma patient, then a second EMT can kneel straddling the patient and hold the patient's head in a neutral position during the intubation. A third rescuer can improve visualization of the vocal cords by performing a Sellick's maneuver in the fashion described earlier (Figure B.13).

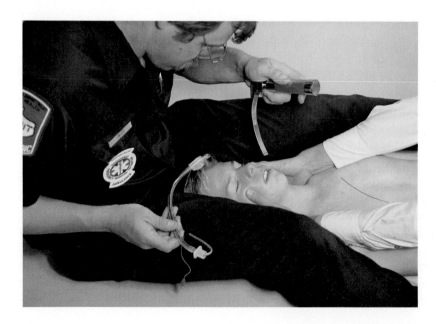

FIGURE B.13 When spinal injury is suspected, the endotracheal intubation technique must be modified. One EMT must straddle the patient and hold the neck in a neutral position. The Sellick maneuver will improve the chances of successful intubation.

Complications of Endotracheal Intubation

As mentioned earlier, pushing the ETT too far through the vocal cords is the most common complication of its use. This causes the tube to pass into the right mainstem bronchus. In this position it will only ventilate the right lung. Even when placed properly, the ETT will migrate if not secured. The EMT must never let go of the tube until it is adequately taped in place. A second complication occurs when the EMT places the endotracheal tube without seeing the vocal cords. Usually, the ETT winds up in the esophagus. In this position it will rapidly inflate the stomach and will not ventilate the lungs at all. Therefore, it is essential that the EMT watch the ETT as it passes through the vocal cords. A third complication of using the ETT is aggravation of a spinal injury. Whenever there is concern about a neck injury, the EMT must intubate without moving the patient's neck from the neutral position.

A fourth complication occurs when too much time is spent placing the tube. The EMT should never spend more than 30 seconds trying to intubate. If it takes longer than this, the EMT should stop and ventilate the patient with 100 percent oxygen for at least 60 seconds before trying again. If after two tries at intubation the tube cannot be passed, then an alternative ventilation technique should be used.

Finally, the laryngoscope and the tip of the ETT can cause damage. If the laryngoscope blade is used as a lever, teeth can be broken. If the tube is blindly pushed forward without the EMT's watching the vocal cords, it can lacerate the pharynx. The advantages and disadvantages of endotracheal intubation are listed in Table B.1.

THE ESOPHAGEAL OBTURATOR AIRWAY

Advanced airway management can also be achieved by using an **esophageal obturator airway (EOA).** The EOA has been used since 1973 to facilitate airway management in cardiopulmonary resuscitation. While there is no doubt that a properly placed endotracheal tube provides the most efficient possible delivery of oxygen to the lungs, some recent studies have demonstrated that the EOA, when properly used, may be as effective as endotracheal intubation.

TABLE B.1   Endotracheal Intubation

Advantages	Disadvantages
Definitive airway	If placed in esophagus
Easy to ventilate	and not recognized,
Prevents aspiration	the patient gets no
Can be left in for long	air
time	Neck manipulation in
Easy to maintain good	patient with possible
seal	neck injury
Some cardiac medica-	Requires frequent prac-
tions can be adminis-	tice to maintain skill
tered through ETT	
Can suction lungs	
through ETT	

Less practice and skill are required to insert the EOA because the EMT does not have to use a laryngoscope to visualize the vocal cords during intubation.

The esophageal obturator airway is a plastic, semirigid tube 34 cm long and 13 mm in diameter (Figure B.14). The lower end is smooth, rounded, and closed. The upper one-third of the tube is designed to function as an airway; it has 16 holes in the wall at the junction of the middle and upper thirds. When properly placed, these holes will lie at the level of the pharynx and provide free passage of oxygen-enriched air to the lungs. The lower two-thirds of the EOA should lie in the esophagus. The balloon surrounding the end of the tube can be inflated to block the esophagus and prevent the regurgitation of stomach contents into the airway.

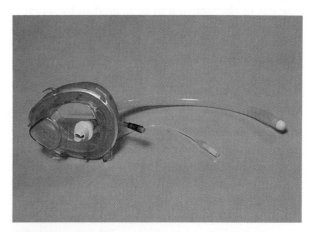

FIGURE B.14 The assembled esophageal obturator airway.

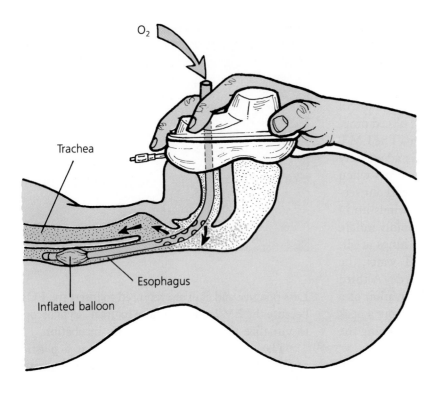

FIGURE B.15 When properly placed, the EOA will allow oxygen-enriched air to pass only from the side holes into the trachea.

The face mask that comes with the EOA is designed to fit snuggly about the patient's nose and mouth to provide a tight seal. Oxygen-enriched air given through the opening in the face mask passes through the upper portion of the airway and then into the lungs through the side holes in the tube because the esophagus is blocked by the inflated balloon (Figure B.15).

Some brands of the EOA are modified by the addition of a gastric decompression tube. This device is called an **esophageal gastric tube airway (EGTA).** The gastric decompression tube, by allowing gas in the stomach to be vented to the outside, decreases gastric distention. In other respects, the EGTA functions in a manner similar to the EOA (Figure B.16).

Inserting the EOA

The EMT must always check first for proper function of the EOA prior to insertion. A 30 cc syringe filled with air should be attached to the valve supplying the obturator balloon. The balloon should be inflated with 20 cc of air and checked for leaks. The balloon is then deflated, and the syringe is left attached. Next, the mask is attached to the tube. It is designed to lock into proper position with a definite snap. The lower two-thirds of the tube should

be well lubricated with a water-soluble gel. Before the EOA is inserted, the EMT must ventilate the patient as well as possible. Several ventilations should be given by the mouth-to-mouth technique or preferably with a bag-valve-mask device giving oxygen-enriched air.

The tube is designed to be placed with the head flexed or in a neutral position. Flexion of the head on the trunk will decrease the risk of inserting the tube incorrectly into the larynx and trachea. In a pa-

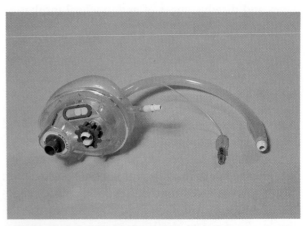

FIGURE B.16 An esophageal gastric tube airway. The gastric decompression tube allows the stomach to be vented of excessive air.

tient who is not suspected of having sustained a neck injury, the head should be flexed forward. In the unconscious trauma patient, the head must be supported in a neutral position by one EMT, while another EMT opens the patient's airway and inserts the tube.

The patient's airway is opened and prepared for intubation by grasping the tongue and mandible between the thumb and index finger and lifting them forward with the left hand (Figure B.17). The EOA with mask attached is grasped with the right hand and inserted along the tongue and against the posterior wall of the pharynx in the midline (Figure B.18a). The EMT does not have to use great force to insert the EOA. Only light to moderate pressure is needed. The EOA is inserted until the mask makes good contact with the face and the bite block lies at the level of the incisor teeth (Figure B.18b).

Using both hands, the EMT holds the face mask firmly against the face and checks the EOA for proper placement. Mouth-to-mask ventilation is given by one EMT, while a second EMT listens for breath sounds over both lung fields with a stethoscope. If the EOA is in the esophagus, breath sounds should be heard over both lung fields. If it has been placed in the trachea, no breath sounds will be heard. If it has been placed in the right mainstem bronchus, breath sounds will be heard only on the left side. If there is un-

certainty about its position, the EOA should be removed, and the patient should be ventilated before another attempt is made to place the EOA properly. If good breath sounds are heard over both lung fields, the esophageal balloon should be inflated with 20 cc of air and the syringe removed to keep the balloon inflated.

With the tube in proper position, the mask still must be held firmly against the patient's face. The EMT stays at the head of the patient using the index finger and thumb to hold the mask to the face

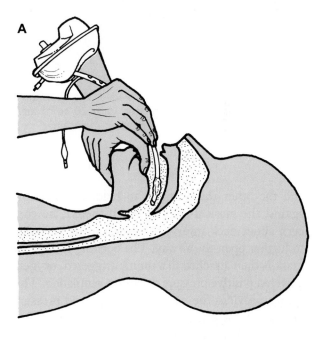

A

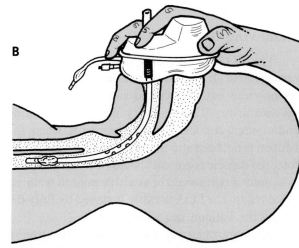

B

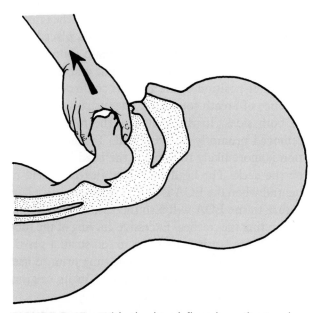

FIGURE B.17 With the head flexed on the trunk, the mandible and tongue are grasped and lifted forward in preparation for EOA insertion.

FIGURE B.18 (a) The EOA is inserted along the tongue (b) until the face mask makes good contact with the face. Only moderate pressure should be required to insert the EOA.

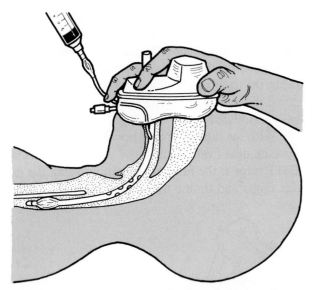

FIGURE B.19 Once properly placed, the esophageal obturator balloon is inflated with 20 cc of air, and a secure fit of the face mask is maintained manually.

and the other three fingers to hold the mandible against the mask (Figure B.19). If there is no concern about neck injury, the head can be extended to further open the airway. The opening in the face mask is then attached to a thumb-triggered, oxygen-powered positive pressure device for ventilation. This device provides the necessary volume and pressure of oxygen for effective ventilation with an EOA. These levels cannot be achieved with a bag-valve-mask system.

Removing the EOA

The EOA is used only for short-term airway management. It should be removed only when the unconscious patient awakens and is able to protect his own airway. There is a very high risk of vomiting and/or regurgitation of gastric contents when the balloon is deflated and the EOA is removed. Therefore, the conscious patient should be turned onto his side, and suction should be available prior to removal. Once ready, the EOA is easily removed by fully deflating the balloon and sliding it out.

If long-term airway management is required in the hospital, the EOA should be replaced by an endotracheal tube. In this circumstance, the EOA must be left in place until the ETT is securely and properly placed.

Contraindications to the Use of an EOA

Under the following circumstances, the EOA should *not* be used:

1. On patients who are awake. EOA placement will cause vomiting and aspiration of vomitus. The EOA should be used only in deeply unconscious patients.
2. On small children. It is commonly recommended that the EOA not be used in children under 16 years of age. Because there is only one size of EOA, it is too large for children and does not work effectively.
3. On patients with known esophageal disease. The EOA may cause serious problems for a patient with esophageal cancer or esophageal varices. If a patient has swallowed a caustic agent such as lye, the EOA may perforate the injured esophagus.
4. On patients with significant upper airway bleeding. Blood from the nose or mouth will pass directly into the lungs once the esophageal balloon is inflated. If the patient accumulates some blood, mucus, or saliva in the upper airway once an EOA is in place, it must be cleared with suction.

Complications of Using the EOA

The most common complication of using the EOA is accidental placement into the trachea rather than the esophagus. Once the EOA is placed, the EMT must listen carefully for breath sounds with the stethoscope over both the right and left chest. Improper position of the EOA is confirmed by the absence of breath sounds on one (usually the right) or both sides. In this instance, the tube must be removed promptly and replaced. Tracheal intubation is more likely to occur if the head is extended on the neck. The head should be flexed or held in neutral when the EOA is inserted. An excessive curvature to the EOA will also increase the likelihood of entering the trachea. Excessive curving of the tube results from storing the EOA in too small a plastic bag, where it stays bent for some time prior to use. The EOA should always be stored in its original packaging to prevent this problem.

Esophageal rupture or tear can also result from the use of this device. The EOA should never be inserted roughly or with excessive force. While the balloon will hold up to 30 cc of air, 20 cc is usually sufficient to block the esophagus, and this smaller volume of air is less likely to injure the esophagus. Furthermore, the EOA should not be stored in a cold ambulance or kept in a cold environment, as it will become stiff and be more likely to injure the esophagus when inserted.

The third complication is inadequate ventilation, despite proper placement of the airway. A major cause of this problem is persistent leakage of air around the face mask. A firm seal of the mask against the face must be maintained at all times during the use of the EOA. Another cause of inadequate ventilation is the delivery of an inadequate volume of air to the airway using a bag-valve-mask delivery system. The proper delivery system is a thumb-triggered, oxygen-powered positive pressure device. The advantages and disadvantages of the EOA are listed in Table B.2.

TABLE B.2 Esophageal Obturator Airway

Advantages	Disadvantages
Can be placed without moving patient's neck	Ineffective unless good seal with face mask is maintained
Can be used in both cardiac arrest and for trauma	Requires frequent practice to maintain skill
Unrecognized tracheal placement will ventilate at least left lung	

YOU ARE THE EMT...

1. What is the difference between endotracheal intubation and the esophageal obturator airway? Even though an EOA is easier than an ETT to use, when should an EOA *not* be used?
2. What must you do to prepare a patient *before* inserting an ETT? What should you do *after* it is inserted?
3. Why is an EOA useful only for short-term airway management? What would you do if the unconscious patient regained consciousness with an EOA in place?
4. How does the addition of a gastric decompression tube modify an EOA?

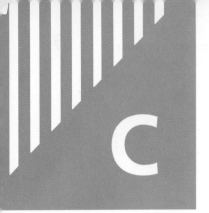

APPENDIX C
Defibrillation by EMTs

OVERVIEW

Defibrillation can be a lifesaving measure in the treatment of sudden cardiac death. Great skill is needed to apply this technique, and training over and above basic EMT training is required. Once trained, "EMT-Ds" must frequently review their skills and update their knowledge in this area. An essential component of an effective prehospital defibrillation program is strict medical control with constant supervision of the performance of the EMT-Ds. In such a setting, the effectiveness of the basic EMS system can be expanded to provide an even more valuable service to the community.

Appendix C begins by defining some of the terms associated with defibrillation. Then the role of the EMT in defibrillation is described. The principles of defibrillation are discussed next — how the heart's electrical system operates, how cardiac arrhythmias are detected, and how the EMT recognizes ventricular fibrillation using the electrocardiogram. Appendix C goes on to describe defibrillation equipment and gives a detailed explanation of how it is used. Some of the problems the EMT may encounter during defibrillation are then discussed, followed by guidelines for maintaining the defibrillation equipment. The last section talks about the requirements and local variations in EMT-D programs.

OBJECTIVES

The objectives of Appendix C are to

- define defibrillation and related terms.
- discuss the EMT's involvement in defibrillation programs, when the EMT uses defibrillation, and the difference between manual and automatic defibrillators.
- understand the principles of defibrillation, including the heart's electrical system, cardiac arrhythmias, and the electrocardiogram.
- become familiar with defibrillation equipment.
- learn the steps of defibrillation.
- recognize the problems that may occur during defibrillation.
- realize the importance of maintaining defibrillation equipment.
- distinguish between the essential requirements and local variations in EMT-D programs.

DEFINITION OF TERMS

Defibrillation is the delivery of an electric current through a person's chest wall and heart for the purpose of ending a lethal cardiac arrythmia called **ventricular fibrillation (VF).** Portable battery-powered devices called **defibrillators** are used to record the cardiac rhythm and to generate and deliver the electric charge (a **countershock**). An **EMT-defibrillation (EMT-D) program** is one in which fully trained EMTs undergo further training and are then certified to perform defibrillation on people in cardiac arrest. In a *manual* EMT-defibrillation program, the EMT must learn to recognize VF when it is recorded, and then to charge and deliver the electrical countershock with a manual defibrillator. In

an *automatic* EMT-defibrillation program, EMTs attach and operate defibrillators that recognize VF automatically. These automatic defibrillators then proceed to charge and deliver the countershock (fully automatic defibrillators), or they advise the EMT that a countershock is needed (semi-automatic, or shock-advisory defibrillators).

THE EMT AND DEFIBRILLATION
Essential Requirements for an EMT-D Program

EMT-defibrillation is a separate skill level over and above the basic EMT training. For an EMT to participate in an EMT-defibrillation program, the following features must be present:

1. Basic certification as an EMT.
2. A medical director who assumes responsibility for all prehospital medical care that involves EMT-defibrillation.
3. Patient care protocols in the form of standing orders, developed and authorized by the medical director.
4. A state-EMS authorized EMT-D training program that includes written and practical testing.
5. A continuing education program that includes regular review of practical defibrillation skills.
6. Defibrillators capable of voice and electrocardiographic recording.
7. Written reports for all prehospital care that involves the use of defibrillators.
8. Satisfactory performance by the EMT-D to the level of training and within the guidelines provided by the program's medical director and confirmed by medical review of every patient.

Rationale for Early Defibrillation by the EMT

Sudden cardiac death is the leading cause of death in the United States for people over the age of 40. Research in prehospital treatment for sudden death has identified several factors essential for a successful resuscitation, among them the following:

1. The collapse is observed by a witness who activates the emergency medical system.
2. The electrical rhythm of the patient's heart is ventricular fibrillation.
3. CPR is begun early, within 4 to 6 minutes of the collapse.
4. A defibrillator is available quickly (within 10 to 15 minutes) to reverse the rhythm of ventricular fibrillation.
5. Additional advanced life support (either paramedics or hospital emergency departments) is available within 15 to 30 minutes to provide further treatment for the patient.

Equipping the EMT with a defibrillator is an extension of the concept that early defibrillation improves the chances that a cardiac arrest patient will survive sudden death. EMT-defibrillation programs have been successful in suburban, rural, urban, and wilderness areas, with and without paramedic prehospital support.

Manual vs. Automatic Defibrillation by EMTs

There is only one difference between manual and automatic defibrillation by EMTs: manual defibrillators require that the EMT recognize lethal cardiac rhythms. Automatic and semi-automatic defibrillators recognize the rhythm for the EMT. In practice, this means that for automatic and semi-automatic programs, the content of the initial training and the continuing education review sessions are simpler and less time-consuming. All other requirements for an EMT-D outlined in this appendix remain the same. Clinical studies have shown that EMTs are equally successful at saving lives, whether using manual or automatic defibrillators. The final choice between manual and automatic defibrillators will be determined by the program medical director. Both automatic and manual defibrillators require close case-by-case medical review of EMT-D field performance.

THE PRINCIPLES OF DEFIBRILLATION

The Electrical System of the Heart

A network of specialized tissue, capable of conducting electrical current, runs throughout the heart muscle. The flow of electrical current through this network causes smooth, coordinated contractions of the heart. These contractions produce the pumping action of the heart (Figure C.1).

If part of the cardiac muscle becomes injured or dies, the electrical system becomes disturbed, and the heart may not continue to beat properly. The patient may not have an adequate blood pressure and may lose consciousness. Sometimes the injured area of the heart begins to fire off uncoordinated electrical impulses. These impulses can produce abnormal beats called **premature ventricular contractions (PVCs).** If several PVCs occur close together, they produce a rhythm called **ventricular tachycardia.** The patient may still have a palpable pulse with ventricular tachycardia. Ventricular tachycardia, however, seldom lasts longer than 60 seconds. The

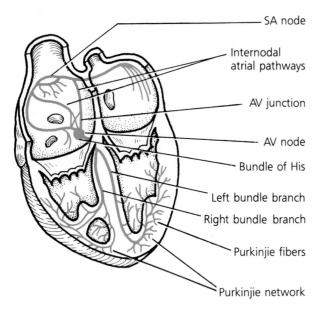

— SA node

— Internodal atrial pathways

— AV junction

— AV node

— Bundle of His

— Left bundle branch

— Right bundle branch

— Purkinjie fibers

— Purkinjie network

FIGURE C.1 The electrical conduction system of the heart.

injured heart muscle continues to beat faster until its oxygen supply is exhausted. At that point the electrical impulses become completely uncoordinated and begin to fire off randomly. Effective pumping of the heart ceases, and no peripheral pulse can be palpated. This rhythm is called ventricular fibrillation (VF). The heart will stay in VF for several minutes until all electrical activity in the heart muscle ceases. This final rhythm of complete electrical inactivity (standstill) is called **asystole** (Figure C.2).

If a defibrillator can be applied to the patient and an electrical shock given to the heart during the time of ventricular fibrillation, there is a good possibility of restoring a more normal electrical activity. This electrical activity may stimulate the cardiac muscle to contract in an organized fashion. The pumping action of the heart will resume, and the pulse will often return (Figure C.3).

Detecting Cardiac Arrhythmias

This section on the electrocardiogram and the visual detection of lethal cardiac rhythms is essential for EMT-D programs that choose to use manual defibrillators. EMT-Ds in programs that choose to use automatic or semi-automatic external defibrillators do not have to learn to recognize the various lethal cardiac rhythms but must be familiar with the basic principles of the ECG.

The Electrocardiogram

An **electrocardiogram (ECG or EKG)** is a recording of the electrical current that flows through the heart (Figure C.4). Portable defibrillators display the electrocardiogram on either a paper strip, a cathode ray monitor screen, or (usually) both.

Each mechanical contraction of the heart is associated with two electrical processes. The first is **depolarization,** during which the electrical charges on the surface of the muscle cell change from positive to negative. The second is **repolarization,** during which the heart returns to its resting state, and the positive charge is restored to the surface.

The body acts as a conductor of electrical current. Any two points on the body may be connected with electrical "leads" to record the electrical activity of the heart. The tracing produced by the electrical activity of the heart, as it depolarizes and repolarizes, forms a series of waves and complexes that are separated by regularly occurring intervals. The waves or deflections of the ECG are called the **P wave,** the **QRS complex,** and the **T wave.** Polarization of the atria produces the P wave. Depolarization of the ventricles produces the QRS complex, or when mechanical contraction of the heart occurs. When the ventricles polarize, the T wave is formed.

The **PR interval** — from the beginning of the P wave to the beginning of the QRS complex — records the time it takes for the electrical signal to go from the atria to the ventricles. The QRS complex, during which the ventricles are rapidly depolarized, should be narrow, no broader than 0.12 seconds, or three of the 1-millimeter boxes on the ECG paper strip.

When the heart is working normally and the heart's pacemaker begins high in the atria, there is a smooth flow of electricity through the heart, which depolarizes the muscle and produces a coordinated pumping contraction called **normal sinus rhythm.** The electrocardiogram of normal sinus rhythm looks like the drawing in Figure C.5.

Visual Recognition of Ventricular Fibrillation

During a cardiac arrest, EMT-Ds who are trained to operate a manual defibrillator must perform a challenging task. They must view the squiggly line moving across a small monitor screen and decide

A Ventricular tachycardia

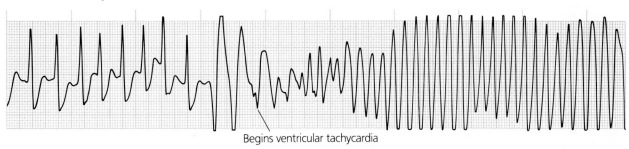

Begins ventricular tachycardia

B Ventricular fibrillation

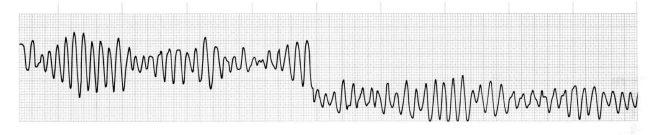

C Asystole

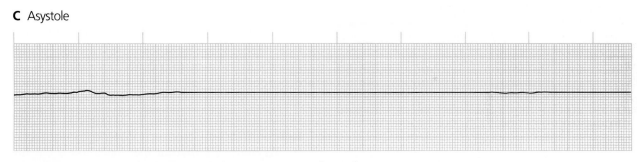

FIGURE C.2 Rhythms of the dying heart. Heart attack produces abnormal cardiac rhythms that can be analyzed on the ECG monitor. (a) Early cardiac disturbance is ventricular tachycardia. (b) Ventricular tachycardia often is followed promptly by ventricular fibrillation, a sign of ineffective cardiac function. (c) If untreated, asystole, or cardiac standstill, will occur.

Shock

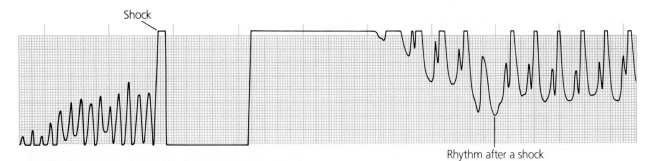

Rhythm after a shock

FIGURE C.3 If an electrical shock is applied to the heart during the time of ventricular fibrillation, normal electrical activity can be restored and effective cardiac contractions can resume.

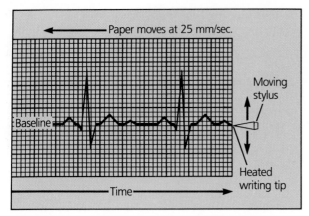

FIGURE C.4 The normal electrocardiogram recorded on a continuously moving strip of paper.

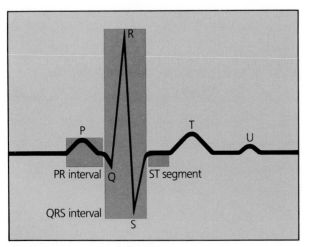

FIGURE C.5 The components of a normal cardiac rhythm.

if the electrical activity of the heart is normal or if VF is present. Ventricular fibrillation is the only heart rhythm that can be treated with defibrillation. For practical purposes, therefore, an EMT-D must be able to identify only two rhythms — ventricular fibrillation and "nonventricular fibrillation." The EMT-D should look at three features of the electrical signal to detect ventricular fibrillation:

1. Overall pattern: The overall pattern should be irregularly shaped, chaotic, and lack any regular repeating features. Narrow QRS complexes are never present with VF.
2. Height: The electrical signal varies in height.
3. Rate: The distance between the peaks of the signal varies greatly.

As shown in Figure C.6, ventricular fibrillation can vary from coarse to fine, but the three features of irregularity in pattern, height, and rate are always present.

Visual Recognition of Other Rhythms

There are only three other rhythms that an EMT-D using a manual defibrillator needs to know: normal sinus rhythm, ventricular tachycardia, and asystole. Normal sinus rhythm has already been described. Ventricular tachycardia is the rhythm produced when the pacemaker for the heart is located in the ventricles. Beats that originate in the ventricles are broad, slurred, and slightly distorted. They are fast, between 140 to 200 beats per minute. When many of them occur one after another, they can produce a rhythm with the characteristics of regular height and regular rate. Therefore, because there is a regularly shaped pattern, with little variation in signal height and rate, the EMT-D can quickly conclude that this is a nonventricular fibrillation pattern (Figure C.7). Ventricular tachycardia must be carefully monitored by the EMT because it can deteriorate rapidly into ventricular fibrillation, often in seconds. When ventricular tachycardia does not quickly deteriorate to VF and the patient is unquestionably in full cardiac arrest, some medical directors instruct EMT-Ds to deliver a shock. This practice, however, must be ordered by the local medical director.

Asystole is a rhythm that looks like a flat line and indicates no electrical activity in the heart (Figure C.8). Defibrillation has no effect on true asystole. In some programs, however, EMT-Ds are instructed to shock a patient with asystole because of a small possibility that the heart does have some undetected ventricular fibrillation remaining and may respond to the shock.

DEFIBRILLATION EQUIPMENT

Defibrillators for Prehospital Use

A number of companies manufacture portable defibrillators specifically for prehospital use by paramedics, EMTs, and other emergency personnel. These devices should have the following features:

1. Rechargeable power source. The defibrillator for EMT use must have a portable energy

A Coarse ventricular fibrillation

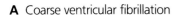
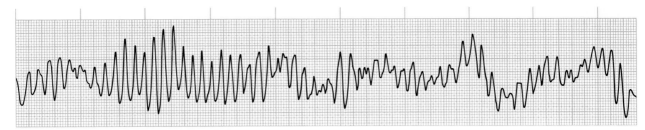

B Fine ventricular fibrillation

FIGURE C.6 Ventricular fibrillation is irregular, chaotic, and lacks regular, repeating features. The signal may vary in height and width. (a) Coarse, ventricular fibrillation and (b) fine ventricular fibrillation.

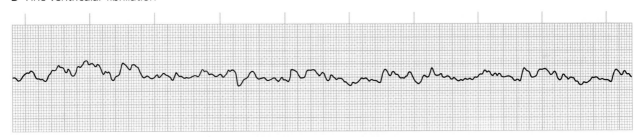

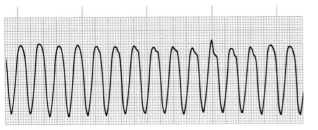

FIGURE C.7 Two examples of ventricular tachycardia. Note the regular pattern with little variation in height and rate.

supply, usually rechargeable lead-acid or nickel-cadmium batteries.

2. Portability. The defibrillator should be light in weight (less than 30 pounds) and designed for easy carrying.

3. Construction for prehospital care. The defibrillators should be environmentally sealed for all weather conditions and resistant to rough usage.

4. Dual-channel voice/electrocardiographic recorders. Defibrillators used in EMT-D programs must be capable of recording both the cardiac rhythm and the verbal report of the defibrillator operators.

A Asystole

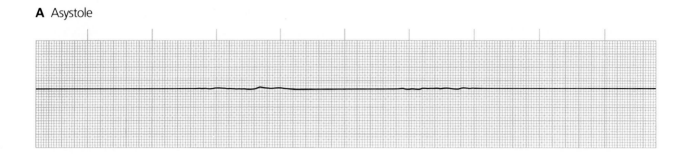

B Asystole with p waves present

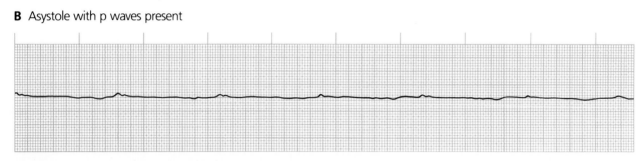

FIGURE C.8   (a) Asystole indicates no electrical activity of the ventricles of the heart. (b) On occasion, P waves indicating some residual electrical activity in the atria may persist with asystole.

Manual Defibrillators

Defibrillators used in manual EMT-defibrillation programs must accurately record the patient's rhythm and then display the rhythm in a clear, easy-to-see manner. This allows the EMT-D to interpret the patient's rhythm for the presence or absence of ventricular fibrillation.

The rhythm can be recorded in two ways, either through standard cardiac monitor electrodes that are attached to the patient's chest or through the two paddles of the defibrillator. To lower the electrical resistance between the patient's skin and the defibrillator paddles, the EMT applies a special gel. Rhythm assessment through the hand-held defibrillator paddles is difficult because artifacts on the ECG tracing frequently occur from motion of the paddles and the monitor cables. Because of this problem, EMT-Ds in manual programs must interpret *only* rhythms recorded through the monitor electrodes attached to the patient's chest, and *never* through the defibrillator paddles.

Most defibrillators for manual EMT-D care simultaneously display the rhythm by two techniques: on a paper rhythm strip and on a cardiac monitor screen. Both of these methods are useful. The paper rhythm strip provides a physical copy of the rhythm for immediate review at the scene and for later review after use of the defibrillator. The cardiac monitor screen allows long periods of monitoring, without an accumulation of large amounts of ECG recording paper.

If the rhythm is ventricular fibrillation, the EMT-D must press the "charge" switch on the defibrillator to allow the power source to charge the capacitors. The EMT-D then delivers the electrical countershock across the chest by pressing appropriate "discharge" or "shock" switches.

Automatic and Semi-Automatic Defibrillators

Both automatic and semi-automatic defibrillators are attached to the patient's chest with two large adhesive pads precoated with an electrode gel (Fig-

DEFIBRILLATOR PAD/PADDLE PLACEMENT

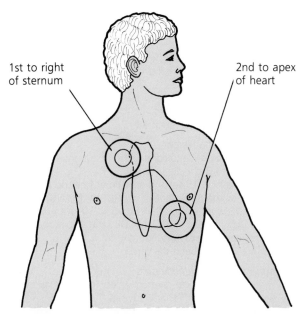

1st to right
of sternum

2nd to apex
of heart

FIGURE C.9 The defibrillator paddles or monitor electrodes are positioned on the anterior chest wall, one to the right of the sternum at the level of the angle of Louis and the second over the apex of the heart.

ure C.9). These pads serve a dual function — to record the patient's rhythm and to deliver the countershock. The electrical signal from the patient's heart is picked up by the adhesive electrodes and then analyzed in the internal circuitry of the automatic defibrillator. With a fully automatic defibrillator, a signal is sent directly to the capacitor to begin to charge if the rhythm is ventricular fibrillation. When the capacitor has reached full charge, the fully automatic defibrillator will then deliver the shock through the two adhesive electrodes. A semi-automatic defibrillator, once it detects VF, will "advise" the operator to press the "shock" button, after which the capacitors are charged and the shock is delivered. The energy levels and the electrical characteristics of the countershocks are virtually identical to countershocks delivered by manual defibrillators.

Energy Levels of Defibrillators

The electrical current delivered by defibrillators is measured in units called **joules** or **watt-seconds.** Manual defibrillators can deliver countershocks from 10 to 360 joules. An EMT-D must select the energy

level determined by local standing orders. In most EMT-D programs an energy level of 200 joules is used, although medical directors may order higher levels for the second or third shocks. Automatic and semi-automatic defibrillators are preset to deliver only one or two energy levels, usually in the 200 to 350 joule range.

PREHOSPITAL DEFIBRILLATION BY EMTs

Standing Orders Versus Telemetry

Standing orders are a direct order from the program medical director to perform certain tasks for a patient under a specific set of circumstances (Figure C.10). Virtually all EMT-D programs use standing orders rather than **telemetric transmission** of an ECG recording to a base station physician. This is because quickness is so important during a cardiac arrest, and because telemetry frequently causes long decision-making delays.

Standing orders must be memorized and practiced by the EMT-D. The EMT-D operates under the authority of the medical director's medical license. When EMT-Ds successfully complete their training course, they receive a certificate of authorization. This certificate is a "prescription" from the medical director that legally authorizes the EMT to use the defibrillator in certain situations and in a prescribed manner. Standing orders define exactly what these certain situations and the prescribed manner are.

The Steps of Defibrillation

Defibrillation should not be thought of as simply the proper operation of the defibrillator. The steps of defibrillation are best understood as parts of three cycles. These cycles are similar for both manual and automatic defibrillators.

Step 1: Assessment Cycles

The defibrillator must be properly attached to the patient in cardiac arrest so heart rhythm can be recorded. With manual defibrillators, the EMT-D assesses the rhythm as it is displayed on the monitor screen and the paper rhythm strip to decide if VF is present. With automatic defibrillators, the internal circuitry of the device assesses the recorded

SAMPLE STANDING ORDERS FOR PATIENT TREATMENT FOR EMTs CERTIFIED IN MANUAL, AUTOMATIC, OR SEMI-AUTOMATIC DEFIBRILLATION

Purpose: The purpose of these orders is to provide prompt defibrillation for patients who have confirmed circulatory arrest due to ventricular fibrillation.

Authorization: In the event of a cardiac arrest, the medical director authorizes you to perform the following:

1. Immediately upon arrival, verify circulatory and respiratory arrest by the absence of consciousness, normal respirations, and carotid pulses.

2. Initiate CPR and the defibrillation protocol.

3. Assessment. Assess the rhythm for the presence of ventricular fibrillation:

   (1) Turn defibrillator POWER on.
   (2) Turn recorder on.
   (3) Begin verbal report.
   (4) Attach monitor leads or defibrillator pads.

   Manual Defibrillators
   (1) Gel defibrillation paddles.
   (2) Charge to 200 joules.
   (3) Start paper chart recorder.
   (4) Place paddles against the chest.
   (5) Inspect the rhythm.

   Automatic Defibrillators
   (1) Clear the patient.
   (2) Switch to AUTO MODE.
   (3) Count to 15 seconds.

   Semi-Automatic Defibrillators
   (1) Clear the patient.
   (2) Press the ANALYZE switch.
   (3) Count to 15 seconds.

4. Treatment. Treat ventricular fibrillation with a maximum of three countershocks. When VF is persistent, deliver up to three shocks without pausing for CPR between shocks, as outlined below:

   Manual Defibrillators
   (1) Deliver shock #1.
   (2) Leave paddles on the chest.
   (3) Recharge to 200 J.
   (4) Clear the patient.
   (5) Reassess the rhythm.
   (6) Deliver countershock #2.
   (7) Leave paddles on the chest.
   (8) Recharge to 200 J.
   (9) Clear the patient.
   (10) Reassess the rhythm.
   (11) Deliver countershock #3.

   Automatic Defibrillators
   (1) Allow the device to continue to assess and treat for up to 3 shocks in a row.
   (2) Whenever a 15-second assessment period occurs without a shock, switch to MANUAL MODE, and resume CPR for 15 to 30 seconds.
   (3) Switch back to AUTO MODE, and allow the device to assess and treat until a total of 3 shocks have been delivered.

   Semi-Automatic Defibrillators
   (1) Push the "shock" switch when the message screen displays "shock advised."
   (2) Repeat "analyze," and repeat "shock" each time the message screen displays "shock advised" until a total of 3 shocks in a row have been delivered.
   (3) Whenever the "shock not advised" message appears, resume CPR for 15 seconds.

5. Manual Defibrillators Only. The rhythm assessment reveals asystole.

   (1) Resume CPR.
   (2) Check lead connections to the patient.
   (3) Check lead connections to the monitor/defibrillator.
   (4) Check calibrations.
   (5) Verify that lead selector switch is in the lead II position, *not* the paddles position.
   (6) Check for possible hidden VF by assessing the rhythm for 5 seconds in lead I, and then 5 seconds in lead III.
   (7) Follow *treatment* orders if VF is observed in any lead.

(*Note:* The details of standing orders may differ from program to program. These sample standing orders are for an EMT-D program that uses only 200-joule shocks, allows a total of three shocks for persistent VF, and does not permit shocks for asystole.)

FIGURE C.10 Sample standing orders for patient treatment for EMTs certified in manual, automatic, or semi-automatic defibrillation.

rhythm and decides whether the electrical signal represents VF. CPR must stop during the assessment cycles.

During an assessment cycle, the EMT follows these steps:

1. Attach monitor leads or defibrillatory pads to the patient's chest.
2. Discontinue CPR.
3. Clear all personnel from contact with the patient.
4. In manual programs, make a visual inspection of the rhythm.
5. In automatic programs, wait for an internal analysis of the rhythm by the automatic defibrillator.

Step 2: Treatment Cycles

Once assessment has occurred and either the EMT-D or the automatic defibrillator has decided that VF is present, the capacitors of the defibrillator must be charged to the selected energy level. Having made sure that no one, including himself, is touching the patient, the EMT delivers the countershock. All EMT-Ds must recognize the sudden movement of the patient that indicates a countershock has been delivered. When using a manual defibrillator, the EMT should follow these steps of the treatment cycle:

1. Apply gel to the paddles.
2. Select the energy level (as determined by standing order or directed by medical control).
3. Charge the defibrillator.
4. Apply the defibrillator paddles to the chest in the proper position (see Figure C.9).
5. Recheck that no personnel are touching the patient.
6. Press the shock delivery controls.
7. Make a visual recognition that a shock has been delivered.

When using an automatic defibrillator, the EMT should follow these four steps of the treatment cycle:

1. Recheck that no personnel are touching the patient.
2. Make an auditory and visual check that charging has occurred.

3. Press the shock delivery switch (semi-automatic device).
4. Make a visual check that the shock has been delivered.

Step 3: CPR Cycles

The importance of CPR must never be forgotten. CPR must be continued at all times, except during the assessment and the treatment cycles. CPR is administered right up to the moment the assessment cycle begins, and it is resumed immediately after the treatment cycle ends. In some programs the medical director will require CPR cycles for a specified period prior to the assessment cycle and also between the treatment cycles. A CPR cycle ends with a pulse check of the patient — if a pulse is present, then the blood pressure is measured to see if the pulse is adequate. If a pulse is absent, the CPR cycles resume until the next treatment or assessment cycles begin.

The EMT should therefore follow these steps of the CPR cycle:

1. Administer proper CPR.
2. Perform CPR for the specified time.
3. Stop CPR for a pulse check.
4. Restart CPR if the pulse is absent.

TROUBLESHOOTING

An EMT-D must learn to recognize the most common problems that can occur while attempting to treat patients in cardiac arrest with a defibrillator. Each of these problems should trigger a mental checklist of possible causes and possible solutions.

Manual Defibrillators

Excessive Artifact

Manual defibrillation is impossible when **excessive artifact** occurs on the monitor screen (Figure C.11). This prevents the EMT-D from analyzing the rhythm and identifying VF. It must be removed. There are several causes of excessive artifact, but probably the most common cause is unsnapped monitor leads, which produces a straight line tracing. The EMT should quickly check to see if the leads are snapped to the adhesive patches.

Cable movement is another problem that can be caused by the following:

A Faulty head attachment

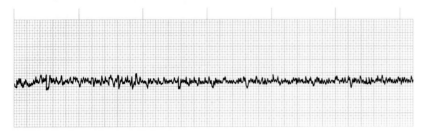

B Muscle tremors

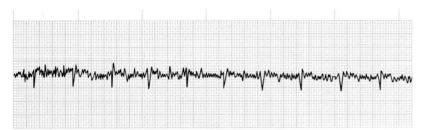

FIGURE C.11 (a) Faulty lead attachment or (b) patient muscle tremors may produce an artifact — an extraneous mechanical or electrical interference with the ECG signal.

1. Patient movement during transport. The rhythm should never be analyzed during transport. The rescue vehicle should be brought to a complete stop to analyze the rhythm and to defibrillate.
2. **Agonal respirations** or muscle tremor. Patients who are dying often gasp irregularly (agonal respirations) or have involuntary muscular twitching. Sometimes the rhythm can be properly assessed between agonal respirations. Otherwise the EMT-D must continue CPR until the agonal respirations cease.
3. Continued chest compressions or ventilations. All contact with the patient must cease while the rhythm is being assessed.

Poor contact between adhesive monitor patches and the patient's skin is yet another problem. The first response of the EMT should always be to push firmly against the monitor patches to see if proper contact can be established. Other common causes include:

1. Hairy chest. A small safety razor should be carried to quickly shave a small area of the chest.
2. Sweaty or wet chest. Patients with severe chest pain who are in cardiac arrest are often covered with perspiration. They may also be wet from rain, or from immersion. Alcohol swabs, 4″ × 4″ gauze, and a small towel to dry off the patient's chest should be available.
3. Small, bony or irregular chest. The monitor leads should be quickly repositioned on the arms or another portion of the chest.
4. Dry or defective monitor patches. The monitor patches can become outdated. They should be replaced. In the meantime, a small amount of the electrode gel can be applied under the patches.

Excessive 60-Cycle Interference

Sixty-cycle interference is usually due to electrical appliances in the vicinity such as electric blankets, televisions, fluorescent lights, clocks, and radios (Figure C.12). Nearby appliances should be unplugged, or the patient should be moved to a different location.

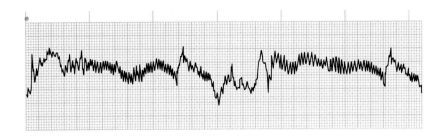

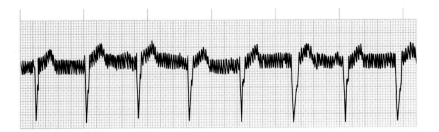

FIGURE C.12 Sixty-cycle interference is usually due to electrical appliances operating in the vicinity of the ECG.

Equipment Problems

Manual defibrillators contain a number of warning signals to indicate low batteries, end of tape cassettes, aborted charges, or other equipment failure. Also, several components of manual defibrillators will occasionally produce problems such as blown fuses, paper recorders that do not run, defective ECG paper stylus, and prolonged charge times. EMT-Ds should become thoroughly familiar with the operating manual of the defibrillator so they can quickly recognize these problems and respond correctly.

Automatic Defibrillators

Inadequate Contact Between the Skin and the Pads

The available automatic and semi-automatic defibrillators are able to measure the impedance between the two adhesive defibrillatory pads. As a result they can detect inadequate contact between the skin and the defibrillatory pad. The EMT-D will receive alarm signals from the device if the defibrillatory pads are not properly connected. Whenever these alarm signals are received, the EMT-D should:

1. Firmly press the defibrillatory pads against the chest.

2. Recheck all cable, pad, and device connections.
3. Consider whether the chest has excessive hair or is too wet, sweaty, or irregularly shaped for proper contact. Respond to these problems as outlined above for manual defibrillators.

Failure to Deliver Defibrillatory Shock When VF Exists

Some of the reasons for this failure include the following:

1. Insufficient time in automatic or analyze mode.
2. Switching out of automatic mode when charging occurs.
3. Movement from CPR, agonal respirations, or touching the patient while the defibrillator attempts to analyze the rhythm.
4. Failure to place the device in the automatic or analyze mode.
5. Failure to press the shock button when a "shock advised" message appears on semi-automatic defibrillators.
6. Equipment problems — usually inadequately charged batteries or batteries that have spontaneously discharged.

MAINTENANCE OF DEFIBRILLATION EQUIPMENT

The entire mechanical integrity of a defibrillator should be checked regularly, following a standard checklist. Manufacturers' recommendations will help determine the items in this checklist. Figure C.13 presents a sample checklist. Several areas need particular attention, among them the following:

Battery Care and Maintenance. The charging and care of batteries is the most demanding feature of equipment maintenance. All defibrillators for prehospital EMT-D use have rechargeable power sources, either lead-acid, nickel-cadmium, or lithium batteries. Nickel cadmium batteries require regular

charge and discharge cycles to maintain optimal performance. Lead-acid batteries must be checked regularly, although their general maintenance is simpler than maintenance of nickel-cadmium batteries. Lithium batteries require no maintenance and have an extremely long shelf life. They are used as a backup power source for emergencies, rather than as a primary power source. EMT-Ds must become thoroughly familiar with the manufacturer's recommendations for battery maintenance of their particular defibrillator.

Defibrillator. The ability of the defibrillator to charge its capacitors and deliver a standard energy level must be checked regularly. Most manufacturers provide a method to measure defibrillator output. The defibrillator is charged to the specified level and then discharged against resistive test plates. Output indicators compare the selected charge level with the actual delivered charge. This procedure can identify problems with the batteries, the capacitor, or the general circuitry.

ECG Monitor Screen/ECG Paper Recorder. The entire circuit from the interface with the patient to the display on the monitor screen and ECG paper recorder must be checked regularly. Monitor leads should be attached either to simulators that many manufacturers provide or to a volunteer. The paper supply must be checked periodically, and a spare roll must always be available. The monitor display should be clear and easily seen, and the paper should run smoothly with a clear tracing produced by the stylus. Calibrations on some defibrillators need to be checked.

Voice/ECG Recorder. The voice/ECG recorder must always be ready to document the events of a cardiac arrest. A voice recording can be used during equipment checks to verify that the tape recorder is working correctly and that a fresh tape cassette is present.

SAMPLE CHECKLIST FOR EQUIPMENT INSPECTIONS

1. Inspect for general mechanical integrity.
2. Check patient monitor leads and cables.
3. Check quality of monitor display.
4. Check all visual and audio indicator signals.
5. Check calibration setting.
6. Run the paper ECG drive and check quality of tracing.
7. Run the tape recorder and check that voice and rhythm are recorded.
8. Check defibrillator cords and the paddle surfaces. Clean if necessary.
9. Make sure batteries are adequately charged.
10. Charge defibrillator and discharge into test load to verify proper energy output.
11. Note time to charge to recommended energy level and compare with manufacturer's recommendations.
12. Check presence and condition of accessories and supplies:
    (1) tape cassette
    (2) ECG paper
    (3) defibrillatory pads
    (4) disposable monitor leads
    (5) electrode gel, paste, or disposable pads
    (6) safety razor blade
    (7) towel, alcohol swabs

FIGURE C.13 Sample checklist for equipment inspections.

EMT-D PROGRAM REQUIREMENTS AND LOCAL VARIATIONS

Essential Requirements

The essential requirements for an EMT-defibrillation program that were presented earlier must be met by every EMT-D program. This is true regardless of setting, population, or type or brand of defibrillator. It must be emphasized repeatedly that the purchase of automatic or semi-automatic external defibrillators does not eliminate any of these requirements. Use of automatic defibrillators in an EMT-D program changes only the final "decision-maker" at the time of shock delivery; the content and complexity of the initial training and continuing education, in addition to all other requirements, remain the same.

Local Variations

A number of features of EMT-D programs do vary locally, however, based on the directives of the states' EMS offices or the local medical directors. Once the essential requirements have been met, local medical directors and state EMS offices have the option to establish local variations that, in their medical judgment, are best for their particular program. Examples of standing orders that demonstrate some of these local variations were presented earlier in Figure C.10. Several others are discussed in the following paragraphs.

Initial Training. If an EMT-D program selects manual defibrillators, EMT-Ds must learn to recognize lethal cardiac rhythms and which rhythms are treated with a defibrillator. As stated previously, this is the cardinal distinction between a manual EMT-D program and an automatic EMT-D program. The initial training for automatic EMT-D programs is consequently simpler and takes less time. Initial classes for manual EMT-D programs range from 10 to 16 hours, depending primarily on the amount of rhythm recognition that is taught. Some program medical directors require only that the EMT-D distinguish between ventricular fibrillation and nonventricular fibrillation; other medical directors believe more advanced rhythm recognition is necessary. In contrast, initial classes for automatic EMT-D programs range from 2 to 6 hours.

Continuing Education. The frequency of continuing education can vary from once a month to once every 6 months. The maximum time between reviews should be 90 days. The content of continuing education must emphasize the practical skills of proper attachment of the defibrillators, proper operation of the device, and close adherence to the standing orders. This general content is identical regardless of whether automatic or manual defibrillators are used. Programs that have selected manual defibrillators, however, must add a component on rhythm recognition to their continuing education program.

Electrical Countershocks. The American Heart Association 1986 recommendations for the initial treatment of persistent ventricular fibrillation are as follows:

1. Countershock of 200 joules
2. Repeat countershock of 200–300 joules
3. Repeat countershock of 200–360 joules
4. Initiation of further advanced cardiac life support in the form of endotracheal intubation and intravenous medications
5. Additional countershocks

EMT-D programs should keep within these general guidelines and permit at least three countershocks for persistent VF, at an initial energy level of 200 joules, and perhaps an increase in energy level for subsequent countershocks. Many EMT-D programs will not have paramedic backup, and consequently intubation and intravenous medications will not be available. In these systems, medical directors should issue standing orders that permit more than three countershocks for persistent ventricular fibrillation.

Stacked shocks. Properly performed CPR must be continued throughout the care of a person in cardiac arrest; it is stopped only during rhythm assessment and the actual delivery of the countershock. A prescribed period of CPR is not necessary prior to the first shock. Instead, CPR should be performed only for the length of time that it takes to attach the monitor leads, gel the defibrillator paddles, and charge the defibrillator. CPR is then stopped, the rhythm is assessed, by either the EMT-D or the automatic defibrillator, and the shock is delivered if indicated. A number of EMT-D protocols "stack" the second and sometimes the third countershocks, a procedure called **stacked shocks.** CPR is not resumed immediately after the first shock. Instead, the EMT-D leaves the automatic defibrillator in automatic mode for continued rhythm assessment and the delivery of one or more shocks if VF persists. With semi-automatic defibrillators, the "analyze" and the "shock" switches are pressed after each shock, without resumption of CPR. Similarly, manual EMT-Ds do not remove the defibrillator paddles from the chest but treat persistent VF with continued shocks without interposed periods of CPR. Other programs may decide to provide a 15- to 30-second period of CPR after each shock.

Shocking Asystole. There is clinical evidence to suggest that on rare occasions, ventricular fibrillation may appear as asystole on the ECG tracing. To avoid the possibility of failure to shock occult ventricular fibrillation, some medical directors permit their EMT-Ds to deliver a countershock during asystole. As a result, some successful conversions of "asystole" to an effective cardiac rhythm have been reported. These successes, however, are extremely rare. No more than one out of every 100 patients in asystole who are shocked will regain a perfusing rhythm. Countershocks during asystole should be permitted only after the EMT-Ds have verified that there is no alternative explanation for the apparent asystole, such as inadequate batteries, incorrect calibrations, or improper monitor connections. Auto-

matic and semi-automatic defibrillators will not deliver a shock during asystole.

YOU ARE THE EMT...

1. What factors must be present in order for defibrillation to be successful in reversing sudden death?
2. What three features are always present in an electrocardiogram showing ventricular fibrillation?
3. Why can't you use a defibrillator for nonventricular fibrillation? Why do some doctors instruct EMTs to use paddles on a patient with asystole?
4. You are unable to identify VF in your patient because of excessive artifact. You have checked the monitor leads and find they have not unsnapped. What other problems could be causing excessive artifact and how should you deal with such problems?

GLOSSARY

Glossary

abandonment failure of the EMT to continue emergency medical treatment.

abdomen (ab-do′mən) the more inferior of the two major body cavities, lying between the thorax and the pelvis and containing the major organs of digestion and excretion.

abdominal catastrophe (ka′tas-tra′fē) a term describing the most severe form of an acute abdomen; the presence of a severe intra-abdominal problem that causes peritonitis.

abdominal cavity the cavity between the diaphragm and the pelvis that contains all the abdominal organs.

abdominal eviscerations (e-vis-er-a′shunz) injuries in which abdominal organs are exposed.

abdominal quadrants (kwod′rantz) four equal parts into which the abdomen is divided; they are separated by two imaginary lines that intersect at right angles at the umbilicus. The quadrants are the right upper, right lower, left upper, and left lower quadrants.

abdominal (**subdiaphragmatic;** sub′di-ă-frag-mat′ik) **thrust maneuver** a series of 6 to 10 manual thrusts to the upper abdomen, just above the umbilicus and well below the xiphoid to relieve upper airway obstruction; also called the Heimlich maneuver.

abduction (ab-duk′shən) motion of a limb away from the midline.

abortion (ə-bor′shən) delivery of the fetus before it is mature enough to survive outside the womb (about 20 weeks), either from natural causes (spontaneous abortion) or induced; also called miscarriage.

abrasion (ə-bra′zhən) loss of skin as a result of a body part being rubbed or scraped across a rough or hard surface.

abruptio (ab-rup′she-o) **placentae** (plə-sen′ti) early separation of the placenta from the wall of the uterus.

abscess (ab′ses) a localized collection of pus in a cavity formed by the disintegration of tissues.

abuse a cause of injury that can take the form of beatings, burns, rape, attempted murder, etc.

acetabulum (as′ĕ-tab′u-ləm) the socket portion of the hip joint, into which the femoral head fits.

acetone (as′ə-tōn) a colorless liquid found in small quantities in normal urine and in larger amounts in diabetic urine; a metabolic end product of the use of fat for routine energy needs.

Achilles (ə-kil′ēz) **tendon** the tendon joining the muscles in the calf of the leg to the bone of the heel.

acid (as′id) any compound of an electronegative element with one or more electropositive hydrogen ions. Acids can cause severe burns.

acidosis (as′ĭ-do′sis) a condition caused by accumulation of acid or loss of base in the body.

A/C joint *See* acromioclavicular joint.

acquired immune deficiency syndrome (AIDS) a fatal disease first noted in 1978 and caused by a virus. It is spread through direct contact with the blood, semen, or oral secretions of infected individuals.

acromioclavicular (ə-kro′mē-o-klə-vik′u-lar) (**A/C**) **joint** joint at the top of the shoulder, formed by bony projections of the scapula and clavicle.

acromion (ə-kro′mē-on) **process** lateral extension of the spine of the scapula; the highest point of the shoulder.

A/C separation a dislocation of the acromioclavicular joint; shoulder separation.

activated charcoal powdered charcoal that has been treated to increase its powers of adsorption; used as a general-purpose antidote.

actual consent consent actually given by a person authorizing the EMT to provide care or transportation.

acute abdomen a term indicating the presence of some abdominal process that causes the sudden irritation of the peritoneum and intense pain.

acute cholecystitis (ko-le-sis-ti′tis) inflammation of the gallbladder.

acute epiglottitis (ep′ĭ-glot-ti′tis) a bacterial infection of the epiglottis. In children it can cause swelling severe enough to cause airway obstruction.

acute myocardial infarction (mi′o-kar′dē-al in-fark′shon) (**AMI**) heart attack; death of the heart muscle caused by lack of oxygen to the muscle.

acute pulmonary edema (pul′mo-ner′ē ĕ-de′mə) severe fluid buildup in the lungs that usually occurs following acute myocardial infarction.

acute symptoms symptoms of sudden onset.

acute urinary retention a condition more common in the older male, often in conjunction with enlargement of the prostate gland, in which the urethal outlet of the bladder is obstructed and the patient is unable to void.

Adam's apple   the firm prominence (more prominent in men than women) in the upper part of the larynx formed by the thyroid cartilage.

addiction (ə-dik′shən)   a state characterized by an overwhelming desire or need (compulsion) to continue the use of a drug and to obtain it by any means whatsoever.

adduction (ə-duk′shən)   motion of a limb toward the midline.

administration set   equipment used for intravenous fluid therapy; consists of a fluid container that holds the solution, tubing, and a drip chamber. *Mini-drip sets* flow with minimum volume infusion; they are designed to keep an IV line open. *Solution sets* deliver large volumes of fluid to be infused over a short period of time.

adrenal (ə-dre′nəl) **glands**   glands which secrete hormones that control salt levels in the blood and some sexual function.

adult onset diabetes (di′ə-bē′tēz)   milder form of diabetes mellitus that affects adults. Insulin is still produced, but at a lower, insufficient level. Many of these patients can control their diabetes by diet alone or with pills that stimulate the pancreas.

advanced life support   the use of adjunctive equipment, cardiac monitoring, defibrillation, intravenous lifeline, and drug infusion.

afterbirth (**placenta**; plə-sen′tə)   a special organ of pregnancy attached to the wall of the uterus through which the fetus receives its nourishment and gets rid of waste products.

agonal (ag′on-al) **respirations**   irregular gasping respirations, sometimes heard in dying patients.

AIDS   *See* acquired immune deficiency syndrome.

air ambulance   an ambulance that is also an aircraft (a helicopter or fixed-wing aircraft).

airborne transmission   a method of disease transmission in which the infective organism is introduced into the air by coughing or sneezing; droplets of mucus that carry bacteria or other organisms are then inhaled by another person.

air embolism (em′bo-lizm) (pl. **emboli**)   bubbles of air released into the blood from rupture of lung alveoli during ascent from the water or flying too high in an unpressurized plane.

air hunger   a distressing dyspnea occurring in paroxysms; found in diabetic coma.

air splint   a precontoured, inflatable plastic type of soft splint. After application, it is inflated by mouth, *never* with a pump.

airway   route for the passage of air in and out of the lungs; describing the upper airway, or air passages above the larynx: the nose, mouth, and throat.

alcohol   a liquid obtained by fermentation of carbohydrates with yeast.

alcoholic hallucinations (hə-lu′sə-nay′shənz)   the awareness or perception of fantastic figures, often walking on the wall or appearing as if to attack the patient; they are a manifestation of the alcoholic withdrawal syndrome.

alcoholism   addiction to alcohol; overuse that affects the individual's health and social and economic functioning.

alkali (al′kə-li)   any compound of an electropositive element with an electronegative hydroxyl ion or similar ion. Alkalis can cause severe burns.

alkaline   having a pH above the normal level of 7.45.

alkalosis (al′kə-lo′sis)   a condition in which excessive breathing, as from hyperventilating, "blows off" too much carbon dioxide. The patient experiences shortness of breath. This response is common in psychological stress.

allergens (al′er-jenz)   agents to which a person is sensitive.

allergic (ə-ler′jik)   suffering from an allergy.

allergy (al′er-ji)   exaggerated reaction to substances, situations, or physical states that have no such effect on the average person.

alopecia (al-o-pe′shĭ-ah)   loss of hair.

alpha (al′fə) **particle**   a positively charged particle emitted from the nucleus of a radioactive atom.

alpha radiation   a form of ionizing radiation that poses little danger; these rays are easily stopped by paper, a few inches of air, or light clothing.

alveoli (al-ve′o-li)   the air sacs of the lungs where the exchange of oxygen and carbon dioxide takes place.

ambulance (am′byu-ləns)   vehicle for emergency medical care, especially designed to provide a driver compartment and a patient compartment large enough for two EMTs and two litter patients, so positioned that at least one patient can be given intensive lifesaving care during transit.

ambulance run report   a permanent run report filled out by the EMT after the patient has been delivered to the emergency department.

ambulance street form   a compact form, frequently printed on a 3 × 5 card, that allows the EMT to record the information needed to make a radio report to the emergency department.

American Standard System   safety system for large cylinders of gas in which gas outlet valves are threaded to accept matching regulator valves so that a regulator cannot be attached to a wrong supply tank.

amino (ə-mē′no) **acids**   organic compounds that form the chief structure of proteins.

amnesia (am-nē′zē-a)   loss of memory.

amniotic (am′nē-ot′ik) **fluid**   a liquid that surrounds the fetus in the uterus and protects it from injury.

amniotic sac   the innermost of the membranes enveloping the fetus in the uterus.

amphetamines (am-fet′ə-mēnz)   stimulants that are taken to produce a general mood elevation, improve task performance, suppress appetite, or prevent sleepiness; common forms are "speed," "uppers," or "Bennies."

amputation am′pyu-tay′shən)   removal of a body part.

anal (ay′nəl) **canal**   the lower end of the alimentary canal.

anaphylactic (an′a-fə-lak′tik) **shock**   severe shock caused by an allergic reaction.

anaphylaxis (an-a-fi-lak′sis)   the most severe form of an allergic reaction resulting in shock.

anatomic (an′ə-tom′ik) **position**   position of a patient standing erect, facing the examiner, arms at the side, and palms facing forward.

anesthesia (an′es-the′zĭ-ah)   the loss of sensation from injury or the administration of drugs.

anesthetic (an′es-thet-ik)   without feeling.

aneurysm (an′yu-rizm)   a weakened, bulging area of a blood vessel.

angina pectoris (an-jī′nə pek-to′ris)   chest pain with squeezing or tightness in the chest caused by an inadequate flow of blood to the heart muscle.

angle of Louis   a bony prominence on the breastbone, just inferior to the junction of the clavicle and sternum and just opposite the second intercostal space.

angulation (an′gyu-lay′shən)   departure from a straight line, as in a broken bone.

anisocoria (an′i-so-ko′rē-ə)   unequal size of the pupils of the eyes.

ankle joint   a hinge joint that allows flexion and extension of the foot on the leg.

anorexia (an-o-rek′sĭ-ah)   loss of hunger or appetite.

anorexia nervosa (ner-vo′sa)   a condition more common in young females in which the patient takes less and less food and may become seriously emaciated and malnourished. It is a manifestation of a severe underlying psychological disorder.

anoxia (an-ok′sĭ-ah)   lack of oxygen.

antecubital fossa (an′tē-kyu′bə-təl fos′ə)   the depression in the anterior region of the elbow.

anterior superior iliac (il′ē-ak) **spines**   the hard bony prominences at the front on each side of the lower abdomen just below the plane of the umbilicus; they form the anterior ends of the iliac crest.

anterior surface   the front surface of the body, facing the examiner.

antibiotic (an′tĭ-bī-ot′ik)   a chemical substance produced by a microorganism, which has the capacity to kill other microorganisms.

antidote (an′tĭ-dōt)   a substance that will counteract poison.

antihistamine (an′tĭ-his-tə-mēn)   a drug that counteracts the effects of histamine and relieves the symptoms of an allergic reaction.

antivenin (an′tĭ-ven′in)   antitoxin (remedy) for a venom.

anus (ay′nəs)   the distal or terminal ending of the alimentary canal.

aorta (ay-or′tə)   the major artery leaving the left side of the heart, which carries freshly oxygenated blood to the body.

aortic (ay-or′tik) **valve**   a valve that guards the aortic opening in the left ventricle of the heart and prevents backflow into the left ventricle.

aorto-coronary (ay-or′to kor′ə-na-rē) **bypass**   an operation to bypass damaged coronary arteries to the heart; a vein from the leg or an artificial vessel is sewn directly from the aorta to a coronary artery beyond the point of obstruction.

Apgar score   a system whereby the status of a newborn baby is assessed in five areas: cardiac rate, respirations, muscle tone, reflex irritability, and color.

aphasic (ă-fa′sĭk)   unable to speak.

apneic (ap-nē′ik)   having no spontaneous breathing.

appendicitis (ə-pen′də-sī′tis)   inflammation of the appendix.

appendix (ə-pen′diks)   a small tubular structure that is attached to the lower border of the cecum in the lower right quadrant of the abdomen.

aqueous (ay′kwē-us) **humor**   the fluid in front of the lens of the eye.

arachnoid (ə-rak′noid)   middle layer of the three layers of tissue that envelop the brain and spinal cord; lies between the dura mater and the pia mater.

arm   part of the upper extremity that extends from the shoulder to the elbow.

arrhythmia (ə-rith′me-ə)   abnormal heart rhythm.

arterial (ar-te′rē-al) **pressure**   the pressure of the blood that flows through the arteries.

arterial pressure points (pulse points)   points where an artery passes over a bony prominence or lies close to the skin; at these points the artery can be palpated and the arterial pulse taken.

arterial rupture   rupture of a cerebral artery.

arteries (ar′ter-ēz)   the tubular vessels that carry blood from the heart to the body tissues.

arterioles (ar-te′rē-ōlz)   small branches of arteries.

arteriosclerosis (ar-te′rē-o-sklə-ro′sis) a disease characterized by a thickening and destruction of the arterial walls, caused by fatty deposits within them; the arteries lose the ability to dilate and carry oxygen-enriched blood.

articular (ar-tik′yu-lər) pertaining to a joint.

articular cartilage (kar′tə-lij) a layer of cartilage covering the ends of bones to form the joint surface.

articulation (ar-tik′yu-lay′shən) joint; the juncture where two bones come in contact.

artificial airway a device that is inserted through the nose or mouth to allow passage of air and oxygen to the lungs.

artificial circulation a means of providing circulation by external chest compression.

artificial respiration *See* artificial ventilation.

artificial ventilation (ven′tə-lay′shən) opening the airway and restoring breathing by mouth-to-mouth or mouth-to-nose ventilation and by the use of mechanical devices.

ascending colon (kō′lən) part of the colon that lies in the vertical position on the right side of the abdomen, extending up to the lower border of the liver.

ascent injuries injuries in ascent from a dive, especially air embolism and decompression sickness.

aspiration (as′pə-ray′shən) taking foreign matter such as vomitus into the lungs during inhalation.

asthma (az′mə) an acute spasm of the smaller air passages; a condition marked by labored breathing and wheezing due to contraction of the bronchi.

asystole (ə-sis-tō-lē) lack of any electric or muscular activity in the heart; lack of a heartbeat.

atom (at′əm) the smallest particle of an element that can enter into a chemical reaction.

atrial fibrillation (ay′tre-əl fi-bri-lay′shən) disorganized, ineffective quivering of the atria, causing an irregular, often rapid ventricular heart rate.

atrial flutter beating of the atria up to rates of 300/minute not associated with equal beating of the ventricles.

atrium (ay′tre-um) either of the two upper chambers of the heart.

auditory (aw′dĭ-to′rē) **nerves** nerves transmitting hearing sensations to the brain.

aura (aw′rah) the first phase of a generalized epileptic seizure. It is a sensation experienced by the patient that a seizure is about to occur.

auscultate (aws′kul-tāt) to listen.

auscultation (aws′kul-tay′shən) listening to sounds within the organs, usually with a stethoscope; a method of taking a patient's blood pressure.

autonomic (aw′to-nom′ik) **(involuntary) nervous system** that part of the nervous system that regulates functions not controlled by a voluntary act of conscious will, such as digestion or sweating.

AVPU scale a scale to measure a patient's level of consciousness. The letters stand for alert, verbal, pain, unresponsive.

avulsion (ə-vul′shən) an injury in which a piece of skin is either torn completely loose from all of its attachments or is left hanging as a flap.

axilla (ak-sil′ə) the armpit.

back blows sharp blows delivered with the EMT's hand over the patient's spine between the scapulae to relieve upper airway obstruction.

bacterial meningitis (men′in-ji′tis) a form of meningitis that carries the risk of transmission.

bacterium (bak-te′re-um) microorganism that causes infection.

bad trip an unpleasant or frightening hallucination caused by drugs.

bag of waters the amniotic sac and its contained amniotic fluid in which the fetus is enveloped within the uterus.

bag-valve-mask resuscitators (re-sus′ĭ-tay′torz) equipment for supplying supplemental oxygen; consists of an inflatable, deflatable bag, a face mask, and a valve that connects the face mask and bag and attaches to the oxygen supply.

bag-valve-mask system method of delivering air with more than 90 percent oxygen; *see* bag-valve-mask resuscitators.

ball-and-socket joint a joint that allows internal and external rotation as well as bending.

barbiturates (bar-bit′u-raytz) drugs that depress the nervous system; they can alter the state of consciousness so that the individual may appear drowsy or peaceful. On the street, barbiturates are commonly known as "Goof Balls."

basal skull fracture fracture of the base of the skull; cerebrospinal fluid may leak from the ear, nose, or a scalp laceration, or there may be hemorrhage from the ear without apparent cause.

base the nonacid part of any salt that combines with acids to form salts; an alkali.

base station any fixed radio hardware containing a transmitter and receiver. For EMS purposes, they will generally be within the class, land mobile service, as defined by the Federal Communications Commission (FCC).

basic life support emergency lifesaving procedures without the aid of mechanical devices whereby first responders can correct respiratory or circulatory failure.

basilar (bas'ĭ-lar) **artery** artery formed by two vertebral arteries that unite at the base of the brain; the basilar artery has connections that link with the two carotid arteries at the base of the brain to form a circle of vessels around the brain stem.

bee sting kit kit with medications for the patient who has severe allergic reactions to bee stings.

belays (bi-lāz') rescue lines.

bends decompression sickness; bubbles of nitrogen that form in the blood vessels when a diver ascends too rapidly.

benign (be-nīn) nonmalignant.

beta cells of the islets (ī'letz) **of Langerhans** (län'ər-häns) specialized cells in the pancreas that produce insulin.

beta particles negatively charged electrons that are given off by the nuclei of radioactive material at fairly high energy levels.

beta radiation a form of ionizing radiation that can penetrate to a greater depth than alpha rays but that are effectively stopped by clothing, glass, or thin metal shielding.

biceps (bī'seps) **muscle** large muscle that covers the front of the humerus.

bile (bīl) a fluid secreted by the liver and transmitted to the small intestine through the bile ducts. It is required for normal fat digestion.

bile ducts (dukts) ducts that convey bile between the liver and the intestines.

biliary (bil'ē-a-rē) **tract** a ductal system through which bile passes from the liver into the intestines.

birth the act or process of being born; separation of the infant from the mother's body.

birth canal the vagina and the lower part of the uterus.

bite an injury caused by the teeth of an animal; the relation of the upper and lower teeth when in contact.

bite block block to put in the patient's mouth to prevent biting of the tongue.

black widow spider a poisonous spider; the female is black with an hourglass-shaped red mark on the underside of the abdomen.

bladder a musculomembranous sac for collecting and storing urine.

blanched skin becomes pale.

blanket drag a method by which one EMT encloses a patient in a blanket and drags the patient to safety.

blood a complex, thick, red fluid composed of plasma, red blood cells (erythrocytes), white blood cells (leukocytes), and platelets.

blood pressure the pressure of the circulating blood against the walls of the arteries.

blood volume the amount of blood within the circulatory system.

bloody show a small plug of blood-stained mucus that forms in the cervix and is expelled when labor begins.

blowout fracture fracture of the orbit (eye socket) or of the bones that support the floor of the orbit.

blunt (closed) abdominal injuries injuries to the abdomen caused by a blunt object like a steering wheel; the skin remains intact.

blunt trauma (trou'mə) injury in which the force of impact is concentrated on a large area of contact between the wounding object and the body; the force of impact is transmitted through the skin, not breaking the skin, but damaging the tissues and organs below the skin.

body (of the sternum) one of three parts of the sternum; (of a vertebra) the front part of a vertebra; a round solid block of bone.

bone the hard form of connective tissue that makes up the skeleton.

bone marrow the central portion of all bones that produces red blood cells.

bony arch the back part of each vertebra; together, the bony arches form a tunnel that runs the length of the spine and protects the spinal cord.

bony rib cage twelve pairs of ribs that extend from their respective thoracic vertebrae around to the front to create the walls of the chest.

botulism (bot'u-lizm) the most severe form of food poisoning; usually results from eating improperly canned food that contains bacterial toxins.

Bourdon gauge flowmeter a pressure gauge on a medical compressed gas cylinder calibrated to record flow rate.

brachial (bra'kē-al) **artery** artery on the inside of the arm between the elbow and the shoulder; used in taking blood pressure and for checking the pulse in infants.

brachial plexus (plek'sus) a network of nerves originating from branches of the spinal nerves; located in the neck and the axilla.

bradycardia (brad'ē-kar'dē-ə) unusually slow but regular beating of the heart.

brain controlling organ of the body; center of consciousness; functions include perception, control of reactions to the environment, emotional responses, and judgment.

brain stem   area of the brain between the spinal cord and cerebrum, surrounded by the cerebellum; controls functions necessary for life, such as respiration.

breath-holding blackout   a blackout that occurs under water because of hypoxia when the swimmer does not realize the need to take a breath.

breech presentation   a delivery in which the baby's buttocks appear first rather than the head.

bridge   the proximal one-third of the nose that is formed by bone. The rest of the nose is made of cartilage.

bronchi (brong'kī)   the two main branches of the trachea that lead into the right and left lungs. Within the lungs they branch into smaller airways. Three major bronchi form in the right lung. Two major bronchi form in the left lung.

bronchioles (brong'ke-ōlz)   the finer subdivisions of the bronchi, less than 1 millimeter in diameter, having smooth muscle and elastic fibers in their walls.

brow   one of two soft areas on a baby's head, located near the front.

brown recluse (rek'lus) **spider**   a poisonous spider with a violin-shaped mark on the head and thorax.

bulb syringe (sə-rin'gə)   a rubber or plastic device of defined capacity (60 cc) used for gentle suction and irrigation in neonates and small infants.

bulimia (bu-lim'ĭ-ah)   a condition in which the patient significantly overeats and then induces vomiting in an effort not to gain weight from the extra food. It is a manifestation of a severe underlying psychological disorder.

bulky hand dressing   dressing and splint for hand injuries.

burn   a lesion caused by heat exposure or exposure to chemicals or electricity.

burp   regurgitation.

butterfly   a steel needle that is used for intravenous fluid therapy.

caffeine (kə-fēn')   a mild stimulant found in coffee and cola drinks.

calcaneus (kal-kay'nē-us) **(os calcis)**   the heel bone.

calcium (kal'sē-um)   an element found in nearly all organized tissues, especially bone.

cancer (kan'sər)   a condition in which tissue develops a malignant neoplasm.

capillaries (kap'i-lar'ēz)   the minute blood vessels that connect the arterioles and venules; their thin walls act as membranes for the interchange of various substances between the blood and tissue fluid.

capillary perfusion (per-fyu'zhən)   the process whereby oxygen and nutrients are brought to every cell, and waste and carbon dioxide are removed.

capillary refill   the ability of the circulatory system to restore blood to the capillary blood vessels after it has been squeezed out by the examiner.

carbohydrate (kar'bo-hi'drayt)   compound derived from alcohols. The starches, sugars, and cellulose, are examples.

carbon dioxide (di-ok'sīd) **(CO$_2$)**   a waste product formed in body tissues by the metabolism of sugars.

carbon dioxide drive   the stimulus to breathing caused by the carbon dioxide level in the arterial blood; regulation of rate and depth of breathing by the carbon dioxide level.

carbon dioxide narcosis (nar-ko'sis)   a condition in which the carbon dioxide in the blood rises to high levels, and the respiratory center becomes narcotized, or depressed.

carbon monoxide (mon-ok'sīd) **(CO)**   a colorless, odorless, poisonous gas formed by the incomplete combustion of carbohydrates; when breathed in, it blocks oxygen transport and use.

cardiac (kar'dē-ak) **arrest**   a sudden ceasing of heart function because the heart has failed to generate an effective blood flow.

cardiac muscle   the muscle of the heart.

cardiac output   the effective volume of blood expelled by either ventricle of the heart per unit of time.

cardiac pacemaker   device that imposes a regular rhythm on the heart by delivering an electrical impulse through wires sewn into the heart muscle.

cardiac tamponade (tam-pŏ-nād')   a condition in which the sac around the heart fills with blood.

cardiogenic (kar'dē-o-jen'ik) **shock**   shock resulting from inadequate functioning of the heart.

cardiopulmonary resuscitation (CPR)   the artificial establishment of circulation of the blood and movement of air into and out of the lungs in a pulseless, nonbreathing patient.

cardiovascular collapse   *See* cardiac arrest.

cardiovascular (kar'dē-o-vas'kyu-lar) **(circulatory) system**   a complex arrangement of connected tubes that include arteries, arterioles, capillaries, venules, and veins; the heart pumps blood through this system.

carotid (kə-rot'id) **arteries**   The principal arteries of the neck. They run upward in the neck and divide into the external and internal carotid arteries to supply the face, head, and brain. They can be palpated on either side of the neck.

carotid artery pulse   pulse that can be felt at the upper portion of the neck where the carotid artery on each side of the neck is close to the skin.

carpal (kar′pal) **bones**   the eight bones of the wrist.

carpometacarpal (kar′po-met′ə-kar′pal) **joint**   the joint between the wrist and the metacarpal bones.

carrier   an animal or a person who may transmit an infectious disease but does not display any symptoms of it; a basic radio signal (wave) generated by a transmitter without voice or other information imposed on it.

cartilage (kar′tĭ-lij)   a form of connective tissue containing a tough, elastic substance; found in joints, at the developing ends of bones, and in some specific areas such as the nose and ear.

case law   law established by judicial decision in particular cases.

cataract (kat′ə-rakt)   opacity of the lens of the eye, so that vision is impaired.

catheterization (kath′ə-tər-ī-zā′shən)   a procedure in which a tube is inserted directly into the bladder to remove urine when a patient is unable to void.

catheter (kath′ə-tər)   a hollow, cylindrical structure that can be inserted into the body to drain or deliver fluids.

catheter over the needle   the most popular type of needle used with intravenous therapy.

catheter through the needle   a type of needle used with intravenous therapy.

cecum (se-kum)   the first part of the large intestine, into which the ileum opens.

cell   a small mass of protoplasm (living matter) bounded by a membrane; the smallest unit of living matter that can function independently.

cellulitis (sel′yu-līt′is)   a spreading redness and swelling of the skin usually caused by infection.

Celsius (sel′sē-əs)   designation of temperature on a thermometer on which 0° is the freezing point and 100° is the boiling point of water; same as centigrade.

centigrade (sen′tə-grād)   designation of temperature on a thermometer on which 0° is the freezing point and 100° is the boiling point of water; same as Celsius.

centralized medical emergency dispatch (CMED)   a special communications operation that monitors and allocates medical control channels among EMS providers.

central nervous system (CNS)   the brain and spinal cord.

cerebellum (ser′ĕ-bel′um)   one of three major subdivisions of the brain, sometimes called the "little brain"; coordinates the various activities of the brain, particularly body movements.

cerebral (ser′ĕ-bral)   pertaining to the brain.

cerebral arteries   arteries that supply blood to the brain.

cerebral concussion (kon-kush-ən)   a jarring injury of the brain resulting in disturbance of brain function. No permanent physical damage occurs to the brain tissue.

cerebral contusion (kon-tu′zhən)   bruising of the brain tissue from a blow to the head that can cause bleeding, swelling, and brain damage.

cerebral embolism (em′bə-lizm)   obstruction of a cerebral arterial artery by a clot that formed elsewhere in the body and traveled to the brain.

cerebral hematoma (hēm′ə-to′mə)   a hematoma, or collection of blood, inside the brain tissue itself.

cerebrospinal (ser′ĕ-bro-spi′nal) **fluid**   fluid that fills the spaces between the arachnoid and the pia mater. The brain and spinal cord essentially float in this fluid.

cerebrovascular (ser′ĕ-bro-vas′kyu-lar) **accident (CVA)**   stroke; a sudden lessening or loss of consciousness, sensation, and voluntary movement caused by rupture or obstruction of an artery in the brain.

cerebrovascular disease   degeneration of the blood vessels in the brain.

cerebrum (ser′ĕ-brum)   the largest of the three subdivisions of the brain, sometimes called the "gray matter"; it is made up of several lobes that control movement, hearing, balance, speech, visual perception, emotions, and personality.

certification (ser′tĭ-fĭ-cay′shən)   formal notice of certain privileges and abilities after completion of certain training and testing.

cervical (ser′vĭ-kal) **collar**   a neck brace that partially stabilizes the neck following injury.

cervical spine   that portion of the spinal column consisting of the seven vertebrae that lie in the neck.

cervical vertebrae (ver′tĕ-bre)   the first seven vertebrae of the spinal column that lie in the neck.

cervix (ser′viks)   the lower and narrow end of the uterus.

chain of evidence   protocol of EMTs assisting law enforcement agencies in collecting evidence; involves not moving or touching items unless for medical reasons, noting torn clothing, and noting and recording all injury sites.

channel   an assigned frequency or frequencies used to carry voice and/or data communications.

chassis (shas′ē) **set**   the transfer of weight of a vehicle to different points on the chassis or frame.

chemical burns burns that occur when any toxic substance comes in contact with the skin. Most chemical burns are caused by strong acids or alkalis.

chemical pneumonia (nu-mo-ne-ə) pneumonia caused by the aspiration of petroleum products or acid gastric juice into the lungs.

Chemical Transportation Emergency Center (CHEMTREC) a center that provides hazardous information warning and guidance if the DOT identification number, the chemical name, or the product name of the hazardous material is given.

chest-thrust maneuver a series of manual thrusts to the chest to relieve upper airway obstruction.

chief complaint the first words out of a patient's mouth in response to a general question such as "What's wrong?" or "What happened?"

chilblains a form of cold exposure that occurs after prolonged exposure to the cold, but freezing of the skin and deeper tissues has not occurred.

child abuse the deliberate, intentional injury of a child physically and/or emotionally.

child molestation (mo-les-ta′shən) sexual abuse of children.

chin-lift maneuver *See* head-tilt/chin-lift maneuver.

cholesterol (ko-les′ter-ol) a fatlike substance found in animal fats and oils that is deposited on the inner walls of some people's arteries; the buildup of these deposits narrows the arteries and limits their ability to dilate, the disease process called arteriosclerosis.

choroid (ko′roid) a layer of blood vessels between the retina and the sclera, which nourishes the eye, especially the retina.

chronic bronchitis (kron′ik brong′kī′tis) chronic irritation of the trachea and bronchi, with attacks of coughing and changes in the lung tissue.

chronic obstructive lung (pulmonary) disease a slow process of disruption of the airways, alveoli, and pulmonary blood vessels, caused by chronic bronchial obstruction.

chronic symptoms symptoms that are slowly progressive.

circulatory overload the administration of an excessive amount of IV fluids.

circulatory (cardiovascular) system a complex arrangement of connected tubes that include arteries, arterioles, capillaries, venules, and veins; the heart pumps blood through this system.

cirrhosis (sir-ro′sis) progressive liver damage, often associated with chronic alcohol abuse.

clammy cold, damp.

clavicle (klav′ĭ-kl) the collarbone. It is attached medially to the sternum and laterally to the scapula.

clinical (klin′e-kl) pertaining to or founded on actual observation and treatment of patients.

clinical sign a physical finding that can be elicited or viewed by the physician or EMT.

clonic (klän′ik) **muscular activity** spasms that occur during a generalized epileptic seizure.

closed (blunt) abdominal injuries injuries to the abdomen caused by a blunt object like a steering wheel; the skin remains intact.

closed chest injuries injuries to the chest in which the skin has not been broken.

closed fracture a fracture in which the bone ends have not penetrated the skin and no wound exists near the fracture site.

closed wound injury in which soft tissue damage occurs beneath the skin but in which there is no break in the surface of the skin.

clothes drag a method by which one EMT can drag a patient to safety by grasping the patient's clothes.

CMED *See* centralized medical emergency dispatch.

CO₂ carbon dioxide.

cocaine (ko′kayn) a powerful stimulant that induces an extreme state of euphoria. Legitimately, it is a potent local anesthetic. On the street, it is commonly known as "coke."

coccyx (kok′siks) the tailbone; the small bone below the sacrum formed by the final three to four vertebrae.

codeine (ko′dēn) a narcotic drug; a depressant.

coffee grounds vomitus (vom′ĭ-tus) vomitus consisting of dark-colored matter, usually digested blood.

colic (kol′ik) an intermittent painful intestinal cramp caused by strong peristaltic waves.

colitis (ko-lī′tis) inflammation of the colon.

Colles' (kol′ēz) **fracture** fracture of the distal radius, producing the silver-fork deformity in which the injured wrist assumes a curvature similar to the side view of a dinner fork.

colloids (kol-loyds) fluids used for intravenous infusion that include Dextran® (large molecules of dextrose that are not metabolized) and Plamanate®.

colon (ko′lon) that part of the large intestine that extends from the ileocecal valve to the rectum.

coma (ko′mə) a state of unconsciousness from which the patient cannot be aroused.

comatose (ko′mə-tos) in a coma.

comminuted (kom′ĭ-nūt′əd) **fracture** a fracture in which the bone is broken into more than two fragments.

communicable (ko-myu′nĭ-kə-bl) infectious or contagious; capable of transmitting disease.

communicable (contagious, infectious) diseases diseases that can be transmitted from one person to another.

complex partial seizure (se′zhur) a partial epileptic seizure in which consciousness may be clouded, or the patient may display automatic behavior such as chewing, fumbling with clothes, or walking aimlessly.

compound (open) fracture any fracture in which the overlying skin has been damaged.

compression (kom-presh′ən) **dressing** a dressing by which pressure is applied to a limb to prevent edema or bleeding.

computer-aided dispatch (CAD) a sophisticated system that enables a dispatcher to input information from an emergency phone call into a computer terminal.

concussion (kon-kush′ən) a jarring injury of the brain resulting in disturbance of brain function.

conduction (kon-duk′shən) loss of body heat by the direct transfer of heat to a colder object as when a warm hand comes in contact with snow or ice.

conductor any substance that allows a current to flow through it; water and most metals are good conductors.

condyles (kon′dīlz) prominences at one or both ends of a bone.

congenital (kon-jen′ĭ-tal) **defect** a physical abnormality or deficiency that is present at birth.

congenital lesion (le′zhun) a weakened portion of the arterial wall that has been present since birth.

congestive (kon-jes′tiv) **heart failure (CHF)** heart disease characterized by breathlessness and sodium and water retention. There may be fluid in the lungs as well as generalized swelling of the body.

conjunctiva (kon′junk-ti′və) the delicate membrane that lines the eyelids and covers the exposed surface of the eye.

conjunctivitis (kon′junk-ti-vi′tis) ("pink eye") inflammation of the conjunctiva of the eye.

connecting nerves nerves that allow sensory and motor impulses to be transmitted from one nerve to another within the central nervous system.

consciousness (kon′shus-nes) the state of being conscious; responsiveness of the mind to the impressions made by the senses.

consent (kon-sent′) To agree. *See* actual consent; implied consent; informed consent.

constipation (kon-sti-pa′shən) difficult, incomplete, or infrequent passage of stools, more common in older individuals who become less physically active.

contact transmission a method of disease transmission, either from direct physical contact between an individual and the infected person or from indirect physical contact between an individual and inanimate objects that may have infectious organisms on them.

contagious (kon-tay′jus) **(communicable or infectious) diseases** diseases that can be transmitted from one person to another.

contaminated (kon-tam′i-nay-ted) soiled, stained, or infected by contact with bacterial or other infectious agents.

contamination the presence of infective organisms on or in objects such as dressings, water, food, or on any body surface.

contraindication (kon′trə-in′di-kay-shən) when a medical procedure, treatment, or medication should not be used.

control console (kän′sōl) typically, a desk-mounted, enclosed piece of equipment that contains the mechanical and electronic controls used to operate a radio base station.

controlled acceleration use of controlled pressure on the accelerator and of acceleration to control the vehicle.

controlled braking the use of the brakes to control the vehicle; controlled application of pressure to the brake pedal.

contusion (kon-tu′zhən) a bruise; injury caused by a blunt object striking the body and crushing the tissue beneath the skin.

convection (kon-vek′shən) loss of body heat by air moving across the body surface to a cooler area.

convulsion (kon-vul′shən) a violent involuntary contraction or series of contractions of the skeletal muscles.

convulsive seizure (se′zhur) a generalized epileptic seizure; also called a tonic-clonic seizure.

core temperature the temperature of the heart, lungs, brain, and other vital organs.

cornea (kor′nē-ə) the transparent tissue layer in front of the pupil and iris of the eye.

cornering negotiation of a curve at the speed best for maintaining good road position when coming out of the curve.

coronary (kor′ŏ-na-rē) **arteries** arteries of the heart.

coronary bypass *See* aorto-coronary bypass.

coroner (kor′o-ner) a public officer whose duty it is to inquire by an inquest into the cause of any death which there is reason to suppose may not be due to natural causes.

costal (kos′tal) **arch**   the fused cartilages of the seventh to tenth ribs, forming the upper limit of the abdomen.

costovertebral (kos′to-ver′te-bral) **angle**   angle that is formed by the spine and the tenth rib. The kidneys lie beneath the back muscles in the costovertebral angle.

counteragent   a drug or agent that opposes the effects of another drug or agent.

counterpressure   pressure countering the pressure that already exists.

countershock   the electric charge generated and delivered by a defibrillator.

countertraction   traction applied against a fixed point of the body.

coverage   the geographic area where reliable radio communications exist. Coverage is usually expressed as the radius in miles from a fixed base station.

CPR   *See* cardiopulmonary resuscitation.

cramp   a painful spasm, usually of a muscle; a gripping pain in the abdominal area; colic.

CRAMS scale   a trauma scoring system (circulation, respiration, abdomen, motor, and speech) used to determine the probability of survival.

cranial (kra′ne-al) **nerves**   12 pairs of peripheral nerves that exit the brain through holes in the skull; they are specialized nerves that control specific functions in the head and face.

cranium (kra′ne-um)   the area of the head above the ears and eyes; the skull. The cranium contains the brain.

crepitus (krep′ĭ-tus)   a grating or grinding sensation when raw, fractured bone ends rub against each other.

crib death   *See* sudden infant death syndrome.

cricoid (kri′koid) **cartilage**   a firm ridge of cartilage that forms the lower part of the larynx.

cricothyroid (kri-kō-thi′roid) **membrane**   a thin sheet of connective tissue (fascia) that connects the thyroid and cricoid cartilages that make up the larynx.

critical burns   the most serious burns. They include burns complicated by respiratory tract injury; third-degree burns involving critical areas or more than 10 percent of the body surface; second-degree burns involving more than 20–25 percent of the body surface; and any otherwise moderate burn in an elderly or critically ill patient.

cross-finger technique   a method of opening a patient's mouth; the EMT crosses his thumb under his index finger and braces both against the patient's lower and upper teeth, respectfully. Then using his fingers, the EMT can pry open the jaws.

croup (kroop)   acute obstruction of the larynx, with barking cough and hoarseness and a harsh, high-pitched breathing sound.

crowning   the phase in labor just before delivery when the baby's head appears in the vaginal opening.

crushing injury   injury resulting from the application of force to body tissue over a relatively long period of time. Crushing can cause soft tissue damage and cut off circulation.

Curies   a unit of measure of radiation from beta particles.

CVA   *See* cerebrovascular accident.

cyanosis (sī′ə-no′sis)   blue color of the skin resulting from poor oxygenation of the circulating blood.

cyanotic   having a bluish color.

cystitis (sis-tī′tis)   inflammation of the bladder.

decompensation (dē-căm′pən-sa′shən)   loss of ability to breathe due to insufficient circulation of blood.

decompression (dē′kəm-pres′shən) **sickness (the bends)**   bubbles of nitrogen that form in the blood vessels when a diver ascends too rapidly. They block the blood vessels, which prevents parts of the body from receiving a normal blood supply.

decongestants (de′kon-jes′tantz)   drugs that reduce congestion or swelling of the mucous membranes.

decontamination (de′kon-tam-ĭ-nā′shən)   removal of a contaminating substance from the person or equipment that was exposed.

dedicated line   a special telephone circuit used for specific point-to-point communications purposes.

defibrillation (de-fib′rĭ-lay′shən)   delivery of an electric current through a person's chest wall and heart for the purpose of ending a lethal cardiac arrythmia called ventricular fibrillation.

defibrillators (de-fib′rĭ-lay′torz)   portable battery-powered devices that are used to record cardiac rhythm and to generate and deliver an electric charge to patients with ventricular fibrillation.

deformity (de-for′mĭ-tē)   distortion (twisting out of the natural shape) of a body part.

degeneration (de-jən-ər-a′shən)   destruction of normal, healthy tissue from disease.

degenerative arthritis (är-thrīt′is)   deterioration of joints.

dehydration (de′hĭ-dray′shən)   loss of body water.

deliberate abortion (ə-bor-shən)   an abortion that is deliberately arranged. The abortion may be self-induced or performed in a hospital or clinic.

delirium (de-lir′ĭ-um)   a mental disturbance marked by hallucinations, cerebral excitement, and physical restlessness, usually lasting only a short time.

delirium tremens (trem′ənz) (**DTs**) a severe, often fatal, complication of alcoholic withdrawal that can occur from one to seven days after withdrawal. They are characterized by restlessness, fever, sweating, confusion, disorientation, agitation, hallucinations, and convulsions.

dementia (de-men′she-ə) a severe emotionally disturbed state, where the patient acts irrationally.

dependency (di-pen′dən-sē) the combined psychological and physical state of an individual in which the usual or increasing doses of a drug are required to prevent the onset of withdrawal symptoms.

dependent lividity (li-vid′ə-tē) a sign of death; blood settling in the skin of a dependent body part, usually the back.

depolarization (de-pol′lə-riz-a′shən) any of two electrical processes involving the heart, during which the electrical charges on the surface of the muscle cell change from positive to negative.

depressants (de-pres′antz) drugs that decrease awareness and the mental capacity to function, slow reflexes, and may decrease the respiratory and heart rates.

depression (de-presh′ən) a psychiatric disorder in which the patient may not want to do anything, even move. The depressed patient may not cooperate or even answer questions.

dermis (der′mis) the inner layer of the skin, containing hair follicles, sweat glands, nerve endings, and blood vessels.

descending colon part of the colon that lies on the left side of the abdomen, extending from a point below the stomach to the level of the iliac crest.

descent injury compression problems caused by outside pressure on the diver's body.

diabetes mellitus (di′ə-bē′tēz mel′ə-tus) a disease in which the body is unable to utilize sugar normally because of a deficiency or total lack of insulin; often called "sugar diabetes."

diabetic (di′ə-bet′ik) one who has diabetes; pertaining to diabetes.

diabetic coma a state of unconsciousness caused by loss of fluid and increased acidity in diabetes.

diabetic ketoacidosis (ke′to-ə-sǐ-do′sis) a condition caused by excessive fluid and sugar loss in the kidneys and an excessive buildup in the bloodstream of acid metabolic products (ketones) caused by the body's use of substances other than sugar for energy.

diagnosis (di′ag-nō′sis) identifying a disease or injury from its signs and symptoms.

diaphoresis (di′ə-fə-rē′sis) sweating.

diaphragm (di′ə-fram) a muscular dome that forms the undersurface of the thorax, separating the chest from the abdominal cavity. Contraction of the diaphragm (and the chest wall muscles) brings air into the lungs. Relaxation allows air to be expelled from the lungs.

diarrhea (di′ə-re-ə) a large number of bowel movements of abnormally liquid character.

diastole (di-as′to-le) relaxation of the heart while the ventricles fill with blood.

diastolic (di′ə-stol′ik) **blood pressure** the lower blood pressure noted during ventricular relaxation as the heart fills with blood.

Dieffenbachia (de′fən-bahk-e-ə) dumbcane; a tropical American herb that when chewed causes the tongue to swell; the swelling may cause obstruction of the airway.

digestion (di-jest′yun) the process of breaking food down to its basic chemical components, which can be absorbed by the intestine.

digestive (di-jes′tiv) **system** the gastrointestinal tract (stomach and intestines), mouth, salivary glands, pharynx, esophagus, liver, gallbladder, pancreas, rectum, and anus.

dilate (dī-layt) swell, become wide.

dilation of the cervix a phase of labor just before delivery in which the cervix of the uterus opens so that the baby's head can pass through into the vagina.

diphtheria (dif-the′re-ə) acute bacterial infection of the throat, tonsils, nose, and sometimes skin, with local pain and swelling.

disentanglement freeing; extricating.

dislocation (dis′lo-kay′shən) disruption of a joint so that the bone ends are no longer in contact.

dispatcher one who transmits calls to service units, sending vehicles and EMTs on emergency assignments.

displaced fracture a fracture that produces deformity of the limb.

disruptive behavior behavior that presents a danger to the patient or others or causes a delay in treatment.

distal (dis′tal) describing structures that are nearer to the free end of an extremity; any location on the trunk that is farther from the midline or from the point of reference named.

distention (dis-ten′shən) bulging or swelling.

diverticulitis (di′ver-tik-yu-lī′tis) inflammation of small pockets in the colon.

diving reflex a sudden reflex involving the vagus nerves that can cause bradycardia or cardiac arrest in people who dive or jump into very cold water.

dizygotic (di′zi-got′ik) **twins**   fraternal twins; they may be of the same sex or of different sexes.

dorsal (dor′sal)   posterior, referring to the back or top.

dorsalis pedis (dor-sa′lis pe′dis) **artery**   artery on the anterior surface of the foot between the first and second metatarsals.

dorsal (thoracic) **spine**   the 12 vertebrae that attach to the 12 ribs; the upper part of the back.

dorsiflex (dor′sĭ-flex)   to move a joint in the posterior direction.

"downer"   a depressant.

dressing   a bandage.

drowning   death by suffocation after being submerged in water.

drug   any substance that is given with the intention of preventing or curing disease or otherwise enhancing the physical or mental welfare of humans or animals. Any drug can produce undesirable side effects or adverse reactions or be used to excess.

drug withdrawal   a physical reaction characterized by anxiety, nausea, vomiting, convulsions, delirium, sweating, or cramps, that occurs when an addict is unable to get drugs.

duodenum (du′o-de′num)   first or most proximal portion of the small intestine, passing from the stomach to the jejunum.

duplex   the ability to transmit and receive traffic simultaneously on a particular channel.

dura mater (du′rə ma′ter)   outermost of the three layers of tissue that envelop the brain and spinal cord.

duty to respond   the responsibility of an ambulance service attached to a government agency to respond to calls within its jurisdiction. A commercial or volunteer service is not so obligated unless such care is advertised or is a requirement of its licensure.

dysfunction (dis-funk′shən)   impaired or abnormal functioning.

dysphagia (dis-fa′jē-ə)   sensation of sticking or discomfort when swallowing.

dyspnea (disp′nē-ə)   difficulty or pain with breathing.

dysuria (dis-u′rē-ə)   sensation of pain, burning, or itching that occurs during urination.

eardrum   a thin, tense membrane forming the greater part of the outer wall of the middle ear and separating it from the outer ear canal.

ecchymosis (ek′ĭ-mo′sis)   a bruise; a discoloration of the skin due to bleeding under and into the skin. Bluish at first, it changes later to a greenish yellow because of chemical changes in the pooled blood.

eclampsia (e-klamp′sē-ə)   convulsions that result from severe hypertension during pregnancy.

ectopic (ek-top′ik) **pregnancy**   development of a fetus in an abnormal location, usually in the Fallopian tube.

edema (ĕ-de′mə)   a condition in which fluid escapes into the tissues from vascular or lymphatic spaces and causes local or generalized swelling.

edema fluid   watery fluid that leaks into the tissues.

ejaculation (e-jak′yu-lay′shən)   act of expelling semen from the penis.

elbow joint   the joint between the humerus and the radius and ulna.

electrical burns   burns caused by exposure to electric current.

electric charge   a definite quantity of electricity.

electric shock   the effects produced by the passage of an electric current through any part of the body.

electrocardiogram (e-lek′tro-kar′de-ə-gram) **(ECG or EKG)**   a recording of the electrical current that flows through the heart. The results are displayed on a paper strip or a cathode ray monitor screen or (usually) both.

electrolytes (e-lek′tro-lītz)   ionic components of salts contained in body fluids and cells.

electrolyte solutions   fluids used for intravenous infusion that contain electrolytes.

electromechanical dissociation (ē-lek′tro-mə-kan′ĭ-kl di-sō-sē-ā′shən)   that form of cardiac arrest in which the electrocardiogram displays an adequate heart rate and rhythm, but the heart is incapable of generating a palpable pulse and blood pressure in the circulation.

electrons (e-lek′tronz)   particles of an atom that have a negative charge.

embolism (em′bo-lizm)   an embolus that causes an obstruction.

embolus (em′bo-lus)   a blood clot or other substance that passes from point to another point in the body through the vascular system.

emergency cardiac care (ECC)   subject addressed at national conferences at which techniques for providing ECC are reviewed and revised as necessary.

emergency delivery pack   a kit kept on the emergency vehicle that contains supplies needed for an emergency delivery of a baby.

emergency medical identification card or **tag**   card carried or tag worn as a bracelet or necklace to warn of any serious medical problem the patient may have.

emergency medical services (EMS) system the combined efforts of several professionals and agencies to provide prehospital emergency care to the sick and injured.

emergency medical technician (EMT) a member of a prehospital emergency medical system who is trained to provide basic life support.

emesis (em′ə-sis) vomiting.

emetic (i-met′ik) medication to induce vomiting.

emphysema (em′fĭ-sē′mə) disease of the lung in which there is extreme dilation of pulmonary air sacs and poor exchange of oxygen and carbon dioxide. It causes rapid, shallow breathing and frequently results in secondary impairment of heart action.

EMS system *See* emergency medical services (EMS) system.

EMT-defibrillation (EMT-D) program one in which fully trained EMTs undergo further training and are then certified to perform defibrillation on people in cardiac arrest.

EMT-intermediate (EMT-I) an EMT who has training in specific aspects of advanced life support such as intravenous therapy, cardiac defibrillation, or advanced airway management.

EMT-paramedic (EMT-P) an EMT who has received extensive training in advanced life support, including intravenous therapy, pharmacology, cardiac monitoring, and defibrillation; advanced airway maintenance, including intubation; and other advanced assessment and treatment skills.

endocarditis (en′də-kar′dīt′is) infection of the valves or the lining of the heart.

endocrine (en′də-krin) **glands** glands that produce hormones that regulate specific bodily functions.

endometrium (en-do-mē′tre-um) the lining of the uterus.

endotracheal intubation (en-do-trāk′kē-əl in′tōō-bay′shən) a method of intubation in which an endotracheal tube is placed through a patient's mouth or nose and directly through the larynx between the vocal cords into the trachea for the purpose of opening and maintaining an airway.

endotracheal tube (ETT) the tube that is placed in the airway during endotracheal intubation.

enhanced 911 system (E911) the most technologically advanced version of the 911 universal emergency telephone service; features include automatic number identification (ANI), automatic call location identification (ALI), and automatic ringback.

envenomation (en-ven′o-ma′shən) the deposit of venom into a victim by a poisonous bite.

enzyme (en′zīm) a protein capable of producing or accelerating some change in a given substance.

epidermis (ep′ĭ-der′mis) the outer layer of skin which is made up of cells that are sealed together to form a watertight protective covering for the body.

epidural (ep′ĭ-du′ral) outside the dura and under the skull.

epidural hematoma (hem′ə-to′mə) a hematoma, or collection of blood, outside the dura mater and under the skull.

epigastric (ep′ĭ-gas′trik) relating to the epigastrium.

epigastrium (ep′ĭ-gas′tre-um) upper-middle region of the abdomen.

epiglottis (ep′ĭ-glot′is) a thin, leaf-shaped valve that allows air to pass into the trachea but prevents food or liquid from entering.

epilepsy (ep′ĭ′lep′se) a condition manifested by seizures, which are caused by an abnormal focus of activity within the brain that produces severe motor responses or changes in consciousness.

epinephrine (ep′ĭ-nef′rin) a hormone used to stimulate the heart and the sympathetic nervous system.

epiphyseal (ep′ĭ-fiz′e-al) **fracture** injury to the growth plate of a long bone in children, which may lead to an arrest of bone growth if it is not properly treated.

epiphyseal plate a transverse cartilage plate near the end of a child's bone, responsible for growth in length of the bone.

epistaxis (ep′ĭ-stak′sis) nosebleed.

erectile (i-rek′tl) **tissue** tissue containing large vascular spaces that fill with blood on stimulation (a process called erection) as in the penis and clitoris.

erythematous (er′ə-them′ə-təs) reddened.

erythrocytes (e-rith′ro-sītz) red blood cells.

esophageal (e-sof′ə-je′al) **gastric tube airway (EGTA)** an esophageal obturator airway with an added gastic decompression tube; it allows gas in the stomach to be vented to the outside, thereby decreasing gastric distention.

esophageal obturator (äb′too-rāt′or) **airway (EOA)** a plastic, semirigid tube that can be inserted in the esophagus; the upper third, which has holes in it, lies at the level of the pharynx and provides free passage of oxygen-enriched air to the lungs.

esophageal reflux (re′fluks) **(heartburn)** a burning pain under the sternum caused by gastric juices that reflux into the lower esophagus and attack its lining.

esophageal varices (var′i-sēz) dilated veins in the wall of the esophagus that develop in patients with liver disease. If these enlarged veins rupture, subsequent bleeding can be fatal.

esophagus (e-sof′ə-gus) a collapsible tube about 10 inches long that extends from the pharynx to the stomach; contractions of the muscle in the wall of the esophagus propel food and liquids through it to the stomach.

ethics (eth′iks) the study of what is good and bad, and of moral duty.

euphoria (yu-fo′rē-ə) a sense of well-being.

evaporation (e-vap′i-ray′shən) the conversion of any liquid to a gas; body heat is lost during evaporation of sweat.

evisceration (e-vis′er-a′shən) the protruding of internal organs through a wound.

excessive artifact (ik-ses′iv är′tə-fakt) problems that prevent the EMT-D from analyzing the rhythm on the monitor screen of a defibrillator.

excretion (eks-krē′shən) eliminating material from the body.

exempt narcotic a drug that can be sold over the counter without a prescription.

expiration (eks′pĭ-ra′shən) exhaling, breathing out, or expelling air from the lungs.

exsanguinate (eks-san′gwin-āt) bleed to death.

extend to straighten (of a joint).

extension the straightening of a limb at a joint.

external bleeding hemorrhage that can be seen coming from a wound.

external chest compression a technique to produce artificial circulation by applying rhythmic pressure and relaxation to the lower half of the sternum, which has the effect of compressing the heart between the sternum and the spine.

external genitalia (jen′ĭ-ta′le-ə) the parts of the genitalia that are outside of the pelvis.

external maxillary artery artery anterior to the angle of the mandible on the inner surface of the lower jaw that contributes much of the blood supply to the face.

extrasystoles (eks′trə-sis′to-les) irregular extra heartbeats.

extremities (eks-trem′ĭ-tez) the arms and legs.

extrication (eks′trĭ-kay′shən) removal from a difficult situation or position; often used to mean removal of a patient from a wrecked car or other place of entrapment.

eye the organ of vision.

face the front part of the head, including eyes, nose, cheeks, mouth, and forehead.

face mask a mask fitted to the face through which gas is delivered to the patient.

Fahrenheit (F) designation of temperature on a thermometer on which 32° is the freezing point and 212° is the boiling point of water.

failure to thrive a condition in which a child does not gain weight or grow properly; a sign of child abuse.

faint psychogenic shock; a temporary loss of consciousness, usually of brief duration and not serious.

Fallopian (fal-lō′pe-an) **tubes** long, slender tubes that extend from the uterus to the region of the ovary on the same side, and through which the ovum passes from ovary to uterus.

false motion motion at a point in a limb where it usually does not occur; a positive indication of bone fracture.

fascia (fash′e-ə) a sheet or band of tough fibrous connective tissue. It lies deep under the skin and forms an outer layer for the muscles.

fat adipose tissue; white or yellowish tissue that forms soft pads in the body and furnishes a reserve supply of energy.

fatty acids acids derived from fats; they contribute to a dangerous level of acidosis in uncontrolled diabetics.

febrile (feb′ril) having fever.

febrile convulsions seizures, usually of short duration and not dangerous, that sometimes accompany high fevers in children.

fecal (fe′kal) pertaining to feces.

fecal impaction (im-pak′shən) a collection of hardened feces in the bowel that produces an obstruction.

femoral (fem′or-al) **artery** the principal artery of the thigh, a continuation of the external iliac artery. It supplies blood to the lower abdominal wall, external genitalia, and legs. It can be palpated in the groin area.

femoral artery pulse pulse that can be felt in the groin where the femoral artery is close to the skin.

femoral condyles (kon′dĭlz) two surfaces at the distal end of the femur that articulate with the superior surfaces of the tibia.

femoral head the proximal end of the femur, articulating with the acetabulum.

femoral neck the heavy column of bone connecting the head and the shaft of the femur.

femoral nerve a major peripheral nerve, lying immediately lateral to the femoral artery in the groin.

femoral shaft the main part of the femur.

femoral vein a continuation of the popliteal vein that becomes the external iliac vein; the major vein draining the thigh.

femur (fe′mur)   the thigh bone; it extends from the pelvis to the knee and is the longest and largest bone in the body.

fender judgment   knowing how much physical operating space a particular vehicle requires when traveling at a given speed.

fetal (fē′tal)   pertaining to the fetus.

fetus (fē′tus)   a developing baby in the uterus or womb.

fibrillation (fi-bri-la′shən)   continuous, uncoordinated quivering of the muscle fibers of the heart; causes uncontrolled and ineffective beating of the heart.

fibula (fib′u-lə)   the outer and smaller of the two bones of the leg, extending from just below the knee to form the lateral portion of the ankle joint.

finger probe   a technique whereby the EMT probes a patient's mouth using the index finger as a hook in an attempt to dislodge a foreign body.

first aid   emergency care and treatment of an injured person before medical help can be secured.

first-degree burns   burns in which only the superficial part of the epidermis has been injured; an example is a sunburn.

first responder   the first person present at the scene of sudden illness or injury.

first stage of labor   the time from the beginning of contractions until the cervix is fully dilated.

flaccid (flas′id)   soft and limp.

flail chest (crushed chest; stove-in chest)   a condition that occurs when three or more ribs are broken each in two places, and the chest wall lying between the fractures becomes a free-floating segment.

flail segment   that segment of the chest wall in a flail chest injury that lies between the rib fractures and moves paradoxically as the patient breathes.

flexion (flek′shən)   bending.

floating ribs   the eleventh and twelfth ribs, which do not connect to the sternum.

flotation device   a device that keeps one from sinking in water, such as a life jacket or vest.

flowmeter   a flow regulator attached to the pressure regulator on emergency medical equipment. It permits the regulated release of gas in liters per minute.

fontanelle (fon′tə-nel′)   area in a baby's head where the skull bones have not yet completely grown together.

foot   the distal portion of the lower extremity, on which one stands and walks.

foot drop   paralysis of the dorsiflexor muscles of the foot and ankle, so that the foot falls and the toes drag on the ground in walking.

foramen magnum (fo-ra′mən mag′nəm)   a large opening in the base of the skull through which the brain connects to the spinal cord.

forearm   the lower portion of the upper extremity, from the elbow to the wrist.

forehead   the part of the face above the eyes.

foreskin   the fold of skin covering the glans penis.

four-person log roll   a method of placing a person on a carrying device, usually on a long spine board or a flat litter, by rolling the patient on one side and then back onto the litter.

fracture   any break in the continuity of a bone.

fracture-dislocation   a two-fold injury in which the joint is dislocated and a part of the bone near the joint also fractures.

frequency (fre′kwən-se)   an abnormally high number of voiding episodes during a 24-hour period; the number of repetitive cycles per second completed by a radio wave.

frontal region   the forehead.

frostbite   a form of cold exposure that occurs after prolonged exposure to the cold and partial or complete freezing of the skin and deeper tissue has taken place.

frostnip   a form of cold exposure that occurs after prolonged exposure to the cold, but freezing of the skin and deeper tissues has not occurred; also called chilblains.

gallbladder (gol′blad′ər)   a pear-shaped sac on the undersurface of the liver that collects bile from the liver and discharges it into the duodenum through the common bile duct.

gallstone   a small hard concretion in the gallbladder or a bile duct, composed chiefly of cholesterol crystals.

gamma radiation   a form of ionizing radiation that can penetrate through the human body, similar to x-rays. Heavy shielding such as lead or concrete is necessary to protect against these rays.

gangrene (gan′grēn)   death of body tissues, usually the result of a loss of blood supply.

gastric (gas-trik) **distention**   inflation of the stomach caused when excessive pressures are used during artificial ventilation or when several breaths are administered quickly in succession.

gastric juice   the digestive fluid secreted by the glands of the stomach; it contains mainly hydrochloric acid, pepsin, and mucus.

gastric lavage (la-vahzh′)   flushing the stomach with fluids to remove ingested toxic substances.

gastritis (gas-trī′tis)   inflammation or irritation of the stomach lining.

gastroenteritis (gas′tro-en-ter-ī′tis) a viral or bacterial infection of the lining of the stomach and/or the intestines.

gastrointestinal system the organs of the stomach and intestines that are involved in the digestion of food and excretion of the solid waste products of digestion.

Geiger (gī′ger) **counter** an instrument used to measure the level of radioactivity in the environment; these instruments are usually designed to detect gamma radiation.

generalized seizure an epileptic seizure involving most of the brain; also called a convulsive or tonic-clonic seizure.

genitalia (jen′i-ta′le-ə) the male and female reproductive systems and the male urethra.

genital (jen′i-tal) **system** the male and female reproductive systems.

genitourinary (jen′ĭ-to-yu′rĭ-nar-ē) **system** the organs of reproduction, together with the organs concerned in the production and excretion of urine.

geriatric (jer′ē-at′rik) a term used to describe the older patient.

geriatric patients elderly patients.

German measles viral illness with fever and rash; can cause birth defects in the fetus if contracted by the mother during the first three months of pregnancy.

germinal layer layer of skin cells that constantly reproduce to replace outer cells that are being shed or rubbed off.

gestation (jes-ta′shən) **period** the usual period for the development of a baby; pregnancy.

glenohumeral (gle′no-hu′mer-al) **joint** the true shoulder joint.

glenoid (gle′noid) **fossa** the recess in the scapula for the articulation of the humeral head laterally forming the glenohumeral joint.

globe the shape of the eye, which is maintained by fluid contained within it.

glucose (gloo′kōs) a sugar.

gonorrhea (gon′o-rē′ə) common venereal disease, a contagious infection of the genital mucous membrane.

Good Samaritan laws laws that prevent an individual who voluntarily helps an injured or suddenly ill person from being legally liable for any errors of omissions in rendering good faith emergency care.

gout (gowt) a hereditary form of arthritis, with excessive uric acid in the blood and recurrent painful attacks of arthritis in one joint.

governmental immunity the doctrine that government agencies are held to be immune from the legal consequences of their actions. Today, more than half the states have abandoned the doctrine of governmental immunity.

great vessels the large vessels entering or leaving the heart, including the aorta, the pulmonary arteries and veins, and the venae cavae.

greater trochanter (tro-kan′ter) a bony prominence on the lateral side of the thigh just below the hip joint to which several muscles are attached.

greenstick fracture an incomplete fracture that passes only partway through the shaft of a bone; occurs only in children.

guarding refusal to use an injured part because motion causes pain; involuntary abdominal muscular contraction reflecting inflammation and pain within the peritoneal cavity.

gunshot wound a form of puncture wound; the amount of damage is directly proportional to the square of the velocity of the bullet.

hair follicles (fol′lĭ-kls) the small organs that produce hair; there is one for each hair, connected with a sebacous gland and a tiny muscle.

hamstring muscles two groups of muscles at the back of the knee.

hard hat a protective helmet worn during any rescue activity, both for the identification of rescue personnel and personal safety.

hard palate (pal′at) a bony plate forming the anterior part of the roof of the mouth.

hay fever a common allergy problem caused by pollen in the air; symptoms include stuffy, runny nose and sneezing.

hazardous material identification number a four-digit identification number displayed on a placard of orange panel on the ends of a tank, vehicle, or rail car transporting hazardous materials, as well as on the shipping paper or packaging of the material.

Hazmat Rule of Thumb a way of determining the size of a danger zone. The EMT holds his arm out straight, with thumb pointing up. The EMT centers his thumb over the hazardous area. The thumb should cover all of the area from view. If not, the EMT is still too close.

head tilt/chin-lift maneuver opening the airway by tilting the patient's head backward and lifting the chin forward, bringing the entire lower jaw with it.

head-tilt maneuver opening the airway by tilting the patient's head backward as far as possible.

heart   a hollow muscular organ that receives blood from the veins and propels it into the arteries.

heart attack   *See* acute myocardial infarction.

heartburn (esophageal reflux)   a burning pain under the sternum caused by gastric juices that reflux into the lower esophagus and attack its lining.

heat collapse (kə-laps′)   a mild form of shock that occurs when the body loses much water and electrolytes through very heavy sweating after exposure to heat; also called heat prostration or heat exhaustion.

heat cramps   painful muscle spasms, usually of the leg muscles, that occur after vigorous exercise.

heat exhaustion   *See* heat collapse.

heat exposure   a dose of excessive energy received by the human organism, either locally or over its entire surface, for which its normal protective mechanisms are insufficient.

heat prostration   *See* heat collapse.

heat stroke   a condition of rapidly rising internal body temperature that occurs when the body's mechanisms for release of heat are overwhelmed. Untreated heat stroke will result in death.

heavy rescue   rescue operations that involve the use of complicated rigging, patient handling under extremely difficult or adverse conditions, breaching of walls, disimpaction of vehicles, and all types of rescue involving buildings with major structural damage.

Heimlich (hīm′lik) **(subdiaphragmatic thrust) maneuver**   a series of 6 to 10 manual thrusts to the upper abdomen, just above the umbilicus and well below the xiphoid, to relieve upper airway obstruction; the abdominal thrust maneuver.

hematemesis (hem′ə-tem′ĕ-sis)   the vomiting of bright red blood.

hematochezia (hem′ə-to-ke′ze-ə)   the passage of bright red blood from the rectum.

hematoma (hem′ə-to′mə)   a lump developing at a wound site from a pool of blood collecting within the damaged tissue; occurs about the broken ends of the bones in all fractures.

hematuria (hem′ə-tu′re-ə)   blood in the urine.

hemiplegia (hem′e-ple′je-ə)   paralysis of one side of the body.

hemithorax (hem′e-tho′raks)   one side (one-half) of the chest.

hemoptysis (he-mop′tĭ-sis)   the coughing up of bright red blood.

hemorrhage (hem′or-ij)   bleeding; blood escaping from arteries or veins.

hemorrhagic (hem′o-raj′ik) **shock**   shock resulting from blood loss.

hemorrhoids (hem′o-roids)   varicose dilation of veins near the rectum.

hemothorax (he′mo-tho′raks)   the presence of blood in the chest cavity within the pleural space, outside the lung.

hepatitis (hep′ə-ti′tis)   an infection of the liver that causes fever, loss of appetite, jaundice, and fatigue. It is caused by chemicals, alcohol, or drugs, or by a virus.

hepatitis A   Type A (viral or infectious) hepatitis that is usually seen in children. It is a liver infection without serious consequences. Adults can be infected by their children or by ingestion of contaminated shellfish or water.

hepatitis B (serum hepatitis)   hepatitis caused by a virus that is spread through blood-to-blood contact (transfusion, needle stick), mucous membrane (saliva or sputum contact), or sexual contact. It is a serious disease with long-term side effects. Signs and symptoms are nausea, vomiting, fatigue, abdominal pain, and jaundice.

hernia   protrusion of a loop of an organ or tissue through an abnormal opening.

heroin (her′o-in)   an opiate narcotic, often abused.

herpes (her′pēz) **virus**   a spreading, recurrent skin eruption caused by infection from the herpes virus.

herpetic whitlow (hər-pet′ik hwit′lō)   a herpes virus infection of the finger.

hiccough (hik′əp)   a sudden inspiration of air that is rapidly checked by closure of the epiglottis of the larynx.

hinge joints   joints that can bend and straighten but cannot rotate.

hip   the joint where the femur articulates with the innominate bone.

hip fractures   fractures of the upper end of the femur.

hives (urticaria) (ur′ti-ka′rē-ə)   an allergic skin disorder marked by patches of swelling and intense itching; caused by contact with something to which the person is allergic.

hollow organs   tubes through which materials pass, such as the stomach, intestines, ureters, and bladder.

hormones (hor′monz)   chemical substances produced in the body by a gland, which have special regulatory effects on the activity of another distant organ.

host   the organism or individual attacked by the infecting agent.

hot line   a dedicated telephone line between two specific points. It is always "open" or under the control of an individual at each end. The line is immediately available by lifting the receiver. Outside access cannot be obtained.

humeral condyles (hyu'mer-al kon'dīlz) bony prominences that form the medial and lateral borders of the upper surface of the elbow joint.

humerus (hyu'mer-əs) the supporting bone of the upper arm that articulates with the scapula to form the shoulder joint and with the ulna and radius to form the elbow joint.

humidification (hyu-mid'i-fi-kay'shən) process of adding moisture during artificial ventilation to prevent pure oxygen from drying patient's mucous membrane surfaces.

hydrochloric (hī-dro-klo'rik) **acid** a normal component of gastric juice.

hydroplaning (hī'dro-play'ning) action of a vehicle skimming over a wet road with tires not directly contacting the surface because they are riding on a film of water.

hyperextension (hī'per-ek-sten'shən) extreme extension or straightening of a limb or body part.

hyperflexion (hī'per-flek'shən) extreme bending.

hyperglycemia (hī'per-glī-se'me-ə) too much sugar in the blood; a factor in diabetic coma.

hypersensitive (hī'per-sen'sĭ-tiv) allergic.

hypersensitive reaction severe allergic reaction with wheezing, cardiovascular collapse, and skin wheals (hives).

hypertension (hī'per-ten'shən) abnormally and persistently high blood pressure.

hyperventilation (hī'per-ven'tĭ-lay'shən) overbreathing to the extent that the level of carbon dioxide in the blood falls way below normal. Symptoms are numbness, tingling of the hands or feet, and, despite rapid breathing, a sense of shortness of breath.

hyphema (hī-fe'mə) bleeding into the anterior chamber of the eye, obscuring the iris.

hypoglycemia (hī'po-glī-se'me-ə) insufficient sugar in the blood; a factor in insulin shock.

hypotension (hī'po-ten'shən) abnormally low blood pressure.

hypothermia (hī'po-ther'me-ə) a condition in which the internal body temperature falls below 95°F after prolonged exposure to freezing or near-freezing temperatures.

hypovolemia (hī'po-vo-le'me-ə) a decrease in the volume of circulating blood or other body fluids.

hypovolemic (low volume) shock shock resulting from loss of body fluid or blood.

hypoxia (hī-pok'se-ə) a deficiency of oxygen reaching the tissues of the body.

hypoxic (hi-pok'sik) oxygen-deficient.

hysteria (his-tēr'e-ə) a neurotic disturbance marked by excitement and self-consciousness, anxiety, symptoms of imaginary illness, and lack of emotional control.

ileocecal (il'e-o-se'kal) **valve** passage through which the contents of the small intestine empty into the large intestine. This valve allows passage of bowel contents in only one direction—into the colon.

ileum (il'e-um) the more distal portion of the small intestine between the jejunum and the colon.

ileus (il'e-us) paralysis of the muscular contractions that propel matter through the intestines.

iliac (il'e-ak) **arteries** two branches of the aorta that carry blood to the lower extremities.

iliac crest the rim of the pelvic bone.

ilium (il'e-um) one of three bones (ilium, ischium, and pubis) that fuse to form the pelvic bones.

immersion (i-mur'shən) **foot** a form of cold exposure that occurs when the feet suffer prolonged exposure to cold but not freezing water; also called trench foot.

immunity (imŏyu'ni-tē) exemptions granted by law to certain individuals or agencies freeing them from the burdens of compensating the injured or damaged individual.

immunization (im'yu-ni-zay'shən) the process by which resistance to an infectious disease is produced.

impaled (im-pay'əld) **foreign object** an object such as a knife or splinter of wood or glass that penetrates the skin and remains in the body.

implied (im-plīd') **consent** consent that is implied by the fact that the individual voluntarily entered a situation.

incomplete abortion (ə-bor'shən) complication of abortion in which portions of the fetus or placenta are left in the uterus.

incontinence (in-kon'ti-nens) the uncontrolled passage of urine or feces.

incubation (in'kyu-bay'shən) **period** the time between exposure of the host to the infectious agent and the appearance of symptoms of that infection.

indirect contact transmission of a communicable disease in which the person infected is not in direct contact with a host or carrier but touches some object that has been contaminated.

infarction (in-fark'shən) death of tissue because its blood supply is lost.

infection (in-fek'shən) the invasion of a host or host tissue by organisms such as bacteria, viruses, or parasites.

infectious (in-fek′shus) **agent**   the cause of an infectious disease, such as a virus, bacterium, or parasite.

infectious (communicable) diseases   diseases that can be transmitted from one person to another.

infectious hepatitis   *See* hepatitis.

inferior portion   that portion of the body or body part that lies nearer the feet than the head.

inferior vena cava (ve′nə ka′və)   one of the two largest veins in the body that carries blood from the lower extremities and the pelvic and abdominal organs into the heart.

infiltration (in-fil-tray′shən)   a condition in which the fluid from intravenous therapy enters the surrounding subcutaneous tissue instead of the vein.

informed consent   consent given by a person who understands the nature and extent of any procedure before agreeing to it and who has sufficient mental and physical capacity to make such a judgment.

infusion (in-fyu′zhən)   the introduction of fluid other than blood or blood products into the vascular system.

inguinal hernia (ing′gwĭ-nal her′nĭ-ah)   a common congenital defect in which a loop of intestine descends into the inguinal canal in the groin.

inguinal ligament   tough fibrous ligament that stretches between the lateral edge of the pubic symphysis and the anterior superior iliac spine.

inhalation (in′hə-lay′shən) **injuries**   injuries resulting from inhaling chemical fumes.

injection (in-jek′shən)   forcing a fluid into, as for medical purposes.

inoculation (ĭ-nok′yu-lay′shən)   introduction of a disease agent such as a vaccine virus into a healthy person to produce a mild form of the disease followed by immunity.

insertion (in-ser′shən)   place of attachment of a muscle.

inspiration (in′spĭ-ray′shən)   inhaling; breathing in, or drawing air into the lungs.

institutional standards   specific rules and procedures of the ambulance service or organization to which the EMT is attached.

insulator (in′su-lay′tor)   material that does not conduct heat; any substance that prevents an electrical circuit from being completed (rubber, for example).

insulin (in′su-lin)   a hormone produced by the pancreas that enables sugar in the blood to enter the cells of the body; insulin from animals and synthetic insulin are used in the treatment and control of diabetes mellitus.

insulin-dependent diabetics   diabetics who have to take one or more injections of insulin every day.

insulin shock   occurs in the diabetic who has taken too much insulin, has taken a regular dose of insulin but has not eaten enough food, or who has exercised excessively and used up all available glucose. Symptoms are sweating, tremor, anxiety, vertigo, and double vision, followed by delirium, convulsion, and collapse.

Interagency Radiological Assistance Plan (IRAP)   a national plan developed to provide professional guidance and assistance in the event of an accident involving radioactive materials.

intercostal (in′ter-kos′tal)   between the ribs.

intercourse (in′tər-kors)   a sexual joining of two individuals during which seminal fluid, prostatic fluid, and sperm pass from the penis into the vagina during ejaculation.

interference (in′tər-fir′əns)   any undesired radio signal on a radio frequency. It may come from another radio transmitter or other sources of electromagnetic radiation.

internal jugular (jug′yu-lar) **vein**   major vein draining the brain.

intervertebral (in′ter-ver′te-bral) **disc**   a cushion between each two vertebral bodies.

intestine (in-tes′tin)   the part of the alimentary canal extending from the stomach to the anus.

intoxicated (in-toks′i-kay′ted)   affected by alcohol or another drug to the point of losing physical and mental control.

intra-abdominal (in′trə-ab-dom′i-nal)   within the abdomen.

intracerebral hematoma   a hematoma, or collection of blood, inside the brain tissue itself.

intracranial (in′trə-kray′ne-al)   within the skull.

intracranial pressure   pressure from the brain swelling inside the rigid bony skull.

intramuscularly   within a muscle.

intraperitoneal (in′trə-per′ĭ-to-ne′al)   within the peritoneal cavity.

intrathoracic (in′trə-tho-ras′ik)   within the chest.

intravascular (in′trə-vas′kyu-lar)   within a vessel.

intravenous (in′trə-ve′nus)   within a vein.

intravenous fluid therapy (IV therapy)   infusion of fluid other than blood or blood products into the vascular system to establish and maintain access to the circulation or to provide fluids in order to maintain an adequate circulatory blood volume.

intravenous line   a polyethylene catheter through which fluids are given directly into a vein.

intubation (in-too-bay′shən)   the placement of a tube in the airway to improve ventilation.

involuntary muscle   muscle that continues to contract rhythmically, regardless of the conscious will of the individual.

involuntary (autonomic) nervous system   that part of the nervous system that regulates functions not controlled by a voluntary act of conscious will, such as digestion or sweating.

ionizing (i′ə-nīz′ing) **radiation**   nuclear radiation that has the ability to alter body cells; there are three forms: alpha, beta, and gamma.

ipecac   *See* syrup of ipecac.

iris (ī′ris)   the muscle behind the cornea that dilates and constricts the pupil, regulating the amount of light that enters the eye.

irrigation (ir′ĭ-gay′shən)   washing by a stream of water or other fluid.

ischemic (is-ke′mic)   lacking oxygen.

ischial (is′ke-al) **tuberosities** (tu′be-ros′i-tez)   the bony prominences felt in the middle of each buttock.

ischium (is′ke-um)   one of three bones (ilium, ischium, and pubis) that fuse to form the pelvic bones. The two pelvic bones, together with the sacrum, form the pelvic ring.

islets of Langerhans (lahng′er-hanz)   glands scattered throughout the pancreas, which produce insulin.

jaundice (jawn′dis)   yellow color of the tissues seen in liver disease.

jaw-thrust maneuver   opening the airway by bringing the patient's jaw forward and pulling the lower lip down.

jejunum (je-joo′num)   that portion of the small intestine that extends from the duodenum to the ileum.

joint (articulation)   the juncture where two bones come in contact.

joint capsule (kap′sl)   a fibrous sac with synovial lining that encloses a joint.

joules (joolz)   a measure of the electrical current delivered by defibrillators.

jugular notch   the superior border of the sternum.

jump kit   a lightweight, durable, waterproof kit used in the immediate care of the patient, usually by the EMT who initially leaves the vehicle while the EMT-driver parks the ambulance and secures the scene.

juvenile (joo′və-nil) **diabetics**   children who have to take insulin every day.

ketoacidosis   *See* diabetic ketoacidosis.

ketones (ke′tonz)   metabolic end products of the use of fat for routine energy needs.

kidneys   the two retroperitoneal organs that excrete the end products of metabolism as urine and regulate the body's salt and water content.

kidney stones   stones that pass from the kidney and into the ureter where they cause excruciating pain until they enter the bladder.

kinetic (ki-net′ik) **energy**   energy in action that produces motion; a mechanism of injury.

knee joint   the articulation between the distal femur and the proximal tibia.

Kussmaul respirations   air hunger, manifested by deep sighing respirations.

labor   the process by which the muscles of the uterus open the birth canal and push the baby down and through so that it can be born.

laceration (las′er-ay′shən)   a cut that may leave a smooth or jagged wound through the skin, subcutaneous tissues, muscles, and associated nerves and blood vessels.

lacrimal (lak′rĭ-mal) **system**   the tear glands and ducts of the eye.

land mobile service   specified by the Federal Communications Commission (FCC); mobile communication service between a base station and mobile stations on land, or between two mobile stations on land.

large intestine (in-tes′tin)   the portion of the digestive tube that extends from the ileocecal valve to the anus. It is made up of the cecum, colon, and rectum.

laryngectomy (lar′in-jek′tə-mē)   surgical removal of the larynx.

laryngoscope (lə-rin′ge-skōp′)   an instrument used to give the EMT-I a direct view of the patient's vocal cords during endotracheal intubation.

laryngospasm (lə-rin′go-spazm)   a severe constriction of the vocal cords.

larynx (lar′inks)   voice box; a structure composed of thyroid cartilage on the top and cricoid cartilage on the bottom. It guards the entrance to the trachea and functions secondarily as the organ of voice.

laser (la′zer)   a device that produces a beam of nonspreading, monochromatic, visible light. High energies are concentrated into a narrow beam.

lateral (lat′er-al)   lying away from the midline.

lateral malleolus (mal-le′o-lus)   the bony prominence at the end of the fibula that, together with the medial malleolus, forms the socket of the ankle joint.

lateral structures   parts of the body that lie at some distance from the midline.

leg the lower extremity; specifically, the lower portion, from the knee to the ankle.

lens the transparent part of the eye, through which images are focused on the retina.

leukemia (loo-ke′me-ə) cancer of the blood; characterized by an abnormal increase in the production of white blood cells and pathological changes in the bone marrow and other lymphoid tissue.

leukocytes (lu′ko-sitz) white blood cells.

levator palpebrae (le-va′tor pal′pĕ-brī) the muscle that lifts the upper eyelid.

licensure formal permission to perform certain acts.

ligaments (lig′ə-mentz) bands of the fibrous joint capsule that connect bones to bones. They also support and strengthen joints.

light rescue rescue operations that involve the transfer of injured patients from uncomplicated motor vehicle accidents and stable buildings using a minimum of equipment.

limb presentation a delivery in which the baby's arm or leg appears first rather than the head.

lips upper and lower fleshy margins of the mouth.

liter (le′ter) basic unit of capacity in the metric system.

litter a type of stretcher for moving or carrying patients.

liver a large solid organ that lies in the upper right quadrant. It produces bile, stores sugar for immediate use by the body, and chemically treats all products of absorption in the gastrointestinal tract.

lividity (lĭ-vid′ə-tē) redness caused by blood pooling in the dependent parts of the body that is seen 15 to 30 minutes after death.

living wills legal documents with specific instructions that the patient does not want to be resuscitated or kept alive by mechanical life support systems.

lobes (lōbz) the dependent fleshy portion of any structure such as the bottom of each ear.

lobulated (läb′yoo-la′ted) consisting of lobes, as, for example, one of the surfaces of the placenta.

localized abdominal tenderness tenderness in a specific part of the abdomen.

lower airway the larynx, the trachea, the major bronchi, and the other air passages within the lung.

lower urinary tract bladder and urethra.

low volume (hypovolemic) shock shock resulting from loss of body fluids or blood.

lucid (lu′sid) **interval** time in which the patient seems normal between periods of unconsciousness.

lumbar (lum′bər) **spine** the lower part of the back formed by the lowest five nonfused vertebrae.

lumbar vertebrae vertebrae of the lumbar spine.

lumbosacral plexus (lum′bo-sa′kral plek′səs) a network of nerves originating from branches of the spinal nerves; they are located in the lower extremity.

lumen (lu′men) the cavity of a tube-shaped organ such as a blood vessel; the inside diameter of an artery.

lungs the organs that aerate the blood; they occupy the lateral cavities of the chest and are separated from each other by the heart and mediastinal structures.

main bronchus (brong′kus) one of the two main branches of the trachea that lead into the left lung and the right lung.

malaria (mə-la′re-ə) parasitic tropical disease with fever in cycles, chills, and fatigue.

malignant (mə-lig′nənt) cancerous.

malingering (mə-lin′ger-ing) faking illness.

malleolus (mal-le′o-lus) (pl. **malleoli**) the rounded projection on either side of the ankle joint.

mandible (man′dĭ-bl) the bone of the lower jaw.

mania (ma′ne-ə) a psychiatric disorder in which the patient may be severely agitated, moving around frantically, speaking rapidly, but never finishing a sentence or a complete thought.

manually controlled resuscitators (re-sus′ĭ-tay′-torz) resuscitators with manual control, used in ambulances.

manubrium (mə-noo′bre-əm) one of three components (manubrium, body, and xiphoid process) of the sternum; the upper quarter of the sternum.

marijuana (mar′ĭ-hwan′ə) extract from the plant top of the flowering hemp plant *cannabi sativa*, that when inhaled as smoke produces euphoria, relaxation, and drowsiness. It is often referred to as "pot."

mask and bag system a system of artificial ventilation in which the oxygen inflow fills a bag that is attached to a mask by a one-way valve.

mastoid (mas′toid) **process** a prominent, hard bony mass at the base of the skull behind the ear.

maxilla (mak-sil′ə) the bone that forms the upper jaw on either side of the face; it contains the upper teeth, the orbit of the eye, the nasal cavity, and the palate.

measles acute viral disease with fever, bronchitis, and red blotchy rash.

mechanism of injury factors involved in producing the injury.

MEDEVAC helicopter an increasingly used method of speeding lifesaving care to patients and of transporting patients with life-threatening injury or illness to treatment facilities using medically equipped helicopters.

medial (me'de-al) lying toward the midline.

medial malleolus (mal-le'o-lus) the bony prominence at the end of the tibia that, together with the lateral malleolus, forms the socket of the ankle joint.

medial structures parts of the body that lie close to the midline.

mediastinum (me'de-as-ti'num) the space between the lungs in which lie the heart, the great vessels, the esophagus, the trachea and major bronchi, and many nerves.

medic-alert a bracelet, necklace, or card stating the patient's medical problems.

medical examiner a public officer who makes postmortem examinations of bodies to find the cause of death.

medicolegal (med'ĭ-ko-le'gal) relating to both medicine and law.

medium rescue rescue operations that involve specialized equipment normally found on a rescue vehicle.

melanin (mel'ə-nin) the pigment in the skin.

melena (me'le-nə) the passage of dark black stools that have the consistency of tar.

meninges (mĕ-nin'jēz) the three layers of tissue that envelop the brain and spinal cord: the dura mater, pia mater, and arachnoid.

meningitis (men'in-ji'tis) an inflammation of the meningeal coverings of the brain; it can be caused by a virus or a bacterium.

meniscus (me-nis'kus) a cushion of cartilage that fills up a space between bones and aids in the gliding motion of the joint.

menstruation (men'stroo-a'shən) a periodic bleeding from the vagina that occurs at approximately four-week intervals, in which the lining of the uterus is shed.

mesentery (mes'en-ter'ē) delicate tissue formed by the peritoneum that suspends the organs within the abdomen from the body walls and carries blood vessels and nerves to all these organs.

metabolic shock shock caused by profound fluid losses from vomiting, diarrhea, or excess urination.

metabolism (me-tab'o-lizm) a series of chemical processes by which the energy needed for life is extracted from food.

metacarpal (met'ə-kar'pal) **bones** (**metacarpals**) the five bones of the hand that extend from the wrist to the fingers.

metatarsal (met'ə-tar'sal) **bones** (**metatarsals**) the five long bones of the foot between the instep and the toes.

microcuries (mi'kro kyoor'ēz) a finer subdivision of curies, a unit of measure of radiation from beta particles.

microwave a term applied to radio waves in the frequency range of 1,000 MHz and upward. The signals are generated by special equipment that depends of line-of-sight placement to operate properly.

middle ear the tympanic cavity with its ossicles.

midline an imaginary vertical line drawn from the midforehead through the nose and the umbilicus to the floor.

midwife a woman who assists in childbirth.

millicuries a finer subdivision of Curies, a unit of measure of radiation from beta particles.

milliliter (mil'ĭ-le'ter) one-thousandth of a liter.

millimeters (mil'ĭ-me-terz) **of mercury** (**mm Hg**) unit of pressure, used in measuring blood pressure.

milliroentgen (mil'ĭ-rent'gen) one-thousandth of a roentgen.

minerals nonorganic substances usually occurring in the earth's crust.

mini-drip sets a type of administration set for intravenous fluid therapy that is designed to keep an IV line open; it flows with minimal volume infusion.

minor burns any third-degree burns that involve less than 2 percent of the body surface or second-degree burns that involve less than 15 percent of the body surface.

minor's consent consent given by person under legal age (usually 21).

miscarriage (mis-kar'ij) (**abortion**) delivery of the fetus before it is mature enough to survive outside the womb (about 20 weeks), either from natural causes (spontaneous abortion) or induced.

mobile relay station a fixed base station established for the automatic retransmission of mobile or portable radio communications.

mobile repeater station a mobile radio station in land mobile service that is authorized to automatically retransmit any radio traffic originated by a hand-held portable, by other mobiles, or by base stations.

mode of transmission (trans-mis'shən) the manner by which an infection is spread: contact, airborne, by vehicles, or by vectors.

moderate burns burns that are less serious than critical burns. They include third-degree burns that involve 2 to 10 percent of the body surface (excluding hands, feet, face, or genitalia); second-degree burns that involve 15 to 25 percent of the body surface area; and first-degree burns that involve 50 to 75 percent of the body surface.

monitor a person who receives, and often records, radio messages without transmitting; to listen to radio messages without transmitting.

monitoring checking constantly on physiological signs (cardiac, respiratory); *see also* monitor.

mononucleosis (mon'o-nu'kle-o'sis) acute viral disease with fever, sore throat, and lymph node swelling.

monozygotic (mon'o-zi-got'ik) **twins** identical twins; they must both be of the same sex.

morphine (mor'fēn) a narcotic drug, a derivative of opium.

motor nerves nerves that transmit impulses to muscles, causing them to move.

mouth the lips, cheeks, gums, teeth, and tongue.

mouth-to-mask ventilation a system of artificial ventilation in which the EMT ventilates the patient with supplemental oxygen through a mask while supplying air from his or her own lungs at the same time.

mouth-to-mouth ventilation artificial ventilation in which the EMT's mouth makes a seal around the patient's mouth as the EMT exhales into the patient's mouth. The patient's nostrils are kept pinched together.

mouth-to-nose-and-mouth ventilation artificial ventilation in which the EMT's mouth makes a seal around an infant's mouth and nose, as the EMT exhales into both, simultaneously.

mouth-to-nose ventilation artificial ventilation in which the EMT's lips make a seal around the patient's nose as the EMT exhales into the patient's nose. The patient's mouth is kept closed, although sometimes the lips are spread apart during exhalation by the patient.

mouth-to-stoma ventilation artificial ventilation for patients who, because of surgical removal of the larynx, have a tracheal stoma. The EMT blows into the tube. Usually the patient's mouth and nose are covered to prevent air from leaking up the trachea.

mucous (myu'kus) **membrane** the lining of body cavities and passages that communicate directly or indirectly with the environment outside the body.

mucus (myu'kus) the opaque, sticky secretion of the mucous membranes that lubricates the body openings.

multigravida (mul'ti-grav'i-də) a pregnant woman who has previously given birth.

multiplex (mul'tĭ-pleks) the ability to transmit simultaneously two or more different types of information in either or both directions over the same frequency.

mumps acute viral disease with fever, swelling, and tenderness of the salivary glands.

muscle pull (strain) a stretched or torn muscle.

musculoskeletal (mus'kyu-lo-skel'ĕ-tl) **system** all the bones, joints, muscles, and tendons of the body, collectively.

musculotendinous unit the portion of fascia that extends beyond the muscle to attach to a bone; it crosses the joint and is responsible for movement of that joint.

mutation (myu-ta'shən) altered heredity of offspring.

myocardial (mi'o-kar'de-al) of the heart muscle.

myocardial contusion a bruise of the heart muscle.

myocardial infarction (in-fark'shən) heart attack; damage or death of an area of the heart muscle.

myocardium (mi'o-kar'de-um) the heart muscle.

narcosis (nar-ko'sis) stupor or anesthesia produced by a narcotic drug.

narcotic (nar-kot'ik) a drug that is a central nervous system depressant and produces stupor, insensibility, or sound sleep.

narcotized (nar'ko-tīzd) a condition in which the respiratory center becomes depressed, with lower than normal activity; it is caused by high levels of carbon dioxide in the blood.

nasal cannula (kan'yu-lə) a tube for insertion into the nose; oxygen can be administered with it, through two small tubular prongs that fit into the nostrils.

nasal mucosa (myu-co'sə) membranes in the nasal passages that contain mucus-secreting glands.

nasal septum (sep'tum) the partition separating the two nostrils; composed of membrane, cartilage, and bone.

nasopharyngeal (na'zo-fə-rin'je-al) **airway** an artificial airway positioned in the nasal cavity with the curvature of the airway following the nasal floor.

nasopharynx (na'zo-far'inks) the part of the pharynx that lies above the level of the soft palate.

near drowning at least temporary survival after submersion in water.

neck of a bone the region below the head of the bone.

necrosis (nĕ-kro′sis) destruction and death of tissues.

negligence (neg′lə′jens) failure to perform an important or necessary technique or performing such a technique in a careless or unskilled manner so as to cause further injury.

neoplasm (ne′ə-plazm) new growth.

nerve root the proximal (nearest) end of a spinal nerve.

nerves branches from the spinal cord and brain; either sensory, motor, or a combination of both.

nervous system the brain, spinal cord, and nerves.

neurogenic (nu′ro-jen′ik) **shock** circulatory failure caused by paralysis of the nerves that control the size of the blood vessels, seen in spinal cord injury.

neurological (nu-ro-loj′ik-l) relating to the branch of medical science that has to do with the nervous system and its disorders.

neuron (nu′ron) a nerve cell; the fundamental functional unit of nervous tissue.

neurosurgical (nu′ro-sur′ji-kl) relating to surgery of the nervous system.

neurotoxic (nu′ro-tok′sik) poisonous to nerve tissue.

neutralize (nu′tral-īz) to render neutral; specifically, the chemical combination of hydrogen and hydroxyl ions to form water, thus rendering each ion harmless.

neutrons particles of an atom that have no electrical charge.

nicotine (nik′ə-tēn) a mild stimulant that is present in tobacco and accounts for the addictive nature of cigarette smoking.

nitrogen (nī′tro-jen) **(N)** a colorless, gaseous element; when released as bubbles of gas under conditions of reduced atmospheric pressure, it can cause serious sickness because of arterial embolization.

nitroglycerine (nī-tro-glis′er-in) a medicine used in treating angina pectoris; it relaxes vascular smooth muscle and increases blood flow and oxygen supply to the heart muscle.

nocturia (nok-tu′re-ə) the necessary passage of urine at night.

Non-A, Non-B hepatitis (hep′ə-tī′tis) viral hepatitis that is usually related to a transfusion or contaminated needle stick; the causative virus is unknown.

nonconductive not transmitting an electrical current or any other source of energy.

nondisplaced fracture a fracture in which there is no deformity of the limb.

normal sinus rhythm the coordinated pumping contractions of a healthy, normal heart.

nose the part of the face that serves as an organ of smell and as part of the respiratory system.

nostril one of the external openings of the nose.

nuclear (nu′kle-ar) relating to the atomic nucleus.

nuclear radiation the products released by radioactivity.

nucleus (nu′kle-us) the central portion of an atom, where most of the mass and all of the positive charge are concentrated.

nutrients (nu′tre-entz) substances that furnish nourishment to the body.

O₂ oxygen.

obesity (o-bēs′ĭ-tē) excessive body weight; an excessive amount of body fat.

obstetrical (ob-stet′re-kal) relating to childbirth.

occipital (ok-sip′ĭ-tal) **region** *See* occiput.

occiput (ok′sĭ-put) the most posterior (back) portion of the cranium (head).

occlusion (o-kloo′shən) blockage.

occlusive (o-kloo′siv) **dressing** a dressing or bandage that closes a wound and protects it from the air.

olecranon (o-lek′rah-non) **process** the superior tip of the ulna which forms most of the elbow joint where the ulna and radius articulate with the humerus.

open (penetrating) abdominal injuries injuries in which a foreign body has entered the abdomen and opened the peritoneum-lined cavity to the outside.

open chest injuries injuries to the chest in which the chest wall has been penetrated by some object such as a knife or bullet.

open (compound) fracture any fracture in which the overlying skin has been damaged.

open wound injury caused by a penetrating object that breaks the skin or the mucous membrane that lines the mouth, nose, anus, or vagina.

opium analgesics (o′pe-um an′l-jez′siks) pain medications that are natural or synthetic derivatives of opium from poppy seeds. They include heroin, morphine, Demerol®, Dilaudid®, and methadone®.

optic (op′tik) **nerve** a cranial nerve that transmits visual sensations to the brain.

oral content contents of the mouth.

orbicularis oculi (or-bik′yu-la′ris ok′yu-li) the circular muscle around the eye whose contraction closes the eyelids.

orbit   the eye socket.

organic brain syndrome   neurological diseases that may cause disruptive or irrational behavior.

organism (or′gə-nizm)   an individual equipped to carry on the activities of life; a living being.

orifices (or′ə-fis-es)   the openings to the body (mouth, nose, anus, vagina).

origin (or′ĭ-jin)   the more fixed end or attachment of a muscle.

oropharyngeal (o′ro-fə-rin′je-al)   pertaining to the oropharynx.

oropharyngeal airway   an artificial airway positioned in the mouth to prevent blockage of the upper airway by the tongue. It permits free passage of air or oxygen and allows easy access for suctioning.

os calcis (os kal′sis) **(calcaneus)**   the heel bone.

osteoporosis (os′te-o-po-ro′sis)   abnormal brittleness of the bones in older people caused by loss of calcium; affected bones fracture easily.

ovaries (o′və-rēz)   female glands that produce sex hormones and ova (eggs).

overdose   an excessive dose of a drug.

ovum (o′vum)   female reproductive cell, which, when fertilized by the sperm, develops a new member of the same species.

oxygen (ok′si-jen) **(O₂)**   a gas that is necessary for breathing and is found free in the air.

oxygen exchange   the process by which oxygen is provided to the blood and carbon dioxide is taken from the blood to be expelled in the expired air.

oxygenated (oksi-je-nay′təd)   supplied with oxygen.

pacemaker   a device generally implanted under a heavy muscle or fold of skin that maintains a regular cardiac rhythm and rate by delivering an electrical impulse through wires that are in direct contact with the heart.

packaging   the physical stabilization and preparation for transport of an ill or injured patient after on-scene emergency medical care has been completed.

pack years   a measure of cigarette smoking: one package of cigarettes per day per year is a one-pack year.

paging   a common alerting system that involves the use of a coded tone radio signal, and sometimes a voice message, transmitted to small individual radio receivers called "beepers."

palate (pal-at)   the roof of the mouth.

pallor (pal′or)   paleness, absence of skin color.

palmar (pal′mar)   pertaining to the palm.

palpate (pal′pāt)   feel; to examine by touch.

pancreas (pan′kre-as)   a large, elongated gland situated transversely behind the stomach, between the spleen and the duodenum; it is a major source of digestive enzymes and produces the hormone insulin, which regulates the metabolism of sugar.

pancreatic (pan′kre-at′ik) **juice**   juice secreted by the pancreas, which contains many enzymes acting in the digestion of fat, starch, and protein; pancreatic juice flows directly into the duodenum through the pancreatic ducts.

pancreatitis (pank′kre-ah-ti′tis)   inflammation of the pancreas.

paradoxical (par′ə-dok′se-kal) **motion**   the motion of the injured segment of a flail chest, opposite to the normal motion of the chest wall.

paralysis (pə-ral′ĭ-sis)   the inability of a conscious patient to move voluntarily.

paranoia (par′ə-noi′ə)   a psychiatric disorder in which the patient may believe that people (including the EMT) are plotting against him, planning to hurt or kill him.

parasite (par′ə-sīt)   an organism that lives within or on another living organism at whose expense it obtains some advantage.

parasympathetic (par′ə-sim′pə-thet′ik) **nervous system**   a part of the autonomic nervous system that causes blood vessels to dilate, slows the heart rate, and relaxes muscle sphincters.

parathyroid (par′ə-thī-roid) **glands**   glands that control calcium levels in the blood, bone, and body fluids.

parietal peritoneum (pə-ri′ĕ-tal per′i-to-ne′um)   the portion of the peritoneum that lines the walls of the abdominal and pelvic cavities and the undersurface of the diaphragm.

parietal pleura (ploor′ə)   a smooth, glistening layer of tissue that lines the chest wall.

parietal regions   the more lateral portions of the cranium that lie between the temporal regions and the occiput.

partial seizure   an epileptic seizure involving a less extensive area of the brain than a generalized seizure.

patch   a special connection between different communication systems—for example, the connection that allows a radio transmission to be carried over a telephone line.

patella (pə-tel′ə)   the kneecap; a specialized bone that lies within the tendon of the quadriceps muscle.

pathologic (path′o-loj′ik) **fracture**   a fracture that occurs from minimal force because the bone is weak or diseased.

pedal edema (ped'l ə-de'mə) fluid that collects in the feet and legs; it may indicate underlying heart disease.

pediatrics (pe'de-at'riks) medical practice devoted to the care of children up to age 15.

pelvic cavity the space within the walls of the pelvis.

pelvic girdle the bony structure formed by the sacrum and the iliac bones that contain the abdominal and pelvic organs.

pelvic inflammatory (in-flam'ah-to're) **disease** an infection in the Fallopian tubes and the surrounding tissue of the pelvis.

pelvic outlet a layer of muscles that form the inferior boundary of the pelvic cavity, with openings for the gastrointestinal tract, the female reproductive system, and the urinary tract.

pelvis a closed bony ring, consisting of the sacrum and two pelvic bones, that connects the trunk to the lower extremities.

penetrating (open) abdominal injuries injuries in which a foreign body has entered the abdomen and opened the peritoneum-lined cavity to the outside.

penetrating chest injury injury in which an object such as a knife or bullet has penetrated the chest wall.

penetrating injury injury in which the force of impact is concentrated on a small point of contact between the skin and the wounding implement. The wounding object penetrates the skin and produces a laceration.

penicillin (pen'ĭ-sil'in) an antibiotic extracted from cultures of certain molds.

penis (pe'nis) the male organ of urinary excretion and copulation (sexual intercourse).

pepsin (pep'sin) the only digestive enzyme produced in the stomach; it initiates the digestion of protein.

peptic (pep'tik) **ulcer** ulcer in the stomach or duodenum caused by the action of pepsin.

perforated tympanic (per'fo-ray'təd tim-pan'ik) **membrane** ruptured eardrum.

perforating (per'fo-ray'ting) **(through and through) wounds** wounds that traverse an entire limb to exit on the opposite side.

perforation (per'fo-ray'shən) a hole made through a part or substance.

perfusion (per'fyu'zhən) the process whereby blood enters an organ or tissue through its arteries and leaves through the veins, providing tissue nourishment and removing wastes.

pericardial (per'ə-kar'de-əl) **sac** the sac that surrounds the heart and the roots of the great vessels.

pericardial tamponade (tam'pon-ad') a condition in which blood or other fluid is present in the pericardial sac outside the heart, exerting an unusual pressure on the heart.

perineum (per'i-ne'um) the pelvic floor and associated structures occupying the pelvic outlet.

periodic symptoms symptoms that recur at intervals.

period of communicability the time during which an infectious agent may be transmitted to a host from another carrier.

peripheral (pe-rif'er-al) **nerves** nerves that carry electrical impulses to and from the cells in the brain.

peripheral nervous system the part of the nervous system that consists of 31 pairs of spinal nerves and 12 pairs of cranial nerves. These peripheral nerves may be sensory nerves or motor nerves.

peristalsis (per'ĭ-stal'sis) the wormlike movement caused by contraction of the muscles in the walls of the gastrointestinal tract that propels food through the digestive tract.

peristaltic (per'ĭ-stal'tik) **contraction** the action of muscles to propel the contents of the intestines.

peritoneum (per'ĭ-to-ne'um) the membrane lining the abdominal cavity (parietal peritoneum) and reflected inward over the abdominal organs (visceral peritoneum).

peritonitis (per'ĭ-to-ni'tis) inflammation of the lining of the abdomen.

peroneal (per'ə-ne'əl) **nerve** a nerve lying below the head of the fibula that controls movement at the ankle and supplies sensation to the top of the foot.

pH a scale used to represent acidity and alkalinity; a pH of 7 is neutral, one less than 7 shows increasing acidity (acidosis), and one greater than 7 shows increasing alkalinity (alkalosis).

phalanges (fah-lan'jez) fourteen bones that form the toes and fingers.

pharyngeal (fah-rin'je-al) relating to the pharynx.

pharygneal suction tips (tonsil tips) large-bore tips that fasten onto suction tubing used to suction the pharynx.

pharynx (far'inks) the throat; the cavity at the back of the nose and mouth.

phenobarbital (fe'no-bar'bi-tal) a barbiturate drug used as a sedative.

phlebitis (fli-bīt'is) inflammation in the vein.

physiologic (fiz'e-o-loj'ik) characteristic of the state or functioning of the body or of a tissue or organ.

physiology (fiz'e-ol'o-je) a branch of biology that deals with the functions and actions of living matter and the physical and chemical factors involved.

pia mater (pi′ə-ma′ter)   innermost of the three layers of tissue that envelop the brain and spinal cord.

pin-indexing safety attachment   a safety system on compressed gas cylinders which consists of a series of pins on the yoke that must be matched with the holes on the yoke attachment of the gas cylinder if a satisfactory connection is to be made.

"pink eye" (conjunctivitis)   inflammation of the conjunctiva of the eye.

pinna (pin′nə)   the external ear.

pit viper   a poisonous snake with a triangular head, fangs, and a heat-sensitive pit between its nostril and eye.

placenta (plə-sen′tə) **(afterbirth)**   a special organ of pregnancy attached to the wall of the uterus through which the baby receives its nourishment and gets rid of waste products. After the birth of the baby, the placenta is expelled through the birth canal.

placenta abruptio (ab-rup′she-o)   premature separation of the placenta from the wall of the uterus that causes serious hemorrhage.

placenta previa (pre′vi-ə)   development of the placenta over the mouth of the uterus; severe hemorrhage results.

plasma (plaz′mə)   a sticky, yellow component of blood that carries the blood cells and nutrients and transports cellular waste material to the organs of excretion.

plasma expanders   fluids used for intravenous infusion that include Dextran (large molecules of dextrose that are not metabolized) and Plasmanate®.

plastic catheter embolus   a complication of intravenous fluid therapy in which the end of the catheter is sheared off by the needle point after venipuncture.

platelets (plat-litz)   tiny disc-shaped elements that are a component of blood; they are essential to the process of blood clot formation—the mechanism that stops bleeding.

plethoric (ple-thor′ik)   dark, reddish-purple skin color due to filling of all visible blood vessels.

pleura (ploor′ə)   layer of smooth, glistening tissue that covers the lungs.

pleural (ploor′al) **space**   the potential space between the parietal pleura and the visceral pleura. It is described as "potential" because under normal conditions the lungs fill this space.

pleurisy (ploor′ə-sē)   a condition in which the normally lubricated pleural surfaces that allow the lungs to move freely become injured or diseased and instead the lung surfaces rub together, causing friction and pain.

pleuritic chest pain   *See* pleuritic pain.

pleuritic (ploo-rit′ik) **pain**   sharp pain with each respiration due to irritation or damage to the pleural surfaces.

plexuses (plek′səs-ez)   complex nerve networks.

pneumatic antishock garment   *See* pneumatic counterpressure devices.

pneumatic (nu-mat′ik) **counterpressure devices**   large air splints for the lower half of the body to provide stability for severe pelvic, hip, and femoral fractures, and to combat shock.

pneumatic trousers   *See* pneumatic counterpressure devices.

pneumomediastinum (nu-mo-me′de-as-ti′num)   the presence of air or gas in the mediastinum, which results in severe dyspnea.

pneumonia (nu-mo′ne-ə)   acute bacterial invasion and infection of the lung.

pneumothorax (nu-mo-tho′raks)   the presence of air within the chest cavity in the pleural space but outside the lung.

pocket mask   mask with an oxygen inlet that allows the EMT to ventilate the patient with air from his own lungs while at the same time supplying supplemental oxygen.

point tenderness   tenderness at the site of injury or disease, which can be located by gently pressing with one finger.

poison   any substance which, when ingested, inhaled, or absorbed, or when applied to, injected into, or developed within the body, in relatively small amounts, by its chemical actions, may cause damage to structures or disturbance of function.

poliomyelitis (po′le-o-mi′ĕ-li′tis)   acute viral disease with fever, headache, gastrointestinal symptoms, stiff neck, and paralysis.

polydipsia (pol′e-dip′se-ə)   frequent drinking of liquid to satisfy continuous thirst; a classic symptom of uncontrolled diabetes.

polyuria (pol′e-u′re-ə)   frequent and copious urination; a classic symptom of uncontrolled diabetes.

popliteal (pop-lit′e-al) **artery**   the continuation of the superficial femoral artery in the popliteal space (posterior surface of the knee).

posterior (pos-ter′e-or)   behind; back.

posterior spinous process   that part of each vertebrae that can be palpated as it lies just under the skin in the midline of the back.

posterior surface   the back surface of the body, away from the examiner.

posterior tibial (tib′e-al) **artery**   artery just posterior to the medial malleolus; supplies blood to the foot.

postictal (post-ik′tal) **state** the third and final phase of a generalized seizure—the period of exhaustion and recovery following a convulsion. The patient's level of consciousness is depressed, and the airway may become obstructed by mucus, vomitus, or the relaxed pharyngeal muscles.

P-Q-R-S-T of pain descriptive of a patient's pain (provokes, quality, region, severity, time).

precordial (pre-kor′de-al) pertaining to the precordium, lying anterior to the heart.

precordial cardiac activity a transmitted impulse felt in the chest wall over the heart; it is not an arterial pulse and is therefore not reliable.

precordium (pre-kor′de-um) chest wall over the heart.

pregnancy (preg′nan-se) period during which a fertilized egg grows and develops in the uterus. Normal pregnancies come to completion at the end of nine months.

premature baby a baby who delivers before 8 months gestation or who weighs less than 5½ pounds at birth.

premature ventricular contractions (**PVCs**) *See* ventricular premature contractions.

presentation (pre′zen-tay′shən) the position in which the fetus lies in the uterus during labor with respect to the mouth of the uterus.

presenting part the part of the baby that is born first, usually the head.

pressure-compensated flowmeter a flowmeter with a float ball incorporated within a tapered calibrated tube. The float rises or falls according to the gas flow within the tube.

pressure point a point where a blood vessel runs near a bone; pressure can be applied to these points to stop bleeding.

pressure regulators regulators attached to medical gas cylinders to reduce pressure to suitable levels.

presumptive negligence violation of a standard of emergency medical care imposed by statute, ordinances, administrative regulation, or case law.

priapism (pri′ə-pizm) a permanent and painful erection of the penis.

primary survey the process of finding and treating the most life-threatening emergencies first.

primigravida (pri′mi-grav′i-də) a woman who is having her first baby.

PR interval the time it takes the electrical signal in the heart to travel from the atria to the ventricles, as measured by an electrocardiogram.

professional standards published recommendations of organizations and societies involved in emergency medical care.

prolapse (pro-laps) **of the umbilical cord** a delivery in which the umbilical cord appears before the baby; the baby's head compresses the cord during birth and cuts off all circulation to the baby.

prominence (prom′i-nens) projection, protrusion.

prostate (pros′tayt) **gland** a small gland that surrounds the male urethra where it emerges from the urinary bladder; it secretes a fluid that is part of the ejaculatory fluid.

prostatic hypertrophy (pros-tat′ik hi-pur′trə-fe) benign enlargement of the prostate gland.

prosthesis (pros-the′sis) an artificial substitute for a missing body part.

protein (pro-tēn) one of a group of complex organic compounds, essential combinations of amino acids; principal constituents of the cell.

protons (pro′tonz) particles of an atom that have a positive electrical charge.

proximal (prok′si-mal) describing structures that are closer to the trunk.

psychiatric (si′ke-at′rik) pertaining to psychiatry, that branch of medicine that deals with the study, treatment, and prevention of mental illness.

psychogenic (si′ko-jen′ik) **shock** the common faint, caused by a temporary reduction in blood supply to the brain.

psychosis (si-ko′sis) a severely disturbed state of mind; a mental disorder characterized by defective or lost contact with reality.

ptyalin (ti′ə-lin) a digestive enzyme in saliva that converts starch to simple sugar.

pubic symphysis (pyu-bic sim′fi-sis) (**symphysis pubis**) the firm fibrocartilaginous joint between the two pubic bones.

pubis (pyu′bis) one of three bones (ilium, ischium, and pubis) that fuse to form the pelvic bones.

pulmonary (pul′mo-ner′ē) of the lung.

pulmonary abscess (ab′ses) an abscess that forms in damaged or diseased lung tissue.

pulmonary arterioles (ar-te′re-alz) small arterial branches in the lungs.

pulmonary artery the major artery leading from the right ventricle of the heart to the lungs.

pulmonary capillaries (kap′i-lar′ez) capillaries in the lungs that are located next to the alveoli (air sacs); here the exchange of oxygen and carbon dioxide takes place.

pulmonary circulation the circulation, sometimes called the lesser circulation, that carries unoxygenated blood from the right ventricle through the lungs and back to the left atrium; as it passes through the lungs, the blood gives up carbon dioxide and absorbs oxygen.

pulmonary contusion (kon-tu′zhən) a bruise of the lung.

pulmonary edema (e-de′mə) abnormal accumulation of fluid in the tissues and air spaces of the lungs.

pulmonary embolism (em′bo-lizm) passage of a clot formed in the venous side of the circulation through that system, through the right side of the heart, and into the pulmonary artery where it becomes lodged.

pulmonary fibrosis (fi-bro′sis) scarring of the lung.

pulmonary veins the four veins that return oxygenated blood from the lungs to the left atrium of the heart.

pulmonary venules (ven′yulz) small veins in the lungs.

pulse the wave of pressure that is created by the heart contracting and forcing blood out the left ventricle and into the major arteries.

pulse point point at which an artery lies close to the surface of the skin.

pulse rate the rate at which the heart is contracting. The normal pulse rate in an adult is 60 to 80 beats per minute; for a child the normal rate is 80 to 100 beats per minute.

pulse volume a rough indicator of the strength of the heart's contractions.

puncture wound a wound resulting from a stab with a knife, ice pick, splinter, or any other pointed object or from a bullet.

pupil the circular opening in the middle of the iris of the eye.

purulent (pyoor′ə-lənt) containing pus.

pus liquid inflammation product made up of white cells and fluid.

P wave the wave on an electrocardiogram that represents depolorization of the atria.

pyloric stenosis (pi-lor′ik ste-no′sis) an obstruction of the outlet of the stomach, a congenital abnormality characterized by excessive growth of the pyloric muscle.

quadriceps (kwod′rĭ-seps) the great extensor muscle of the front of the thigh, divided into four parts.

QRS complex the wave on an electrocardiogram that represents depolarization of the ventricles.

rabies (ray′bez) an acute viral infection of the central nervous system, transmitted by the bite of a rabid animal.

"raccoon eyes" a sign of skull fracture in which ecchymosis develops under the eyes.

rad radiation absorbed dose; a unit of measure of radiation from gamma and x-rays.

radial artery one of the major arteries of the arm; it can be palpated at the base of the thumb.

radial artery pulse pulse that can be felt at the wrist, just at the base of the thumb, where the radial artery is close to the skin.

radial nerve nerve carrying sensation to the greater portion of the back of the hand and controlling extension of the hand at the wrist.

radial nerve palsy (pawl′ze) an injury to the radial nerve in which the patient is unable to extend the wrist or fingers; produces "wrist drop."

radial styloid (stī′loid) bony prominence felt on the lateral (thumb) side of the wrist.

radiant energy any energy that is radiated from any source: electromagnetic waves, radio waves, visible light, x-rays, or nuclear radiation.

radiation the sending forth of light, short radio waves, ultraviolet, or x-rays; loss of body heat from a person standing in a cold room because warmer objects give off heat to a cooler environment.

radioactivity the spontaneous release of energy by particles that make up atoms.

radio-telephone switch station (RTSS) scanning capability built into a radio system that automatically selects a clear channel from among several VHF frequencies.

radium (ray′de-um) a radioactive element that is used in clinical therapy.

radius the bone on the thumb side of the forearm.

rales (rahlz) the sound of air bubbling through fluid in the alveoli and bronchi, much like sand falling on an empty tin can.

rape sexual intercourse by force.

recessed (re′sesd) in a hollow or cavity.

recompression (re′kom-presh′ən) restoration of pressure after the patient has been in a condition of greatly lowered pressure, as, for example, occurs from too rapid an ascent by a diver.

recompression chamber a pressure chamber so constructed that air under greater than atmospheric pressure can be given to a patient with the "bends" or to one who needs oxygen under pressure.

record of live birth a recording of the birth of a live baby, with the exact time of birth.

rectosigmoid (rek′to-sig′moid) **colon** lower part of the large intestine that joins the rectum.

rectum (rek-tum) the lowermost end of the large intestine.

referred pain pain felt on a distant body surface associated with the same area of the spinal cord as the organ causing the pain.

reflex (re′fleks)   the sum total of any involuntary activity; *see also* reflex arc.

reflex arc   the neural arc used in a reflex action such as pulling the hand away from a hot stove; it involves sensory, short-circuiting internuncial, and motor nerves.

regularity   a characteristic of the pulse, occurring at constant intervals.

regurgitation (re-gur′jĭ-ta′shən)   a "burp" of air and fluid that comes back up as a result of the stomach's being too full.

rehabilitation (re′hə-bil′i-tay′shən)   restoration of the patient to self-sufficiency.

renal (re′nal)   pertaining to the kidney.

renal colic   excruciating pain caused by obstruction of the ureter by a kidney stone, as the ureter tries to pass the stone by peristalsis.

renal pelvis   a cone-shaped collecting area that connects the ureter and the kidney.

repolarization (re-po′lər-i-za′shən)   one of two electrical processes of the heart, during which the electrical charges on the surface of the muscle cell change from positive to negative.

reproductive (re′pro-duk′tiv) **process**   the process of conception, pregnancy, and birth.

rescue   to free from danger of death or destruction by prompt and vigorous action. Rescue is classified as light, medium, and heavy.

rescue vehicle   a vehicle with equipment for providing rescue services; should accompany the ambulance.

reservoir (rez′er-vwar)   a place where infectious organisms live and multiply, such as in stagnant water or a sewer.

resistance (re-zis′tans)   the ability of an organism to remain unaffected by infectious agents.

Resource Coordination Centers   special communications operation that monitors and allocates medical control channels among EMS providers.

respiration (res′pi-ray′shən)   breathing.

respiratory center   the area in the brain stem that senses the level of carbon dioxide and controls respiration.

respiratory distress   difficulty in breathing.

respiratory shock   shock caused by an insufficient amount of inspired oxygen.

respiratory system   all the structures of the body that contribute to normal respiration or breathing.

respiratory tract   the organs and structures of respiration, chiefly the nose, larynx, trachea, bronchi, bronchioles, and lungs.

resuscitation (re-sus′i-tay′shən)   restoring to life or consciousness, using assisted breathing to restore ventilation and cardiac massage to restore circulation.

retina (ret′i-nə)   the light-sensitive area of the eye where images are projected; a layer of cells at the back of the eye that changes the light image into electrical impulses, which are carried by the optic nerve to the brain.

retrograde (ret′ro-grayd) **amnesia**   loss of memory for the events that preceded an injury.

retrolental fibroplasia (re′tro-len′tal fi′bro-play′se-ə)   a disease of the eye in newborn infants in which an opaque fibrous membrane develops behind the lens of the eye; caused by high oxygen concentration.

retroperitoneal (re′tro-per′i-to-ne′al)   behind the peritoneum.

retroperitoneal space   the space between the posterior parietal peritoneum and the posterior abdominal wall, containing the kidneys, adrenal glands, ureters, duodenum, ascending and descending colon, pancreas, and large vessels and nerves.

rhonchi (rong′kī)   whistling, snoring sounds in breathing.

ribs   the paired arches of bone, twelve on either side, that extend from the thoracic vertebrae toward the anterior midline of the trunk.

rigid splints   splints made from firm material and applied to sides, front, and/or back of an injured extremity to prevent motion at the injury site.

rigor mortis (rig′ər mor′tis)   a sign of death noted by the resistance felt from a patient's body when an attempt is made to move it. It is best seen by trying to straighten a flexed extremity.

roentgen (rent′gen)   the amount of radiation that will produce one unit of ionization in one cubic centimeter of dry air under standard temperature and pressure conditions.

rotation (ro-tay′shən)   a turning around on an axis; internal rotation: to the inside; external rotation: to the outside.

rubella (roo-bel′ə)   German measles.

rubeola (roo-be′o-lə)   measles.

Rule of Nines   a way to calculate the amount of body surface burned; the body is divided into sections, each of which constitutes approximately 9 percent of the total body surface area.

rupture (rəp′chər)   a break or tear of an organ or tissue.

sacroiliac (sa′kro-il′e-ak) **joint**   the joint formed by the articulation of the sacrum and ilium.

sacrum (say′krum)   One of three bones (sacrum and two pelvic bones) that make up the pelvic ring.

safe residual (ri-zij′oo-wəl) the point on the pressure gauge of a medical compressed gas cylinder at which the cylinder is replaced with a new cylinder.

saliva (sə-li′və) a secretion of water, protein, and salts, secreted into the mouth by salivary glands; makes food easier to chew and begins breaking starch down for digestion.

salivary glands glands that produce saliva to keep the mouth and pharynx moist.

SCAB *See* self-contained breathing apparatus.

scalp the skin covering the cranium, usually bearing hair.

scanner a radio receiver in which the frequency being received is automatically and instantaneously changed until a frequency carrying some message traffic is detected. At that time, the receiver locks on to that frequency until the message is completed. The process is then repeated.

scapula (skap′yu-lə) the shoulder blade.

sciatic (si-at′ik) **nerve** the major nerve to the lower extremities.

sclera (skle′rə) the white portion of the eye; the tough outer coat of the eye which gives protection to the delicate, light-sensitive inner layer.

scleral icterus (skle′rəl ik′tər-əs) yellow color in the sclera of the eye indicating jaundice.

scoop (split frame) stretcher narrow stretcher that is first separated lengthwise, and then the two halves are slipped under the patient from each side. The halves are closed with locking brackets.

scrotum (skro′tum) a pouch of thickened skin hanging at the base of the penis, containing the testicles and their accessory ducts and vessels.

sebaceous (se-bay′shus) **glands** glands that produce an oily substance called sebum, which discharges along the shafts of the hairs.

sebum (se′bum) oily substance secreted by the sebaceous glands which seals the epidermal cells.

secondary survey the final step in the assessment process in which the EMT carefully examines the patient from head to toe, looking for wounds and deformities and observing whether the patient feels pain or sensation.

second-degree burns burns in which the epidermis and a varying extent of the dermis are burned; these burns are characterized by blister formation.

second stage of labor the time from the full dilation of the cervix until the baby is born.

seizure (se′zhur) a manifestation of epilepsy that varies from severe convulsions to simply "blacking out" for a few seconds. Seizures are classified according to the degree and location of abnormal electrical activity in the brain.

self-blood-glucose monitoring a method for diabetics to measure the amount of sugar in their blood. A drop of blood from the fingertip or ear lobe is placed on a strip of chemically treated paper. The color the paper turns is compared with a color chart. The readings are in milligrams per deciliter of blood.

self-contained breathing apparatus (SCAB) a complete unit for delivery of air to a rescuer who enters a contaminated area; contains a mask, controls, and air supply.

Sellick's maneuver a technique whereby one EMT pushes on the cricoid cartilage to help a second EMT visualize the vocal cords during endotracheal intubation.

semen (se′men) seminal fluid ejaculated from the penis and containing sperm.

semiconscious partly conscious.

seminal (sem′i-nal) **fluid** semen.

seminal vesicles storage sacs for sperm and seminal fluid, which empty into the urethra at the prostate.

senile (se′nīl) **dementia** loss of mental faculties occurring as a result of the aging process.

sensitivity (sen′si-tiv′i-te) allergy.

sensory (sen′so-rē) **nerves** nerves that carry sensations of touch, taste, heat, cold, pain, or other modalities.

sepsis (sep′sis) blood poisoning; the presence in the blood or other tissues of harmful microorganisms or their poisons.

septic (sep′tik) **shock** shock caused by infection that damages the walls of blood vessels.

septum (sep′tum) a dividing wall or membrane between body spaces or masses of soft tissue; a wall that divides the heart into the right and left sides.

serum hepatitis (se′rum hep′ə-ti′tis) hepatitis B; hepatitis caused by a virus that is spread through blood-to-blood contact (transfusions, needle stick), mucous membrane (saliva or sputum contact), or sexual contact. It is a serious disease with long-term side effects.

sexual abuse molestation or rape, often accompanied by physical abuse.

shaft of a bone the long, straight, cylindrical midportion.

shock a state of collapse of the cardiovascular system; the state of inadequate perfusion when it involves the entire body.

shock position position with the legs elevated and the knees straight so that blood drains from the enlarged vessels in the legs and returns to the heart for active circulation.

shoulder girdle   the proximal portion of the upper extremity, made up of the clavicle, the scapula, and the humerus.

shoulder separation   A/C separation; a dislocation of the acromioclavicular joint.

side effect   an effect of a drug other than the one for which it is given.

SIDS   *See* sudden infant death syndrome.

signs   something that the EMT observes in a patient, such as bleeding or the patient's blood pressure.

silver fork deformity   wrist injury from a fall on the outstretched hand in which the injured wrist assumes a curvature similar to the profile of a dinner fork.

simple partial seizure   a partial epileptic seizure in which the seizure activity is limited to one or more extremities or one side of the body.

simplex   single-frequency operating capability; radio transmissions can occur in either direction but not simultaneously in both; one party transmits, and the other receives.

sinuses   (sī'nus-ez)   a general term for spaces, such as the channels for venous blood in the cranium or the air cavities within the cranial bones.

sinusitis   (si'nu-si'tis)   inflammation of a sinus.

size-up   a term used by firefighters that means to gather rapidly the facts about the situation, analyze the problem, and decide how to handle it.

sixty-cycle interference   a problem that prevents the EMT-D from analyzing the rhythm on the monitor screen of a manual defibrillator because of interference from electrical appliances in the vicinity.

skeletal   (skel'e-tal) **muscle**   striated muscles that are attached to bones and usually cross at least one joint.

skeleton   (skel'e-ton)   the skeletal system; the supporting framework of the human body, composed of 206 bones.

skin   the outer covering of the body, consisting of the dermis and the epidermis and resting on subcutaneous tissue. It forms the largest organ of the body and serves to isolate the body from its environment, protect it from bacterial invasion, control temperature, retain fluids, and furnish information about the external environment to the brain through its nerve endings.

skull   the bones of the head, collectively.

sling   a triangular bandage or material that is tied around the neck and is used to support the weight of the injured upper extremity.

small intestine   the portion of the digestive tube between the stomach and the cecum, consisting of the duodenum, jejunum, and ileum.

smooth muscle   nonstriated, involuntary muscles; they constitute the bulk of the gastrointestinal tract and are present in nearly every organ to regulate automatic activity.

soft palate   (pal'at)   a fold of mucous membrane and muscle that extends posteriorly into the throat. It is designed to hold food that is being chewed within the mouth and to initiate swallowing.

soft splint   air splint or splint made from soft material that provides gentle support.

solar radiation   radiation from the sun.

solid organs   solid masses of tissue where much of the chemical work of the body takes place, as in the liver, spleen, pancreas, and kidneys.

solution sets   a type of administration set for intravenous fluid therapy that is designed for delivering large volumes of fluid to be infused over a short period of time.

somatic   (so-mat'ik) **nervous system**   part of the nervous system that regulates functions over which there is voluntary control.

somnolent   (som'no-lent)   sleepy.

source of infection   the origin of the infection or infectious agent; it may be a person, object, or any substance carrying bacteria, viruses, or parasites.

sovereign immunity   a doctrine in English common law, now abandoned, that individuals were deprived of a remedy when their injury or damage was caused by the negligence of the king or other members of the royal family.

Spanish Windlass   a tourniquet consisting of a bandage tied around a body part and twisted by a stick passed under it.

spasm   (spazm)   a sudden, violent, involuntary contraction of a group of muscles.

"speed"   amphetamines.

sperm   male cell that fertilizes the ovum.

sphincter   (sfingk-ter) **muscles**   circular muscles that encircle a duct, tube, or opening in such a way that their contraction constricts the opening.

sphygmomanometer   (sfig'mo-mə-nom'e-ter)   an instrument used to measure blood pressure.

spinal canal   a tunnel formed by the back part of each vertebra that encloses and protects the spinal cord.

spinal column   the central supporting bony structure of the body.

spinal cord   an extension of the brain, composed of virtually all the nerves carrying messages between the brain and the rest of the body. It lies inside of and is protected by the spinal canal.

spinal nerves   31 pairs of peripheral nerves that exit the spinal cord by passing between the vertebrae. They conduct sensory impulses from the skin and other organs to the spinal cord. They also conduct motor impulses from the spinal cord to the muscles that are present in that segment of the body.

spine   a column of 33 vertebrae extending from the base of the skull to the tip of the coccyx.

spine board   a wooden board primarily used for extrication and transportation of patients with actual or suspected spinal injuries; also serves as a litter.

spleen (splēn)   a large glandlike organ in the upper left quadrant of the abdomen; its major function is the normal production and destruction of blood cells.

splinting   immobilizing an injured part by means of a device applying rigid support.

split-frame (scoop) stretcher   narrow stretcher that is first separated lengthwise and then the two halves are slipped under the patient from each side. The halves are closed with locking brackets. These stretchers are not adequate for spinal immobilization.

spontaneous (spon-tay′ne-us) **abortion**   an abortion that occurs for no known reason.

spontaneous pneumothorax (nu′mo-tho′raks)   the presence of air in the chest cavity from the rupture of a congenitally weak area on the surface of the lungs.

sprain   a joint injury in which the joint is partially and temporarily dislocated, and some of the supporting ligaments are either stretched or torn.

sputum (spu′tum)   matter, especially mucus, that is expectorated from the lungs.

squelch   several types of radio receiver circuits used for suppressing, though not eliminating, unwanted radio signals or radio noise.

stacked shocks   delivery of a second and sometimes a third countershock during defibrillation immediately after the first countershock has been delivered.

standard of care   the manner in which an individual must act or behave when giving care.

standing orders   a direct order from the program medical director to perform certain tasks for a patient under a specific set of circumstances.

Star of Life   emblem displayed on the sides, rear, and roof of vehicles that meet federal specifications as licensed ambulances.

state of consciousness   the degree of consciousness or unconsciousness of the patient.

status epilepticus (stay′tus ep′i-lep′tik-us)   a series of epileptic seizures that follow one after the other, with no return of full consciousness between them.

sterilize (ster′i-līz)   to make sterile or free from bacterial contamination.

sternoclavicular (ster′no-klə-vik′yu-lar) **joint**   the joint formed by the articulation between the sternum and the clavicle.

sternocleidomastoid (ster′no-kli-do-mas′toid) **muscles**   muscles on either side of the neck that allow movement of the head.

sternum (ster′num)   the breastbone.

stethoscope (steth′o-skōp)   instrument used in the determination of blood pressure and in the detection of heart, breath, and bowel sounds.

stimulants (stim′yu-lantz)   drugs that excite the mind and cause rapid heart rate, increased blood pressure, rapid breathing, and a sense of euphoria or well-being.

stimulus (stim′yu-lus) (pl. **stimuli**)   something that rouses or attempts to rouse the patient to activity.

sting   injury caused by venom of a plant or animal.

Stokes stretcher   a basket stretcher shaped like an oblong plastic shell, useful in removing patients from heights or over difficult terrain or debris.

stoma (sto′mə)   an opening or mouth.

stomach   the expansion of the alimentary canal between the esophagus and the duodenum, which receives food, stores it, and provides for its movement into the small bowel.

stomach ulcers   lesions on the mucous surfaces of the stomach.

stool   the fecal discharge from the bowels.

stove-in chest   *See* flail chest.

straddle slide   a method of placing a patient on a long spine board by straddling both board and patient and sliding the patient onto the board.

strain   muscle pull; a stretched or torn muscle.

street drugs   drugs acquired "on the street" by addicts from pushers or other addicts, not prescribed by a physician.

stress fracture   one that occurs when the bone is subjected to frequent, repeated stresses such as running or marching long distances.

stretcher   a carrying device making it possible for two persons to lift and carry a patient who is lying down; used to transport patients to, from, and in an ambulance.

striated (stri′ayt-əd) **muscle**   muscle that has characteristic stripes, or striations, under the microscope; voluntary, skeletal muscle.

stridor (stri′dər)   a high-pitched sound heard on inspiration; a common sign of croup.

strobe light   lightweight portable light that attaches to the EMT's arm or belt. They enable EMTs to see each other and for oncoming vehicles to see them.

stroke   a sudden lessening or loss of consciousness, sensation, and voluntary movement caused by rupture or obstruction of an artery in the brain.

styloid (stī′loid) **processes**   bony prominences at the ends of the radius and ulna that form the socket for the wrist joint.

subatomic particle   a particle smaller than an atom.

subcutaneous (sub′kyu-tay′ne-us)   under the skin.

subcutaneous emphysema (em′fi-se′mə)   the presence of air in soft tissues, causing a very characteristic crackling sensation on palpation.

subcutaneously   under the skin.

subcutaneous tissue   tissue, largely fat, that lies directly under the dermis and serves as an insulator of the body.

subdiaphragmatic (sub-di′ə-frag-mat′ik) **thrust (Heimlich) maneuver**   a series of 6 to 10 manual thrusts to the upper abdomen just above the umbilicus and well below the xiphoid to relieve upper airway obstruction; also called the abdominal thrust maneuver.

subdural (sub-du′ral)   beneath the dura and outside the brain.

subdural hematoma (hem′ə-to′mə)   a hematoma, or collection of blood, beneath the dura mater and outside the brain.

substance abuse   the intentional misuse or overuse of any material that can be ingested, injected, or otherwise taken to produce an effect greater than or different from that experienced with the normal use of the agent.

substernal (sub-ster′nal)   under the breastbone.

sucking chest wounds   wounds of the chest wall through which air passes into and out of the pleural space with each respiration.

suctioning (suk′shən-ing)   aspirating (sucking out) gas or fluid by mechanical means.

sudden infant death syndrome (SIDS)   death from unknown cause occurring during sleep in an otherwise healthy infant; also called crib death.

suffocate (suf′o-kayt)   stop breathing; have one's breathing blocked; suffer from lack of oxygen.

suicidal (soo′i-sīd-l)   describing a patient who may be threatening to kill himself.

suicide (soo′i-sīd)   self-inflicted death.

sunstroke   *See* heat stroke.

superficial temporal (tem′po-ral) **arteries**   arteries supplying the scalp, palpable just anterior to the ears at the temporomandibular joints.

superior (su-pe′re-or)   toward the head; lying higher in the body.

superior portion   that portion of the body or body part that lies nearer the head than the feet.

superior vena cava (ve′nə ka′və)   one of the two largest veins in the body that carries blood from the upper extremities, head, neck, and chest into the heart.

supine (su′pīn)   lying on the back or with the face upward.

supracondylar (su′prə-kon′de-lar) **fracture**   fracture of the distal end of the humerus in which the fracture line extends across the bone just above the condyles.

sutured (soo′chərd)   describing a wound that was closed or repaired by stitching the opposing surfaces with a fibrous material.

swathe (swäth)   a bandage that passes around the chest, securing the injured arm to the chest.

sweat glands   the glands that secrete sweat.

sympathetic nervous system   a part of the autonomic nervous system that causes blood vessels to constrict, stimulates sweating, increases the heart rate, causes the sphincter muscles to constrict, and prepares the body to respond to stress.

symphysis (sim′fĭ-sis)   a joint formed of cartilage and fibrous tissue that allows only limited movement.

symphysis pubis (pyu′bis) **(pubic symphysis)**   the firm fibrocartilaginous joint between the two pubic bones.

symptom (simp′tum)   something the patient tells the EMT, such as "I feel dizzy."

syncope (sĭn′ko-pē)   fainting.

synovial (sĭ-no′ve-al) **fluid**   fluid produced by the synovium that nourishes and lubricates the articular cartilage of a joint.

synovium (sĭ-no′ve-um)   the inner surface of the joint capsule.

syphilis (sif′i-lis)   acute bacterial venereal disease with hard sores, secondary skin eruptions, late complications of heart and brain.

syringe (sir′inj)   an instrument for injecting liquids into or withdrawing them from any vessel or cavity.

syrup of ipecac (ip′ə-kak)   preparation of the dried root of a shrub found in Brazil and other parts of South America that can cause vomiting.

systemic (sis-tem′ik)   generalized throughout the body, such as fever, chills, and weakness.

systemic circulation   circulation, sometimes called the greater circulation, that carries oxygenated blood from the left ventricle of the heart throughout the body and back to the right atrium.

systemic hypothermia a systemic lowering of the body temperature below 95°F.

systole (sis′to-le) the contraction of the heart muscle, which forces blood out the left ventricle and into the aorta.

systolic blood pressure the higher blood pressure noted at the moment of ventricular contraction of the heart.

systolic pressure *See* systolic blood pressure.

tachycardia (tak′e-kar′de-ə) rapid but regular beating of the heart; high pulse rate.

tachypnea (tak-ĭp-ne′ah) a significant increase in the rate of respiration.

talus (ta′lus) the ankle bone.

tarsal (tahr′sal) **bones** seven bones (the talus, calcaneus, and five other bones) that make up the rear portion of the foot.

tarsal plate a firm framework of connective tissue that gives shape to the upper eyelid.

tear ducts ducts located on the inner side of the eye along the upper and lower lids that drain the tears into the nose.

tear glands lacrimal glands that produce tears that act to lubricate the eye and to flush out foreign material from the eye.

tears a fluid that acts as a lubricating substance to keep the eye from drying and flushes foreign material from the eye.

telemetric transmission orders relayed from a program medical director to medical personnel in the field via radio transmission.

temples (temporal regions) the lateral portions of the cranium.

temporal artery the artery located on either side of the face that supplies the scalp; it can be palpated just anterior to the ear at the temporomandibular joint.

temporal regions (temples) the lateral portions of the cranium.

temporomandibular (tem′po-ro-man-dib′yu-lar) **joint** the joint formed by the articulation between the mandible and the cranium, just in front of the ear.

tendons (ten′dunz) tough, ropelike cords of fibrous tissue that attaches skeletal muscles to bones.

tension pneumothorax (nu′mo-tho′raks) a condition in which air continuously leaks out of the lung into the pleural space, increasing pressure within the space with every breath the patient takes.

terminal disease disease that is known to end in death.

testes (tes′tēz) male reproductive glands.

testicles (tes′tĭ-klz) **(testes)** male genital glands containing specialized cells that produce hormones and sperm.

tetanus (tet′ə-nus) an infectious disease in which muscle spasm causes "lockjaw," arching of the back, and seizures.

tetanus prophylaxis (pro′fə-lak-sis) treatment to prevent tetanus, a potentially fatal infectious disease characterized by extreme body rigidity and muscle spasms.

thermal (ther′mal) **burn** burn caused by heat; the most common type of burn.

third-degree burns burns that extend through the dermis and into or beyond the subcutaneous fat.

third stage of labor the time from the birth of the baby until the delivery of the placenta.

Thomas (traction) splint holds a lower extremity fracture or dislocation immobile and allows steady longitudinal pull on the extremity.

thoracic (tho-ras′ik) **cage** the chest.

thoracic (dorsal) spine the 12 vertebrae that attach to the 12 ribs; the upper part of the back.

thoracic vertebrae the 12 vertebrae that lie between the cervical vertebrae and the lumbar vertebrae.

thorax (tho′raks) the chest; the upper part of the trunk between the neck and the abdomen.

thrombosis (throm-bo′sis) clotting of the blood.

thrombus (throm′bus) a clot plugging a vessel.

through and through (perforating) wounds wounds that traverse an entire limb to exit on the opposite side.

thyroid (thī′roid) **cartilage** a firm prominence of cartilage that forms the upper part of the larynx; the Adam's apple.

thyroid gland a ductless gland lying on the upper part of the trachea; it produces the thyroid hormone thyroxin, which controls the general metabolism of the body.

tibia (tib′e-ə) the larger of the two bones of the leg; the shin bone.

tibial (tib′e-əl) **crest** the lower end of the tibia from its point of insertion in the quadriceps tendon down to the ankle joint.

tibial plateau (pla-to′) the upper end of the tibia, which forms the interior surface of the knee joint.

tibial tuberosity a prominence on the tibia for the insertion of the quadriceps tendon.

tinnitus (ti-nī′tus) ringing in the ear.

tolerance (tol′er-ans) an individual's increasing resistance to the usual effects of a drug, resulting from its continued administration, as in the case of a drug addict.

tone an audio signal or carrier wave of controlled amplitude and frequency that is used for equipment control purposes or to selectively signal a receiver, such as activating a pager.

tongue-jaw-lift maneuver a technique of opening the patient's mouth by grasping the tongue and lower jaw between the thumb and fingers and lifting them forward.

tonic-clonic (ton'ik klahn'ik) **seizure** a generalized epileptic seizure involving most of the brain; also called a convulsive seizure.

tonic muscular contractions sustained, rigid muscular contractions that cause odd posturing of the body and occur during a generalized epileptic seizure.

tonsil tips (pharyngeal suction tips) large-bore tips that fasten onto suction tubing used to suction the pharynx.

topographic (top'o-graf'ik) **anatomy** the superficial landmarks of the body.

topography (to-pog'rah-fē) external features of the body.

torso (tor'so) the human trunk.

tourniquet (toor'nĭ-ket) a device, such as a bandage, twisted tightly around an extremity with a stick. Used to stop bleeding that cannot be controlled by any other means.

toxic (tok'sik) poisonous.

toxins (tok'sinz) poisons.

trachea (tra'ke-ə) the windpipe; the main trunk for air passing to and from the lungs.

tracheal stoma an opening in the neck that connects the trachea directly to the skin.

traction the action of drawing or pulling on an object.

traction splint holds a lower extremity fracture or dislocation immobile and allows steady longitudinal pull on the extremity.

tragus (tra'gus) the small rounded fleshy protuberance immediately at the front of the ear canal.

tranquilizers (tran'kwi-līz'erz) drugs that calm and quiet the patient without affecting the state of consciousness.

transfusion the introduction of whole blood or blood products into the vascular system.

transmission the manner by which an infection is spread: contact, airborne, by vehicles, or by vectors.

transverse colon the part of the colon that runs transversely across the upper part of the abdomen.

transverse presentation a delivery in which the baby is lying sideways inside the uterus.

trauma (traw'mə) a wound or injury, either physical or psychological.

trench foot a form of cold exposure that occurs when the feet suffer prolonged exposure to cold but not freezing water; also called immersion foot.

Trendelenburg position the shock position, achieved by elevating the foot of the long spine board.

triage (tre-ahzh') sorting of patients to determine priority of care to be rendered to each when the number of casualties is greater than what the emergency facilities can handle.

triceps (tri'seps) **muscle** the muscle in the back of the upper arm.

trochanters (tro-kant'terz) prominences on a bone where tendons insert; specifically, two protuberances, greater and lesser, on the femur.

tuberculosis (tu-ber'kyu-lo'sis) **(TB)** a chronic bacterial disease that usually affects the lungs. Signs and symptoms are cough, fatigue, weight loss, chest pain, and coughing up of blood.

tuberosities (tu'be-ros'i-tēz) prominences on a bone where tendons insert.

T wave the wave on an electrocardiogram that represents repolarization of the ventricles.

tympanic (tim-pan'ik) **membrane** eardrum.

UHF (ultrahigh frequency) those radio frequencies between 300 and 3,000 MHz.

ulcer (ul'ser) a lesion on the surface of the skin or a mucous surface, caused by the superficial loss of tissue, usually with inflammation.

ulcerative colitis (ul'ser-ay'tiv ko-lī'tis) chronic ulceration in the colon.

ulna (ul'nə) the inner and larger bone of the forearm, on the side opposite the thumb.

ulnar (ul'nar) **artery** one of the major arteries of the arm; it can be palpated at the medial wrist at the base of the fifth finger.

ulnar nerve controls sensation over the fifth and fourth fingers; controls most of the muscular function of the hand.

ulnar styloid (sti'loid) bony prominence felt on the medial (little finger) side of the wrist.

ultraviolet light those invisible rays of the spectrum that are beyond the violet rays.

umbilical (um-bil'i-kal) **cord** ropelike connection between the placenta and the fetus; before birth the fetus receives nourishment from the placenta and passes waste back to it through blood vessels in this cord.

umbilicus (um-bil'ĭ-kus) the navel; a small depression in the abdominal wall marking the point where the fetus was attached to the umbilical cord.

unconscious (un-kon'shus) having lost consciousness.

unilateral on one side.

universal dressing dressing made of thick, absorbent material, measuring 9 × 36 inches and packed folded into a compact size.

"upper" a stimulant.

upper airway air passages above the larynx: the nose, mouth, and throat.

uremia (yu-re'me-ə) a toxic condition caused by waste products of metabolism accumulating in the blood as a result of failure of kidney function.

ureters (yu-re'terz) small, hollow tubes that carry urine from the kidneys to the bladder.

urethra (yu-re'thrə) the membranous canal conveying urine from the bladder to outside the body.

urethral discharge any material that passes out of the male urethra other than urine or semen.

urinary bladder a musculomembranous sac for collecting and storing urine.

urinary system the organs that control the discharge of certain waste materials filtered from the blood and excreted as urine.

urine (yu'rin) a fluid waste product of the body, excreted by the kidneys, passed through the ureters, stored in the bladder, and discharged through the urethra.

urticaria (ur'ti-ka're-ə) hives; an allergic reaction characterized by bumps on the skin.

uterus (yu-ter-us) the muscular organ that holds and nourishes the fetus; it opens into the vagina through the cervix.

vaccine (vak'sēn) a preparation of killed microorganisms or living organisms that is administered to produce or increase immunity to a disease.

vagina (və-ji'nə) a muscular, distensible tube connecting the uterus with the external female genitalia; it receives the penis during intercourse.

vaginal discharge bloody discharge that occurs approximately once a month in healthy, nonpregnant women after puberty and before menopause. Any other discharge is abnormal.

vagus (vay'gus) **nerve** the tenth cranial nerve, which serves the larynx, lungs, heart, esophagus, stomach, and most of the abdominal viscera.

Valium (val'e-um) a drug used as a tranquilizer and muscle relaxant.

vallecula (va-lek'yoo-lə) the space between the base of the tongue and the epiglottis.

vasa deferentia (va'sə def'er-en'sha) the spermatic ducts of the testicles.

vascular (vas'kyu-lar) relating to or containing blood vessels.

vascular volume the capacity of the veins.

vector transmission a method of disease transmission in which the infective organism is transmitted to an individual by animals.

vehicle transmission a method of disease transmission in which the infective organism is introduced directly into the body through the ingestion of contaminated food or water or by the infusion of contaminated drugs, fluid, or blood.

veins tubular vessels that carry blood from the capillaries and venules into the right atrium of the heart.

vena cava (ve'nə ka'və) one of the two large veins conducting blood to the right upper chamber of the heart. Inferior vena cava: the venous trunk returning blood from the lower extremities and the pelvic and abdominal viscera. Superior vena cava: the venous trunk returning blood from the upper extremities and the head, neck, and chest.

venereal (ve-ne're-al) **disease** a disease transmitted by sexual contact.

venipuncture (ven'i-punk'chər) the site on an extremity, where the needle for intravenous fluid therapy is inserted into a vein.

venom (ven'um) poison secreted by animals and deposited in bite wounds.

venous (ve'nus) **pressure** the pressure of blood that flows through the veins.

venous tourniquet a constricting band placed about and below the site of injection to block the flow of blood in the veins but not the arterial flow.

ventilation (ven'ti-lay'shən) exchange of air between the lungs and the air of the environment; breathing.

ventilator a device to aid breathing.

ventricle (ven'tri-kl) either of the two lower chambers of the heart.

ventricular extrasystoles additional beats of the ventricle interspersed with the regular rhythm.

ventricular fibrillation (VF) a type of arrythmia in which the major pumping chambers of the heart undergo continuous, uncoordinated muscular quivering; the most common arrhythmia causing cardiac arrest.

ventricular premature contractions extra heartbeats arising in a damaged ventricle; can produce ventricular tachycardia.

ventricular tachycardia a type of arrythmia in which the heart beats so fast that there is not enough time for the pumping chambers to fill adequately between beats.

venturi mask a breathing unit that provides a specific concentration of oxygen through a delivery tube connected to a standard face mask.

venules (ven′yulz) small veins into which blood passes from the capillaries.

vertebrae (ver′te-bre) the 33 bones of the spinal column; there are 7 cervical, 12 thoracic, 5 lumbar, 5 sacral, and 4 coccygeal vertebrae.

vertebral arteries two cerebral arteries that supply blood to the brain; they unite at the base of the brain to form the basilar artery.

vertex (ver′teks) **presentation** a normal delivery in which the baby's head appears first.

vertigo (vur′ti-go) dizziness.

VHF (very high frequency) those radio frequencies between 30 and 300 MHz. The VHF spectrum is further divided into "high" and "low" bands.

viral meningitis (men′in-ji′tis) meningitis, or inflammation of the meningeal coverings of the brain, caused by a virus; the viral form of meningitis is usually transmitted via food or water.

virulence (vir′yoo-ləns) the degree to which an organism survives when exposed to light and air.

virus (vi′rus) the specific agent of a type of infectious disease; specifically, a group of microbes that can pass through fine filters that bacteria cannot pass through. An incomplete organism, it cannot sustain life alone but is an obligate intracellular parasite and lives with the cells of the host or organism attached.

viscera (vis′er-ə) the internal organs of the body.

visceral (vis-er-al) **peritoneum** the portion of the peritoneum that covers the surface of all the abdominal organs.

visceral pleura (ploor′ə) a smooth, glistening tissue that covers the lungs.

vital signs signs of life; pulse, respiration, blood pressure, and temperature.

vital statistics age, sex, and kin of the patient.

vitamins organic substances that occur in many foods and are necessary for normal metabolism in the body.

vitreous (vit′re-us) **humor** the fluid behind the lens of the eye.

voice box the larynx.

void to urinate

voiding urinating.

voluntary muscle muscle under direct voluntary control of the brain, which can be contracted or relaxed at will; skeletal muscle.

voluntary nervous system *See* somatic nervous system.

vomiting (vom′it-ing) disgorging the contents of the stomach through the mouth.

vomitus (vom′i-tus) material that is vomited.

vulva (vul′və) the external female genitalia.

watt-seconds a measure of the electrical current delivered by defibrillators.

wheal (hwēl) a raised area on the skin resulting from an allergic reaction.

wheezes (hwēzes) whistling sounds made in breathing.

whooping cough acute bacterial disease with violent attacks of coughing and high-pitched whooping.

withdrawal physical or psychological removal of oneself from a situation.

wrist joint between the forearm and hand.

wrist drop weakness in the wrist or fingers produced by injury of the radial nerve.

xiphoid (zif′oid) **process** one of three components (manubrium, body, and xiphoid process) of the sternum; the narrow, cartilaginous lower tip of the sternum.

x-rays electromagnetic waves that penetrate various substances and can also affect a photographic plate; used in diagnosis and therapy.

zygoma (zi-go′mə) the quadrangular bone of the cheek, articulating with the frontal bone, the maxilla, the zygomatic process of the temporal bone, and the great wing of the sphenoid bone.

INDEX

Index

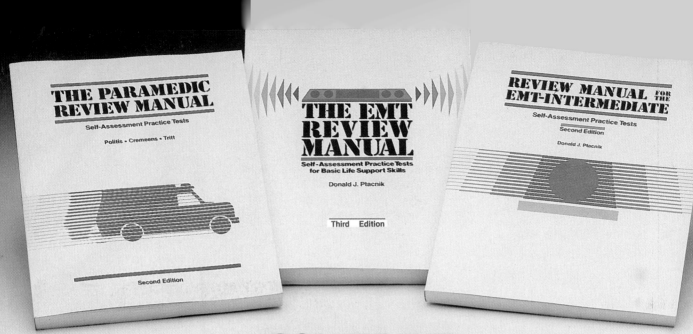

CONTINUE YOUR PROFESSIONAL GROWTH...

Prepare for Exams with EMT Review Manuals

These review manuals–for the Basic, Intermediate, and Paramedic levels–will help EMT students prepare for certification exams and help EMS professionals prepare for recertification. Each manual provides self-assessment practice and testing. Available from the American Academy of Orthopaedic Surgeons (AAOS), these manuals will help you increase your scores on EMT examinations at the same time as they help you improve your professional skills.

Each of the review manuals includes:
- Multiple-choice practice questions
- Answers with complete rationales
- All major DOT course topics
- Examination review guidelines
- Test-taking procedures

There are three convenient ways to order your review manuals:
- Complete the order form below (or a photocopy), and mail with your check or money order made payable to AAOS.
- Call AAOS toll-free 1-800-626-6726 and charge to your VISA or MasterCard.
- Send your institutional purchase order to AAOS Customer Service, 222 S. Prospect Ave., Park Ridge, IL 60068 (please include the order form below).

AAOS will pay shipping and handling on all prepaid orders (check, money order, or VISA/MasterCard).